KU-571-973

Clinical Examination

Royal Liverpool University Hospital – Staff Library

Please return or renew, on or before the last date below. Items can be renewed twice, if not reserved for another user. Renewals may be made by telephone: 0151 706 2248 or email: library.service@rlbuht.nhs.uk.
There is a charge of 10p per day for late items.

2 1 SEP 2010

0 2 JUL 2013

25.7.13

2 0 NOV 2013

1 1 OCT 2010

9 JAN 2015

13 Dec 2010

25 OCT 2018

23/12/20

2 8 JUN 2011

0 1 JUL 2013

Dedication

June, Daniel, Marc, Morris and Nancy
(Owen Epstein)

Harry, George, Josephine, Tom, Ted, Elsie and Ella
(David Perkin)

Anna, Alastair and Fiona
(John Cookson)

Dr Natasha Kapur, my wife and fellow physician. My children
Rohan and Karan.
(Roby Rakhit)

Dr Natasha Arnold, my wife and fellow physician, who shares our
passion for looking after the whole of the patient and is proud
to be called a generalist.
(Andrew Robins)

Sioban, Calum, Kieran and Brendan.
(Ian Watt)

To Rosemary, my wife for her loving support
(Graham Hornett)

Commissioning Editor: **Laurence Hunter**
Development Editor: **Janice Urquhart, Pru Theaker**
Project Manager: **Nancy Arnott**
Illustration Manager: **Gillian Richards**
Illustrator: **Marion Tasker, MTG and Chartwell**

Clinical Examination

Fourth Edition

Owen Epstein MB BCh FRCP

Consultant Physician and Gastroenterologist,
Royal Free Hospital NHS Trust, London, UK

G. David Perkin BA MB FRCP

Emeritus Consultant Neurologist,
Charing Cross Hospital, London, UK

John Cookson MD FRCP

Dean of the Undergraduate School,
Hull York Medical School, University of York, York, UK

Ian S. Watt BSc MB ChB MPH FFPH

Professor of Primary Care,
Hull York Medical School, University of York, York, UK

Roby Rakhit BSc MD FRCP

Consultant Cardiologist and Honorary Senior Lecturer,
Royal Free Hospital, London, UK

Andrew Robins MB MSc MRCP FRCPCH

Consultant Paediatrician,
Whittington Hospital NHS Trust, London, UK

Graham A. W. Hornett MA MB BChir FRCGP

General Practitioner with a Special Interest in ENT,
Surrey Primary Care Trust, UK

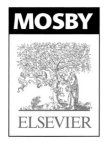

MOSBY

ELSEVIER

Edinburgh   London   New York   Oxford   Philadelphia   St Louis   Sydney   Toronto   2008

MOSBY
ELSEVIER

© 1992 Gower Medical Publishing
© 1997 Times Mirror International Publishers Limited
© 2008, Elsevier Limited. All rights reserved.

No part of this publication may be reproduced, stored in a retrieval system, or transmitted in any form or by any means, electronic, mechanical, photocopying, recording or otherwise, without the prior permission of the Publishers. Permissions may be sought directly from Elsevier's Health Sciences Rights Department, 1600 John F. Kennedy Boulevard, Suite 1800, Philadelphia, PA 19103-2899, USA: phone: (+1) 215 239 3804; fax: (+1) 215 239 3805; or, e-mail: *healthpermissions@elsevier.com*. You may also complete your request on-line via the Elsevier homepage (http://www.elsevier.com), by selecting 'Support and contact' and then 'Copyright and Permission'.

First edition 1992
Second edition 1997
Third edition 2003
Fourth edition 2008
  Reprinted 2009

ISBN 9780723434542

British Library Cataloguing in Publication Data
A catalogue record for this book is available from the British Library

Library of Congress Cataloging in Publication Data
A catalog record for this book is available from the Library of Congress

Note
Knowledge and best practice in this field are constantly changing. As new research and experience broaden our knowledge, changes in practice, treatment and drug therapy may become necessary or appropriate. Readers are advised to check the most current information provided (i) on procedures featured or (ii) by the manufacturer of each product to be administered, to verify the recommended dose or formula, the method and duration of administration, and contraindications. It is the responsibility of the practitioner, relying on their own experience and knowledge of the patient, to make diagnoses, to determine dosages and the best treatment for each individual patient, and to take all appropriate safety precautions. To the fullest extent of the law, neither the Publisher nor the Authors assume any liability for any injury and/or damage to persons or property arising out or related to any use of the material contained in this book.

ELSEVIER your source for books, journals and multimedia in the health sciences
www.elsevierhealth.com

Working together to grow
libraries in developing countries
www.elsevier.com | www.bookaid.org | www.sabre.org

ELSEVIER   BOOK AID International   Sabre Foundation

The
publisher's
policy is to use
**paper manufactured
from sustainable forests**

Printed in China

Preface

The fourth edition of *Clinical Examination* comes at a time of momentous change in medical practice. Gone are the white coats with their dog-eared pockets overflowing with all the paraphernalia of bedside examination. The stethoscope, once peeping subtly from a pocket, in now draped like a necklace, as much a fashion statement as a tool of the trade. The spiral-bound notebook is giving way to the personal digital assistant, the pen for a stylus and keyboard, and the evocative sound of the bleep is making way for the ringtones and soundscape of the mobile phone. In the consulting room, the fraying patient file, with its often illegible testimony of the patient's medical journey, is making way for the electronic patient record, displayed in legible type, and instantly retrievable from cyberspace.

The modern era is also blurring the traditional boundaries which once clearly demarcated the doctor-patient relationship. Where once the nurse primarily tended for patients' physical and emotional needs, highly trained practice nurses and nurse specialists now carry stethoscopes and undertake clinical roles previously considered wholly doctor owned. With improved telecommunication, fax, Internet and email, even medical receptionists and secretaries have to learn to respond to patients' questions, concerns and needs. To all this is added the panoply of new investigations including MRI, spiral CT scanning, virtual colonoscopy, virtual bronchoscopy and coronary angiography, wireless capsule endoscopy, minimal access surgery and a whole new frontier of genetic profiling and targeted biological therapies.

Where does this leave *Clinical Examination*? In this new edition, the authors have reasserted the centrality and importance of the face-to-face consultation in this fast-changing medical landscape. Perhaps it is more important than ever for all those engaged in direct patient care to remain closely connected with the patient's story and physical examination. There is no debate about the value of skilled history taking and physical examination and its importance in directing the patient journey and problem solving. Indeed, as patients become more knowledgeable about health and illness, communication skills and the ability to engage in a professional two-way discourse become increasingly important. The changing emphasis in the clinical encounter is recognized throughout this edition with the first two chapters emphasizing the Calgary-Cambridge schema of gathering information, examining the patient, explaining, planning and closing the consultation. For the first time, each chapter has been peer reviewed by both a primary care and hospital doctor and two general practitioner authors have contributed chapters to the book. Where necessary, changes have been made to reflect the increasing primacy of general practice and the emergence of overlapping roles in modern healthcare practice.

The principles that underpinned the first edition remain intact. Each of the systems chapters is introduced with an overview of clinical anatomy and physiology. This provides a backdrop for describing history taking and the normal and abnormal examination, and the book spans the age range from infancy to old age. The text is lavishly illustrated to provide a multimedia reading experience and the use of colour coded icon boxes, including a new 'red flag' box, provides quick access to summarized information and a revision resource for the 'night before' exams. The first two chapters introduce the reader to history taking, the general examination and the principles of problem-orientated records. The subsequent chapters are systems-based and include the skin, nails and hair, ears, nose and throat, respiratory, cardiovascular and abdominal systems, the female and male genitalia, bones joints and muscle, neurology and finally, the examination of infants and children.

Over a decade, *Clinical Examination* has established its position as a leading text for medical students, postgraduates, nurses, physiotherapists and a range of other healthcare professionals. Clinical tutors have found the book and its illustrations a particularly helpful source for teaching and learning. This latest edition consolidates its position as a rich resource to help learn and teach clinical skills in a rapidly changing modern era.

Acknowledgements

We wish to thank the following individuals and organisations for generously providing illustrative material:

Dr Philip Bardsley, Dr Russell Lane, Dr Mike Morgan, Dr P. H. McKee and Dr John Wales; Joan Slack, Dept of Clinical Genetics, Royal Free NHS Trust (Figs 2.3–2.7, 2.9–2.16); Dr Les Berger, Dept of Radiology, Royal Free NHS Trust (Figs 2.36, 2.37, 7.16a); Dr Malcolm Rustin (Figs 3.12, 3.15, 3.23–3.26, 3.30, 3.31, 3.70–3.72); King's College Hospital (Figs 3.13, 3.14, 3.16, 3.37, 3.39–3.43, 3.45–3.47, 3.54, 3.65, 3.73, 3.74) for slides reproduced from Anthony du Vivier: Atlas of Clinical Dermatology (Gower Medical Publishing UK, 1986); Professor Tony Wright (Figs 4.9, 4.12, 4.13); Dr James Entwhistle for Figs 5.5–5.10; Dr C. Richards for Fig. 5.13; Dame Margaret Turner-Warwick et al (Figs 5.2, 5.11, 5.12, 5.14, 5.20, 5.29) for slides reproduced from Clinical Atlas of Respiratory Diseases (Gower Medical Publishing UK, 1989); Professor Robert H. Anderson and Dr Sally P. Allwork (Figs 6.4, 6.6, 6.7) for slides reproduced form Cardiac Anatomy (Gower Medical Publishing UK, 1980); Dr James S. Bingham (Figs 8.37, 8.43–8.46, 9.14, 9.15, 9.29) for slides reproduced from Sexually Transmitted Diseases (Gower Medical Publishing UK, 1984); Dr Paul A. Dieppe et al (Figs 10.8, 10.9, 10.38, 10.42, 10.50–10.52, 10.64, 10.66, 10.69, 10.75, 10.77, 10.78, 10.80, 10.81, 10.91) for slides reproduced from Atlas of Clinical Rheumatology (Gower Medical Publishing UK, 1986); Mr David Spalton et al (Figs 11.24–11.28, 11.30–11.39, 11.52, 11.62, 11.64, 11.65) Atlas of Clinical Ophthalmology (Gower Medical Publishing UK, 1984).

The figures listed below were derived with permission from the following sources:

Fig. 11.13 from R. B. Strub and F. William Black: The Mental Status Examination in Neurology (F A Davis Co); Figs 11.16, 11.17, 11.19, 11.24–11.26, 11.28–11.41, 11.43–11.45, 11.50, 11.52, 11.62, 11.65) from David Spalton: Atlas of Clinical Ophthalmology (Gower Medical Publishing UK, 1984); Fig. 11.41 (right) from Haymaker, Webb: Bing's Local Diagnosis in Neurological Diseases, 15th edn (St Louis, The C V Mosby Co, 1989); Figs 11.46 and 11.47 from J. S. Glaser: Neuro-ophthalmology (Harper & Row); Figs 11.48 and 11.49 from R. John Leigh and David S. Zee: The Neurology of Eye Movement (F A Davis Co); Fig. 11.106 from Drs J. W. Lance and J. G. McLeod: A Physiological Approach to Clinical Neurology (Butterworths); Fig. 11.103 from Lord Walton of Detchant: Introduction to Clinical Neuroscience, 2nd edn (Baillière Tindall Ltd); Fig. 11.96 from Professor R. S. Snell: Clinical Neuroanatomy for Medical Students, 2nd edn (Little, Brown & Co); Figs 11.104 and 11.105 from Dr V. B. Brooks: Neural Basis of Motor Control (Oxford University Press); Fig. 11.134 from 'Somaesthetic Pathways' Br Med Bull, 33, 113–120, 1977; Fig. 11.142 from Professor Ian A. D. Bouchier CBE and J. S. Morris; Clinical Skills, 2nd edn (W B Saunders); Figs 11.150–11.152 from Dr F. Plum: Diagnosis of Stupor and Coma, 3rd edn (F A Davis Co). Figs 12.1, 12.15–12.26 and 12.27 from Dr Caroline Fertleman, UCL Medical School; Figs 12.3a and b, 12.29, 12.30a–12.30j, 12.30l–12.30n, 12.31, 12.32, 12.35–12.37 from Dr Heather Mackinnon, Whittington Hospital. Growth charts reproduced with kind permission of Castlemead Publications, Welwyn Garden City; Figs 12.11 and 12.33 with kind permission from Dr T. Lissauer: Illustrated Textbook of Paediatrics (Mosby); Figs 12.42 and 12.45 from Clement Clarke.

Contents

User guide to icon boxes

 Differential diagnosis

summarise the common cause of clinical abnormalities

 Emergency

outline the implications for history and examination of certain clinical emergencies

 Examination of elderly people

guide the reader through the particular difficulties encountered when examining the elderly

 Questions to ask

list the key questions to ask the patient to help reach a diagnosis

 Red flag

represent those symptoms and signs which should be taken particularly seriously and acted on urgently to rule out potentially serious pathology; they are also useful in guiding a directed history/ examination if time is short

 Review

summarise the most important points to remember about the examination of each body system

 Risk factors

give the basic information on the risk factors associated with a particular disease

 Symptoms and signs

provide the core clinical features of the diseases and disorders

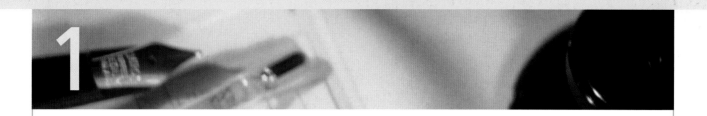

Consultation, medical history and record taking

The ability to take an accurate medical history from a patient is one of the core clinical skills and an essential component of clinical competence. The medical interview or consultation influences the precision of diagnosis and treatment, and studies have indicated that over 80% of diagnoses in general medical clinics are based on the medical history. It is estimated that a doctor might perform 200,000 consultations in a professional lifetime. All of which supports the need to learn and develop effective interviewing technique.

The success of the medical consultation depends not only on the doctor's clinical knowledge and interview skills but also on the nature of the relationship that exists between doctor and patient. For this reason, increasing emphasis is being placed on communication skills alongside history-taking in medical training in order to enhance the doctor–patient relationship and promote more effective consultations. How we communicate is just as important as what we say. The patient needs to feel sufficiently at ease to disclose any problems and express any concerns, and to know they have been understood by the doctor. The patient also needs to reach a shared understanding with the doctor about the nature of any illness and what is proposed to deal with it. As well as being more supportive for patients, good communication skills make history-taking more accurate and effective.

In any consultation, the doctor has a number of tasks to perform. Ideally, these should be undertaken in a structured way so as to maximise the efficiency and effectiveness of the process. A number of consultation models exist but an increasingly influential model is the

Calgary–Cambridge approach. This identifies five main stages in a consultation within a framework that provides structure and emphasises the importance of building a good doctor–patient relationship.

This chapter primarily addresses the first two stages: initiating the session and gathering information. It outlines the basics of taking a medical history within a framework that is patient-centred and emphasises effective communication. In addition, it describes an approach to recording information from the consultation in the clinical record.

The consultation

The medical consultation is the main opportunity for the doctor to explore the patient's problems and concerns and to start to identify the reasons for their ill health. Traditionally, medical history-taking has been based on a conventional medical model and assumed that disease can be fully accounted for by deviations from normal biological function. It gave little consideration for the social, psychological and behavioural dimensions of illness. Consequently, if a patient presented with a history of headaches, for example, the doctor's questions would be focused mainly on trying to identify the abnormalities of pathophysiology that were causing the symptoms, such as 'Where does it hurt?', 'When did the headaches start?', 'What helps relieve the headaches?'.

Whilst abnormalities of pathophysiology are largely common to everyone with the same disease, not everyone with the same disease experiences it in the same way. The experiences of each person are unique because their social, psychological and behavioural perspectives are unique, and interact with abnormal pathophysiology to cause each patient to experience illness in a very individual way. Thus, more recent approaches to medical consultation stress not just assessment of biomedical abnormality but also assessment of psychosocial issues. Questions to identify psychosocial perspectives could include: 'What most concerns you about your headaches?', 'What do

Review

The Calgary–Cambridge schema

- initiating the session
- gathering information
- physical examination
- explanation and planning
- closing the session

your headaches stop you from doing?', and 'What do you think would help these headaches?'.

Unless a doctor can reflect on a patient's psychosocial concerns, they risk failing to accurately diagnose the problem and may ultimately fail to effectively manage the patient's illness. The amount of distress an individual experiences refers not only to the amount of pathophysiological damage but also to what the illness means to them and how it relates to their circumstances. Individuals who have suffered personal upset or are worried may feel ill even when no demonstrable disease is present. Good doctors have always known this, but there is now increasing emphasis in medical history-taking that it should be geared to exploring not just the symptoms of the body's dysfunction but also the individual's perspective of the symptoms. Models of history-taking are becoming increasingly patient-centred and seek to assess both the main components of ill health – the biomedical component and the psychosocial component.

STARTING THE CONSULTATION

There are three main aspects to initiating the session: preparation, establishing initial rapport, and identifying the patient's problems and concerns.

Preparation

In preparing for a consultation, you should plan for an optimal setting in which to conduct the interview. In general practice or in the outpatient department, the consulting room should be quiet and free from interruptions. Patients often find that the clinical setting stokes up anxiety and thought should be given to making the environment welcoming and relaxing. For example, arrange the patient's seat close to yours (Fig. 1.1), rather than confronting them across a desk (Fig. 1.2).

Hospital wards can be busy and noisy, and it may be difficult to prevent your consultation being overheard and maintain confidentiality. If possible, therefore, try and find a quiet room in which to talk to the patient. If you consult with a patient at the bedside, sit in a chair alongside the bed, not on the bed, and ensure the patient

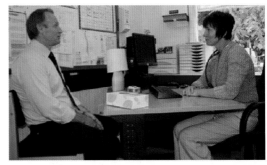

Fig. 1.2 A less than satisfactory seating arrangement. For the more sensitive or nervous patient, it will seem as though an additional barrier has been placed between him and the doctor, hindering the exchange of information.

is comfortable and able to engage with you without straining (Fig. 1.3).

Time management is important when preparing for the consultation. Ideally you should aim to avoid appearing rushed, and ensure that you set aside adequate time. Time constraints are often outside a clinician's immediate control and one has to be pragmatic and comply with clinic appointment times. On the ward, rest periods and mealtimes are generally regarded as sacrosanct by the nursing staff, and it is usual courtesy to ask permission from them before encroaching on a patient's time.

The patient's first judgement of any healthcare professional is influenced by dress, which plays a role in establishing the early impression in the relationship. Whilst fashions change, most patients have clear expectations of what constitutes appropriate dress and it is advisable to adopt a dress code that projects a professional image. This may vary according to setting and patient group. For example, children may feel more at ease with a doctor who adopts a slightly more informal appearance. In addition to dress, you need to pay attention

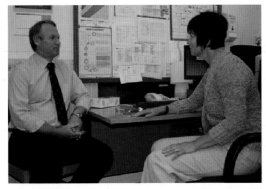

Fig. 1.1 The preferred seating arrangement when interviewing the patient: you are physically closer to the patient, without any barrier.

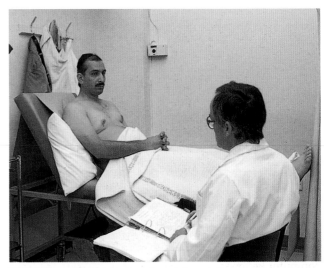

Fig. 1.3 For the bedside interview sit in a chair alongside the bed. Ensure that the patient is comfortable and is able to look at you without straining.

to personal hygiene; make sure, for example, that your hands and nails are clean.

Initial rapport

On first meeting a patient it is important to establish rapport and put the patient at ease. It's a chance for you to demonstrate from the outset your respect, interest and concern for them. You should greet the patient, introduce yourself and clarify your role, giving the patient an outline of what your intentions are. It may sometimes be appropriate to give an idea of how long the interview might take.

> 'Hello, my name is Jean Smith. I'm a medical student here at St Elsewhere and I wonder if I could speak to you about your condition? Your doctor, Dr Brown, has asked me to speak to you.'

Communication consists not only of verbal discourse but also includes body language, especially facial expression and eye contact. The first contact should also be used to obtain or confirm the patient's name and to check how they prefer to be called. Some people like to be addressed by their first name, whilst others may prefer the use of their surname.

Identifying the problems and concerns

Begin by asking the patient to outline their problems and concerns by using an open-ended question (e.g. 'Tell me, what has brought you to the doctor today?'). Open-ended questions are designed to introduce an area of enquiry but allow the patient opportunity to answer in their own way and shape the content of their response. Closed questions require a specific 'yes' or 'no' response.

Remember that patients often have more than one concern they wish to raise and discuss. The order of their problems may not relate to their importance from either the patient's or doctor's perspective. It is therefore particularly important in this opening phase not to interrupt the patient as this might inhibit the disclosure of important information. Research has shown that doctors often fail to allow patients to complete their opening statements uninterrupted and yet, when allowed to proceed without interruption, most people do so in less then 60 seconds.

Once the problems have been identified, it is worth reflecting on whether you have understood the patient correctly; this can be achieved by repeating a summary back to them. It is also good practice to check for additional concerns: 'Is there anything else you would like to discuss?' You may write down a summary of the patient's comments, but constantly maintain eye contact and avoid becoming too immersed in writing (or using a computer keyboard). An example of what you may have written at this stage is shown in the 'symptoms and signs' box below.

Symptoms and signs
Written summary of patient problems

H.M., aged 57, housewife
- Increasing breathlessness for 3 months
- Night-time shortness of breath for 3 weeks
- A dry cough for the last 6 days
- Can no longer attend dance lessons

Gathering information: the history

EXPLORATION OF THE PATIENT'S PROBLEMS

You now need to explore each of the patient's problems in greater detail from both biomedical and psychosocial perspectives. Gathering information on the patient's problems is one of the most important tasks to be mastered in medicine. The doctor must use a range of skills to encourage the patient to tell their story as fully as possible whilst maintaining a degree of control and maintaining a structure in the collection of information. As the history emerges, the doctor must interpret the symptom complex. The manner in which the interview is conducted, the demeanour of the doctor and the type of questions asked may have a profound effect on the information revealed by the patient. Obtaining all the relevant information from the patient can be crucial in helping to formulate a correct diagnosis.

It is important that the patient feels that their welfare is central to the doctor's concern, that their story will be listened to attentively, and that their information and views will be highly valued. Remember that most patients have no knowledge of anatomy, physiology or pathology and it is very important to use appropriate language and avoid medical jargon.

Symptoms and signs
Five fundamental questions you are trying to extract for the history

- From which organ(s) do the symptoms arise?
- What is the likely cause?
- Are there any predisposing or risk factors?
- Are there any complications?
- What are the patient's ideas, concerns and expectations?

During the interview it is usual to use a combination of open-ended and closed questions. Normally, open questions are more commonly asked at the start of the interview with closed questions asked later, as information gathering becomes more focused in an attempt to elicit more detail.

Questions to ask

Examples of open and closed questions

Open questions
- Tell me about your headaches.
- What concerns you most about your headaches?

Closed questions
- Is the headache present when you wake up?
- Does the headache affect your eyesight?

It is also useful to summarise a reflection of the information you have gathered at various times in the consultation: 'So Mrs Smith, if I have understood you correctly, your headaches started two months ago and were initially once a week but now occur almost every day. You feel them worse over the back of the head.' This is helpful not just because it allows you an opportunity to check whether you have understood the patient correctly, but can also provide a stimulus for them to give further information and clarification.

BIOMEDICAL PERSPECTIVE

Questions on the biomedical perspective should seek to clarify the sequence of events and help inform an analysis of the cause of the symptoms.

Symptoms from an organ system have a typical location and character: chest pain may arise from the heart, lungs, oesophagus or chest wall but the localisation and character differs. Establish the location of the symptom, its mode of onset, its progression or regression, its character, aggravating or relieving factors and associated symptoms.

Symptoms and signs

Symptoms helping distinguish different sources of chest pain

- Myocardial ischaemia – pressure, crushing, pressing retrosternal pain
- Pleuritic and chest wall pain – localised, sharp, distinct exacerbation with deep inspiration
- Gastro-oesophageal reflux pain – burning retrosternal discomfort (heart burn) arising from behind the sternum

For the assessment of pain, use the framework shown in the pain assessment box. The quality of the pain is important in determining the organ of origin. Patients often find it difficult to describe the quality of their symptom, so, if necessary, assist them by offering a list of possible adjectives (e.g. cramping, griping, dull, throbbing, stabbing or vice-like). Ask whether medication

has been necessary to alleviate the pain, whether the pain interferes with work or other activities and whether the pain wakes the patient from sleep. It is difficult to assess pain severity. Offering a patient a numerical score for pain, from '0' for no pain to '10' for excruciating pain, may provide a quantitative assessment of the symptom.

Symptoms and signs

Pain assessment

- Type
- Site
- Spread
- Periodicity or constancy
- Relieving factors
- Exacerbating factors
- Associated symptoms

PSYCHOSOCIAL PERSPECTIVE

Information on psychosocial implications of a problem requires questions to be asked about a person's ideas, concerns, expectations and the effect of the problem on their quality of life. For example, if you wanted to explore a patient's psychosocial perspectives of their headaches, potential questions include those listed in the 'questions to ask' box.

Questions to ask

To explore a patient's psychosocial perspectives of their headaches

- What concerns you most about the headaches?
- What do you think is causing the headache?
- Is there some specific treatment you had in mind?
- How do the headaches affect your daily life?

Some people find it difficult to talk about their feelings and concerns and you need to be alert to verbal and nonverbal cues which might add insight to their thoughts and ideas. Following up on such cues can help facilitate further enquiry and might feel less threatening than more direct questions: 'You mentioned that you were frightened that your headaches could be serious. Did you have specific cause you were worried about?'.

It is, of course, important to assess the impact of a problem on daily living by grading severity. For example, if the patient has intermittent claudication, ask how far the patient can walk before pain forces a rest. If breathlessness is a problem, ascertain whether the symptom occurs on the flat, climbing stairs, doing chores in the home or at rest. Gathering such information will allow a clearer understanding of the impact and meaning of an illness for each individual. Combining information on psychosocial perspectives with biomedical information adds to the diagnosis and provides a foundation to plan management.

BACKGROUND INFORMATION

The information gathered about patient's problems needs to be set in context and individualised. The doctor must understand and recognise the patient's background, how this impacts on the problem(s), and why the patient has sought help at this particular time. Such contextual information requires enquiry into a person's family history, their personal and social history, past medical history as well as their drug and allergy history.

Family history

The family history may reveal evidence of an inherited disorder. Information about the immediate family may also have considerable bearing on the patient's symptoms. Social partnerships, marriage, sexual orientation and close emotional attachments are complex systems which exert profound influences on health and illness. A useful starting point might be to ask if the patient has a regular partner or is married. If so, ask about their health status or any recent change in health status. If the patient has children, determine their ages and state of health. Enquire whether any near relatives died in childhood and if so, from what cause. When there is suspicion of a familial disorder, it is helpful to construct a family tree (Fig. 1.4). If the pattern of inheritance suggests a recessive trait, ask whether the parents were related – in particular whether they were first cousins.

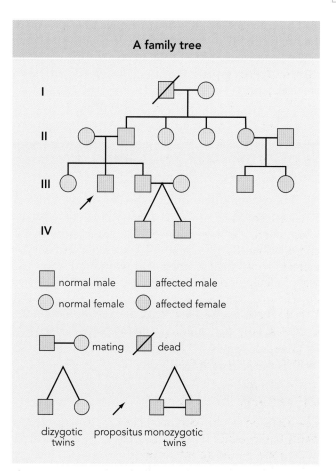

Fig. 1.4 A standard family tree.

	Differential diagnosis
	Common disorders expressed in families

- Hyperlipidaemia (ischaemic heart disease)
- Diabetes mellitus
- Hypertension
- Myopia
- Alcoholism
- Depression
- Osteoporosis
- Cancer (bowel, ovarian, breast)

Personal and social history

Just as with families, interactions with wider society can exert powerful influences on health and well being. We know, for example, that major health inequalities relate closely to social class and income, with socially and financially deprived individuals experiencing poorer health than people on higher incomes. A detailed social history includes enquiries about schooling, past and present employment, social support networks, and leisure. At this point, it is also convenient to ask about the use of tobacco and alcohol – the quantity smoked and the number of units drunk each week.

Education Enquire about the age at which the patient left school and whether they attained any form of higher education or vocational skill. In addition to providing useful background information, this information provides a context for assessing diseases and disorders causing intellectual deterioration and social function.

Employment history Enquire about working conditions as this may be very important if there is suspicion of exposure to an occupational hazard.

Patients may attribute symptoms to work conditions, e.g. a headache from working in front of a computer screen. Other problems such as depression, chronic fatigue syndrome and general malaise may also be blamed on working conditions. Although these associations may be prejudicial or coincidental, avoid dismissing them too

	Differential diagnosis
	Occupational disease

- Asbestos workers, builders: asbestosis, mesothelioma
- Coal miners: coal worker's pneumoconiosis
- Gold, copper and tin miners: silicosis
- Farmers, vets, abattoir workers: brucellosis
- Aniline dye workers: bladder cancer
- Healthcare professionals: hepatitis B

readily. Frequent job changes or chronic unemployment may reflect both socioeconomic circumstances and the patient's personality. It is useful to enquire about specific stress in the workplace, such as bullying or the fear of unemployment.

Tobacco consumption Patients usually give a fairly accurate account of their smoking. Ask what form of tobacco they consume and for how long they have been smoking. If they previously smoked, when did they stop and for how long did they abstain?

Alcohol consumption Unlike smoking, alcohol history is often inaccurate with a tendency to underestimate intake. Many patients consider beer and wine to be less alcoholic than spirits. Establish the type of alcohol the patient consumes and assess their intake in units.

Symptoms and signs
Units of alcohol equivalents

1 unit is equal to
- $^{1}/_{2}$ a pint of beer
- 1 glass of sherry
- 1 glass of wine
- 1 standard measure of spirits

If the patient is vague, ask how long a bottle of wine or spirits might last or the amount they drank over a specific recent time period (e.g. yesterday or over the last week). Alcohol-dependent patients often deny when questioned about alcohol consumption and a third party history from friends and family is often revealing and

Risk factors
Travel-related risks

Viral diseases
- hepatitis A, B and C
- yellow fever
- rabies
- polio

Bacterial diseases
- salmonella
- shigella
- enteropathogenic *Escherichia coli*
- cholera
- meningitis
- tetanus
- Lyme disease

Parasite and protozoan diseases
- malaria
- schistosomiasis
- trypanosomiasis
- amoebiasis

helpful. Certain questions may reveal dependency without asking the patient to specify consumption. Ask about early morning nausea, vomiting and tremulousness, which are typical features of dependency. Ask whether they ever drink alone, when they first wake up in the morning, or during the course of the day as well as in the evenings. Do they have alcohol-free days?

Foreign travel

Ask the patient about recent foreign travel. If so, determine the countries visited and, if the patient has returned from an area where malaria is endemic, ask about adequate prophylaxis for the appropriate period.

Home circumstances

At this stage in the interview, it is useful to ascertain how the patient was coping until the onset of the illness. The issue is particularly relevant for elderly patients and individuals with poor domestic and social support networks. Do they live alone? Do they have any support systems provided by either the community or family? If the patient's condition has been present for some time, determine the effect on daily living. For example, in a patient with chronic obstructive pulmonary disease: Is work still possible? Can the patient climb stairs? If not, what provisions are required for maintaining independence? Can the patient attend to personal needs such as bathing, shaving and cooking? What assistance may be on hand during the day or at night? What effects does the illness have on the financial status of the family?

PAST MEDICAL HISTORY

Patients recall their medical history with varying degrees of detail and accuracy. Some provide a meticulous history, whilst others need reminding. You can jog a patient's memory by asking if they have ever been admitted to hospital or undergone a surgical procedure, including caesarean sections in women. If the patient mentions specific illnesses or diagnoses, explore them in more detail. For example, if a patient mentions migraine, ask for a full description of the attacks so that you can decide whether or not the label is correct.

Drug history

Many patients do not know the names of their medication and it is useful to ask for the labelled bottles or a written medicines list. Remember to ask about nonprescription medicines: NSAIDs commonly cause dyspepsia and codeine-containing analgesics cause constipation. Ask about the duration of medication. Remember that iatrogenic disease is very common and always consider drug-related side effects in the differential diagnosis. Ask women of reproductive age about their choice of contraceptive and postmenopausal women about hormone replacement therapy. Ask about, and record, drug allergies.

At this point, it is useful to enquire sensitively about the use of illicit drugs. This will be influenced by the patient's age and background; few 80-year-olds smoke pot or eat magic mushrooms! Broach the subject by first asking about marijuana, LSD and amphetamine derivatives. If the response suggests exposure, enquire about the use of the harder drugs such as cocaine and heroin.

Systems review

The other major element of background information gathering is to undertake a review of the body's main systems. A systems review can provide an opportunity to identify symptoms or concerns that the patient may have failed to mention in the history. Before focusing on individual systems ask some general questions about the patient's health. Is the patient sleeping well? If not, is there a problem getting to sleep or a tendency to wake in the middle of the night or in the early hours of the morning? Has there been weight loss, fevers, rashes or night sweats? The questions surrounding the presenting complaint will often have completed the systematic enquiry for that organ and there is no need to repeat questions already asked; simply indicate 'see above' in the notes. Develop a routine to avoid missing out a particular system.

CARDIOVASCULAR SYSTEM

Chest pain

Determine the location of any chest pain, its quality and its periodicity. Find out if there are specific triggering factors. Does the pain radiate? If the patient describes an exercise-induced pain, remember that angina can be confined to the throat, jaw or medial aspect of the left arm rather than centring on the chest.

Dyspnoea

Ask about breathlessness. Does this occur after climbing one or more flight of stairs, after walking on the flat and after what distance? Does the patient become short of breath on lying flat (orthopnoea) or does the patient wake up breathless in the middle of the night (paroxysmal nocturnal dyspnoea)?

Ankle swelling

Has the patient noticed any ankle swelling? Is it confined to one leg, or does it affect both? Is the swelling persistent or only noticeable towards the end of the day?

Palpitations

Patients may recognise abnormal heart rhythm, particularly one that is rapid or irregular. Try to establish whether the abnormal rhythm is regular or irregular and for how long it lasts. Can the patient give you an idea of the frequency by beating out the rhythm with a hand? Do any other symptoms appear such as dizziness, fainting or loss of consciousness at or around the time of the palpitation?

RESPIRATORY SYSTEM

Cough

Cough is difficult to quantify, particularly if dry. Does the cough wake the patient from sleep? If productive, assess the volume of sputum produced, using a standard measure like an egg cupful as a reference point. Is the sputum mucoid (white or grey) or purulent (yellow or green)?

Haemoptysis

If the patient has coughed up blood, ask whether this is blood staining of the sputum or more conspicuous frank bleeding. Is it a recent event, or has it happened periodically over a more prolonged period? Did it follow a particularly violent bout of coughing? Was it a definite cough or was it vomited (haematemesis)? Was it associated with pleuritic chest pain or breathlessness?

Wheezing

Is the wheezing constant or intermittent, and are there trigger factors such as exercise? If the patient is using bronchodilators, determine the dosage and the frequency of use.

Pain

If the patient complains of localised chest pain, ask whether the painful area is tender to touch as might be expected with chest wall pain. Is the pain worse on inspiration? This is a characteristic symptom of pleural, or pleuritic, pain.

GASTROINTESTINAL SYSTEM

Change in weight

Ask the patient if there has been any recent weight loss or gain. If there is uncertainty about weight change, ask the patient whether they have noticed any alteration in the fit of clothes or belts.

Flatulence and heart burn

Does the patient complain of flatulence or burping? Is there heart burn, and, if so, is it aggravated by postural change such as bending? Does the mouth suddenly fill with saliva (waterbrash)?

Dysphagia

Has there been difficulty in swallowing? Does this affect solids more than liquids or both equally? Is the difficulty swallowing progressive or fluctuant and unpredictable? Can the patient identify a site where they believe the obstruction occurs (this correlates poorly with the site of the relevant pathology).

Abdominal pain

Ask about abdominal pain. Determine its site, quality and relationship to food. Does it appear soon after a meal, or 3 to 4 hours later? Is there any relationship to posture? Can the pain disappear for weeks or months or is it more persistent? Does the pain cause night waking?

Vomiting

Ask the patient about nausea and vomiting. Is the vomiting violent (projectile) or does it represent effortless passive regurgitation of stomach contents? Is the vomiting lightly bloodstained or does it look like coffee-grounds, suggesting partly altered blood? Are items of food eaten some hours before still recognisable? Is there recognisable (green) bile in the vomit?

Bowel habit

Many patients believe they are constipated simply because they do not have a daily bowel action. If the patient has always experienced a bowel movement three times a week, and there has been no recent change, there is little likelihood of pathology. A change in bowel habit can refer to frequency, consistency of stool or both. Has the appearance of the stool altered? Are they black (suggestive of melaena) or pale and difficult to flush (suggestive of steatorrhoea)? If there has been a change in bowel habit, ask the patient what drugs they are taking. A common cause of constipation is the use of codeine-containing analgesics. Has there been rectal bleeding or mucous discharge? Finally, ask about incontinence or soiling of underwear. Although this is not uncommon, particularly in parous women, few patients volunteer this symptom.

GENITOURINARY SYSTEM

Frequency

Determine the daytime (D) and night-time (N) frequency of micturition. The findings can be recorded as: D 6–8, N 0–1.

Has there been an increase in the actual volume passed (polyuria) or, alternatively, a sense of urgency with small volumes passed on each occasion? Does the patient wake at night to void urine and is this associated with increased thirst (polydipsia) and fluid intake?

Pain

Ask whether there is pain either during or immediately after micturition. Has the patient noticed a urethral discharge? Is the urine offensive, cloudy or bloodstained?

Altered bladder control

Determine if there has been urgency of micturition, with or without incontinence. Does the patient have urinary incontinence without warning? Does coughing or sneezing cause incontinence? Has the urinary stream become slower, perhaps associated with difficulty in starting or stopping (terminal dribbling)? Does the patient have the desire to empty the bladder soon after completing micturition?

Menstruation

Ask about menstrual rhythm. Are they regular and predictable? Use a fraction notation to summarise the duration of menstruation and the number of days between each period (e.g. 7/28). Are the periods heavy (menorrhagia) or painful (dysmenorrhoea)? Have they changed in quality or quantity?

Sexual activity

Although sexual dysfunction is common, few patients volunteer this information and questions about sexual activity need to be asked sensitively. Ask whether they have a sexual partner and whether they are able to achieve a satisfactory physical relationship. Ask whether the partner is male or female. Does the patient practise 'safe sex'? Has the patient ever had a sexually transmitted disease? In addition, ask whether intercourse is painful or whether the patient is concerned about a lack of sexual activity, whether due to loss of libido or to actual impotence. Prompting in this manner might prompt the patient to volunteer information on libido, potency and pain.

NERVOUS SYSTEM

Headache

Most people experience headache. A useful distinguishing feature is whether the headaches are unusual in either frequency or character. Follow the enquiry you use for other forms of pain but, in addition, ask if the pain is affected by head movement, coughing or sneezing. This might suggest pain arising from the sinuses. If the patient mentions migraine, ask the patient to describe the headaches in detail.

Loss of consciousness

Has the patient lost consciousness? Avoid terms like blackouts even if the patient tries to use them. Enquire about prodromal warning symptoms, whether they have been witnessed and whether they have led to incontinence, injury or a bitten tongue. Do the episodes occur only in certain environments or can they be triggered by certain activities (e.g. rising rapidly from a lying or sitting position)? How does the patient feel after the attack? Patients recover rapidly from a simple faint but after an epileptic seizure, patients often complain of headache and may sleep deeply for several hours. If the patient mentions epilepsy, ask about the exact nature of the attacks. There may be specific symptoms accompanying the attack that assist in making an accurate diagnosis.

Dizziness and vertigo

Dizziness (or giddiness) is a common complaint, describing an ill-defined sense of disequilibrium most often without any objective evidence of imbalance. This symptom is usually episodic, although some patients describe a more continuous feeling of dizziness. If the symptom is paroxysmal, does it occur in particular environments or with particular actions? For instance, dizziness associated with hyperventilation attacks can occur with anxiety in crowded places, whereas patients with postural hypotension will notice dizziness triggered by sudden change of posture from lying or sitting to standing. Only use the term 'vertigo' if the patient describes a sense of rotation, either of the body or the room or environment. Again, detail any triggering factors. In benign positional vertigo, the symptom is induced by lying down in bed at night on one particular side or movement of the head from side to side.

Speech and related functions

The history will already have provided information about the patient's speech. If there is a speech impediment, is this a problem of articulation, or does the patient use wrong words, with or without a reduction in total speech output? Note the patient's handedness, which should include questions about the limb used for a variety of skilled tasks, rather than just writing. Enquire from either the patient or a third party whether there has been difficulty understanding speech. Has there been any change in reading or writing skill?

Memory

The patient may not complain of memory disturbance and, if this becomes evident, determine whether this applies to recent events, to events further back in the patient's youth, or to both. Is the memory problem persistent or does the patient have fluctuating memory loss? Impaired memory is a common symptom, although further enquiry may suggest that it is not interfering with quality of life or social functioning.

CRANIAL NERVE SYMPTOMS

Vision

Ask about any visual disturbances. Do these take the form of visual loss or positive symptoms such as scintillations or shimmerings? Most patients assume that the right eye is concerned with vision to the right and the left eye with vision to the left. Consequently, few will cover-test during attacks of visual disturbance to determine whether the problem is monocular or binocular. Ask whether the patient has cover-tested before labelling the account of the visual symptoms. Is the visual disturbance transient and reversible, or continuous? Is it accompanied or followed by headache?

Diplopia

If the patient has experienced double vision (diplopia), determine whether the images were separated horizontally or in an oblique orientation. Can the patient describe in which direction of gaze the diplopia is most evident? Is it relieved by covering one eye or the other?

Facial numbness

Can the patient outline the distribution of any facial sensory loss? Does the involvement include the tongue, gums and the buccal mucosa.

Deafness

Has the patient become aware of deafness? A useful reference point is to ask about difficulties using the telephone or listening to the radio/television. Is the hearing loss bilateral or unilateral? Is there a history of chronic exposure to environmental noise or a family history of deafness? Is the hearing particularly troublesome when there is an increased level of background noise? Is the hearing problem accompanied by any ringing sound in the ear (tinnitus)?

Oropharyngeal dysphagia

Has the patient problems with swallowing? Does this principally affect fluids, solids or both? Is there spluttering and coughing associated with swallowing?

Limb motor or sensory symptoms

Is the problem confined to one limb, the limbs on one side of the body, the lower limbs alone or all four limbs? Does the patient describe loss of sensation or some distortion of sensation (e.g. a feeling of tightness round the limb)? If the patient complains of weakness, enquire whether it is intermittent or continuous and, if the latter, whether it is progressing. Does the weakness mainly affect the proximal or the distal part of the limb? Has the patient noticed muscle wasting or any twitching of limb muscles?

Loss of coordination

Few patients with a cerebellar syndrome will describe their problem as loss of coordination. Some will complain of clumsiness, others will simply refer to the problem as weakness. When assessing the loss of limb coordination, it is useful to ask the patient about everyday activities such as writing, fastening buttons and using eating utensils. Ask the patient about the sense of balance. Does the patient tend to deviate to a particular side or in either direction? Has the patient had falls as a consequence of any imbalance?

ENDOCRINE HISTORY

The history may provide clues to endocrine disease. Diabetes mellitus is characterised by weight loss, polydipsia and polyuria. An overactive thyroid is suggested by recent onset heat intolerance, weight loss with increased appetite, irritability and palpitations. An underactive thyroid is suggested by constipation, weight gain, altered skin texture, recent-onset cold tolerance and depression.

MUSCULOSKELETAL SYSTEM

Has the patient experienced bone or joint pain? Has joint pain been accompanied by swelling, tenderness or redness? Is the pain confined to a single joint or is it more diffuse? Does the pain predominate on waking or does it appear as the relevant joint is used (e.g. in walking)? Is there a history of trauma to the affected joint and is there a family history of joint disease?

SKIN

Has the patient noticed any rashes? What is the truncal and appendicular distribution? Was the rash accompanied by itching? Is there a potential occupational risk of a chemical contact dermatitis? Enquire about recent change in cosmetics which might have provoked a skin reaction. Have metal bracelets or necklaces caused the rash (nickel allergy)? Does the patient wear protective gloves when using washing up liquid?

DOCUMENTING THE FINDINGS

It is essential that all the relevant information from the patient interview is accurately recorded in the notes. Deciding what is relevant can be difficult, but, if in any doubt, err on the side of inclusion. A specimen case history is illustrated in Figure 1.5.

PARTICULAR PROBLEMS

The patient with depression or dementia

It is useful to couple these clinical problems as both can cause the patient to appear withdrawn and uncommunicative. Patients with depression may dwell on symptoms such as insomnia and appetite loss and there may be a reluctance to discuss mood or mood change. Determine whether there has been any suicidal intent. Patients with dementia initially retain some insight and in particular may have reasonable memory of distant events. However, recent recall, orientation for 'person, place and time' and logical thought patterns may be obviously dysfunctional. A characteristic feature of Alzheimer's dementia is loss of insight and failure of the patient to recognise their memory loss. This contrasts with senile dementias in which the patient is often concerned at their memory loss. When depression or dementia interferes with history-taking, family, friends and carers become crucially important in the assessment.

In addition, the history may only be complete with a visit to the patient's home.

The hostile patient

If a patient is hostile to your attempts to take a history, back off with dignity and use the experience to try and analyse the reasons for the reaction. The reaction may reflect anger at being ill, separated from family and work, and the doctor or student provides an easy target for the emotion. You may wish to conclude the interview, although you may feel it reasonable to question the patient gently about their anger and use the encounter to restore trust and confidence, allowing you to explore the history more formally. If the hostility persists, terminate the interview and discuss the problem with the family. Involve another member of the medical or nursing staff to act as witness.

History-taking in the presence of students

Occasionally, patients find the presence of a group of students intimidating or an infringement of confidentiality. Although most often an explanation of their presence will satisfy the patient, it may be appropriate to leave the consultation and allow the patient to continue the consultation privately (Fig. 1.6).

Time considerations

The limited time allocated to a consultation might preclude a full history-taking, and part of the expertise of a skilled consulter is the ability to adapt and manage the interview in the face of time or other constraints. The interview should be efficiently choreographed to maximise the patient's communication of important and relevant information. Judgement about which information is relevant can be difficult, and sometimes seemingly insignificant details can subsequently prove important to patient management. It is important to be competent and familiar with the approaches outlined in this and following chapters even if time constraints make it difficult to apply. It is also important to recognise which symptoms and signs necessitate prompt or urgent action. To help with this, *Emergency* boxes and *Red flag* boxes can be found throughout the book. *Emergency* boxes identify those clinical situations in which immediate action is necessary, whereas *Red flag* boxes identify symptoms and signs that necessitate urgent referral for assessment and investigation.

Recording the medical interview

Almost every encounter between doctor (or student) and patient involves recording information. The initial record will include a detailed history and examination, the problem list and plans for investigation and treatment. Whenever the results of investigations become available, this new information is added to the record and, at each

Patient history

Mrs G. W. 76-year-old female
Date of birth: 11/1/36 Retired shop assistant

Date: 1/6/07

Patient's problems:
(1) Constipation
(2) Stomach pain

History of patient's problems:
(1) Constipation: Started on 7/4/07. Normally bowels open once a day, but didn't go for 6 days. Subsequently has been going once every 2–4 days.
(2) Stomach pain: Pain started at the same time. Site of pain is in the left iliac fossa. Patient thought it was due to 'straining'. Episodes of pain are of sudden onset and are a 'sagging dull ache'.They last 1 hour and occur anything between 2–3 times a day to once every 3 days. There are no alleviating or exacerbating factors. Pain unrelated to eating or defecation and there are no preceding events. Pain appears not to fluctuate.

Patient went to visit GP after 6 days constipation. GP felt a mass on abdominal palpatation which on bimanual examination was thought to be of ovarian origin. Patient referred to the gynaecological outpatient department.

Patient does not understand why GP has referred her to hospital. Hopes the hospital can just prescribe a laxative and discharge her. Her children have arranged a holiday for her and her husband in one month's time and she does not want to miss it.

Social history:
Retired at age of 60 as shop assistant. Married. Husband is a retired bus driver. Alive and well. Live together in own terraced house. Self-sufficient. No pets.

Smoking:
Ex-smoker, 4–5 a day for 5 years as a teenager.

Alcohol:
Only on Christmas Day and birthdays.

Past obstetric history:
Menarche – 12   Menopause – 50 Gravidity 3 Parity 3

(1) Female 41   Spontaneous vaginal delivery full term (7 lb)
(2) Female 38   Spontaneous vaginal delivery full term (8 lb 4 oz)
(3) Female 35   Spontaneous vaginal delivery 39 weeks (6 lb 8 oz)

Past medical history:
Hypertension for last 6 years treated by GP with atenolol. No previous operations.

Drug history: Atenolol

Allergies: None known

Travel abroad: Never

Family history

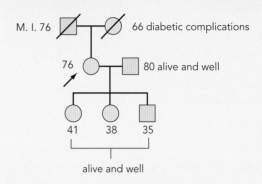

No family history of TB.

Systems review

General:
No weight change, appetite normal, no fevers, night sweats, fatigue or itch.

Cardiovascular system:
No chest pain, palpitations, exertional dyspnoea, paroxysmal nocturnal dyspnoea, orthopnoea or ankle oedema.

Respiratory system:
No cough, wheeze, sputum or haemoptysis

Gastrointestinal system:
No abdominal swelling noticed by patient, no nausea or vomiting, no haematemesis. Bowels open once every 2–3 days. Stool normally formed. No blood or slime. No melaena.

Genitourinary system:
No dysuria, haematuria. Frequency: D 2–3, N1. No vaginal discharge. Not sexually active.

Nervous system:
No fits, faints or funny turns. No headache, paraesthesiae, weakness or poor balance.

Musculoskeletal system:
No pain or swelling of joints. Slight stiffness in morning.

Summary:
A 76-year-old hypertensive woman, referred to gynaecological outpatients with a short history of constipation and stomach pain. She has no other previous medical history.

Fig. 1.5 A specimen case history taken from a student's notes. Note the brief summary at the end, the writing of which gives useful practice in the art of condensing a substantial volume of information.

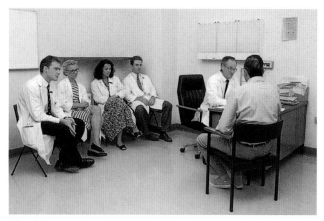

Fig. 1.6 The patient has to face not only the doctor but a number of students. Some patients will have difficulty coping with a 'mass audience'.

follow-up visit, progress and change in management are recorded. The medical record chronicles the patient's medical history from the first illness through to death. Over a lifetime, patients present with distinct episodes of acute disease and chronic, intractable or progressive conditions. A number of doctors and healthcare professionals may contribute to the medical record. In addition, this multi-authored document may follow the patient whenever he or she moves home.

There is an onus on the author of each medical entry to recognise the historical importance of each record and to ensure that the entry conveys a clear and accurate account which can be easily understood by others.

The medical record has other uses: it is the prime resource used in medical audit, a practice widely adopted for quality control in medical practice, and it provides much of the evidence used in medicolegal situations; under judicial examination, your professional credibility relies solely on the medical record if your memory fails. Medical records are also a valuable source of data for research.

As medical care becomes more specialised and complex and increasingly dependent on teamwork, it has become necessary to standardise the approach to clinical record-keeping. The problem-orientated medical record (POMR) is a widely accepted framework for both standardising and improving the quality of medical records. The system encourages a logical approach to diagnosis and management and addresses the problem of maintaining order in the multidisciplinary, highly specialised practice of modern medical care. The problem-orientated approach to medical records was first advocated in 1969 by Lawrence Weed and remains relevant today. However, it is probably more widely used in hospital practice than general practice. There is also increasing use of computers to record medical interviews with software packages that provide a rigid template for recording consultation notes. Nevertheless many of the principles underlying the POMR provide useful insights and guidance to those learning about how to maintain good medical records.

PROBLEM-ORIENTATED MEDICAL RECORD

The accuracy of information gathered from a patient during the course of an illness influences the precision of the diagnosis and treatment. The POMR stresses the need to gather all the information, biomedical, psychosocial, demographic, symptoms and signs and special tests, and uses this 'database' to construct a list of problems. This problem list not only provides a summary of the 'whole' patient but also offers a resource for planning management and encourages you to look for relationships between problems, allowing an integrated overview of the patient to emerge. Moreover, it distinguishes problems needing active management from problems that may be of only historical significance. The problem list does not provide a perspective of the relative importance of each problem: this must rely on discussion with the patient and the skill of clinical judgement. The database and problem list evolve through the course of an illness and changes with each subsequent presentation.

In addition to the problem list, the POMR provides a framework for standardising the structure of follow-up notes (Fig. 1.7); this stresses changes in the patient's symptoms and signs and the evolution of clinical assessment and management plans. The POMR also provides a flow sheet that records sequential changes in clinical and biochemical measurements.

THE HISTORY

For generations, there has been little change in the method of recording information from the history. The interview is the focal point of the doctor–patient relationship and establishes the bonding necessary for the patient's care. The history guides the patient through a series of questions designed to build a profile of the individual and his or her problems. By the end of the first interview you should have a good understanding of the patient's personality, social habits and clinical problems. Additionally, you will have considered a differential diagnosis that may explain the patient's symptoms.

A new history and examination are recorded in the notes whenever a patient presents with a fresh problem. Some information may remain unchanged over long periods (previous illness, family history, education and occupation). If these were accurately recorded at the time of the first presentation, there is no need to re-enter them unless there has been change.

Remember, at some time in the future the medical history may provide an important source of information, particularly if a patient is admitted to hospital with, for example, intense pain, altered consciousness or severe breathlessness and is therefore unable to provide a history. In these circumstances, a detailed systematic record may provide crucial information. A routine systems enquiry also prompts your patient to remember

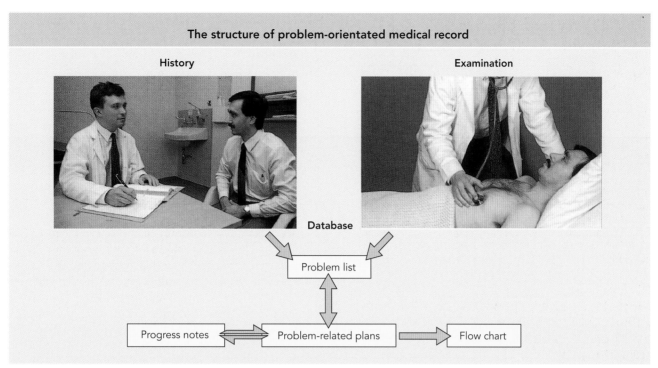

The structure of problem-orientated medical record

History   Examination

Database

Problem list

Progress notes ⇔ Problem-related plans ⇒ Flow chart

Fig. 1.7 Structure of the problem-orientated medical record (POMR).

events or illnesses that may otherwise have been overlooked.

THE EXAMINATION

The examination may confirm or refute a diagnosis suspected from the history and by adding this information to the database you will be able to construct a more accurate problem list. Like the history, the examination is structured to record both positive and negative findings in detail.

THE PROBLEM LIST

The problem list is fundamental to the POMR. The entries provide a record of all the patient's important health-related problems, both biomedical and psychosocial. The master problem list is placed at the front of the medical record and each entry is dated (Fig. 1.8). This date refers to the time of the entry, not the date when the patient first noted the problem (this can be indicated in brackets alongside the problem). The dates entered into the problem list not only provide a chronology of the patient's health-related problems but also a 'table of contents' which serves the medical record. Using the entry date as a reference, there should be no difficulty finding the original entry in the notes. In addition to providing a summary and index, the problem list also assists the development of management plans.

Setting up the problem list

Divide the problems into those that are active (i.e. those requiring active management) and those that are inactive

(problems that have resolved or require no action but may be important at some stage in the patient's present or future management). An entry of 'Peptic ulcer (2006)' in the 'inactive' column will provide a reminder to someone considering the use of a nonsteroidal anti-inflammatory (NSAID) drug in a patient presenting at a later date with arthritis. The problem list is dynamic and the page is designed to allow you to shift problems between the active and inactive columns (Fig. 1.9).

Your entries into the problem list may include established diagnoses (e.g. ulcerative colitis), symptoms (e.g. dyspnoea), psychosocial concerns (e.g. concern that they will die of stomach cancer like their brother), physical signs (e.g. ejection systolic murmur), laboratory tests (e.g. anaemia), family and social history (e.g. carer for partner, unemployment) or special risk factors (e.g. smoking, alcohol or narcotic abuse). The diagnostic level at which you make the entry depends on the information available at a particular moment. Express the problem at the highest possible level but update the list if new findings alter or refine your understanding of the problem. The problem list is designed to accommodate change; consequently, it is not necessary to delete an entry once a higher level of diagnosis (or understanding) is reached. For example, a patient may present with the problems of jaundice, anorexia and weight loss. This information will be entered into the problem list (Fig. 1.8). If, a few days later, serological investigation confirms that the patient was suffering from type A viral hepatitis, this new level of diagnosis can be entered on a new line in the block reserved for active problem 1 (Fig. 1.9). Other problems explained by the diagnosis (anorexia and weight loss)

Initial problem list					
Patient's name:			Hospital no:		
No.	Active problems	Date	Inactive problems		Date
1	jaundice (Jan '07)	9/1/07			
2	anorexia (Dec '06)	9/1/07			
3	weight loss	9/1/07			
4	recurrent rectal bleeding	9/1/07			
5	smoking (since 1980)	9/1/07			
6	unemployed (Nov '06)	9/1/07			
7	stutter	9/1/07			
8	brother died of colon cancer – patient concerned he may have similar condition (Dec '06)	9/1/07			
9			duodenal ulcer (1996)		9/1/07
10					

Fig. 1.8 Problem list entered on 9 January 2007.

should be amended with an arrow and asterisk to indicate the connection with the solved problem. At this point, viral hepatitis represents the highest level of diagnosis. Once the disease has resolved, an arrow to the opposite 'inactive' column will indicate the point during follow-up that the doctor noted return of the liver tests to normal (Fig. 1.9). Unexpected problems may become evident in the course of investigation (e.g. hypercholesterolaemia) and these are added to the problem list.

The problem list should be under constant review to ensure that the entries are accurate and up-to-date.

INITIAL PROBLEM-RELATED PLANS

The POMR offers a structured approach to the management of a patient's problems. By constructing the problem list you will have clearly defined problems requiring active management (i.e. investigation and treatment), so it should be reasonably easy to develop a management plan (Fig. 1.10) by considering four headings (see below); all or only some of these headings may be applicable to a particular problem.

Diagnostic tests (Dx)

Enter the differential next to each problem. Adjacent to each of the possible diagnoses, enter the investigation

that may aid the diagnosis. There are a large number of special tests that may be applicable to a particular problem; therefore, it is useful to evolve a general framework for investigation and to adapt this to each problem. You can construct a logical flow of investigations by considering bedside tests, side-ward tests, plain radiographs, ultrasound, blood tests and specialised imaging examinations (Fig. 1.11).

Monitoring tests (Mx)

Monitoring information charts the patient's progress. Consider whether a particular problem can be monitored and, if so, document the appropriate tests and the frequency with which they should be performed to provide a meaningful flow of information.

Treatment (Rx)

Consider each problem in turn with a view to deciding on a treatment strategy. If drug treatment is indicated, note the drug and dosage. Include a plan for monitoring both side effects and the effectiveness of treatment.

Education (Ed)

An important component of your patient's management is education and sharing information and decisions. Patients are able to cope better with their illness if they

			Updated problem list			
Patient's name:				Hospital no:		
No.	Active problems		Date	Inactive problems		Date
1	jaundice (Jan '07) → type A hepatitis*		9/1/07	resolved		14/2/07
2	anorexia (Dec '06) →*1		9/1/07			
3	weight loss →*1		9/1/07			
4	recurrent rectal bleeding → haemorrhoids		9/1/07 13/1/07	haemorrhoid banding		1/2/07
5	smoking (since 1980)		9/1/07			
6	unemployed (Nov '06)		9/1/07			
7	stutter		9/1/07			
8	brother died of colon cancer – patient concerned he may have similar condition (Dec '06)		9/1/07	resolved		Jan 2007
9				duodenal ulcer (1996)		9/1/07
10	hypercholesterolaemia		13/1/07			

Fig. 1.9 Problem list updated to 14 February 2007, indicating the diagnosis of hepatitis A on 13 January and return of liver tests to normal by 14 February. The anorexia and weight loss are readily explained by the hepatitis; these problems are arrowed to indicate the relationship to problem 1 (hepatitis*). Note that the haemorrhoids were diagnosed on 11 January and this problem became 'inactive' when banding was performed on 1 February. The patient's fears re colon cancer resolved when the diagnosis and causes of symptoms were explained. When the biochemical tests were returned on 13 January, hypercholesterolaemia was diagnosed for the first time and this was entered into the problem list on the same day. On 14 February, four unresolved problems remained.

understand its nature, its likely course and the effect of treatment, and management is most effective when patients are involved in decisions about their care. By including this heading in your plans, you will be reminded of the need to talk to your patient about the illness and involve them in decisions, and encouraged to develop an educational plan for your overall management strategy.

PROGRESS NOTES

The POMR provides a disciplined and standardised structure to follow-up notes. These should be succinct and brief, focusing mainly on change. There are four headings to guide you through the progress note (Fig. 1.12).

Subjective (S)

Record any change in the patient's symptoms and, when necessary, comment on compliance with a particular regimen (e.g. stopping smoking) or tolerance of drug treatment.

Objective (O)

Record any change in physical signs and investigations that may influence diagnosis, monitoring or treatment.

Assessment (A)

Comment on whether the subjective and objective information has confirmed or altered your assessment and plans.

Plan (P)

After making the assessment, and in discussion with the patient, consider whether any modification of the original plan is needed. Structure this section according to the headings listed earlier (Dx, Mx, Rx and Ed).

If there is no subjective or objective change from one visit to the next, simply record 'No change in assessment or plans'.

FLOW CHARTS

Clinical investigations and measurements are often repeated to monitor the course of acute or chronic illness.

Problem-related plans		
	Problem	**Differential diagnosis**	**Investigation**

	Problem	Differential diagnosis	Investigation
Dx	jaundice	acute hepatitis	liver tests, prothrombin time hepatitis screen (A, B and C) auto-antibodies (SMA, ANA, AMA)
		alcohol	mean cell volume, gamma-GT
		drugs	check with family doctor
		obstructive jaundice	ultrasound liver
	anorexia	see jaundice	urea and electrolytes
	weight loss	see jaundice	basal weight
	recurrent rectal bleeding	haemorrhoids	full blood count
		polyp or colon cancer	proctoscopy
			colonoscopy or barium enema
	smoking		chest radiograph

	Problem	Monitor
Mx	jaundice	twice weekly liver tests
	anorexia	monitor diet and caloric intake
	weight loss	twice weekly weight
	recurrent rectal bleeding	haemoglobin weekly

	Problem	Treatment
Rx	jaundice	bed-rest
	anorexia	encourage calorific intake (favourite foods)
	weight loss	special high calorific drink supplements
	recurrent rectal bleeding	treat cause (haemorrhoids or tumour) seek surgical opinion
	smoking	encourage relaxation and stress management
	unemployed	arrange meeting with social worker
	concern recancer	discuss concerns, advise refindings of tests and reassure

	Problem	Education
Ed	jaundice	discuss differential diagnosis
	anorexia	explain association with jaundice
	smoking	discuss dangers, techniques for coping
	rectal bleeding	explain need for colonic investigation

Fig. 1.10 Example of a problem-related plan after the creation of a problem list (Dx, diagnostic tests; Mx, monitoring tests; Rx, treatments; Ed, education.)

For example, patients presenting with diabetic ketoacidosis require frequent checks of blood sugar, urea, electrolytes, blood pH, urine output and central venous pressure. In chronic renal failure, the course of the disease and its treatment is monitored by repeated measurements of blood urea and electrolytes, creatinine, creatinine clearance, haemoglobin and body weight. A flow sheet is convenient for recording these data in a format that, at a glance, provides a summary of trends and progress (Fig. 1.13). Graphs may be equally revealing (Fig. 1.14) and are now often prepared automatically in computerised notes.

ADVANTAGES OF THE POMR

Whilst the POMR may not be followed in all health care settings, its underlying principles represent qualities that are relevant to medical record systems in general. The POMR encourages all the members of the healthcare team to standardise their approach to record-keeping. This, in turn, enhances communication and guarantees that everybody involved in the patient's care can contribute to the medical biography. Furthermore, careful structuring of the problem list, care plans and follow-up notes encourages logical, disciplined thinking and ensures that the record is comprehensive and accurate. The POMR approach to record-keeping counteracts the tendency for the 'weight' of a single problem to overwhelm and to distract from other subsidiary but potentially important problems.

Peer review and medical audit have become an integral part of quality assurance and continuing medical education. The structure of the POMR exposes the clinician's and patient's thoughts and their decision-

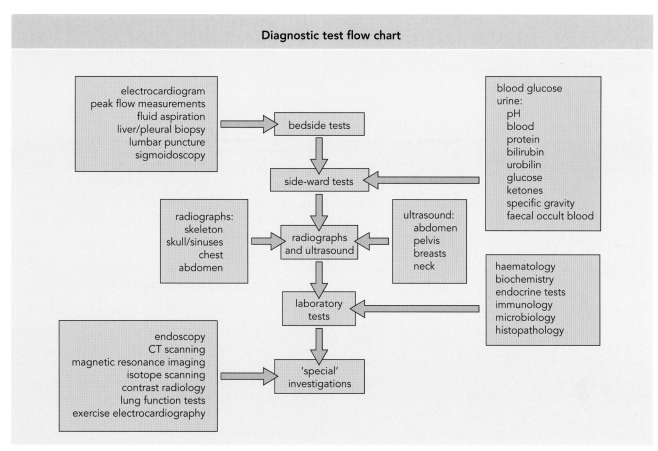

Diagnostic test flow chart

electrocardiogram
peak flow measurements
fluid aspiration
liver/pleural biopsy
lumbar puncture
sigmoidoscopy
→ bedside tests

blood glucose
urine:
  pH
  blood
  protein
  bilirubin
  urobilin
  glucose
  ketones
  specific gravity
  faecal occult blood

side-ward tests ←

radiographs:
  skeleton
  skull/sinuses
  chest
  abdomen
→ radiographs and ultrasound ← ultrasound:
  abdomen
  pelvis
  breasts
  neck

laboratory tests ← haematology
biochemistry
endocrine tests
immunology
microbiology
histopathology

endoscopy
CT scanning
magnetic resonance imaging
isotope scanning
contrast radiology
lung function tests
exercise electrocardiography
→ 'special' investigations

Fig. 1.11 Flow diagram to help plan diagnostic tests.

Progress notes

date

11/1/07   S – nauseated, fatigued

O – less jaundiced
liver less tender
taking adequate calories and fluid
ultrasound liver/biliary tract: normal
A – seems to be improving
no obstruction
P – check liver tests tomorrow
phone laboratory for hepatitis markers

13/1/07   S – feels considerably better, appetite improving
O – transaminase levels and bilirubin falling
IgM antibody to hepatitis A positive
sigmoidoscopy: bleeding haemorrhoids
hypercholesterolaemia
A – resolving hepatitis A
rectal bleeding in young patient likely
to be haemorrhoids
P – reassess patient, explain hepatitis A
consider discharge if next set of liver tests
show sustained improvement; ask surgeon
to consider treating haemorrhoids
recheck cholesterol in 3 months
reassure re no evidence of cancer found

Fig. 1.12 Example of follow-up notes.

making processes. This, in itself, is educational for both the clinician and others reading the notes, and makes the system particularly suited to the process of audit. The pressure to record meticulous and detailed information is also of intrinsic value to research workers embarking on retrospective or prospective clinical studies. Perhaps most importantly, the POMR helps to maintain a perspective of the 'whole' patient, thereby providing an overview of physical, psychological and social problems and their interaction in health and disease.

CONFIDENTIALITY

Clinical notes contain confidential information and it is important that you protect this confidentiality. Ensure that there is control over access to the medical record and that only individuals directly involved in the patient's care should read or write in the notes. Computerised notes should be password protected. In certain circumstances special security may be necessary. Patients with HIV infection and AIDS and individuals attending sexually transmitted or psychiatric clinics may have a separate set of clinical notes that are maintained distinct from the general medical records. Access to these classified records is usually restricted to doctors working in that department and the notes never leave the area of the specialist unit.

Flow sheet						
Date	9.1.07	11.1.07	13.1.07	14.1.07	7.2.07	14.2.07
Tests						
Bilirubin (<17)	233	190	130		28	10
AST (<40)	1140	830	500		52	23
ALT (<45)	1600	650	491		61	31
Albumin (35–45)	41	40	41		42	43
Pro-time (s)	14/12	14/12	13/12	d i s c h a r g e d	13/12	12/12
Haemoglobin (11.5–16.2)	12.1	12.3	12.1		12.2	12.6
Blood urea (3.5–6.5)	3.1	4.2	4.8		6.0	6.2
Blood glucose (3.5–6.5)	5.5	6.8	5.0		5.6	6,0
Hepatitis screen			IgM Hep A +ve			
Cholesterol (3.5–6.8)			8.1			8.4

Fig. 1.13 Example of a flow sheet.

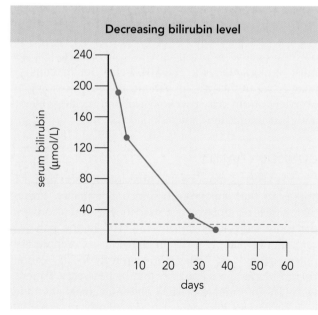

Fig. 1.14 Example of the use of a graph to illustrate changes in serum bilirubin levels following acute type A hepatitis.

Examination of elderly people

History-taking

There are special problems when recording a history from elderly patients. Consider the following:

Hearing loss
- Common in the elderly
- May be helped by hearing aid
- Important to speak clearly and slowly
- Face the patient and avoid extraneous sound
- If necessary, write questions in bold letters

Visual handicap
- Cataracts, glaucoma and macular degeneration are common in the elderly
- Ensure the room is well lit
- Engage an assistant or carer to help patients move in and out of the consulting room and examination area

Dementia
- Often occurs in patients who appear physically fit
- Forgetfulness, repetition and inappropriate answers characterise responses
- Family members, friends and carers often note the development of dementia

Important aspects of a history from elderly patients include:
- State of the domestic environment and general living conditions
- Provision of community and social services
- Family support structures
- Economic status and pension provision
- Mobility (at home and in the local environment)
- Detailed drug history and compliance
- Provision of laundry services
- Legal will

Review

The history

- Welcome
- Note the patient's body language
- Begin with an open-ended question
- Take a history of the presenting complaints(s) – both biomedical and psychosocial perspectives; use closed questions to answer the following:
  - which organ system?
  - likely cause?
  - predisposing factors?
  - complications
- Social history
- Medical history
- Education
- Employment
- Medicines, drugs and tobacco
- Alcohol consumption
- Foreign travel
- Home circumstances
- Family history
- Systems review
  - cardiovascular
  - respiratory
  - gastrointestinal
  - genitourinary
  - nervous
  - endocrine
  - musculoskeletal
  - skin and hair

2

The general examination

The dividing line between the history and examination is artificial. The examination really begins from the moment you set eyes on the patient. During the course of the history you will examine the patient's intellect, personality, family and genetic background, as well as gather information on the presenting complaint and medical history. In addition, you will have the opportunity to assess speech, orientation for person, place and time, and mood (affect). Throughout the history and examination you should sense information from the patient's unspoken body language. These physical signs are rarely taught, although the patient's body language may provide many useful signs. The patient's facial expression and tone of voice often impart more information than verbal communication. Hunched shoulders, a slow gait and poor eye contact may convey a reluctant patient, unable or unwilling to confront or expose anxieties or fears. Facial expression, tone of voice and body attitude may signal depression, even if the patient does not complain of feeling depressed. Try to look, listen and then write, this will give you the opportunity to see, as well as listen to, the patient's complaints.

The formal physical examination follows on from the history and calls on your major senses of sight, touch and hearing. Inspection, palpation, percussion and auscultation form the foundation of the physical examination and this formula is repeated each time you examine an organ system. The otoscope and ophthalmoscope extend your vision into the ear and eye, respectively, whereas the stethoscope provides an amplification system to help you listen to the heart, lung and bowel sounds. With the help of technology, we are now able to extend our vision deep into the body: radiographs (including computerised axial tomography scanning), ultrasound, magnetic resonance imaging and fibreoptics greatly broaden our powers of observation.

The physical examination begins with a general examination and is followed by examination of the skin, head and neck, heart and lungs, abdominal organs, musculoskeletal and neurological systems. With practice it is possible to perform the 'routine' examination in

10–15 min, although if you discover an abnormality, considerably more time will be spent refining the findings. From the outset you should aim to choreograph an economical, aesthetic and complete examination.

General examination

The general examination permits you to obtain an overview of the general state of health and provides an opportunity to examine systems that do not fall neatly into a regional examination. For the patient, the general examination is also a gentle introduction to the more intense systems examination to follow.

FIRST IMPRESSIONS

The examination commences as the patient walks into the consulting room or as you sit down at the bedside to take a history. At this first encounter, even before you initiate the history, decide whether the patient looks well or not and whether there is any striking physical abnormality. You will also gain an immediate impression of dress, grooming and personal hygiene.

As the patient approaches you in the consulting or examination room, observe the posture, gait and character of the stride. Diseases of nerves, muscles, bones and joints are associated with abnormal gaits and postures. You should quickly recognise the slow shuffling gait and 'pill rolling' tremor of Parkinson's disease or the unsteady broad-based gait of the ataxic patient. Patients with proximal muscle weakness may have difficulty rising from the waiting room chair and their gait may have a waddling appearance. Patients with osteoporosis lose height as the vertebrae progressively collapse: you may be struck by the typically stooped (kyphotic) appearance and 'round shoulders' of these patients. Take note if the patient walks with a stick or some form of additional physical support. A white stick indicates partial or complete blindness. The gait also conveys body language: the patient may have a spring in the step, make rapid eye

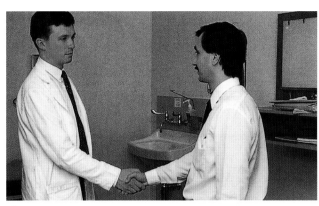

Fig. 2.1 The handshake serves as a gentle introduction to the physical contact that will occur during the formal physical examination.

contact and immediately offer a firm handshake. This contrasts with the patient with drooping shoulders and a slow (but otherwise normal) step who avoids eye contact.

When making your initial acquaintance with the patient, a warm handshake serves a number of functions (Fig. 2.1). The touching of hands may reassure the patient and serve as a gentle and symbolic introduction to the more intimate physical contact of the examination that follows the history. Before shaking hands, glance momentarily at the hand to ensure that you will not be grabbing a prosthesis or deformed hand. A well-made prosthesis may cause considerable embarrassment as you suddenly realise that the hand you are shaking is hard and lifeless. You may also note other abnormalities such as a potentially painful rheumatoid hand or missing fingers. The grip of the handshake usually provides some useful information. A normal grip conveys different information from a weak, lethargic handshake, which may imply distal muscle weakness, general ill-health or depression. The handshake is a useful physical sign in patients with myotonia dystrophica, a rare autosomal dominant inherited disease of muscle. A feature of this disease is the abnormally slow relaxation of the grip on completion of the handshake. The syndrome is also characterised by premature frontal balding, testicular atrophy and cataracts.

On first contact with the patient, you may be struck by an unusual physical stature. Unusually short stature may reflect constitutional shortness, a distinct genetic syndrome or the consequence of intrauterine, childhood or adolescent growth retardation. Unusually tall stature is most often constitutional, although hypothalamic tumours in childhood or adolescence may cause excessive growth hormone release, resulting in abnormally rapid linear growth and gigantism. If excess growth hormone release occurs after the bony epiphyses have fused, body shape changes (acromegaly). Severe malnutrition and obesity are readily recognised on the first encounter with a patient.

In hospitalised patients, posture may provide helpful information. Patients with acute pancreatitis find some

relief lying with knees drawn towards the chest. Patients with peritonitis lie motionless, as any abdominal wall movement causes intense pain. The pain of acute pyelonephritis or perinephric abscess might be partly relieved by lateral flexion to the side of the pathology. In acute pericarditis, the patient finds modest relief by sitting forward; and in left ventricular failure, patients breath more easily when lying propped up on three or four pillows (this is termed orthopnoea).

Formal examination

On completion of the history, prepare the patient for the formal examination. Always remain sensitive to the apprehension most patients feel when laid out naked on the examination couch or bed. Imagine yourself in that position, confronted by a near stranger who is about to inspect, palpate, percuss and auscultate your body – a daunting thought. The history should already have provided you with the opportunity to build a confident professional relationship with the patient. It is a cultural and established fact that it is quite acceptable for a doctor to undertake a comprehensive physical examination, although remain sensitive to some cultural norms where same-sex examinations might be preferable. This acceptance usually extends to medical students who can be reassured that most patients welcome students and recognise their need to learn the examination technique. Explain the necessity of undertaking a full physical examination. The examination adds information to the clinical database and a thorough examination provides considerable reassurance to the patient.

Differential diagnosis
Growth failure

Genetic
- Achondroplasia
- Turner's syndrome
- Down's syndrome

Constitutional
- Family members who have short stature

Endocrine
- Hypopituitarism
- Hypothyroidism

Systemic disease
- Crohn's disease
- Ulcerative colitis
- Renal failure

Malnutrition
- Intrauterine growth retardation
- Marasmus
- Kwashiorkor

The examination requires full exposure: men and women should be asked to remove superficial clothing and vests or undershirts. For a chest examination, women should be asked to remove their bra. Ensure a clean and presentable examination gown is available in the examination room for the patient to don before you enter the room. When a patient of the opposite sex is to be examined, always ask the chaperone to check whether the patient is ready.

SETTING

A separate examination room or adequate screening should be provided to ensure privacy while the patient is undressing and being examined. The room should be comfortably warm. Ensure that there are fresh sheets (either linen or disposable) and a clean blanket for cover. The examination couch should be positioned to allow you to examine from the patient's right side and there must be good general illumination. You should be fully equipped to undertake the examination without disruption. Ensure you have a working penlight torch and stethoscope. Close at hand there must be a sphygmomanometer, ophthalmoscope, otoscope, tongue depressors and disposable gloves (for genital and rectal examination). Basic equipment for the neurological examination should be available. This includes a patellar hammer, tuning fork, cotton wool buds, an appropriate object for testing pin-prick responses, test tubes to fill with hot and cold water for temperature testing, and hat pins with red and white tops to assess visual fields. A cupful of drinking water should also be available, as you may ask the patient to swallow a mouthful to check for a thyroid goitre or other neck swelling.

As you approach the patient, re-establish both verbal and eye contact. You may ask the patient whether they feel comfortable and are prepared for the examination. Start the examination with the patient supine and the head and shoulders raised to approximately 45° above the horizontal. Most modern examination couches and hospital beds are designed to allow easy adjustment of the upper body. Most of the examination takes place with the patient comfortably resting in this position (Fig. 2.2). Three further adjustments will be made in the course of the examination. When auscultating the mitral area of the heart it is helpful to roll the patient towards the left lateral position as this brings the apex closer to the stethoscope. To examine the neck, posterior chest, back and spine you will ask the patient to sit forward. For assessing the abdomen, reposition the patient to lie flat, as this provides optimal access for the abdominal examination. Plan the examination to ensure the most economical movements for both you and the patient.

Following the history, reflect on which physical signs may help you confirm or refine your initial assessment. Anticipation of physical signs will help you to direct and focus the examination. For example, if a patient complains of breathlessness, you may anticipate anaemia or

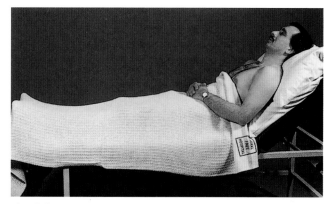

Fig. 2.2 The position of the patient at the start of the examination.

respiratory or cardiac disease, therefore, you should gear the examination towards determining which of these possibilities is responsible for the symptoms.

Begin with an inspection of overall appearance.

Symptoms and signs
Observation of general appearance

- Does the patient look comfortable or distressed?
- Is the patient well or ill?
- Is there a recognisable syndrome?
- Is the patient well nourished?
- Is the patient well hydrated?

Recognisable syndromes and facies

When inspecting the face, you might be struck by a single sign such as a red eye or the characteristic facies associated with discrete syndromes.

THE EYE

The history might be helpful in distinguishing possible causes of the red eye. Ask about duration, previous attacks, pain (and its character), photophobia and possible direct causes of traumatic damage. It is useful to

Questions to ask
Red eyes

- Is red eye painful or painless?
- Is vision affected? Can the patient read ordinary print with the affected eye(s)?
- Is there foreign body sensation?
- Is there photophobia?
- Is there a discharge other than tears?
- Was there trauma?
- Are you a contact lens wearer?

distinguish the sensation of a foreign body from less specific symptoms such as 'grittiness' and 'itching'. A foreign body sensation feels as if there is something in the eye and is associated with some difficulty opening the eye. This symptom is characteristic of an active corneal process causing the red eye.

Differential diagnosis

Main causes of red eye

- Conjunctivitis (infective, allergic, toxic)
- Keratitis (infective, foreign body, sicca syndrome)
- Acute closed angle glaucoma
- Iritis
- Subconjunctival haemorrhage

Begin the examination by inspecting the eyes. In lid and conjunctival disorders, there is no foreign body sensation or photophobia and the patient sits in a brightly lit room without discomfort. In bacterial conjunctivitis the patient complains of pussy discharge (especially in the morning on waking) and this might be seen on inspection. A foreign body sensation (rather than gritty or itchy sensation) is typical of active corneal disease. In infectious keratitis the patient has difficulty keeping the affected eye open, and a similar sign occurs with contact lens abrasion. Patients with iritis may present with difficulty keeping the eye open and some photophobia but without the complaint of a foreign body sensation. In acute angle closure glaucoma the patient often clutches the affected eye and complains of associated headache and malaise. Visual acuity may be affected in red eye and should be assessed. The pinhole test helps distinguish refractive errors from other causes of visual loss. In refractive visual disturbances (e.g. myopia), vision is improved when

peering through a small hole. In nonrefractive disorders, improvement does not occur.

Next, use a penlight to inspect the pupils and anterior segment. In angle closure glaucoma the pupil may be fixed in mid-dilation and may not respond to light. In corneal abrasion, acute keratitis and iritis, the pupil might be pinpoint. A purulent discharge suggests bacterial conjunctivitis or keratitis. The pattern of redness might be helpful. Diffuse injection of both the palpebral and bulbar conjunctivae suggests primary conjunctival disorders (bacterial, viral, allergic, toxic or associated with dry eyes). In contrast, more serious disorders such as keratitis, iritis and angle closure glaucoma present with a 'ciliary flush' with injection most marked at the limbus (the sclerocorneal junction). A white spot or opacity on the cornea indicates keratitis and further slit-lamp examination with fluorescein is required to delineate the lesion. Hypopyon is seen as a layer of pus in the anterior chamber and is associated with infectious keratitis, acute iritis and endophthalmitis and is an ophthalmic emergency. Hyphaema refers to the presence of a layer of blood in the anterior compartment and is usually caused by injury. Subconjunctival haemorrhage is painless and characterised by demarcated areas of extravasated blood which resolves in 1–2 weeks.

Red flag – urgent referral

Indications for emergency referral to ophthalmology

- Unilateral red eye which is painful with nausea and vomiting (e.g. acute glaucoma)
- Associated loss of vision
- Corneal infiltrate or hypopion

Symptoms and signs

Quick testing of visual acuity

- Assess ability of each eye to read newspaper print
- Pinhole test
- Snellen chart

Symptoms and signs

Penlight inspection of the red eye

- Does the pupil react to light?
- Is the pupil smaller than expected or pinpoint?
- Is there a purulent discharge?
- What is the pattern of the redness?
- Is there a corneal 'white spot'?
- Is there hypopyon or hyphema?

FACIES AND SYNDROMES

Certain diseases are readily identified by a distinctive combination of physical characteristics. There are a large number of recognisable congenital syndromes that were probably diagnosed during childhood and should not present as an undiagnosed problem to physicians caring for teenagers or adults. In addition, only a proportion survives into adulthood. There are several recognisable genetic or chromosomal syndromes that may present to clinicians caring for adults; examples include Down's syndrome (trisomy 21; Fig. 2.3), Turner's syndrome (Fig. 2.4), Marfan's syndrome (Fig. 2.5), tuberous sclerosis (Figs 2.6, 2.7), albinism (Fig. 2.8), the fragile X chromosome (a common genetic cause of mental subnormality in which affected males have unusually large testes), Peutz–Jeghers syndrome (Figs 2.9–2.11), Waardenburg's syndrome (Fig. 2.12), familial hypercholesterolaemia (Figs 2.13–2.17) and neurofibromatosis. Other readily recognisable syndromes include the endocrine disorders

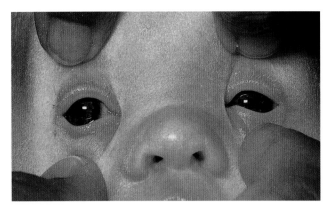

Fig. 2.3 Down's syndrome: epicanthic folds, Brushfield's spots and hypertelorism (increased interorbital distance).

Symptoms and signs

Down's syndrome (trisomy 21)

- Facies – oblique orbital fissures, epicanthic folds, small ears, flat nasal bridge, protruding tongue, Brushfield's spots on iris
- Short stature
- Hands – single palmar crease, curved little finger, short hands
- Heart disease (endocardial cushion defects)
- Gap between first and second toes
- Educationally subnormal

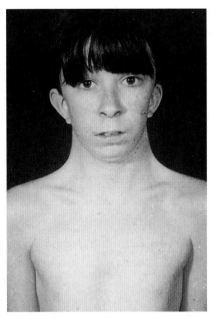

Fig. 2.4 Turner's syndrome: typical facial appearance, webbed neck and widely spaced nipples.

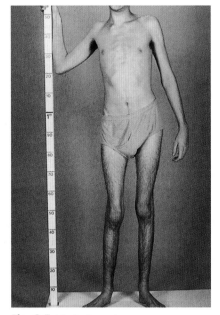

Fig. 2.5 Marfan's syndrome.

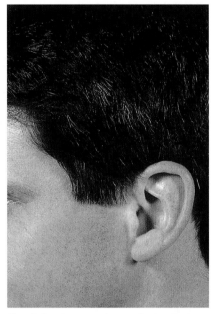

Fig. 2.6 Tuberous sclerosis: flecks of white hair.

Symptoms and signs

Turner's syndrome (XO karyotype)

- Failure of sexual development
- Short stature
- Facies – micrognathia (small chin), low-set ears, fish-like mouth, epicanthic folds
- Short, webbed neck with low hairline; widely spaced nipples (shield-shaped chest)
- Heart disease (coarctation)
- Short fourth metacarpal or metatarsal
- Abnormally wide carrying angle of the elbow

Symptoms and signs

Marfan's syndrome

- Arm span greater than height
- Above average crown-to-heel height
- Long slender fingers
- Hyperextensible joints
- Kyphoscoliosis and anterior chest wall deformity
- High-arched palate
- Aortic incompetence and dissecting aortic aneurysms
- Subluxation or dislocation of the lens

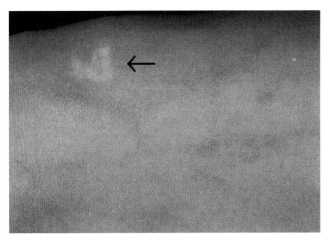

Symptoms and signs

Tuberous sclerosis (Bourneville's disease, autosomal dominant chromosome 9)

- Epilepsy
- Cognitive impairment (67%)
- Skin lesions (facial adenoma sebaceum, shagreen patch, fibromas near toenails and eyebrows)
- Flecks of white hair
- Retinal haemorrhages

Fig. 2.7 Tuberous sclerosis: shagreen patch.

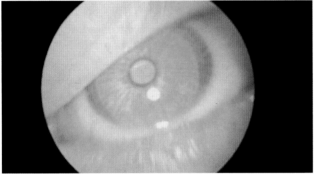

Symptoms and signs

Oculocutaneous albinism (autosomal recessive)

- Hypomelanosis or amelanosis of skin
- White hair
- Photophobia, nystagmus
- Hypopigmented fundus and translucent iris

Fig. 2.8 Albinism: typical translucent iris.

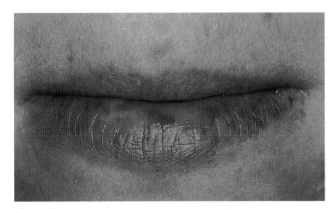

Fig. 2.9 Peutz–Jeghers syndrome: freckles on lips.

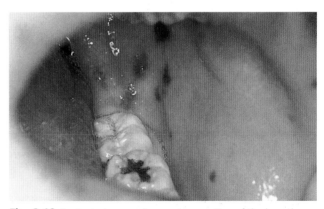

Fig. 2.10 Peutz–Jeghers syndrome: pigmentation of the buccal mucosa.

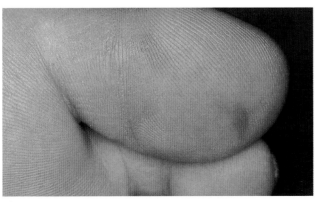

Fig. 2.11 Peutz–Jeghers syndrome: pigmentation of the big toe.

Symptoms and signs

Peutz–Jeghers syndrome (autosomal dominant)

- Pigmented macules (1–5 mm in diameter)
- Occur in profusion on lips, buccal mucosa and fingers
- Gastric, small intestinal and colonic hamartoms polyps that sometimes give rise to abdominal pain, bleeding and intussusception

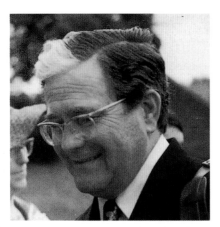

Fig. 2.12 Waardenberg's syndrome: typical white forelock.

Symptoms and signs

Waardenberg's syndrome (autosomal dominant)

- Cochlear deafness
- Frontal white lock of hair
- Wide-set eyes
- Different coloured irises (heterochromia)
- White eyelashes
- Piebaldism

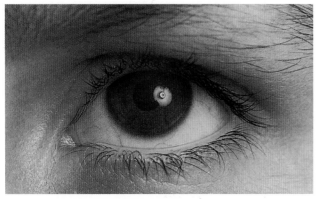

Fig. 2.13 Familial hypercholesterolaemia: corneal arcus senilis.

Symptoms and signs

Familial hypercholesterolaemia (autosomal dominant)

- Xanthelasmas, skin xanthomas
- Tendon xanthomas
- Arcus senilis
- Marked artherosclerosis
- Ischaemic heart disease, peripheral vascular disease

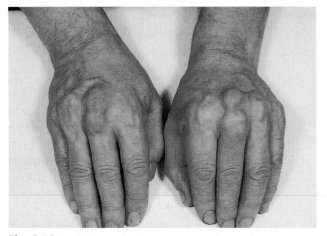

Fig. 2.14 Familial hypercholesterolaemia: tendon xanthomas.

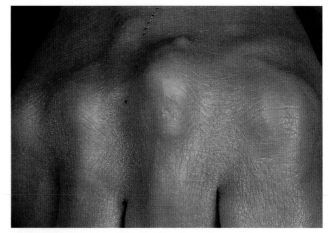

Fig. 2.15 Familial hypercholesterolaemia: tendon xanthomas.

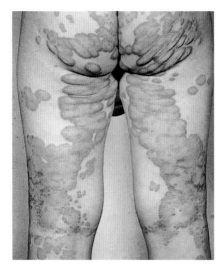

Fig. 2.16 Familial hypercholesterolaemia: skin xanthomas.

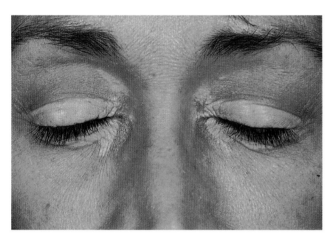

Fig. 2.17 Familial hypercholesterolaemia: xanthelasmata around the eyelids.

and major organ failure (liver, heart, lungs and kidneys).

Endocrine syndromes

The endocrine glands are scattered throughout the body (Fig. 2.18). It is practical to consider the examination of the endocrine glands in the context of the overall general examination. Both over- and underactivity of the endocrine glands can be suspected from the patient's facies, body build and skin colour; endocrinopathies are often readily recognised in the course of the general examination.

Distinct clinical syndromes occur in diseases of the thyroid, parathyroid, adrenal and pituitary glands. An overview of the structure and function of each of these organs will help your clinical assessment and syndrome recognition.

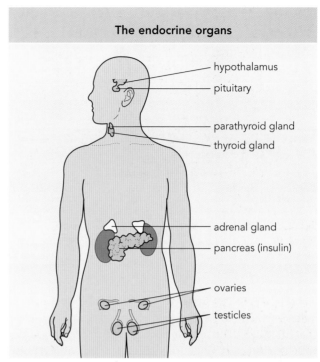

The endocrine organs

- hypothalamus
- pituitary
- parathyroid gland
- thyroid gland
- adrenal gland
- pancreas (insulin)
- ovaries
- testicles

Fig. 2.18 The positions of the main endocrine organs.

The thyroid gland

Structure and function

The thyroid gland develops from a ventral pouch of the fetal pharynx. This pouch evolves into the thyroid gland by migrating caudally to a resting place in front of the trachea. The migration may leave thyroid remnants along the embryonic tract which extends from the back of the tongue (where a residual lingual thyroid 'rest' may occur). A midline thyroglossal cyst may develop if the migration tract fails to obliterate.

The thyroid gland consists of two lateral lobes joined by an isthmus. The gland lies in front of the larynx and trachea with the isthmus overlying the second to fourth tracheal rings (Fig. 2.19). The lateral lobes extend from the side of the thyroid cartilage to the sixth tracheal ring. Two nerves lie in close proximity to the thyroid gland: the recurrent laryngeal nerve runs in the groove between the trachea and the thyroid; and the external branch of the superior laryngeal nerve lies deep to the upper poles. In thyroid cancer, these nerves may be invaded and damage may occur in the course of thyroid surgery.

THYROXINE SYNTHESIS AND SECRETION

The anterior pituitary hormone, thyroid stimulating hormone (TSH), stimulates the synthesis of thyroxine

Thyroid anatomy

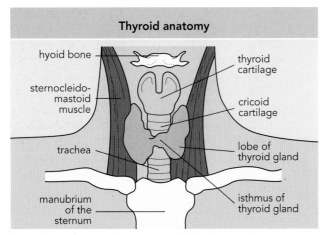

Fig. 2.19 Anatomy of the thyroid gland and surrounding structures.

(T_4) (Fig. 2.20). The functioning unit of the thyroid is the follicle, which consists of epithelial cells lining a central colloid space. The epithelial cells concentrate iodide, which is oxidised to iodine and incorporated with tyrosine to form mono-iodotyrosine and di-iodotyrosine. These two iodinated tyrosines are combined in the colloid to form either tri-iodothyronine (T_3) or tetra-iodothyronine (T_4). The two active hormones, T_3 and T_4, are stored in the colloid and bound to a specific binding protein (thyroglobulin). The protein-bound hormones are taken back up into the follicle epithelium by endocytosis. In the cells, the colloid droplets are disrupted by proteolytic enzymes, allowing the release of T_3 and T_4 into the circulation where most circulate bound to thyroid binding globulin (TBG). Free hormone levels dictate the metabolic effects of T_4. T_4 is synthesised only in the thyroid but T_3 can also be produced from conversion of circulating T_4 in the liver, the kidney and other tissues. The hepatic conversion of T_4 results in two species of T_3: an active T_3 and an inactive reverse T_3.

Clinical examination of the thyroid gland and function

Although considered part of the general examination, the thyroid gland is usually examined when examining the head and neck (see Ch. 4).

Like any other organ, the thyroid examination relies on inspection, palpation, percussion and auscultation. Examine the thyroid gland with the patient sitting forward in bed or seated in a chair.

Ensure complete exposure of the neck and upper chest. Inspect the thyroid from the front of the neck. The normal thyroid gland is neither visible nor palpable. An enlarged thyroid, or goitre, is seen as a fullness on either side of the trachea below the cricoid cartilage, or as a distinct, enlarged, nodular organ with one or both lobes easily visible (Figs. 2.21–2.23). If the lobes are visible,

Biosynthesis of thyroxine

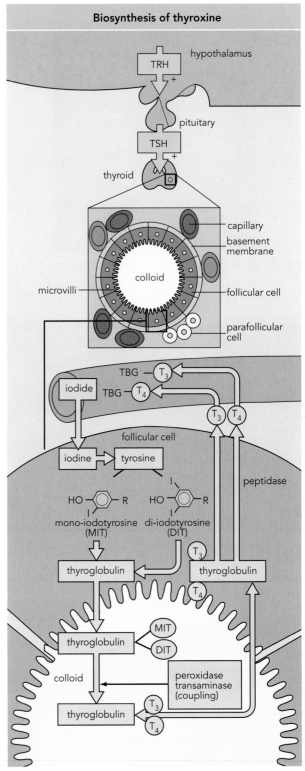

Fig. 2.20 The hypothalamus secretes thyroid releasing hormone (TRH) which stimulates the anterior pituitary to produce thyroid stimulating hormone (TSH). This stimulates the synthesis of thyroxine (T_4) in the follicles. Iodide taken up into the follicular cell is oxidised to iodine and then incorporated into tyrosine to form mono-iodotyrosine (MIT) and di-iodotyrosine (DIT), which binds with thyroglobulin and is secreted into the colloid where T_3 and T_4 are synthesised. These are taken back into the follicular cells taken up by endocytosis where the T_3 and T_4 are split from thyroglobulin and released into the circulation, where they are bound to T_4 binding globulin (TBG).

determine whether they look symmetrical or irregular. Ask the patient to sip a little water and hold it in the mouth. When you give the instruction to swallow, watch for the characteristic upward movement of the goitre as the pharyngeal muscles contract. This test helps distinguish a thyroid mass from other neck masses (e.g. enlarged lymph nodes, which hardly move with swallowing). The midline remnant of the thyroid (thyroglossal cysts or thyroid remnants) also moves with swallowing.

Next, explain to the patient that you wish to feel the front of the neck for the thyroid gland. Position yourself to the right and slightly behind the patient. Feel for the left and right lobes with the finger pulps of both hands (Fig. 2.24). Ensure a gentle examination, as your hands are positioned in a throttling posture; reassure the patient by standing to the side rather than at the rear so that you remain in the patient's peripheral field of vision. Assess the texture (hard or soft, single or multiple nodules),

symmetry and extent of the goitre. A soft, smooth goitre may be more easily seen than felt. It is unusual for the goitre to be tender unless the enlargement is caused by acute inflammatory thyroiditis. In the course of thyroid palpation, again ask the patient to take a sip of water and to swallow when you indicate. As the patient gulps, you should feel the goitre move beneath your fingers. Complete the palpation by feeling for the carotids, which may be encased by a malignant thyroid gland. Thyroid carcinoma may spread to local neck lymph nodes, so it is important to conclude the palpation by checking for palpable regional lymph nodes.

The thyroid gland may also enlarge in a downward direction behind the manubrium sterni. This retrosternal goitre may extend deeply into the superior mediastinum and may even cause compression symptoms (i.e. breathlessness and dysphagia). Retrosternal extension can be assessed by percussing over the manubrium and upper sternum (Fig. 2.25). Normally, this area resonates, yet when there is retrosternal enlargement the percussion note is dull. Auscultate the gland for bruits by applying the diaphragm of the stethoscope to each lobe in turn (Fig. 2.26). Ask the patient to stop breathing for a moment while you listen on either side for a bruit. A soft bruit is characteristic of the smooth symmetrical hyperthyroid goitre of Graves' disease.

Clinical assessment of thyroid function

T_4 has a number of important metabolic effects and over- or underactivity results in characteristic clinical syndromes that may readily be recognised. Diagnosis of hyperthyroidism is confirmed by measuring the serum levels of T_4 and T_3, whereas in hypothyroidism the serum TSH level is elevated and T_4 is subnormal.

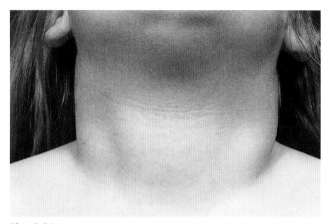

Fig. 2.21 Smooth goitre appearing as fullness in the anterior neck.

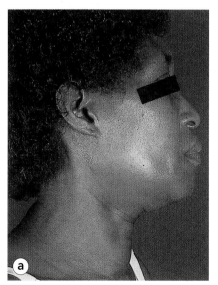
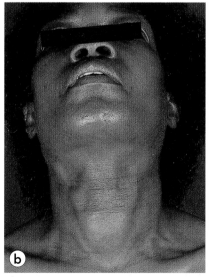

Fig. 2.22 Readily visible multinodular thyroid goitre.

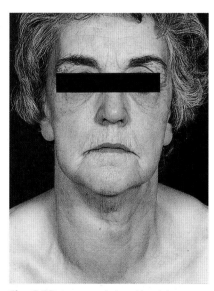

Fig. 2.23 Asymmetrical multinodular goitre.

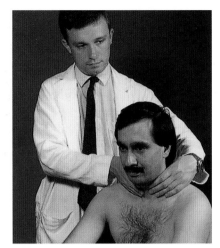

Fig. 2.24 Position for palpation of the lateral lobes of the isthmus of the thyroid.

? Questions to ask
Hyperthyroidism

- Have you lost weight recently?
- Has your appetite changed (e.g. increased)?
- Have you noticed a change in bowel habit (e.g. increased)?
- Have you noticed a recent change in heat tolerance?
- Do you suffer from excessive sweating?
- Does your heart race or palpitate?
- Have you noticed a change in mood?

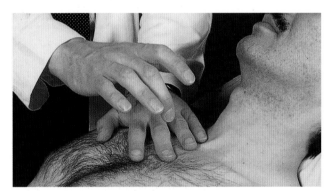

Fig. 2.25 A retrosternal goitre is suggested by dullness to percussion over the manubrium sterni.

Symptoms and signs
Hyperthyroidism

- Weight loss, increased appetite
- Recent onset of heat intolerance
- Agitation, nervousness
- Hot sweaty palms
- Fine peripheral tremor
- Bounding peripheral pulses
- Tachycardia, atrial fibrillation
- Lid retraction and lid lag
- Goitre, with or without overlying bruit
- Brisk tendon reflexes

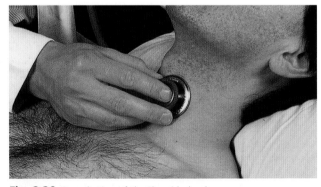

Fig. 2.26 Auscultation of the thyroid gland.

masquerades as classical hypothyroidism. In both young and older thyrotoxic patients, you may be alerted to the diagnosis by a history of weight loss, recent intolerance to hot weather, sweating, palpitations, abnormal irritability and nervousness and increased bowel frequency. Most hyperthyroid patients feel warm and sweaty, have a tachycardia, staring eyes (caused by lid retraction) and abnormally brisk tendon reflexes. A fine peripheral tremor is common in thyrotoxicosis. This can be demonstrated by placing a sheet of paper on the back of the outstretched hand and watching the tremor, which is amplified by the sheet of paper 'trembling' (Fig. 2.27). Although similar signs of hyperthyroidism may occur in the young and old, Graves' disease is more readily recognisable from the characteristic facial appearance and associated physical signs.

HYPERTHYROIDISM

Hyperthyroidism occurs most commonly in young women presenting with smooth diffuse goitres (Graves' disease). However, in elderly people, hyperthyroidism may be caused by an autonomous 'toxic' adenoma and, rarely, a functioning carcinoma. Rarely factitious hyperthyroidism caused by excessive T$_4$ intake

GRAVES' DISEASE

The facies in Graves' disease is dominated by a staring appearance caused by retraction of the upper eyelid. Normally, during a relaxed forward gaze, the upper lid protects the eye by lying in a horizontal position which crosses the eye in a plane just above the upper pole of the pupil. In Graves' disease, autonomic overactivity causes increased tone and spasm of levator palpebrae

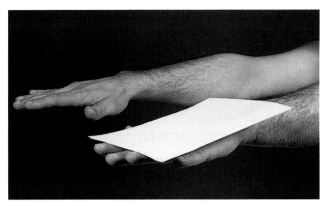

Fig. 2.27 Place a sheet of paper on the outstretched fingers to demonstrate the fine tremor of hyperthyroidism.

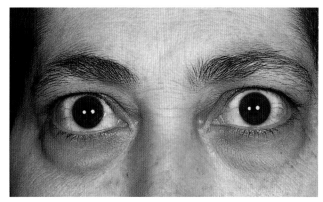

Fig. 2.28 Bilateral lid retraction in a patient with Graves' disease. Note that the upper lid is positioned well above the pupil and the palpebral fissure is widened.

Symptoms and signs		
Hyperthyroidism in Graves' disease and toxic nodular goitre		
	Graves' disease	**Nodular goitre**
Sex	female >> men	female = men
Eye signs	very common, exopthalmos	less severe
Goitre	diffuse, overlying bruit	may be multinodular
Heart	tachycardia, atrial fibrillation	also angina, congestive heart failure
Weight	may lose weight	often profound weight loss

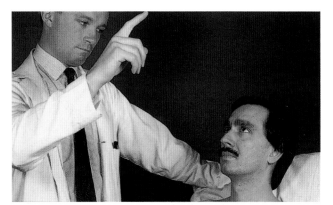

Fig. 2.29 Lid lag. With the patient sitting, position yourself on the patient's right side. Watch how the lid moves with the downward movement of the eye as the patient follows your finger moving from a point approximately 45° above the horizontal to a point below this plane. Normally there is perfect coordination as the lid follows the downward movement of the eye.

superioris. This causes retraction of the upper lid, which exposes most, if not all, of the iris, exposing sclera above the iris and creating the typical staring appearance (Fig. 2.28). Spasm of the muscles supplying the upper lid also results in an abnormal following reflex. Normally, if you ask a patient to follow the movement of an object (e.g. your fingertip) (Fig. 2.29) from a point above eye level to a vertical point below eye level, you will note that as the eye moves, the upper lid follows the upper margin of the pupil in a fully synchronised downward movement. In hyperthyroidism, this coordination is lost and the movement of the upper lid lags well behind the pupil (this is termed 'lid lag') (Fig. 2.30).

In progressive Graves' disease, abnormal connective tissue (especially hyaluronic acid) is deposited in the orbit and external ocular muscles. The globes are pushed forward, resulting first in proptosis and in the more severe form, exophthalmos (defined as >18 mm protrusion). To examine for exophthalmos, seat the patient in a chair and inspect the globes from above by looking over the forehead or from the side of the profile (Fig. 2.31).

A Hertel exophthalmometer can be used to make an accurate baseline measurement of the degree of exophthalmos and this measurement is used to monitor progression and regression. Other eye signs of Graves' disease include ophthalmoplegia caused by weakness and infiltration of the external ophthalmic muscles. These patients complain of double vision (diplopia) and on examination there is a loss of gaze symmetry. Conjunctival oedema (chemosis) may also occur. The eye signs can be either bilateral or unilateral (Fig. 2.32), although, in the latter, always consider a space-occupying lesion of the orbit. Other features of Graves' disease include finger clubbing, onycholysis (separation of the nail from its bed), pretibial myxoedema (brawny swelling of lower legs), and periostitis (inflammation of the periosteum).

A rare complication of hyperthyroidism is thyroid storm. This is an exaggerated manifestation of hyperthyroidism and is life threatening. While thyroid storm can develop in patients with longstanding untreated hyperthyroidism, it is more often precipitated by an acute

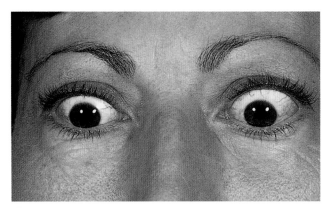

Fig. 2.30 In hyperthyroidism the downward movement of the lid lags behind the movement of the bulb as it follows your finger through an arc.

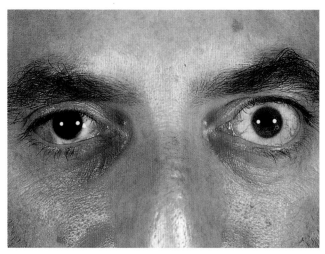

Fig. 2.32 Graves' disease: unilateral eye condition.

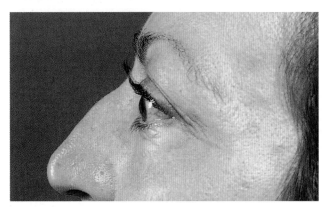

Fig. 2.31 Graves' disease: proptosis of the eye.

	Emergency
	Features of thyroid storm

- Thermoregulation dysfunction
- CNS effects (agitation, delirium, psychosis, epilepsy, coma)
- Gastrointestinal dysfunction (diarrhoea, vomiting, abdominal pain)
- Cardiovascular features (tachycardia, high output cardiac function)

	Symptoms and signs
	Graves' disease (autoimmune hyperthyroidism)

- Diffuse goitre with audible bruit
- Pretibial myxoedema, finger clubbing
- Onycholysis (Plummer's nails)
- Lid retraction, lid lag
- Proptosis, exopthalmos
- Conjunctival oedema (chemosis)

	Symptoms and signs
	Assessment of severity of Graves' ophthalmopathy

Class	Signs / symptoms
0	no symptoms or signs
I	signs but no symptoms
II	soft tissue involvement
III	proptosis
IV	extraocular muscle involvement
V	corneal involvement
VI	visual loss (optic nerve damage)

event such as thyroid or nonthyroid surgery, trauma, infection or an acute iodine load.

HYPOTHYROIDISM

Hypothyroidism presents insidiously; the diagnosis may be readily apparent on general examination. Suspect hypothyroidism in patients complaining of unexplained lethargy, weight gain, newly noted cold intolerance, constipation, generalised hair loss and pain in the hand suggestive of a carpal tunnel syndrome. Poor memory and general intellectual deterioration may also be presenting features. While taking the history you might have noticed on unusually coarse voice. The disorder may occur at any age, although it is most common in elderly individuals. There are a number of possible causes to consider. On first sight you may notice the characteristic puffy facial appearance, the pale 'waxy' skin and diffuse hair loss from the scalp and eyebrows. Look for other signs to confirm your clinical suspicion of myxoedema (Fig. 2.33). The delayed relaxation phase of the Achilles tendon jerk is especially helpful (Fig. 2.34).

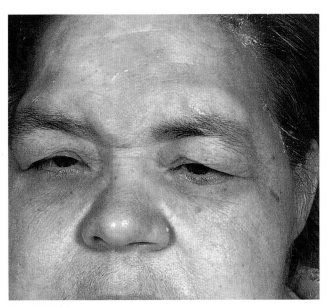

Fig. 2.33 Myxoedema.

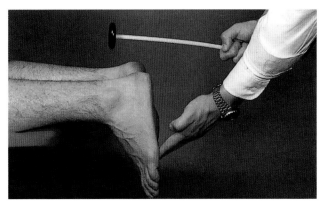

Fig. 2.34 The ankle jerk in hypothyroidism. Although all the reflexes show a distinct slowing of the relaxation phase of the tendon reflex, the sign is best observed and felt with the Achilles tendon jerk. Ask the patient to kneel on a chair or examination couch with the feet hanging over the edge. Expose the Achilles tendon and percuss with a patellar hammer while gently resting one hand on the sole of the foot. Watch and feel for the delayed return of the foot to its resting position after the reflex contraction that follows the tendon tap.

Questions to ask

Hypothyroidism

- Has your weight changed?
- Has your bowel habit changed (e.g. constipation)?
- Is your hair falling out?
- Have you noticed a change in weather preference (e.g. cold intolerance)?
- Has there been a change in your voice (e.g. hoarse)?
- Do you suffer from pain in your hands (e.g. carpal tunnel syndrome)?

Differential diagnosis

Hypothyroidism

Congenital
- Congenital absence
- Inborn errors of thyroxine metabolism

Acquired
- Iodine deficiency (endemic goitre)
- Autoimmune thyroiditis (Hashimoto's disease)
- Postradiotherapy for hyperthyroidism
- Postsurgical thyroidectomy
- Antithyroid drugs (e.g. carbimazole)
- Pituitary tumours and granulomas

The parathyroid glands

Structure and function

There are usually four parathyroid glands (two superior and two inferior). Ninety per cent of parathyroid glands lie in intimate contact with the thyroid gland, although in 10% of patients the inferior glands lie in an aberrant position. These pea-sized glands usually lie embedded in the posterior aspect of the upper and lower poles of the thyroid or superficially on the surface of the thyroid.

PARATHYROID HORMONE

Parathyroid hormone (PTH) is synthesised in a precursor form known as pre-pro-PTH, which is first cleaved to

Symptoms and signs

Hypothyroidism

- Constipation, weight gain
- Hair loss
- Angina pectoris
- Hoarse croaky voice
- Dry flaky skin
- Balding and loss of eyebrows (beginning laterally)
- Bradycardia
- Xanthelasmas (hyperlipidaemia)
- Goitre (especially with iodine deficiency)
- Effusions (pericardial or pleural)
- Delayed relaxation phase of tendon reflexes
- Carpal tunnel syndrome

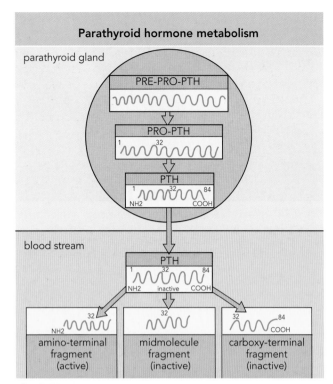

Fig. 2.35 Parathyroid hormone (PTH) metabolism. A large precursor molecule (PRE-PRO-PTH) is cleaved to form an 84 amino acid molecule PTH which is secreted into the blood stream. The molecule, which has an amino carboxy terminal, is cleaved to smaller fragments. Only fragments with the first 32 amino terminal amino acids are metabolically active.

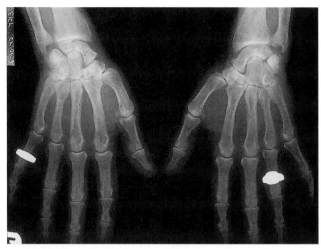

Fig. 2.36 Hyperparathyroidism: a radiograph of the phalanges may show subperiosteal erosions and bone cysts.

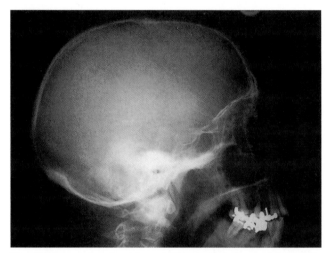

Fig. 2.37 Hyperparathyroidism: skull radiograph shows thinning of the cortex and small osteolytic areas, known as 'pepper pot' skull.

pro-PTH and then cleaved again to the 84 amino acid polypeptide, PTH (Fig. 2.35). PTH secretion is regulated by the level of calcium in the blood; hypocalcaemia stimulates its release. In the circulation, the 84 amino acid PTH is cleaved to smaller fragments, most of which are inactive; the only active fragment is that containing the first 32 amino acids. The hormone's prime effect is on the renal tubule, where it stimulates calcium resorption from the tubular fluid and phosphate excretion in the urine. PTH also stimulates calcium resorption from bone.

HYPERPARATHYROIDISM

Hyperparathyroidism is usually detected by finding an abnormally high serum calcium level on routine blood testing or in patients presenting with renal colic caused by stones. Hyperparathyroidism may be caused by hyperplasia or one or more autonomous adenomas (often associated with the multiple endocrine neoplasia syndromes). In chronic renal failure, longstanding stimulation may result in loss of feedback and an autonomous secretion of PTH leading to hypercalcaemia (this is known as tertiary hyperparathyroidism). The clinical syndrome may be difficult to recognise, because the symptoms ('moans') dominate the signs ('stones and bones'). The patient complains of tiredness and lethargy,

excessive thirst (polydipsia), and symptoms of increased urine output (nocturia and frequency). There may be profound changes in the mental state and, in severe cases, drowsiness and even coma may occur. The patient may complain of gastrointestinal symptoms, including nausea and constipation. Renal stones are common and the patient may present with severe acute unilateral renal angle pain radiating towards the groin. On examination, there may be proximal muscle weakness (due to a myopathy), a thin opaque ring around the limbus of the cornea, and bone pain or radiological evidence of hyperparathyroidism (Figs 2.36, 2.37).

HYPOPARATHYROIDISM

Surgical damage or removal of three or four parathyroid glands during neck surgery (usually thyroidectomy) is the most common cause of hypoparathyroidism. Rarely, autoimmune destruction may cause hypoparathyroidism. The serum calcium level is low (in the presence of a normal serum albumin). The major symptoms of acute hypoparathyroidism are paraesthesiae around the mouth, fingers and toes. Abnormal nerve and muscle irritability can be elicited with Chvostek's (Fig. 2.38) and Trousseau's signs (Fig. 2.39). In chronic hypoparathyroidism, the physical effects develop slowly. The symptoms include tiredness, fatigue, muscle cramps and epilepsy. Premature cataracts should also alert you to the possibility of underlying chronic hypoparathyroidism.

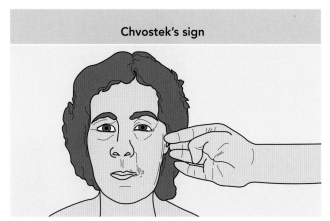

Fig. 2.38 Chvostek's sign. Tap over the facial nerve in front of the ear – this causes a momentary twitch of the corner of the mouth on the same side as the irritable facial muscles contract.

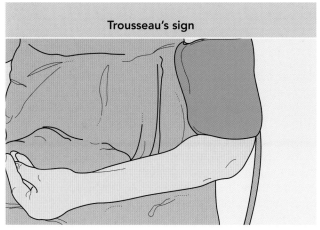

Fig. 2.39 Trousseau's sign. Inflate a sphygmomanometer cuff to above systolic pressure. Within approximately 4 minutes there is characteristic 'carpopedal' spasm of the hand. There is opposition of the thumb, extension of the interphalangeal joints and flexion of the metacarpophalangeal joints. This posture reverses spontaneously when the cuff is deflated.

The adrenal glands

Structure and function

The high fat content of the adrenal glands gives the organ a distinctive yellow colour. The adrenals lie on the upper poles of the kidneys abutting the diaphragm. Each gland weighs approximately 4 g and has a rich arterial blood supply from vessels derived from the aorta and renal and phrenic arteries. A single adrenal vein drains from the hila of the glands to the inferior vena cava on the right and to the renal vein on the left. The gland has an outer cortex derived from mesoderm and central medulla, which is derived from neuroectoderm.

The cortex comprises 90% of the gland and consists of three distinct layers: the subcapsular zona glomerulosa, the middle zona fasciculata and the zona reticularis, which lies adjacent to the medulla (Fig. 2.40).

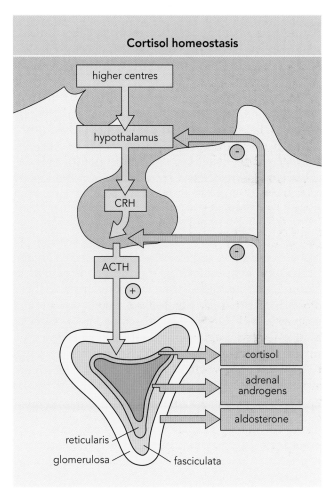

Fig. 2.40 Secretion of cortisol is stimulated by adrenocorticotrophin (ACTH) secretion, which is under the influence of hypothalamic cortisol releasing hormone (CRH). Both ACTH and CRH are under negative feedback control by circulating cortisol. Aldosterone is secreted from the zona glomerulus by the stimulatory effect of angiotensin II.

HORMONE REGULATION

The adrenal cortex synthesises three steroid hormones: mineralocorticoids, glucocorticoids and androgens. Aldosterone is produced in the cells of the zona glomerulosa. Aldosterone secretion is primarily regulated by the renin–angiotensin system, which in turn is influenced by the intravascular volume (Fig. 2.41). In contrast to the glucocorticoids, mineralocorticoid metabolism is not influenced by adrenocorticotrophic hormone (ACTH). When adrenal failure is secondary to pituitary failure, mineralocorticoid function is preserved, whereas glucocorticoid function is impaired. Aldosterone promotes the entry of sodium into cells and the secretion of potassium from cells; consequently, the overall effect of aldosterone is to cause sodium retention and potassium loss. This effect on renal tubular cells plays a central role in the regulation of sodium, potassium and water balance. Aldosterone-producing tumours of the adrenal cortex cause Conn's syndrome, which is characterised by hypertension, oedema (due to sodium and water retention) and hypokalaemia.

The cells of the zona fasciculata and reticularis synthesise cortisol and adrenal androgens. Glucocorticoid synthesis and secretion is under the direct control of ACTH secreted by the anterior pituitary. The secretion of ACTH is itself regulated by the release of hypothalamic corticotrophin releasing hormone (CRH). There is a feedback loop between the hypothalamus and pituitary on one side of the axis and the adrenal on the other. Although ACTH stimulates glucocorticoid and adrenal androgen synthesis and secretion, cortisol (and exogenous corticosteroids) inhibits ACTH secretion by impairing the release of CRH and directly inhibiting ACTH release from the anterior pituitary.

The hormones of the adrenal cortex have a circadian rhythm: blood levels of cortisol and aldosterone are highest on waking and lowest at and around midnight. Glucocorticoids promote the conversion of protein to glucose (gluconeogenesis) and inhibit the peripheral use of glucose. The corticoids increase blood pressure and support kidney function by increasing the glomerular filtration rate. Diagnosis of adrenal disease is based on measurement of ACTH, blood cortisol and the adrenal response to ACTH stimulation.

HYPERADRENALISM (CUSHING'S SYNDROME)

Excessive glucocorticoids (either endogenous or exogenous) cause a significant change in body appearance which can be readily recognised as Cushing's syndrome. A cushingoid appearance is most commonly caused by treatment with exogenous steroids. The most characteristic

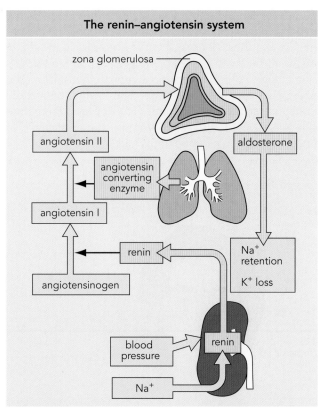

The renin–angiotensin system

Fig. 2.41 Renin–angiotensin system. Renin is secreted from the juxtaglomerular apparatus of the kidney in response to reduced serum sodium or reduced renal blood pressure. Renin converts angiotensinogen to angiotensin I, which is in turn converted to angiotensin II by angiotensin converting enzyme (ACE) from the lung. The angiotensin II stimulates aldosterone release from the zona glomerulosa cells of the adrenal gland.

feature is the rounded, 'moon-shaped' face (Fig. 2.42), an obese body (Fig. 2.43) and thin limbs (Fig. 2.44). A typical cushingoid appearance may also occur in chronic alcoholism and, in this setting, it is called pseudo-Cushing's syndrome. The diagnosis is suspected if the physical appearance of Cushing's syndrome occurs against a background of excessive alcohol consumption. The physical and biochemical abnormalities of pseudo-Cushing's syndrome regress when alcohol is discontinued.

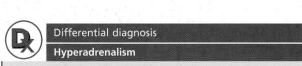

Differential diagnosis

Hyperadrenalism

- Iatrogenic, exogenous steroids
- Bilateral adrenal hyperplasia
- Benign autonomous adrenal adenoma
- Malignant adrenal adenocarcinoma
- Nonmetastatic tumour effect (e.g. lung cancer producing ACTH-like peptide)
- Alcoholism causing pseudo-Cushing's syndrome

Symptoms and signs

Cushing's syndrome

- Round, moon-shaped plethoric facies
- Hirsutes
- Acne
- Hypertension
- Buffalo hump on neck (fatty deposit)
- Central distribution of fat
- Proximal muscle weakness and wasting
- Purple skin striae

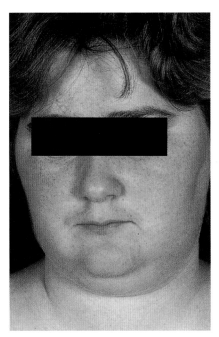

Fig. 2.42 Cushing's syndrome: plethoric 'moon-shaped' facies.

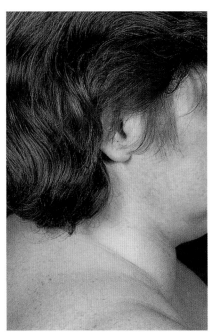

Fig. 2.43 Cushing's syndrome: typical buffalo hump. Recognised as fullness below the hairline, rather than an actual hump.

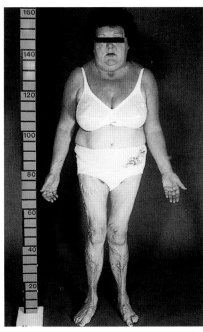

Fig. 2.44 Cushing's syndrome: proximal muscle wasting and central distribution of fat.

HYPOADRENALISM AND ADDISON'S DISEASE

In acute adrenal failure, the clinical features may be nonspecific and puzzling. The patient usually presents with malaise, weakness, nausea, vomiting and abdominal pain with an acute change in bowel habit (constipation or diarrhoea). The most helpful physical sign is the profound drop in blood pressure when the patient quickly changes position from lying to standing (postural hypotension). Collapse and prostration may occur. As a result of a mineralocorticoid deficiency, serum potassium levels are often elevated.

In chronic, progressive adrenal failure there are usually clinical clues to the diagnosis. Increased pigmentation develops in the skin (especially sun-exposed areas, pressure points, areolae and skin creases) (Fig. 2.45) and mucous membranes (seen best in the buccal mucous membrane). In Addison's disease, patients may also develop characteristic symmetrical patches of depigmented skin (vitiligo). Vague abdominal pain, altered bowel habit, weight loss and weakness also occur. Like the acute disease, postural hypotension is a helpful clinical sign which, later in the course of the disease, may dominate the patient's symptoms.

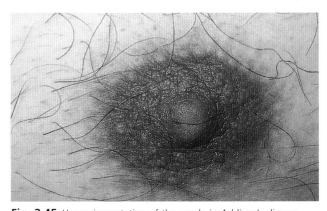

Fig. 2.45 Hyperpigmentation of the areola in Addison's disease.

 Differential diagnosis

Hypoadrenalism

Acute
- Rapid withdrawal after exogenous steroid treatment
- Failure to increase steroid dose when steroid-dependent patient is subjected to physiological stress
- Septicaemia (especially meningococcus)

Chronic
- Autoimmune (Addison's disease)
- Tuberculosis
- Carcinomatosis with adrenal invasion

Symptoms and signs

Presenting features of acute adrenal (Addisonian) crisis

- Profound dehydration, postural hypotension, shock
- Severe nausea and vomiting associated with unexplained weight loss
- Acute abdominal pain
- Unexplained hypoglycaemia
- Unexplained fever
- Hypernatraemia, hyperkalaemia, uraemia, hypercalcaemia, eosinophilia
- Hyperpigmentation of vitiligo

The pituitary gland

Structure and function

The pituitary gland is suspended from the hypothalamus by the infundibulum and lies in the pituitary fossa at the base of the skull (Fig. 2.46). The hypothalamus communicates with the anterior pituitary (or adenohypophysis) via a unique portal blood system which transports chemical stimuli to the anterior pituitary. A different form of communication occurs with the posterior pituitary (or neurohypophysis). The supraoptic and paraventricular nuclei of the hypothalamus synthesise antidiuretic hormone (ADH) and oxytocin and these hormones flow along the axons to nerve endings in the posterior pituitary, where they are released into the circulation so that they can assert their distant effects.

Hormones synthesised and secreted by the anterior pituitary include follicle stimulating hormone (FSH), luteinising hormone (LH), growth hormone, prolactin, TSH and ACTH. These hormones are regulated by the secretion of specific releasing factors produced in the hypothalamus and transported to the pituitary by the hypothalamic–pituitary portal circulation (Fig. 2.47). The regulation of the anterior pituitary hormones is controlled by the balance between the stimulating effects of the release factors and the inhibitory feedback from the target circulating hormone. There are also inhibitory hypothalamic hormones (somatostatin and dopamine). Prolactin release is inhibited by hypothalamic dopamine; this neurotransmitter is secreted into the portal circulation, causing tonic inhibition of prolactin release (Fig. 2.48).

Hypothalamic osmoreceptors and volume receptors sense blood osmolality and effective circulating volume and regulate the secretion of ADH from the posterior pituitary. ADH reduces free water clearance by the distal

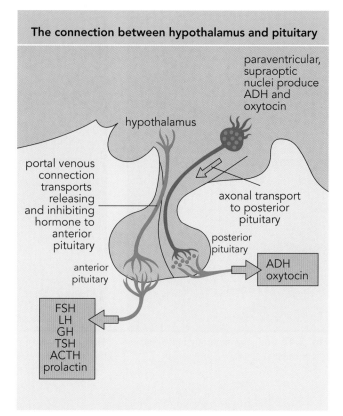

The connection between hypothalamus and pituitary

Fig. 2.46 The hypothalamus connects to the anterior pituitary by a portal venous network which carries releasing and inhibiting hormones to stimulate the release of hormones into the circulation. By contrast, the posterior pituitary hormones are synthesised in the supraoptic and paraventricular nuclei of the hypothalamus and transported to the posterior pituitary along axons which discharge directly into the systemic circulation.

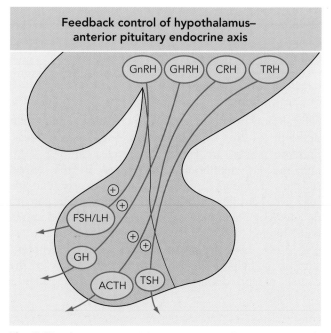

Fig. 2.47 Regulation of the hypothalamic–anterior pituitary endocrine axis.

Regulation of prolactin secretion

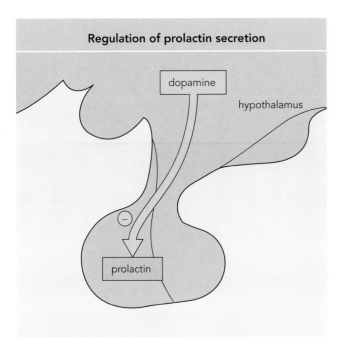

Fig. 2.48 Prolactin secretion from the anterior pituitary is inhibited by the tonic secretion of dopamine from the hypothalamus.

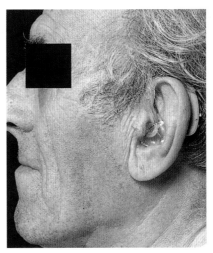

Fig. 2.49 Acromegaly: typical facial appearance.

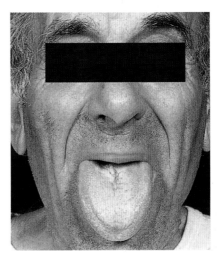

Fig. 2.50 Acromegaly: large tongue.

tubules of the nephron, resulting in concentration of the urine and water conservation. Oxytocin from the posterior pituitary causes uterine contraction during childbirth. In addition, the hormone promotes milk ejection during lactation by stimulating contraction of the smooth muscles surrounding the mammary gland ducts.

Pituitary tumours may cause overstimulation syndromes or destruction of the gland and deficiency syndromes. Both over- and understimulation cause recognisable clinical syndromes that can be identified on general examination. Remember that pituitary tumours may be associated with other endocrine adenomas, especially parathyroid adenomas, which cause hypercalcaemia. Diagnosis of pituitary disease depends on the responsiveness of stimulatory influences (e.g. effect of administration of hypothalamic releasing hormones or insulin-induced hypoglycaemic stress).

SYNDROMES ASSOCIATED WITH OVERPRODUCTION OF PITUITARY HORMONES

Acromegaly

Acidophil (or more rarely chromophobe) tumours of the anterior pituitary may cause inappropriate release of growth hormone, resulting in gigantism if the epiphyses have not fused and acromegaly in adults when fusion has occurred. Acromegalic patients may present complaining that their shoes, gloves or rings no longer fit or that they are aware of a change in facial appearance. There may also be symptoms suggestive of visual field

defects. Ask for a previous photograph to compare physical features. On physical examination, a typical syndrome reflects the overgrowth of bone and other tissues resulting from growth hormone hypersecretion (Figs 2.49–2.51).

Hyperprolactinaemia

Disruption of the tonic inhibition of prolactin release by dopamine results in the syndrome of hyperprolactinaemia. The syndromes associated with the overproduction of prolactin may be dominated by either the effect of the prolactin or the destructive effect of the pituitary tumour. Breast secretion (galactorrhoea) may develop in both women and men. The usual presenting symptom in women is alteration in the menstrual pattern (usually oligomenorrhoea or amenorrhoea). Men may present with impotence or with symptoms of pituitary expansion and malfunction (headaches, visual defects, hypothyroidism, hypoadrenalism).

Symptoms and signs
Acromegaly

- Coarse, prominent facial features
- Prognathoid jaw
- Prominent nose and forehead
- Thickened lips and large tongue
- 'Spade-shaped' hands
- Excessive sweating and greasy skin
- Kyphosis
- Hypertension
- Bitemporal hemianopia develops
- Carpal tunnel syndrome
- Impaired glucose tolerance

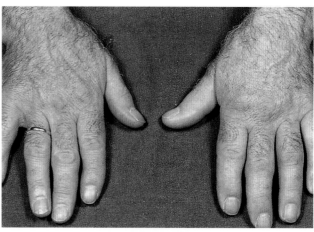

Fig. 2.51 Acromegaly: spade-shaped hands.

Symptoms and signs
Prolactinaemia

Women	Men
• Present earlier	• Present later
• Galactorrhoea (<30%)	• Galactorrhoea
• Infertility	• Impotence
• Menstrual disorders	• Signs of pituitary tumour
	• Visual field defects
	• Anterior pituitary failure

Symptoms and signs
Hypopituitarism

Women	Men
• Amenorrhoea, infertility	• Loss of libido or
• Vaginal atrophy,	impotence, infertility
dyspareunia	• Soft atrophic testes and
• Atrophic breasts	loss of secondary sexual
• Loss of axillary and	characteristics
pubic hair	
• TSH deficiency, mild to moderate hypothyroidism	
• ACTH deficiency:	
– weakness	
– postural hypotension	
– pallor	
– hypoglycaemia	

SYNDROMES ASSOCIATED WITH PITUITARY HYPOFUNCTION

Hypopituitarism

The syndrome of hypopituitarism may become recognisable if the pituitary is destroyed by a tumour, granulomatous disease (e.g. sarcoidosis, tuberculosis, histiocytosis X), trauma or after a postpartum haemorrhage (Sheehan's syndrome). Secondary pituitary failure may also occur with disease of the hypothalamus. The clinical features progress in a characteristic sequence. Growth and luteinising hormone failure occurs first, followed by FSH and TSH, and finally ACTH (Fig. 2.52).

Impaired ADH secretion causes a typical syndrome known as cranial diabetes insipidus. Patients have inappropriate polyuria and produce a dilute urine, even when deprived of water for prolonged periods. Often there is no obvious cause for the isolated defect. Head injury or cranial surgery may be complicated by posterior pituitary damage and diabetes insipidus. Other rare causes include pituitary tumours (e.g. destructive adenomas, craniopharyngiomas, metastases), granulomatous diseases (e.g. sarcoidosis, eosinophilic granulomas), infections (e.g. bacterial meningitis, tuberculosis) and familial disease. The symptoms of cranial diabetes insipidus can be confused with compulsive water drinking (i.e. when water deprivation causes appropriate urine concentration) and nephrogenic diabetes insipidus (i.e. when water deprivation is associated with dilute urine and high serum levels of ADH).

Nutrition

Nutritional status may be an important marker of disease and the progression or regression of a disorder. Poor nutrition is readily treatable and nutritional support can hasten recovery and protect against complications. Malnutrition may seriously impair immunological and healing responses and attention to nutritional status may positively influence the course of disease. In contrast, obesity is also associated with morbidity, so weight loss in these individuals can be advantageous.

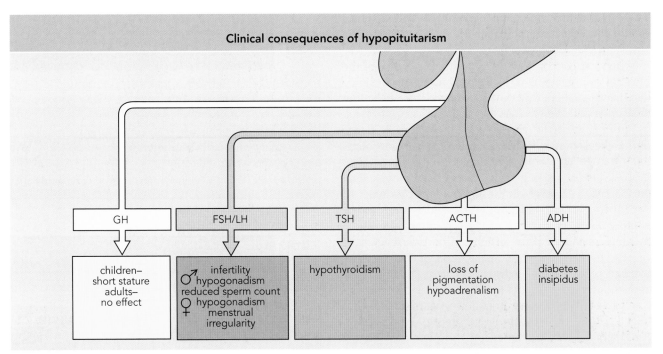

Fig. 2.52 Clinical consequences of pituitary failure. Diabetes insipidus is a rare manifestation of the hypopituitary syndrome (GH, growth hormone; FSH, follicle stimulating hormone; LH, luteinising hormone; TSH, thyroid stimulating hormone; ACTH, adrenocorticotrophin; ADH, antidiuretic hormone).

ASSESSMENT OF NUTRITION

The clinical assessment of nutritional status includes overall appearance, weight, height, muscle and fat bulk, and vitamin, mineral and haematinic status.

Either at the beginning or conclusion of the first examination, you should weigh the patient and measure the height. This provides useful baseline information, as standard growth charts are available to help you judge whether the patient falls within the normal range of weight for height (Fig. 2.53). Always adopt a standard procedure for weighing the patient. In the outpatient department, it is customary to weigh the patient in socks and basic clothing. Patients in hospital can be weighed either naked or with a light linen gown. Ensure that all subsequent weighings are performed in a standard manner. Standard weight charts indicating expected percentiles and norms for height assume that the patient has been weighed naked. Body mass index (BMI) is the preferred method for assessing weight as it considers both weight and height. This is calculated from the formula:

$$weight~(kg)/height~(m)^2$$

The normal BMI range is 20–25.

Standardise the method for measuring height. The height measurement is usually made on the vertical height ruler attached to the scale. Ensure that the patient stands bolt upright with heels firmly on the surface and back flush against the rule. Measure the height by sliding the height marker to touch the crown. The sitting height

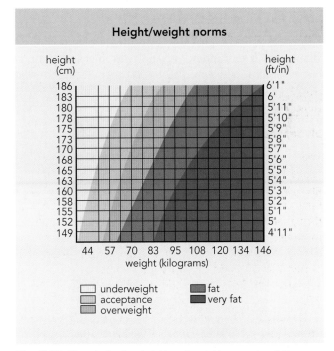

Fig. 2.53 Chart indicating height and weight norms in adults.

is also useful; from the teens to adulthood, this height should be near 50% of the total height. In osteoporosis, the collapse of vertebrae causes shortening, which is reflected in a reduction of the sitting height. Arm span may occasionally be helpful. Ask the patient to extend the arms and hands fully and measure the distance between the tips of the middle fingers. This distance should equal the linear height. In Marfan's syndrome, the arm span exceeds the height.

When the patient is exposed during the course of the physical examination, take the opportunity to evaluate whether the patient is of usual body build, unusually thin or overweight. Weight loss and 'wasting' are suggested by indrawing of the cheeks and unusual prominence of the cheek-bones, head of humerus and major joints, the rib cage and bony landmarks of the pelvis (Fig. 2.54). Muscle wasting may exaggerate the skeletal prominence. Atrophy of the deltoid muscles may be particularly striking. Hypoalbuminaemia may cause white nails (leukonychia) and loss of capillary osmotic pressure results in pedal oedema. Iron deficiency may cause spooning of the nails (koilonychia). Other features of nutritional deficiency include inflammation and cracks at the angle of the mouth (angular stomatitis), a smooth tongue lacking in papillae (atrophic glossitis) (Fig. 2.55) and skin rashes (e.g. pellagra) (Fig. 2.56). Although a visual assessment provides a relatively accurate assessment of general nutritional status, more objective measures, both clinical and biochemical, are necessary – especially when it is important to establish a baseline for nutritional support and when progress needs monitoring.

MIDARM MUSCLE CIRCUMFERENCE

This measurement provides an estimate of muscle and fat status. The standard position for measurement is the midpoint between the tip of the olecranon and

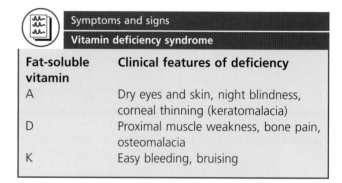

Symptoms and signs

Biochemical and immunological markers of malnutrition

- Haemoglobin (iron, B_{12}, folate deficiency)
- Low serum albumin
- Low serum transferrin
- Reduced creatinine (reflects reduced muscle bulk)
- Creatinine : height ratio reduced
- Reduced white cell count
- Impaired delayed cell-mediated immunity (skin tests)

Symptoms and signs

Vitamin deficiency syndrome

Fat-soluble vitamin	Clinical features of deficiency
A	Dry eyes and skin, night blindness, corneal thinning (keratomalacia)
D	Proximal muscle weakness, bone pain, osteomalacia
K	Easy bleeding, bruising

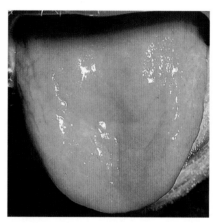

Fig. 2.55 Smooth shiny tongue of atrophic glossitis (especially iron deficiency).

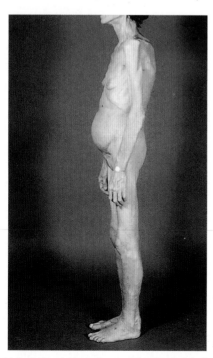

Fig. 2.54 Malnutrition in liver disease. Muscle wasting is readily recognised by the prominence of the skeleton due to loss of muscle bulk and fatty tissue.

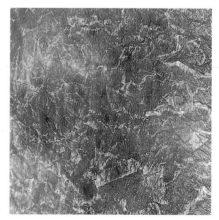

Fig. 2.56 Pellagra: photosensitive 'crazy paving' skin rash.

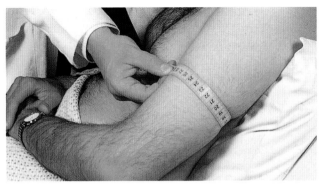

Fig. 2.57 Measurement of the midarm muscle circumference.

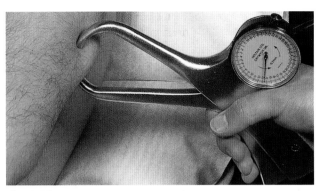

Fig. 2.58 Measurement of triceps skinfold thickness.

acromial process. The patient's arm should be relaxed and flexed to a right angle. Take the measurement by wrapping the tape-measure around the upper arm midpoint (Fig. 2.57), taking care not to pull too tight or to leave excessive slackness. Take three measurements at the same point and calculate the average. The measurement is itself a useful baseline measure for follow-up purposes. In addition, the single measurement can be compared with percentiles in standard age and sex charts.

TRICEPS SKINFOLD THICKNESS

In adults, the skin overlying the triceps muscle can be lifted and subcutaneous tissue can be distinguished from the underlying muscle bulk. This fold of skin and subcutaneous tissue (the fat fold) provides an indirect assessment of fat stores. Measure the fat fold thickness from the patient's rear and make the measurement at the same midarm landmark used for measuring the midarm muscle circumference. It is useful to mark this point so that you can lift the skinfold between your thumb and index finger and position the jaws of the calipers on either side of the midarm mark on the raised skinfold (Fig. 2.58). As with the tape measurement of midarm muscle circumference, ensure that the caliper jaws are neither too tight nor too loose. Repeat the measurement three times and take the average to compare with standard tables.

Clinical assessment of vitamin status

Vitamins are essential cofactors obtained from the diet. Reduced dietary intake may result in recognisable deficiency syndromes. Specific deficiencies of the fat-soluble vitamins (A, D and K) occur in patients with chronic steatorrhoea due to chronic cholestasis and malabsorption syndromes complicated by steatorrhoea.

Deficiencies of water-soluble vitamins occur in all forms of malnutrition. The syndromes are especially prevalent in malnutrition due to famine, malnourished alcoholic patients, patients on chronic renal dialysis and

Symptoms and signs
Water-soluble vitamin deficiency

B₁ (thiamine)
- Wet beriberi
  - peripheral vasodilatation
  - high output cardiac failure
  - oedema
- Dry beriberi
  - sensory and motor peripheral neuropathy
- Wernicke's encephalopathy
  - ataxia, nystagmus, lateral rectus palsy
  - altered mental state
- Korsakoff's psychosis
  - retrograde amnesia
  - confabulation

B₂ riboflavin
- Inflamed oral mucous membranes
- Angular stomatitis
- Glossitis, normocytic anaemia

B₃ niacin
- Pellagra
- Dermatitis (photosensitive)
- Diarrhoea
- Dementia

B₆ pyridoxine
- Peripheral neuropathy
- Sideroblastic anaemia

B₁₂
- Megaloblastic, macrocytic anaemia
- Glossitis
- Subacute combined degeneration of the cord

Folic acid
- Megaloblastic, macrocytic anaemia
- Glossitis

C
- Scurvy
  - perifollicular haemorrhage
  - bleeding gums, skin purpura
  - bleeding into muscles and joints
- Anaemia
- Osteoporosis

in underdeveloped countries where processing of staple foods reduces vitamin content.

Clinical assessment of hydration

Fluid and electrolyte balance is carefully regulated. The intake of fluid and electrolytes is closely matched by loss in urine, stool and sweat. Dehydration can occur if there is a mismatch between fluid intake and loss. Ill patients may be anorexic and fail to take in the minimal fluid intake necessary to maintain fluid balance; the kidney may lose its ability to regulate the quality and quantity of urine; and there may be excessive gastrointestinal fluid loss (diarrhoea and vomiting) or abnormal sweating (pyrexia).

The history may be helpful when assessing hydration. Dehydration rapidly provokes thirst, the first clinical symptom of dehydration. Ask patients whether they feel abnormally thirsty and whether they have noticed a dry, parched mouth. Physical signs of dehydration are usually only apparent with moderate to severe dehydration. Inspect the tongue and note whether the mucosa is wet and glistening. Touching the tongue may help you assess its moistness. Look at the eyes, which should have a glistening, shiny appearance; this sparkle is lost as dehydration develops. With moderate dehydration, the eyes may appear sunken into the orbits; the pulse rate may increase to compensate for intravascular volume loss. Blood pressure falls in hypovolaemic patients and the demonstration of postural hypotension is a cardinal sign of significant intravascular fluid loss. In addition, the capillary refill time can be used to assess the circulatory effects of volume depletion.

With marked dehydration skin turgor is lost. This can be demonstrated by gently pinching a fold of skin on the neck or anterior chest wall, holding the fold for a few moments (Fig. 2.59) and letting it go. Well-hydrated

Symptoms and signs

Measuring the capillary refill time

- Patient's hand placed level with heart
- Distal phalanx of the middle finger compressed for 5 seconds
- Release pressure
- Measure time to regain normal colour (refill time)
  - normal filling time is 2–3 seconds (2–4 seconds on the elderly)

skin immediately springs back to its original position, whereas in dehydration the skinfold only slowly returns back to normal. This sign is unreliable in elderly patients whose skin may have lost its normal elasticity. Urine output falls and the urine is concentrated. In severe dehydration, the patient may be profoundly hypotensive and anuric, and renal failure caused by tubular necrosis may occur.

Clinical assessment of shock

The clinical presentation of shock varies both with the type and the cause, but there are several common features. Any patient suspected of developing shock should have continuous assessment of the peripheral and central circulation. In the earliest phase (preshock), the pulse rate rises and the blood pressure may be maintained by peripheral vasoconstriction, resulting in cool peripheries, skin pallor and reduced capillary refill time. Blood pressure measurement is very helpful in assessing shock, and postural (orthostatic) hypotension antedates the development of recumbent hypotension (systolic BP <90 mmHg or a drop of 40 mmHg in previous hypertensive patients). Once the blood pressure has fallen, oliguria

Symptoms and signs

Measurement of postural change in blood pressure

- Lie the patient supine for 2 min
- Record pulse rate and blood pressure in supine position
- Ask the patient to stand upright
- Wait 1 min
- Measure standing heart rate and blood pressure at 1 and 3 min
- Heart normally increases by 8–12 beats/min
- Systolic blood pressure drops by 3–4 mmHg
- Diastolic blood pressure increases by 3–7 mmHg
- Postural hypotension when systolic drops by 20 mmHg and/or diastolic drops by 10 mmHg

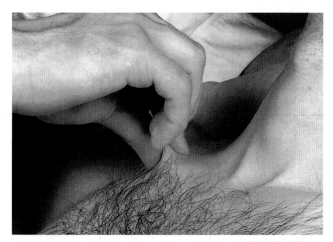

Fig. 2.59 To test for moderate to severe dehydration, assess skin turgor by lifting the skin, pinching it and observing the rate at which it springs back to its normal position.

develops. Cerebral hypoperfusion results in altered mental state, characterised initially by agitation and progressing to confusion, delirium, obtundation and coma. Initially patients might hyperventilate, causing a short, transient respiratory acidosis, but this is soon replaced by metabolic acidosis reflecting renal hypoperfusion and impaired clearance of lactate by the liver, kidney and muscle.

Differential diagnosis

Shock

- Hypovolaemic shock
  - GI bleeding
  - trauma
  - ruptured aneurysm
  - burns
  - haemorrhagic pancreatitis
  - fractures (e.g. neck of femur)
  - diarrhoea and vomiting
- Cardiogenic shock
  - acute myocardial infarction
  - acute arrythmias
  - acute rupture of valve cusp
  - pericardial tamponade
- Distributive shock
  - Gram-negative sepsis
  - toxic shock syndrome
  - anaphylaxis
  - Addisonian crisis
  - spinal cord/major brain injury

Red flag – urgent referral

Assessment of shock

- Rise in pulse occurs early
- Reduced pulse volume/pressure
- Orthostatic hypotension
- Recumbent hypotension
- Cool, pale peripheries
- Delayed capillary refill time
- Dry mucous membranes
- Oliguria
- Altered mental state
- Signs of metabolic acidosis

Colour

Once you have assessed nutrition and hydration, look at the patient's 'colour'. Look for pallor or plethora, central and peripheral cyanosis, jaundice and skin pigmentation.

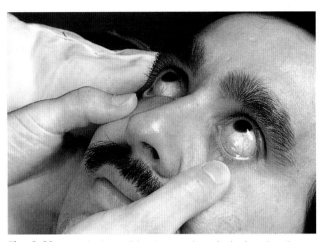

Fig. 2.60 Evert the lower lid to inspect the palpebral conjunctiva for pallor.

PALLOR

The cardinal sign of anaemia is pallor. Severe anaemia may be readily recognised by a pale facial appearance and shortness of breath on exertion. The red colour of arterial blood is easiest to assess where the horny layer of the epidermis is thinnest; this includes the palpebral conjunctiva, nail bed, lips and tongue. Inspect the palpebral conjunctiva by gently everting the lower eyelid (Fig. 2.60). The palpebral conjunctiva is normally a healthy red colour but, in anaemia, it appears a pale pink.

Experience will teach you to distinguish normal from abnormal. Conjunctival pallor should be accompanied by pallor of the nail bed and palmar skin creases (only assess this if the hands are warm). Pallor is an unreliable sign in cold or shocked patients because peripheral vasoconstriction causes skin and conjunctival pallor even when not associated with blood loss.

PLETHORA

This refers to a ruddy 'weather beaten' facial appearance where the skin has an unusually red or bluish (cyanosed) appearance. Facial plethora is usually caused by an abnormally high haemoglobin concentration (polycythaemia). This is usually caused by chronic cyanotic lung disease in which hypoxia stimulates erythropoietin release from the macula densa of the proximal renal tubule cells. This hormone stimulates the marrow to increase red cell production with consequent increase in haemoglobin concentration. The plethora causes a bloated facial appearance and, together with the cyanosis, these patients have a typical 'blue bloater' appearance.

Polycythaemia rubra vera is a myeloproliferative disorder that causes very high haemoglobin levels and plethora occurs in the absence of hypoxic cyanosis. The conjunctiva has a characteristic 'plum' colour and on fundoscopy the increased blood viscosity causes the venules to assume a thickened 'sausage-shaped' appearance.

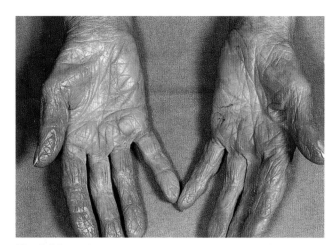

Fig. 2.61 Peripheral cyanosis; note the bluish discoloration of the fingers.

CYANOSIS

Cyanosis refers to a bluish or purplish discoloration of the skin or mucous membranes caused by excessive amounts of reduced haemoglobin in blood. At least 5 g/dl of reduced haemoglobin is necessary for cyanosis to appear. In peripheral cyanosis, the extremities are cyanosed (Fig. 2.61) but the tongue retains a healthy pink colour. This is caused by any condition resulting in slowing of the peripheral circulation. In cold weather, there is reflex peripheral vasoconstriction with slowing of the circulation, allowing more time for the extraction of oxygen from haemoglobin. A similar mechanism accounts for peripheral cyanosis in heart failure, peripheral vascular disease, Raynaud's phenomenon and shock. A reduction in arterial oxygen saturation results in central cyanosis. The extremities are cyanosed and the tongue and mucous membranes also have a bluish or purple discoloration. Central cyanosis may develop in any lung disease in which there is a mismatch between ventilation and perfusion. In right-to-left shunts caused by congenital heart disease, the admixture of venous blood to the systemic circulation causes cyanosis.

JAUNDICE

Skin pigmentation influences the ease with which jaundice can be detected. The yellow discoloration is most easily recognised in fair-skinned individuals and is more difficult to detect in darkly pigmented patients. Bilirubin has a high affinity for elastic tissue. This, together with the sclera's white colour, makes the sclera the most sensitive area for looking for the yellow discoloration of jaundice.

Mild jaundice is best seen in natural daylight. Expose the sclera by gently holding down the lower lid and asking the patient to look upwards. With progression, the yellow discoloration becomes obvious on the truncal skin. In chronic, severe obstructive jaundice, the skin develops a yellow-green appearance. Eating

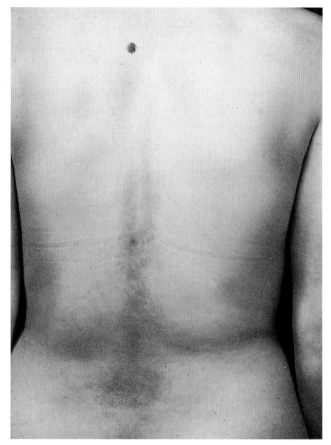

Fig. 2.62 Typical skin pigmentation in chronic cholestasis (primary biliary cirrhosis).

large amounts of carrots or other carotene-containing vegetables or substances causes carotenaemia, which can be confused with jaundice. The yellow discoloration is prominent in the face, palms and soles but, in contrast to jaundice, the sclera remains white.

PIGMENTATION

Sunburn is the most common cause of increased pigmentation and this should be readily distinguished from the history. In iron overload (haemochromatosis), the skin colour may appear slate grey. A silver-grey colour develops in silver poisoning (argyria). In chronic cholestasis (e.g. primary biliary cirrhosis), skin hyperpigmentation may develop, especially over pressure points (Fig. 2.62). A marked increase in pigmentation occurs after bilateral adrenalectomy for adrenal hyperplasia. This condition (Nelson's syndrome) is caused by unopposed pituitary stimulation. Addison's disease may also be associated with deepening pigmentation, especially skin creases and pressure points.

Oedema

Fluid movement between the intravascular and extravascular space occurs through the walls of capillaries.

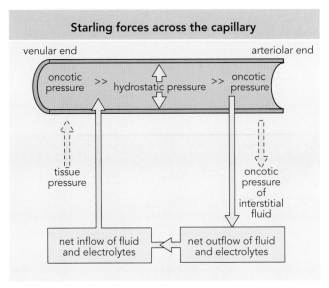

Fig. 2.63 The Starling forces across the capillary bed. At the arteriolar end the hydrostatic and interstitial oncotic pressures exceed the plasma oncotic pressure, resulting in efflux of fluid and electrolytes. At the venular end plasma oncotic pressure exceeds hydrostatic pressure, resulting in net influx.

The efflux of fluid across the capillary wall is governed mainly by the hydrostatic pressure transmitted by the arterial blood pressure through the precapillary arteriole, and also by the capillary permeability and the opposing osmotic (oncotic) pressure exerted by the serum proteins (especially albumin). In addition, the oncotic pressure of the interstitial fluid may contribute to the efflux of intravascular fluid. The reabsorption of interstitial fluid is driven primarily by the plasma oncotic pressure, the hydrostatic pressure in the interstitial space (known as the tissue pressure) and the fall in hydrostatic pressure at the venular end of the capillary. These forces (known as the Starling forces) determine the movement of fluid and electrolytes between the intravascular and interstitial compartments (Fig. 2.63).

Any imbalance of the Starling forces will cause expansion of the interstitial space. In heart failure, the increased central venous pressure causes increased capillary pressure, reduced resorption and oedema; renal hypoperfusion also stimulates the renin–angiotensin system, which, in turn, causes inappropriate sodium and water retention, and further contributes to oedema. When serum albumin levels fall there is a loss of plasma oncotic pressure. This favours the movement of fluid into the interstitial space. The consequent fall in intravascular volume causes activation of the renin–angiotensin system, which adds further to fluid retention and oedema. Hypoalbuminaemia occurs in nephrotic syndrome (albuminuria, hypoalbuminaemia, hyperlipidaemia and oedema), liver failure, malabsorption syndromes, protein-losing enteropathy, severe burns and malnutrition.

In liver disease complicated by portal hypertension, there is pooling of blood in the splanchnic bed with increased splanchnic capillary pressure. The pooling results in a fall in the effective intravascular volume, which, in turn, activates the renin–angiotensin system. These factors all contribute to the fluid retention that complicates portal hypertension. Ascites complicating portal hypertension usually only develops when there is hypoalbuminaemia and a fall in oncotic pressure (Fig. 2.64).

Inflammation increases capillary permeability, allowing movement of albumin and other colloidal proteins as well as fluid into the interstitial space. The increase in interstitial oncotic pressure encourages the shift of fluid and electrolytes out of the capillaries into the interstitium. This causes the swelling that invariably accompanies the inflammatory response. Lymph is particularly rich in protein and, when lymphatic flow is obstructed, the abnormal accumulation of lymph in the interstitial space increases the interstitial oncotic pressure, with consequent retention of interstitial fluid.

The distribution of excess fluid depends on its underlying cause, the shifting effect of gravity and the capacity of the tissue in which it accumulates. In congestive heart failure, patients often notice marked ankle swelling (dependent oedema) which becomes more noticeable as the day wears on and appears to resolve through the night. In the upright posture, increased capillary pressure is transmitted to the lower limbs: this favours the regional accumulation of excess fluid in the loose connective tissue around the ankles. At night, the recumbent position causes redistribution of the transcapillary and gravitational forces so that by early morning the oedema is most prominent in the sacral region and appears to have resolved from around the ankles. When the left ventricle fails, interstitial oedema accumulates in the lungs, causing pulmonary oedema. The fluid settles in the most dependent (basal) areas of the lung, causing the basal alveoli to collapse during expiration. The opening of these collapsed alveoli during inspiration can be heard with a stethoscope as 'crackles'. Facial and periorbital tissue is particularly compliant. In superior vena caval obstruction and chronic renal failure, facial 'puffiness' is prominent, especially on waking. Anasarca refers to the gross, generalised oedema that accompanies profound hypoproteinaemic states.

SYMPTOMS OF OEDEMA

If the oedema is generalised, patients may notice tight-fitting shoes, frank swelling of the legs or an unexplained increase in weight. There may be associated symptoms linked to underlying diseases such as heart failure and liver, kidney, bowel or nutritional disease. Localised oedema may be obvious if there is venous thrombosis, regional lymphatic obstruction or a painful, inflamed area of swelling. Fluid accumulation in the pleural space (hydrothorax or pleural effusion) may cause breathlessness. Ascites may be noticed as an increase in girth, weight gain or the eversion of the umbilicus.

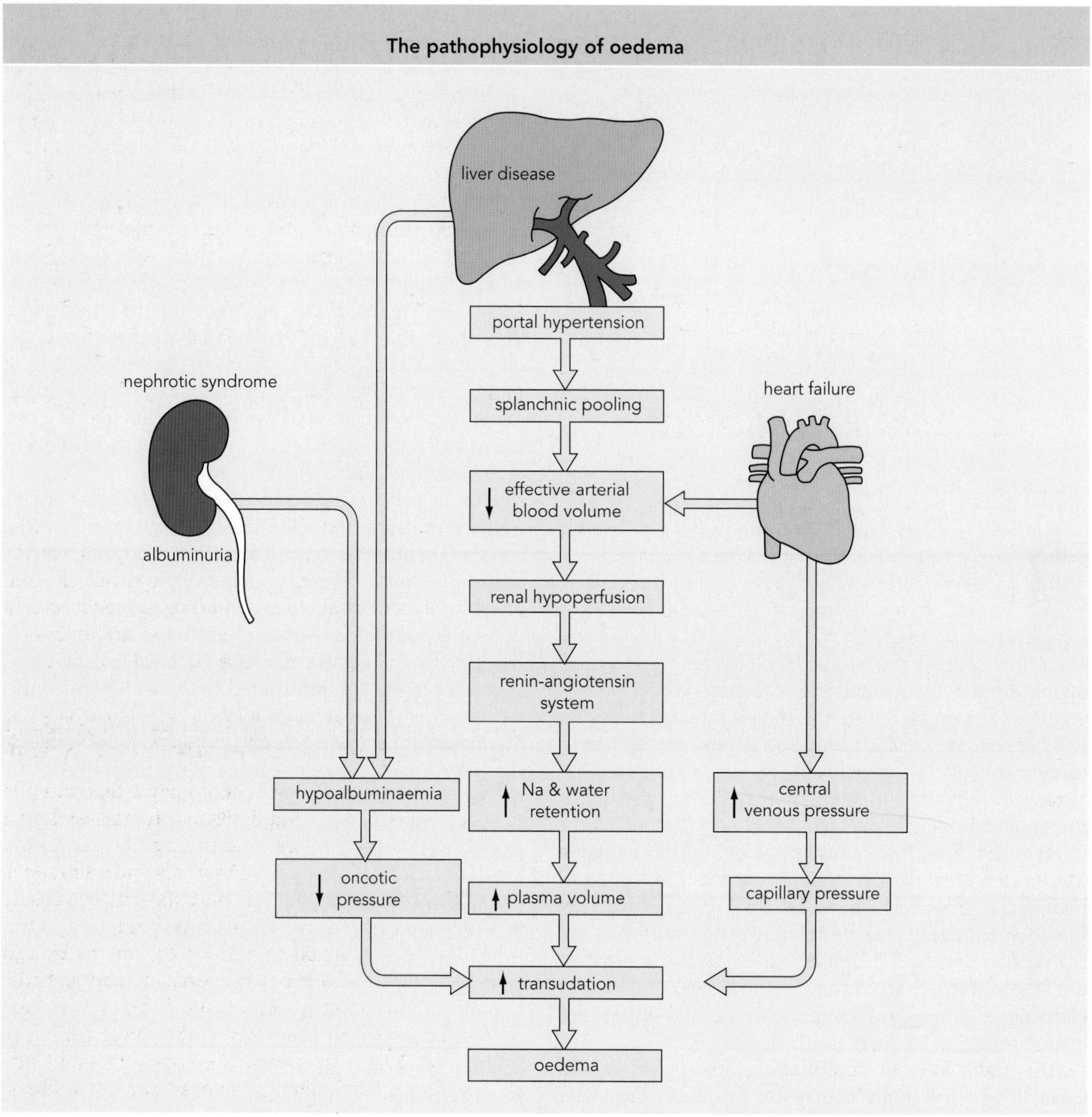

The pathophysiology of oedema

Fig. 2.64 The formation of oedema in liver disease with portal hypertension, cardiac failure and nephrotic syndrome.

SIGNS OF OEDEMA

In ambulant patients, generalised oedema is readily demonstrated in the tissue space behind the medial malleolus. Fluid accumulates in the loose connective tissue of this dependent area; the skin between the medial malleolus and Achilles tendon is normally concave but with fluid accumulation it becomes flattened and then convex. You may notice a skin impression made by tight-fitting socks. In longstanding oedema, the skin may become shiny, thin, and even ulcerated due to poor local tissue circulation. Mild pedal oedema may not be obvious on inspection. Palpation is, however, a sensitive test for

oedema. Press the ball of your thumb or the tips of your index and middle fingers into the posterior malleolar space and maintain moderate pressure for a few seconds. The skin has a 'boggy' feel. The extrinsic pressure will squeeze oedema fluid away from the pressure point. On removing your thumb or fingers, the finger impression remains imprinted in the skin for a short while before fading as the oedema redistributes. Repeat the compression test more proximally to assess the upper margin of oedema (Fig. 2.65).

In the recumbent posture, oedema is less obvious around the ankles and most prominent over the sacrum and lower back. This is often forgotten when examining

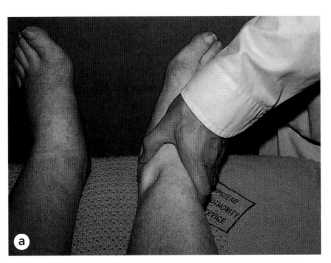
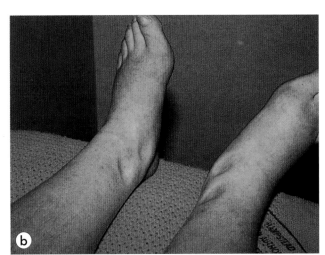
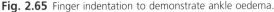

Fig. 2.65 Finger indentation to demonstrate ankle oedema.

patients confined to bed. Ask the patient to sit well forward in bed and expose the lower back and sacral region. Press the thumb or fingers into the skin over the midsacrum. Like pedal oedema, abnormal fluid retention is indicated by the residual impression left at the pressure point. In anasarca, the signs of oedema extends to the thighs, scrotum and anterior abdominal wall. Anasarca occurs in hypoproteinaemic states (especially nephrotic syndrome, malnutrition and malabsorption), severe cardiac or renal failure and when there is a generalised increase in capillary permeability (e.g. severe allergic reactions).

The veins of the lower legs have valves that protect the vessels from the pressure effect of the column of blood from the right ventricle. Damaged and incompetent valves in the deep and perforating veins of the lower limb cause a marked increase in hydrostatic pressure to the lower limb veins, causing varicose veins and pedal oedema. Localised oedema may occur in deep venous thrombosis of the leg veins. The affected limb becomes swollen and if there is thrombophlebitis and rapid muscle swelling, the calf muscle may be tender to palpation (Homan's sign).

Lymphatic oedema has a high protein content and the oedema is localised to the area drained by the lymphatics. The swelling is pronounced and on palpation the skin has an indurated, thickened feel. This 'brawny' oedema is the clinical hallmark of lymphoedema (filariasis is a common cause of brawny oedema in certain tropical countries). Surgical removal of axillary lymph nodes in the treatment of breast cancer commonly results in troublesome lymphoedema of the arm.

Ascites is characterised by abdominal distention (especially in the flanks) and, on examination, there is shifting dullness. Look for signs of abdominal disease such as peritoneal infection, peritoneal carcinomatosis or liver disease with portal hypertension (e.g. splenomegaly or liver flap). Removing a small volume of ascitic fluid is often helpful in reaching a diagnosis. A bloodstained sample suggests malignancy; cytology, pH, protein content, neutrophil count and Gram and direct stains for tuberculosis can facilitate a rapid diagnosis. Pleural effusions are readily detected on clinical examination and chest radiograph (see Ch. 5). Like ascites, an aspiration sample can provide valuable diagnostic information.

Temperature and fever

In all warm-blooded animals, core body temperature is set within closely regulated limits and is stabilised by a combination of convection, conduction and evaporation. The major regulatory organ for heat loss and retention is the extensive vascular plexus in the subcutaneous tissue. Although metabolism produces most of the body heat, ventilation and ingestion of hot or cold substances also make a small contribution to heat exchange in the body. Vasodilatation of skin vessels allows dissipation of heat transferred from the deep organs. Sweating facilitates heat loss through evaporation; the eccrine sweat glands are innervated by cholinergic sympathetic nerve fibres. Conservation of heat by adrenergic autonomic stimuli reduces blood flow through the subcutaneous vascular plexus. The integrated response to temperature regulation is under the control of the hypothalamus.

MEASURING TEMPERATURE

Temperature may be measured by placing a thermometer under the tongue, in the rectum or under the axilla. If you use a mercury thermometer, shake it to ensure that the mercury is well below 37°C and leave for at least 90s. Electronic temperature sensors are now widely available, providing more rapid stabilisation.

NORMAL TEMPERATURE

Temperature depends on the site of measurement. The mouth, rectum and axilla are common sites. 'Normal' oral temperature is usually considered to be 37°C. Rectal temperature is 0.5°C higher than the mouth and the axilla 0.5°C lower. Remember that 'normal' temperature is not set at a precise level and there are small variations between individuals (which may range from 35.8 to 37.1°C). There is also a distinct diurnal variation: oral temperature is usually about 37°C on waking in the morning, rising to a daytime peak between 6.00 and 10.00 p.m. and falling to a low point between 2.00 and 4.00 a.m. In menstruating women, ovulation is accompanied by a 0.5°C increase in body temperature. Daily temperature measurement can be used as an accurate marker of ovulation.

FEVER

Abnormally high body temperature is an important physical sign. Pathological temperatures often show an exaggerated diurnal pattern with evening high points and the lowest temperatures in the early morning. Fever may be caused by microbes, immunological reactions, hormones (e.g. T_4 and progesterone), inability to lose heat (e.g. absence of sweat glands and scaling of the skin – ichthyosis), drugs (e.g. penicillin and quinidine) and malignancy (e.g. Hodgkin's disease and hypernephroma).

Sequential recording of temperature may show a variety of patterns (Fig. 2.66). These patterns are neither specific nor sensitive signs of individual diseases. Typhoid fever may show a 'stepwise' increase in temperature associated with a relative bradycardia. Occasionally, patients with Hodgkin's disease have a Pel–Ebstein fever, characterised by 4–5 days of persistent fever, followed by a similar period when the temperature hovers around the normal baseline. Abscess and collections of pus often present with a high spiking fever.

CHILLS AND RIGORS

High fever may be accompanied by a subjective sensation of chill, which may be accompanied by goose pimples, shivering and chattering of the teeth. As the fever subsides, the defervescence is accompanied by hot sensations and intense sweating. When shivering is extreme, the presentation is dominated by the rigors. Severe rigors and spiking fevers are characteristic of biliary and renal bacterial infections and malaria.

Differential diagnosis
Rigors

- Biliary sepsis (Charcot's triad)
  - jaundice
  - right hypochondrial pain and tenderness
  - fever and rigors
- Pyelonephritis
- Visceral abscesses
- Malaria

HYPOTHERMIA

Hypothermia usually occurs with prolonged exposure to winter cold. Predisposing factors include old age, myxoedema, pituitary dysfunction, Addison's disease and abuse of drugs or alcohol. Patients are pale, the skin feels cold and waxy and the muscles are stiff. Consciousness is depressed and when the temperature drops to below 27°C, consciousness is lost. A special low-reading thermometer is required to establish the baseline temperature. The most convenient measuring device is a rectal probe (thermocouple) which provides real-time temperature measurement.

Differential diagnosis
Hypothermia

- Environmental exposure
- Hypothyroidism
- Increased cutaneous heat loss – burns, toxic epidermal necrolysis
- Drugs (alcohol, opiates, barbiturates, phenothiazines, lithium)
- Altered thermoregulation (sepsis, hypothalamic disease, spinal cord injury)

The lymphatic system

Examination of the lymphatic system

As the lymphoreticular system is widespread, it is convenient to consider its examination in the general

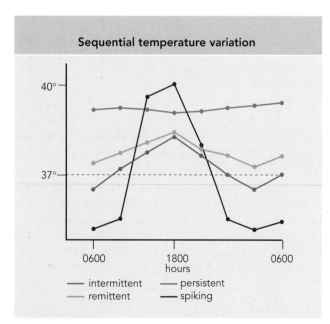

Fig. 2.66 Temperature may be described as intermittent, remittent, persistent or spiking.

Primary and secondary lymphoid tissue

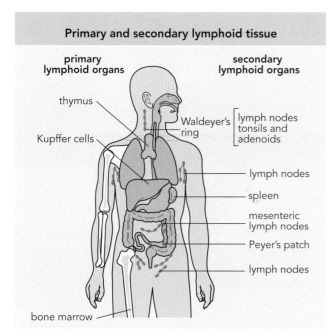

Fig. 2.67 The primary lymphoid organs include bone marrow (which produces B lymphocytes) and the thymus (which produces T lymphocytes). The secondary lymphoid organs provide a 'base camp' for interaction between lymphocytic subtypes and antigens (i.e. macrophages, antigen presenting cells, T and B lymphocytes). The immune response is generated in the secondary lymphoid tissues.

The lymphatic drainage system

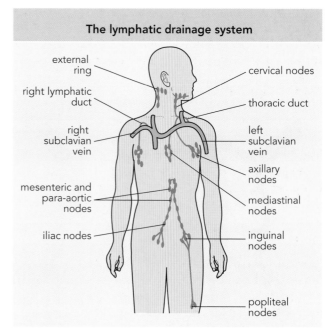

Fig. 2.68 Regional drainage of the lymphatic system. The right upper quadrant drains via the right thoracic duct into the right subclavian vein. The remainder of the lymphatic network drains into the left subclavian vein via the thoracic duct.

examination. You may choose to examine for enlargement of the lymph nodes (lymphadenopathy) as part of the preliminary general examination, although most clinicians integrate the examination into the regional examination of the head and neck, chest and abdomen.

Structure and function of the lymphatic system

The lymphatic system drains the interstitial space, facilitates antigen presentation, produces antibodies and phagocytes, and provides a pathway for chylomicron absorption from enterocytes. It comprises the lymphatic ducts, lymph nodes, spleen, tonsils, adenoids and the thymus gland (Figs 2.67, 2.68). Lymphoid tissue is also present in the Peyer's patches of the terminal ileum. The lungs contain significant islands of lymphoid tissue and the hepatic reticuloendothelial cells are an integral component of the lymphoreticular system.

A network of lymphatic ducts accompanies the blood vessels; these lymphatics transport lymph from the interstitial tissues to the lymph nodes. Lymph is an opalescent fluid derived from the protein-rich fluid, enriched with lymphocytes, which bathes the interstitial space. The lymphatic vessels drain distinct regions of the body into groups of regional lymph nodes. Efferent lymph vessels leave the regional nodes, converging to form larger vessels. Ultimately, the larger lymphatic vessels converge into two main lymph vessels – the lymphatic trunk drains the right upper body into the right subclavian

vein, with the remainder of the body ultimately draining to the thoracic duct, which drains into the left subclavian vein (Fig. 2.68). Fat from the small intestine is not absorbed into the portal circulation. Triglyceride in the enterocyte is coated with protein to form chylomicrons and these are absorbed into mesenteric lymphatics which drain through the thoracic duct into the systemic circulation.

The lymph nodes are comprised of lymphocyte-rich lymphoid follicles and sinuses that are lined with reticuloendothelial cells (histiocytes and macrophages). The follicles in the cortex of the node have a germinal centre populated by rapidly dividing B lymphocytes and macrophages. The germinal centre is surrounded by a cuff of T lymphocytes. Antigens from a distant region drain through the lymphatic vessels into the regional nodes, where they are presented to the lymphocytes, which respond by proliferating into antibody-producing B lymphocytes or antigen-specific T lymphocytes (Fig. 2.69).

Lymphadenopathy may be caused by proliferation of cells in response to antigen challenge. Abnormal cells may populate the nodes. Malignant transformation of the lymphoid cells in lymphomas may cause lymphadenopathy. The glands may become populated by leukaemic cells or metastatic carcinoma. In the lipid storage diseases, lipid-laden macrophages may infiltrate and enlarge the nodes.

Before setting out to examine the lymphatic system, it is important to know the regional arrangement of the major groups of superficial nodes (Fig. 2.68).

Anatomy of the lymph node

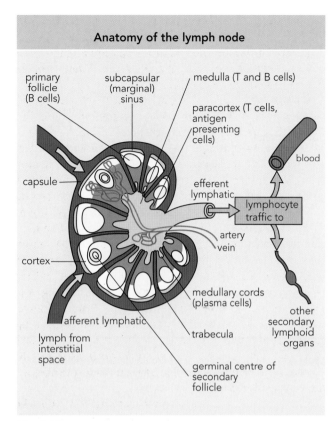

Fig. 2.69 Structure of the lymph node.

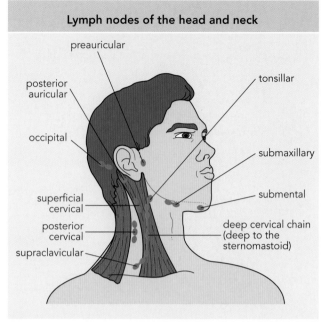

Lymph nodes of the head and neck

Fig. 2.70 Horizontal ring of facial nodes and the vertical chain of cervical neck nodes.

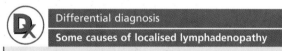

Differential diagnosis
Some causes of localised lymphadenopathy

- Local acute or chronic infections
- Metastatic carcinoma (especially breast, lung, head and neck, kidney)
- Hodgkin's disease

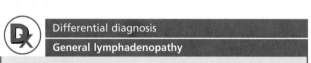

Differential diagnosis
General lymphadenopathy

- Lymphoma
- Acute and chronic lymphatic leukaemia
- Viral infections (HIV/AIDS, infectious mononucleosis, cytomegalovirus)
- Bacterial infections (tuberculosis, brucellosis, syphilis)
- Toxoplasmosis
- Sarcoidosis
- Phenytoin pseudolymphoma, serum sickness
- Autoimmune diseases (systemic lupus erythematosus, rheumatoid arthritis)

The lymph nodes of the head and neck are grouped in an encircling examination and vertical arrangement (Fig. 2.70). The circle of nodes drains the superficial structures of the head and neck. This ring of nodes includes the submental, submandibular, preauricular (superficial parotid), posterior auricular (mastoid) and occipital nodes. The vertical nodes also drain the deep structures of the head and neck. The deep cervical chain extends along the internal jugular vein from the base of the skull to the root of the neck (deep to sternocleidomastoid) and then to the thoracic and right lymphatic ducts. A chain of superficial cervical nodes lies along the external jugular vein, draining the parotid glands and the inferior portion of the ear. This chain drains into the deep cervical nodes. The tip of the tongue drains to the submental nodes, the anterior two-thirds to the submental and submandibular nodes, and then to the lower deep cervical nodes; the posterior tongue drains to the tonsillar nodes at the upper limit of the deep cervical chain.

The lymphatics of the hand and arm drain to the axillary and infraclavicular group of nodes (Fig. 2.71). The epitrochlear node is the most distal node in the arm. The anterior chest wall (and breast) drains medially to the internal mammary chain and laterally to the axillary and brachial nodes. The lung parenchyma and visceral pleura drain to the hilar nodes, whereas the parietal pleura drains to the axillary nodes (this is why the axilla is palpated in the course of the lung examination). The lymphatics of the lower limb drain to the popliteal nodes and then up to the vertical group of superficial inguinal nodes lying close to the upper portion of the great saphenous vein (Fig. 2.72). The perineum, scrotal skin, penis, lower vagina and vulva, and lower trunk and the back below the umbilicus drain into the horizontal group lying below the inguinal ligament. The tests drain to the para-aortic nodes, whereas the female genitalia drain to pelvic, intra-abdominal and para-aortic nodes.

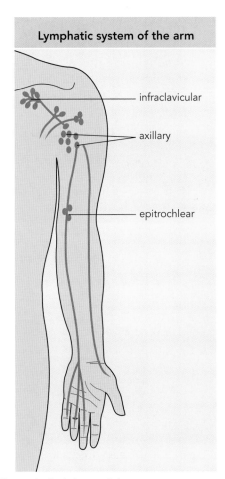

Lymphatic system of the arm

infraclavicular

axillary

epitrochlear

Fig. 2.71 Lymphatic drainage of the arm.

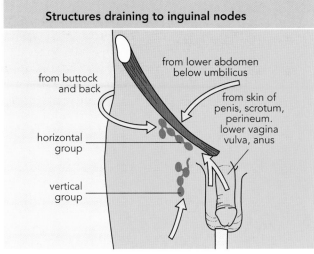

Structures draining to inguinal nodes

from buttock and back

from lower abdomen below umbilicus

from skin of penis, scrotum, perineum. lower vagina vulva, anus

horizontal group

vertical group

Fig. 2.72 Inguinal nodes drain the lower limbs, lower trunk, penis, scrotum, perineum, lower vagina and anus.

Examination of the lymph nodes

Examination of the lymph nodes involves inspection and palpation. Large nodes may be clearly visible on inspection. Infected nodes are enlarged and tender (lymphadenitis) and the overlying skin may be red and inflamed. When superficial lymphatic vessels leading to a group of nodes are inflamed (lymphangitis), the channels can be seen as thin red streaks leading from a more distal site of inflammation.

Use your fingertips to palpate the regional nodes. Feel for the node by applying moderate pressure over the region and moving your fingers in an attempt to feel a node or nodes slipping under your fingers. Normal nodes are not palpable. If you feel nodes, assess their size (length and width), consistency (soft, firm, rubbery, hard or craggy), tenderness and mobility to surrounding nodes and tissues. Whenever you discover an enlarged node, inspect the draining area in an attempt to find a source. Painful, tender nodes usually indicate an infected source that may be hidden from obvious view (e.g. infected cracks between toes). Malignant lymph nodes (either primary or secondary) are not usually tender. Malignant nodes vary in size from tiny, barely palpable structures to large glands 3–4 cm in size. Malignant lymph nodes may feel unusually firm (often described as 'rubbery') or hard and irregular. Fixation to surrounding tissue is highly suspicious of malignancy. Matted glands may occur in tuberculous lymphadenitis.

Often, in the course of routine examination, you will discover one or more small, mobile, nontender 'pea-sized' lymph nodes. The 'significance' of these 'shotty' nodes may be difficult to assess. Before embarking on a major exercise to diagnose the cause of the lymphadenopathy, it is reasonable to re-examine the node a few weeks later. If there is no change in symptoms and signs or gland size over this period, it is reasonable to consider the node a relic of a previous illness.

On completion of the lymphoreticular examination, it should be clear whether the lymphadenopathy is localised or generalised. This, in turn, helps with the differential diagnosis. If there is widespread adenopathy, consider HIV infection and AIDS, lymphomas and leukaemia.

HEAD AND NECK NODES

First, examine the nodes encircling the lower face and neck. Sit the patient forward. You may choose to examine these nodes from the front (Fig. 2.73) or back (Fig. 2.74). Both left and right sides can be examined simultaneously using the fingers of your left and right hands. Palpate the nodes in sequence, starting with the submental group in the midline behind the tip of the mandible. Next, feel for the submandibular nodes midway and along the inner surface of the inferior margin of the mandible. Feel for the tonsillar node at the angle of the jaw, the preauricular nodes immediately in front of the ear, the postauricular nodes over the mastoid process and, finally, the occipital nodes at the base of the skull posteriorly.

Follow this examination with palpation of the vertical groups of neck nodes. It may be helpful to flex the

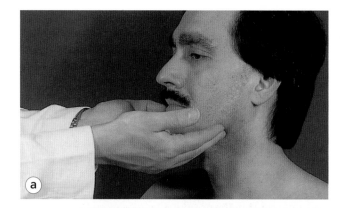

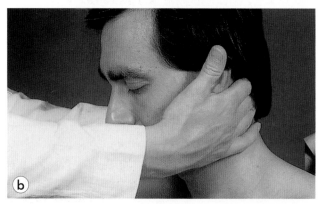

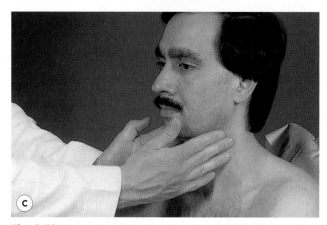

Fig. 2.73 Examination of the lymph nodes of the head and neck from the patient's front: (a) submandibular nodes, (b) occipital nodes, (c) deep cervical nodes.

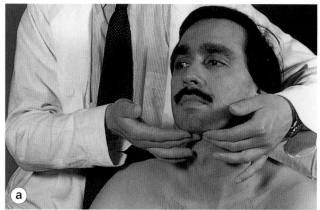

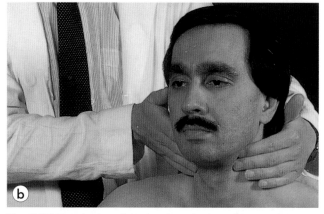

Fig. 2.74 Examination of the lymph nodes from the posterior: (a) submandibular nodes, (b) cervical nodes.

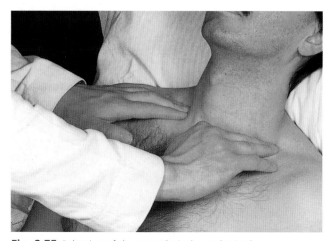

Fig. 2.75 Palpation of the supraclavicular nodes in the supraclavicular fossa.

patient's neck slightly to relax the strap muscles. Feel for the superficial cervical nodes along the body of sternocleidomastoid (Fig. 2.70). The posterior cervical nodes run along the anterior border of trapezius. The deep cervical chain is difficult to feel as the nodes are deep to the long axis of sternocleidomastoid; explore for these nodes by palpating more firmly through the body of this muscle. Conclude the examination by probing for the supraclavicular nodes which lie in the area bound by the clavicle inferiorly and the lateral border of sternocleidomastoid medially (Fig. 2.75). A palpable left supraclavicular node (Virchow's node) should always alert you to the possibility of stomach cancer.

EPITROCHLEAR AND AXILLARY NODES

To palpate the epitrochlear node, passively flex the patient's relaxed elbow to a right angle. Support this position with one hand while feeling with your fingers for the epitrochlear nodes which lie in a groove above and posterior to the medial condyle of the humerus (Fig. 2.76). The axillary group includes anterior, posterior, central, lateral and brachial nodes. Examine the axillary nodes from the patient's front. The technique for examining this region is described in Chapter 8.

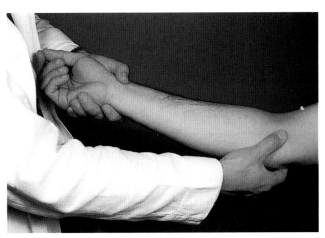

Fig. 2.76 Palpation of the epitrochlear nodes which lie in a groove above and posterior to the medial condyle of the humerus.

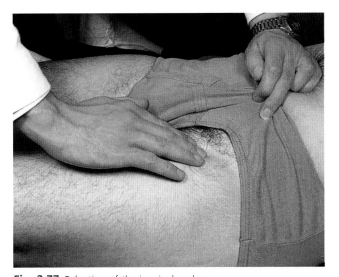

Fig. 2.77 Palpation of the inguinal nodes.

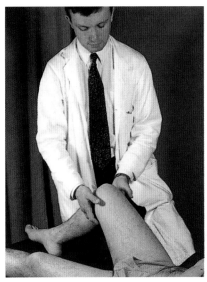

Fig. 2.78 Palpation of the popliteal nodes.

INGUINAL AND LEG NODES

Examine these nodes with the patient lying down (Fig. 2.77). The superficial inguinal nodes run in two chains. Palpate the horizontal chain which runs just below the line of the inguinal ligament and the vertical chain which runs along the saphenous vein. Relax the posterior popliteal fossa by passively flexing the knee. Explore the fossa for enlarged popliteal nodes by wrapping the hands around either side of the knee and exploring the fossa with the fingers of both hands (Fig. 2.78).

Remember that the spleen and liver are important components of the lymphoreticular system. Both may enlarge in lymphoreticular diseases. The examination of these organs is covered in Chapter 6.

Examination of elderly people

Nutrition in the elderly

- Elderly at special risk of nutritional compromise
- Contributory factors:
  - socioeconomic
  - inability to shop
  - loneliness
  - loss of smell, taste and teeth

- Age-related norms for height, weight, midarm muscle circumference and triceps skinfold thickness unavailable for elderly people
- Nutrition best assessed by careful dietary assessment (using third party to validate information)
- Assessment of hydration affected by loss of elastic tissue in skin

General examination
- First impressions
- Clinical syndromes (including endocrinopathies)
- Nutritional status
- Hydration
- 'Colour'
- Oedema
- Temperature
- Lymphoreticular examination

Skin examination
- Skin inspection
- Palpation
- Description of lesions
- Hair
- Nails

Ear, nose and throat examination
- Inspection of outer ear and ear drum, test hearing and balance
- Inspection of nose and palpation/percussion of sinuses
- Inspection of lips, teeth, tongue, oral cavity and pharynx, inspection and palpation of salivary glands
- Palpation of regional lymph nodes

Cardiovascular examination
- Hands (splinters, clubbing)
- Pulses
- Blood pressure
- Jugular blood pressure
- Heart (inspect, palpate, auscultate)
- Lungs (basal crackles, effusions)
- Abdomen (liver pulsation)
- Extremities (peripheral circulation, oedema)

Respiratory examination
- Hands (clubbing, cyanosis, CO_2 retention)
- Blood pressure (pulsus paradoxus)
- Neck (JVP, trachea)

- Lungs (inspect, palpate, percuss, auscultate)
- Heart (evidence of cor pulmonale)

Abdominal examination
- Hands (flapping tremor, nails, palms)
- Jaundice and signs of liver failure
- Parotids
- Mouth and tongue
- Chest (gynaecomastia, spiders, upper body of liver)
- Abdomen (inspect, palpate, percuss, auscultate)
- Groins
- Rectal examination

Male genitalia
- Sexual development
- Penis
- Scrotum
- Testes and spermatic cord
- Inguinal region

Female breasts and genitalia
- Sexual development
- Breast (inspection, palpation)
- Vulva (inspection, palpation)
- Vagina (inspection, palpation)
- Uterus and adnexae (palpation)

Musculoskeletal examination
- Proximal and distal muscles (inspection, palpation)
- Large joints
- Small joints
- Spine

Neurological examination
- Psychological profile
- Mental status
- Cranial nerves
- Motor and sensory examination (central and peripheral), cerebellar examination
- Autonomic nervous system

3

Skin, hair and nails

This chapter aims to familiarise you with the clinical features of skin disease and illustrates some of the more common skin disorders.

The relatively sparse distribution of hair in the human species contrasts starkly with most other mammals and reflects an evolutionary event that must, in some way, have been advantageous. Perhaps human nakedness provided a strong stimulus for developing alternative 'coats' and from this emerged the creative attributes that characterise the species.

The environment in which we live is harsh, variable and unpredictable. In contrast, the efficiency with which the body operates is set within narrow limits of temperature and hydration. Skin has evolved to encapsulate, insulate and thermoregulate. Recently, other functions have been recognised: the skin is an important link in the immune system, and the Langerhans cells of the dermis are closely related to monocytes and macrophages and are probably important in delayed hypersensitivity reactions and allograft rejection. Skin also has an important endocrine function, being responsible for the modification of sex hormones produced by the gonads and adrenals. In addition, skin is the site of vitamin D synthesis.

Structure and function

SKIN

The skin comprises two layers: the epidermis, derived from embryonic ectoderm, and the dermis and hypodermis, derived from mesoderm.

Epidermis

This layer consists of a modified stratified squamous epithelium and arises from basal, germinal columnar keratinocytes that evolve as they migrate towards the surface through a prickle cell layer (where the cells acquire a polyhedral shape) and a granular cell layer (where the nucleated cells acquire keratohyalin granules) and eventually form the superficial keratinised layer (horny layer of the stratum corneum) where the cells lose their nuclei and form a tough superficial barrier (Fig. 3.1). The migratory cycle from the basal to horny layer takes approximately 30 days, with the cornified cells shedding from the surface some 14 days later. Abnormalities of this transit time may lead to certain skin diseases such as psoriasis, in which the migration rate is greatly accelerated. Epidermal cells are linked by structures known as desmosomes. The epidermis rests on a thin basement membrane and is anchored to the dermis by hemidesmosomes and other anchor proteins such as laminin, basement membrane proteoglycan and type IV collagen. These and other proteins are of importance in the pathogenesis of diseases occurring at the epidermal–dermal junction (e.g. bullous pemphigoid and epidermolysis bullosa).

Melanocytes develop among the basal cells. These cells are derived from neural crest cells and synthesise melanin pigment which is transferred to keratinocytes through dendritic processes. Melanin is responsible for skin and hair pigmentation. The pigment protects the skin from the potentially harmful effects of ultraviolet irradiation. Skin colour is determined by the total number, size and distribution of melanin granules, not the number of melanocytes. Hereditary failure to synthesise melanin results in albinism.

Dermis

This layer provides the supporting framework on which the epidermis rests and consists of a fibrous matrix of collagen and elastin set in a ground substance of glycosaminoglycans, hyaluronic acid and chondroitin sulphate (Fig. 3.1). The skin appendages are set in the dermis. Nerves, blood vessels, fibroblasts and various inflammatory cells also populate this layer. The dermis is divided into two layers: the papillary dermis apposes the undulating dermal–epidermal junction, whereas the reticular dermis lies beneath, forming the bulk of collagen, elastic fibres and ground substance. Dermal fibroblasts synthesise and secrete the dermal collagen subtypes (I and III) and elastin. If there is disruption of dermal elastin,

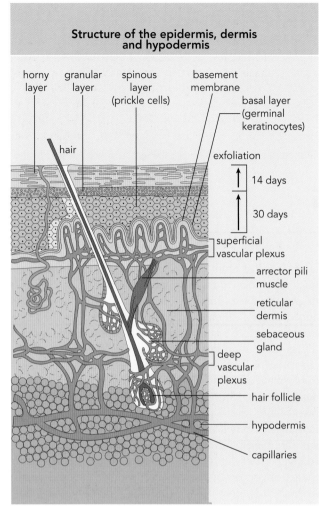

Structure of the epidermis, dermis and hypodermis

horny layer · granular layer · spinous layer (prickle cells) · hair · basement membrane · basal layer (germinal keratinocytes) · exfoliation · 14 days · 30 days · superficial vascular plexus · arrector pili muscle · reticular dermis · sebaceous gland · deep vascular plexus · hair follicle · hypodermis · capillaries

Fig. 3.1 Section through full thickness of skin showing the structure of the epidermis, dermis and hypodermis.

disorders such as wrinkles and a loose skin syndrome (cutis laxa) occur.

Hypodermis

The dermis rests on the hypodermis, which is the subcutaneous layer of fat and loose connective tissue. This layer serves both as a fat store and an insulating layer.

SKIN APPENDAGES

Sebaceous glands

Skin sebaceous glands can function throughout life, although activity is latent between birth and puberty. These glands are partly responsible for the production of vernix caseosa which covers and waterproofs the fetus during the latter stages of gestation. The glands become particularly active during puberty. The secretion is holocrine (i.e. caused by complete degeneration of the acinar cells) and is stimulated by androgens and opposed by oestrogens. Sebaceous glands are absent from the palms and soles and are concentrated on the face, scalp,

midline of the back and the perineum. Sebum contains triglyceride, scalene and wax esters and functions to waterproof and lubricate the skin, as well as inhibiting the growth of skin flora and fungi. Skin disorders such as acne vulgaris and rosacea occur in areas where sebaceous glands concentrate.

Apocrine and eccrine glands

The apocrine glands are concentrated in the axillae, areolae, nipples, anogenital regions, eyelids and external ears. These glands become functionally active at puberty and are responsible for an odourless secretion which is acted on by skin flora, causing characteristic body odour to develop. The eccrine sweat glands are widely distributed and are extremely important in heat regulation and fluid balance. Whereas the eccrine cells secrete an isotonic fluid, the duct cells modify the fluid to render it hypotonic. Secretion and its modification are under cholinergic and hormonal control. Sweating in response to temperature change is under hypothalamic control.

HAIR

In most mammals, hair is important in the control of temperature. In humans, however, hair is mainly important as a tactile organ which also has a sensual function, important in both sexual attraction and stimulation. Hair covers all of the body except the palms, soles, prepuce and glans and inner surface of the labia minora. During gestation the fetus is covered by a fine coat of lanugo hair which is lost shortly before birth, except for the scalp, eyebrows and lashes. Hair may be vellus, which is short, fine and unpigmented, or terminal hair, which is thicker and pigmented. Puberty is characterised by the development of coarse, pigmented hair in a pubic, axillary and facial distribution.

Hair is formed by specialised epidermal cells that invaginate deep into the dermal layer. Hair develops from the base of the hair follicle where the papilla, a network of capillaries, supports the nutrition and growth of the hair. Hair growth is cyclical: the active growth phase is termed anagen; involution of the hair, catagen; and the resting phase, telogen.

The hair shaft consists of a cuticle, cortex and medulla. The arrectores pilorum muscles anchor in the papillary dermis and insert into the perifollicular tissue (Fig. 3.1). Contraction of these muscles causes goose pimples (cutis anserina) to occur. Hair colour is determined by the density of melanosomes within the cortex of the hair shaft; none is present in white hair, whereas grey hair has a reduced number. Red hair has different melanosomes to black hair, both chemically and structurally.

THE NAIL

Nail is a specialised skin appendage derived from an epidermal tuck that invaginates into the dermis. The highly keratinised epithelium is strong but flexible and

Structure of nail

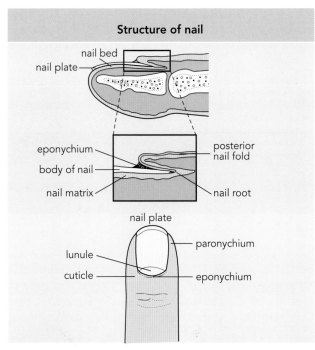

Fig. 3.2 Structure of nail.

provides a sharpened surface for fine manipulation, clawing, scraping or scratching.

The nail has three major components: the root, the nail plate and the free edge (Fig. 3.2). The proximal and lateral nail folds overlap the edges of the nail and a thin cuticular fold, the eponychium, overlies the proximal nail plate. The lunule is the crescent-shaped portion of the proximal nail formed by the distal end of the nail matrix. The free margin of the distal nail is continuous along its undersurface with the hyponychium, a specialised area of thickened epidermis. The nail plate lies on the highly vascularised nail bed, which gives the nail its pink appearance. The paronychium is the soft, loose tissue surrounding the nail border; it is particularly susceptible to bacterial or fungal infection infiltrating from a breach in the eponychium (a paronychia). Fingernails grow approximately 0.1 mm per day, with more rapid growth in summer compared with winter.

Symptoms of skin disease

The history should evaluate possible precipitating factors and determine whether the skin problem is localised or a manifestation of systemic illness.

The skin is readily examined and for this reason the history often assumes less importance than with other systems. However, a thorough history may unearth crucial information to aid diagnosis. Attempt to gain some insight into the patient's social conditions, as overcrowding and close physical contact are important when considering infectious disorders such as scabies and impetigo. Enquire in some depth about possible precipitating factors, especially contact with occupational

or domestic toxins or chemicals. Ask whether waterproof gloves are worn when washing dishes or dusting and cleaning the home. Question the patient about recent exposure to medicines, especially antibiotics which often cause skin rashes. Cosmetics are an important cause of skin sensitisation so enquire about the use of new soaps, deodorants and toiletries. Ask about hobbies (e.g. gardening, model building and photographic developing), foreign travel and insect bites. Ascertain whether or not the skin complaint is seasonal.

Questions to ask

Skin history

- Was the onset sudden or gradual?
- Is the skin itchy or painful?
- Is there any associated discharge (blood or pus)?
- Where is the problem located?
- Have you recently taken any antibiotics or other drugs?
- Have you used any topical medications?
- Were there any preceding systemic symptoms (fever, sore throat, anorexia, vaginal discharge)?
- Have you travelled abroad recently?
- Were you bitten by insects?
- Any possible exposure to industrial or domestic toxins?
- Any possible contact with sexually transmitted disease or HIV?
- Was there close physical contact with others with skin disorders?

Differential diagnosis

Systemic diseases causing pruritus

- Intrahepatic and extrahepatic biliary obstruction (cholestasis)
- Diabetes mellitus
- Polycythaemia rubra vera
- Chronic renal failure
- Lymphoma (especially Hodgkin's disease)

Systemic disorders may also present with skin symptoms. Infectious diseases often present with skin rashes or lesions. Ask about a recent sore throat, as streptococcal infection may be accompanied by typical rash (scarlet fever), painful red nodules on the extensor surface (erythema nodosum) or guttate psoriasis. In a cutaneous candidal infection, the patient often complains of an itchy rash and sore tongue or, in women, a vaginal discharge. *Candida albicans* infection often follows a course of broad-spectrum antibiotics. Skin rashes developing in sun-exposed areas (in the absence of strong sunburn, known as photosensitive rashes) should raise the possibility of systemic lupus erythematosus, porphyria or drugs. If the patient complains of skin lesions around the genitalia, enquire about possible contact with sexually transmitted disease. AIDS may present with the nodular lesions characteristic of Kaposi's sarcoma or thrush affecting the mucosa or skin. Therefore, it is important to take a history of risk factors (e.g. male homosexuality, high-risk heterosexual contact, blood transfusion and intravenous drug abuse). Skin itching (pruritus) in the absence of an obvious rash should alert you to an underlying systemic disorder.

Topical steroids and other topical substances are commonly prescribed to treat a variety of skin lesions. Always ask about topical treatment as this may alter the appearance of a skin lesion, making the diagnosis more difficult.

Symptoms of hair disease

HAIR THINNING

Balding (alopecia) worries patients and you will often be asked to assess scalp hair loss. Male pattern baldness is common; the patient will note the slow onset of hair loss with the hairline receding from the frontal and temporal scalp and crown. Ask about a family history of baldness as male alopecia is an expression of autosomal dominance and may begin early in life. After the menopause, many women note thinning of the hair (Fig. 3.3); this is often associated with growth of facial hair.

Questions to ask

Hair history

- Was the hair loss sudden or gradual?
- Does the loss occur only on the scalp or is the body hair involved as well?
- Is the baldness localised or general, symmetrical or asymmetrical?
- Is there a family history of baldness (especially in men)?
- What drugs have you taken recently?
- Any recent illnesses, stress or trauma?
- Are there other systemic symptoms (e.g. symptoms of hypothyroidism)?

Hair loss may also be a feature of disease and the characteristics of the alopecia may be helpful. Patients complaining of localised alopecia (alopecia areata) (Fig. 3.4) may have an autoimmune disease (e.g. Hashimoto's thyroiditis with myxoedema). Patients with stress or anxiety neurosis may nervously pluck hair from the scalp,

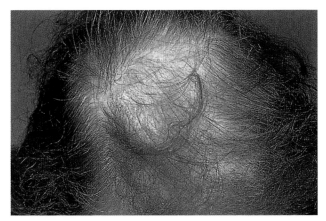

Fig. 3.3 Alopecia.

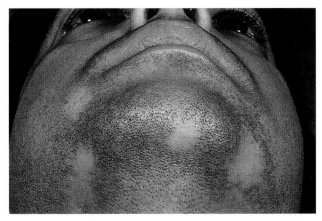

Fig. 3.4 Alopecia areata characterised by localised patches of hair loss.

causing a local area of thinning or baldness. Severe illness and malnutrition, as well as sudden psychological shock, may be associated with hair loss, which usually recovers once the stress has been resolved.

ABNORMAL HAIR GROWTH

Remember to warn patients undergoing cytotoxic treatment for cancer that they can expect generalised hair loss. Failure to develop axillary and pubic hair at the expected time of puberty should alert you to the possibility of pituitary or gonadal dysfunction.

Abnormal facial hair growth (hirsutism) is a distressing symptom in women. It is important to recognise that a certain degree of facial hair growth occurs naturally in postpubertal women. There are racial differences: physiological hirsutism is least apparent in Japanese and Chinese women and most apparent in women of Mediterranean, Middle Eastern, Indian and Negroid extraction. The unexpected occurrence of hirsutism, especially if accompanied by other symptoms and signs of virilism, should alert you to the possibility of a hormonal imbalance.

Questions to ask

Hirsutism

- Is there a family history of hirsutism?
- Are your menstrual periods normal or absent (or scanty)?
- Is there a history of primary or secondary infertility?
- Do you experience visual disturbances or headaches (pituitary disease)?
- What medications do you take (e.g. phenytoin, anabolic steroids, progestogens)?

Differential diagnosis

Hirsutism

- Racial variation in hair distribution
- Hormonal imbalance
  - polycystic ovaries
  - ovarian failure or menopause
  - virilising adrenal tumours
- Drugs
  - phenytoin
  - progestogens
  - anabolic steroids
  - ciclosporin

Symptoms of nail disease

Whereas examination of the nails may be very revealing, nail-related symptoms are usually nonspecific. Patients may relate symptoms suggestive of bacterial infection along the nail edge; these include intense pain, swelling and often a purulent discharge. Complaints of brittleness, splitting or cracking provide little diagnostic information. Ask specifically about skin disease that may affect the nail, such as psoriasis, severe eczema, lichen planus or a susceptibility to fungal skin infection.

Examination of the skin, hair and nails

EXAMINING THE SKIN

When examining the skin, there is a tendency to focus on the local area noticed by the patient. Nonetheless, you should consider the skin as an organ in its own right and, like any other examination, the whole organ should be examined to gain maximum information. The patient should be stripped to the underwear, covered with a gown or blanket and the examination area should be well lit (preferably natural daylight or fluorescent light).

Inspection and palpation

Scan the skin, looking for skin lesions and noting both position and symmetry. Remember to expose hidden areas like the axillae, inner thighs and buttock with its natal cleft. Many skin lesions can be diagnosed by their appearance and localisation. Unlike any other organ system, the examination relies almost entirely on careful inspection and meticulous use of descriptive terminology.

Measurement of the length and breadth of skin lesions is useful, especially when monitoring progression or regression. A broad beam torch or electric light helps to define the outline of the border of a skin lesion; a thin beam is helpful if you wish to check whether or not a lesion transilluminates. A fluid-filled but not solid lesion emits a red glow when the torch light shines through it. A Wood's lamp helps to distinguish a fluorescing lesion; by shining the lamp at a suspect lesion, it may be possible to show the characteristic blue-green fluorescence of fungal infections.

Skin colour

Skin colour varies between individuals and races and is usually even and symmetrical in distribution. Normal variations occur in freckling and sun-exposed areas. During pregnancy, there may be darkening of the skin overlying the cheek bones (melasma) and the areolae surrounding the nipple (chloasma).

Abnormal skin colour

Generalised changes in skin colour occur in jaundice, iron overload, endocrine disorders and albinism. The yellow tinge of jaundice is best observed in good daylight, appearing initially as yellowing of the sclerae and then as a yellow discoloration on the trunk, arms and legs. Jaundice is less apparent in unconjugated as opposed to conjugated hyperbilirubinaemia. In longstanding, deep obstructive jaundice, the skin may turn a deep yellow-green. Remember that people eating large quantities of carrots or other forms of vitamin A may develop yellow skin pigmentation (carotenaemia) and that the absence of scleral discoloration distinguishes this syndrome from jaundice.

Iron overload (haemosiderosis and haemochromatosis) causes the skin to turn a slate-grey colour. The astute observer may recognise this metabolic disease by the characteristic skin pigmentation. Addison's disease (autoimmune adrenal destruction) is characterised by darkening of the skin, occurring first in the skin creases of the palms and soles, scars and other skin creases. The mucosa of the mouth and gums also becomes pigmented. Striking pigmentation also arises after bilateral adrenalectomy for adrenal hyperplasia: this syndrome (Nelson's syndrome) is caused by unopposed pituitary overstimulation. In hypopituitarism, the skin is soft, pale and wrinkled.

Albinism is an autosomal recessive disorder caused by failure of melanocytes to produce melanin. The skin and hair are white and the eyes are pink because of a lack of pigmentation of the iris, and there may also be nystagmus.

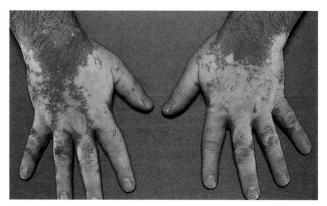

Fig. 3.5 Depigmented skin (vitiligo): white discoloration of brown hand.

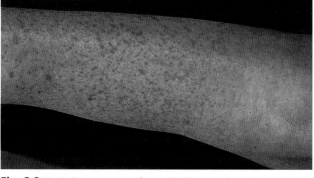

Fig. 3.8 Typical appearance of petechial haemorrhage in a patient with thrombocytopenia.

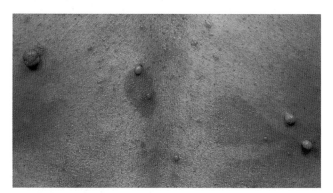

Fig. 3.6 Café-au-lait patches with neurofibromas.

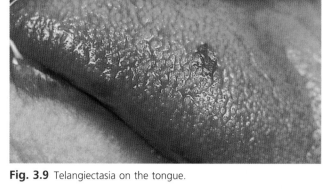

Fig. 3.9 Telangiectasia on the tongue.

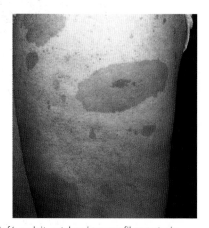

Fig. 3.7 Café-au-lait patches in neurofibromatosis.

Telangiectasia refers to fine blanching vascular lesions caused by superficial capillary dilatation (Fig. 3.9).

Localised skin lesions

Careful descriptions of size, shape, colour, texture and position of lesions are helpful in skin diagnosis. Try to ascertain a primary and secondary description of the skin lesion. To establish the primary nature of the skin lesion decide whether the lesion is flat, nodular or fluid-filled. Flat circumscribed changes in colour are termed macules if less than 1 cm or patches if more than 1 cm. If the lesion is raised and can be palpated, assess whether the mass is a papule, plaque, nodule, tumour or wheal. If a circumscribed elevated lesion is fluctuant and fluid-filled, describe whether it is a vesicle, bulla or pustule (Fig. 3.10). If possible, describe the arrangement of the lesions; that is, whether linear, annular (ring-shaped) or clustered. In shingles (herpes zoster), the rash occurs in the distribution of one or more skin dermatomes.

Add to the primary description any secondary characteristics such as superficial erosions, ulceration, crusting, scaling, fissuring, lichenification, atrophy, excoriation, scarring, necrosis or keloid formation.

Palpation is used to decide whether a lesion is flat, raised or tender. Compression may be helpful (e.g. demonstration of the characteristic arteriolar dilatation of spider naevi occurring in decompensated liver disease) (Fig. 3.11). Use the back of your hand to assess

Common localised abnormalities of skin pigmentation include vitiligo (Fig. 3.5), café-au-lait spots (Figs 3.6, 3.7), pityriasis versicolor and idiopathic guttate hypomelanosis. Erythema of the skin is caused by capillary dilatation; when pressure is applied the red lesion blanches and reforms. When examining a patient, you may notice an erythematous flush in the necklace area which is caused by anxiety. Purpura is the term used for red-purplish lesions of the skin caused by seepage of blood from skin blood vessels. Unlike erythema, these lesions do not blanch with pressure. If the lesions are small (<5 mm) they are called petechiae (Fig. 3.8), whereas larger lesions are purpura. Traumatic bruises are called ecchymoses.

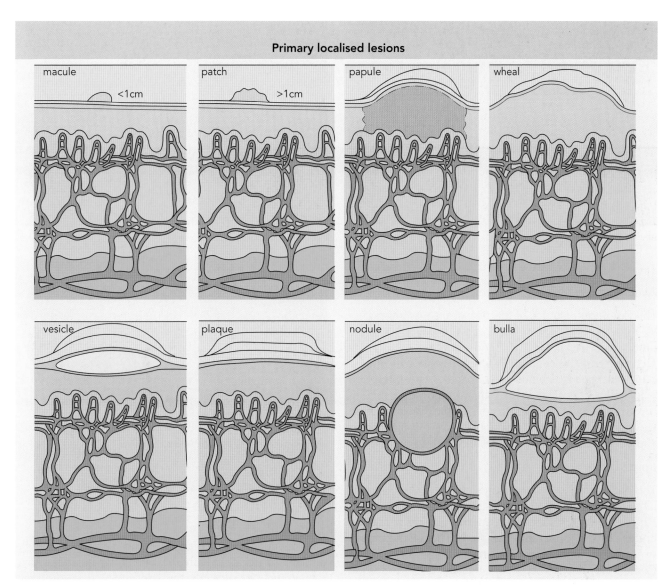

Fig. 3.10 Primary localised skin lesions.

Fig. 3.11 Spider naevi in hepatocellular disease.

temperature. Inflamed lesions (e.g. cellulitis) are hotter than surrounding tissue, whereas skin overlying a lipoma (subcutaneous fat tumours) is cooler than adjacent tissue. Skin turgor may be used as a measure of moderate to severe hydration. Pinch a small area of skin between index finger and thumb. Hold firmly for a few seconds and then release. Healthy, well-hydrated skin immediately springs back into its resting position. In significant dehydration or when skin elastic tissue is lost (e.g. ageing), the skin behaves like putty and only slowly reshapes to its resting position. Skin oedema can be demonstrated by pressing your thumb or fingers into the skin, maintaining the pressure for a short while and then releasing. Your thumb or finger impression will remain indented in the skin if there is excessive fluid ('pitting' oedema).

Although most disorders can be diagnosed from their appearance, special techniques such as microscopy of skin biopsies or skin scrapings, immunofluorescent staining and culture of specimens may be required to confirm diagnosis.

Common skin lesions

Skin lesions are often readily recognisable and you should be able to distinguish some common conditions.

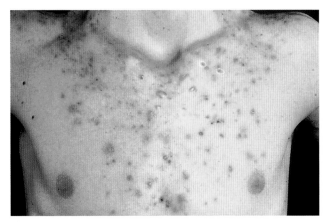

Fig. 3.12 Papules, pustules and scarring in acne vulgaris.

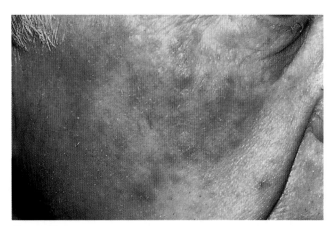

Fig. 3.13 Rosacea: papules and pustules occur on the face.

Acne vulgaris

This common disorder of the pilosebaceous unit occurs at puberty. Plugging of the duct, increased sebum production, bacterial growth and hormonal changes all predispose to the condition. Acne presents with greasy skin, blackheads (comedones), papules, pustules and scars (Fig. 3.12). The lesions are common and vary in severity and most teenagers recognise the problem before visiting the doctor. The disorder affects the face, chest and back. Acne usually subsides in the third decade.

Rosacea

This facial rash usually presents in the fourth decade, although in women it may present after the menopause. Papules and pustules erupt on the forehead, cheeks, bridge of the nose and the chin. The erythematous background highlights the rash (Figs 3.13, 3.14). Comedones do not occur, distinguishing the condition clinically from facial acne. Occasionally, the rash may be localised to the nose. Eye involvement is characterised by grittiness, conjunctivitis and even corneal ulceration. There appears to be vasomotor instability and patients flush readily in response to stimuli such as hot drinks, alcohol and spicy foods. If this disorder is treated with potent topical corticoids there may be a temporary response, but a marked relapse occurs on cessation of treatment. It is important to check carefully whether or not steroids have been applied and to dissuade your patient from using this treatment (like acne vulgaris, antibiotics are the treatment of choice).

Drug reactions

Drugs are probably the most common cause of acute skin disease and your history must include a complete history of all drugs the patient may have been exposed to over the preceding month. Antibiotics such as ampicillin, penicillin and sulphonamides commonly cause drug rashes. It may be difficult to distinguish between a drug reaction and the manifestations of the disease under treatment. In addition, drug reaction may closely mimic skin diseases. Diagnosis may be further confused in

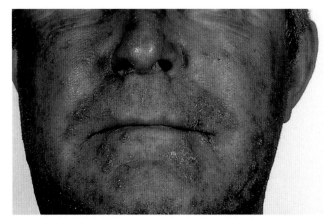

Fig. 3.14 Rosacea: lesions occur on the nose, cheeks and chin.

patients taking more than one drug, because it may be difficult to decide which the offending agent is. Also, remember that drugs may cause secondary skin eruptions: broad-spectrum antibiotics may encourage the growth of candida, which, in turn, can present as a 'drug-related' skin rash. Drug reactions may occur within minutes or hours of taking the medication but there may also be delays of up to 2 weeks for the reaction to manifest. This may even follow the discontinuation of the drug (well known with ampicillin). It is important to recognise different expressions of drug sensitivity.

 Differential diagnosis

Skin lesions associated with drug sensitivity

- Toxic erythema
- Exfoliative dermatitis
- Urticaria
- Angioneurotic oedema
- Erythema nodosum
- Erythema multiforme
- Fixed drug reaction
- Photosensitive drug reactions
- Pemphigus

Toxic erythema

Profuse eruptions affect most of the body. Red macules appear and overlap and coalesce to give the appearance of diffuse erythema (Fig. 3.15). The erythematous skin desquamates as it heals. This condition is most often caused by ampicillin but also by sulphonamides (including co-trimoxazole), phenobarbital and infections.

Exfoliative dermatitis

Also known as erythroderma, this form of dermatitis is characterised by diffuse erythema and desquamation of the epithelium. If severe, the patient may lose both heat and fluids. Many drugs are implicated, although barbiturates, sulphonamides, streptomycin and gold are especially predominant.

Questions to ask
Exfoliative dermatitis

- Is there any loss of hair or nails?
- Have you ever had psoriasis or eczema?
- What drugs have you taken recently (barbiturates, sulphonamides, phenylbutazone, streptomycin)?
- Do you have a fever?

Urticaria

This presents with intense itching and localised swellings of the skin that may occur anywhere on the body. Typically, wheals occur that are red at the margins with paler centres (Fig. 3.16). The characteristic feature of the rash is its tendency to disappear within a few hours. Angio-oedema usually occurs in association with urticaria and is characterised by swelling of the face and hands.

Erythema nodosum

Symmetrical in distribution, the acute crops of painful, tender, raised red nodules usually affect the extensor surfaces, especially the shins but also the thighs and upper arms (Figs 3.17, 3.18). Over 7–10 days, the lesions change colour from bright red through shades of purple to a yellowish area of discoloration. Erythema nodosum is caused by vasculitis, may be recurrent, and is most commonly associated with sulphonamides, oral contraceptives and barbiturates.

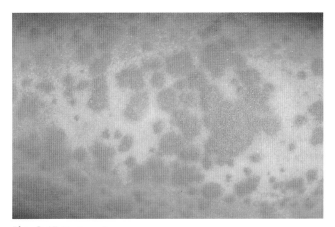

Fig. 3.15 Toxic erythema.

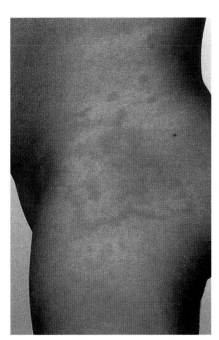

Fig. 3.16 Urticaria: lesions vary in size and shape.

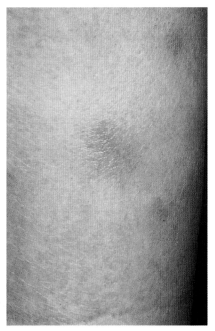

Fig. 3.17 Erythema nodosum: painful, smooth red nodules on the lower leg.

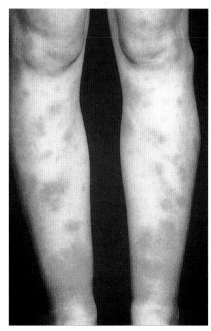

Fig. 3.18 Erythema nodosum: the nodules are raised and tender.

Differential diagnosis

Erythema nodosum

Infections
- Streptococcal infections
- Tuberculosis
- Leprosy
- Syphilis
- Deep fungal diseases

Drugs
- Sulphonamides
- Barbiturates
- Oral contraceptives

Systemic diseases
- Sarcoidosis
- Inflammatory bowel disease

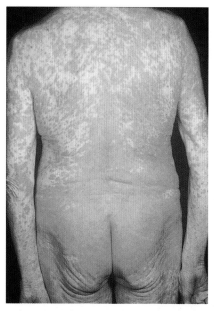

Fig. 3.19 Erythema multiforme: the lesions are widespread on this patient.

Erythema multiforme

This is characterised by symmetrical, round (annular) lesions occurring especially on the hands and feet but which may extend more proximally (Figs 3.19, 3.20). Central blistering may occur, giving the appearance of 'target' lesions. In severe forms, bullae may appear. This skin disease occurs with drugs, vaccination and, frequently, with a herpes simplex infection.

Stevens–Johnson syndrome

This is a severe blistering form of erythema multiforme with blistering and ulceration affecting the mucous membranes of the mouth and often affecting the eyes and nasal and genital mucosa (Fig. 3.21).

Fixed drug eruption

This presents with one or more red blotches that may become swollen and even bullous. The rash always recurs in the same anatomical site: usually the mouth, a limb or genital area. The rash fades, leaving an area of skin discoloration (Fig. 3.22). Associated with many drugs but especially phenolphthalein (common in laxatives), sulphonamides, tetracycline and barbiturates.

Photosensitive drug rashes

This rash occurs in sun-exposed areas (face, necklace region and extensor surfaces of limbs). It may appear as erythema, oedema, blistering or an eczematous rash.

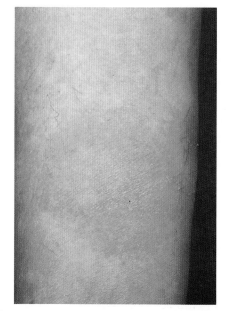

Fig. 3.20 Erythema multiforme.

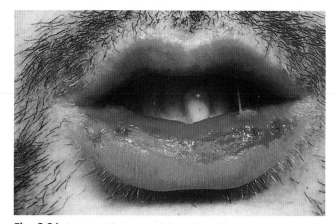

Fig. 3.21 Stevens–Johnson syndrome: ulceration is present on the lips and in the mouth.

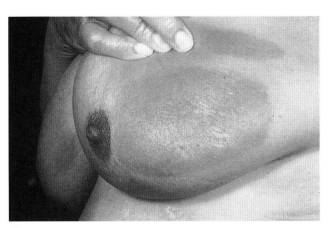

Fig. 3.22 Fixed drug eruption, with hyperpigmentation of the breasts.

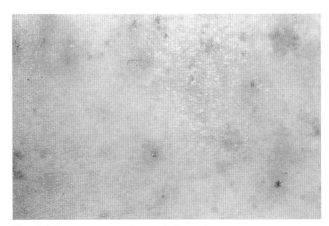

Fig. 3.23 Eczema: note the vesicle formation.

Differential diagnosis
Photosensitive skin reactions

Drugs
- Tetracyclines
- Sulphonamides
- Phenothiazines
- Psoralens
- Hydroxychloroquinones

Systemic disorders
- Pellagra (nicotinic acid deficiency)
- Systemic lupus erythematosus
- Porphyria cutanea tarda
- Erythema multiforme

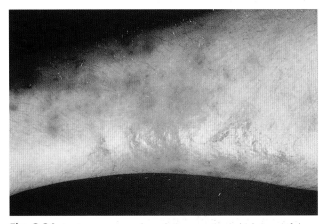

Fig. 3.24 Acute eczema: red exudative eruption which is painful.

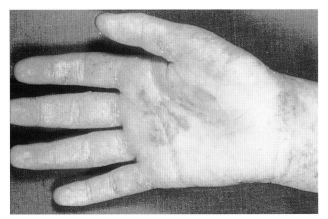

Fig. 3.25 Chronic eczema: the skin is dry and scaly.

Eczema

This common skin abnormality is caused by a number of different mechanisms and the disease may be acute, subacute or chronic, all of which may coexist. Itching is a major symptom. Acute eczema is characterised by oedema, vesicle formation (Fig. 3.23), exudation (weeping) (Fig. 3.24) and crusting. In chronic eczema there are dry, scaly, hyperkeratotic patches and thickening and fissuring of the skin (Fig. 3.25). The appearance of eczema is often modified because the patient scratches, causing secondary changes such as excoriation and secondary infection. The boundaries of an area of chronic eczema are less well defined than psoriasis and this may be a helpful sign in the differential diagnosis (Fig. 3.26).

Discoid (nummular) eczema Unlike other forms of eczema, this subtype has a well-defined, coin-shaped (L. nummularius = of money) outline and may be confused with psoriasis. However, nummular eczema tends to occur on the back of the fingers and hands. It also weeps and does not have the characteristic scales typical of psoriasis.

Atopic eczema This usually presents in infancy, although it does occasionally present for the first time in adulthood. There is normally a family history of eczema or some other atopic disorder (e.g. asthma, hay fever, urticaria). The rash is symmetrical, usually starting on the face

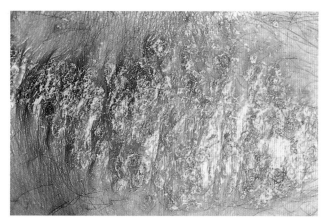

Fig. 3.26 Typical appearance of eczematous lesion. Note that the boundary is less distinct than plaques of psoriasis.

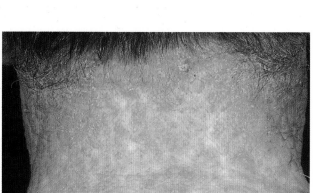

Fig. 3.27 Contact dermatitis caused by shampoo.

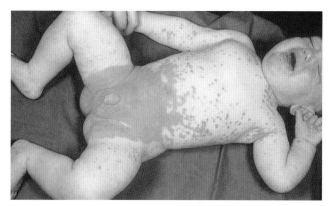

Fig. 3.28 Seborrhoeic dermatitis in an infant.

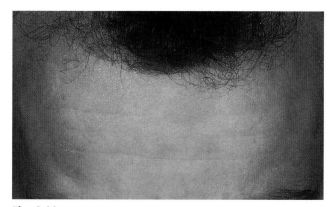

Fig. 3.29 Seborrhoeic dermatitis occurs most commonly on the face.

and migrating to the trunk and limbs (where it tends to affect the flexures of the elbows, knees, wrists and ankles).

Contact dermatitis This variant of eczema is caused by an exogenous irritant (Fig. 3.27). The lesion may be a primary irritant phenomenon, occurring almost predictably when skin contact is made with a concentrated toxic agent, or an allergic contact dermatitis which only occurs in patients who generate a delayed (type IV) immune response to a substance in contact with the skin. The distribution of the eczema may provide an important clue to the nature of the topical irritant. Individuals who regularly immerse their hands in water containing detergents or other sensitising substances will present with the rash restricted to the hands. Jewellery may cause an allergic contact dermatitis; nickel is an important sensitising agent. Rubber, dyes, cosmetics and industrial chemicals are common allergens implicated in this immune-mediated form of eczema. Plants such as primulas and chrysanthemums have also been implicated.

Seborrhoeic dermatitis This is an eczematous condition occurring in infants (Fig. 3.28), adolescents and young adults. There is erythema and scaling with a symmetrical rash (Fig. 3.29). Secondary infection may occur, altering

the appearance of the primary lesion. The scalp is most commonly involved and the condition is distinguished from dandruff by the associated erythema of the skin due to inflammation. Other regions involved include the central areas of the face, eyelid margins, nasolabial folds, cheeks, eyebrows and forehead. Involvement of the outer ear occurs (otitis externa). The vulva may also be affected.

Pompholyx Pompholyx is another variant of eczema affecting the hands and feet (Figs 3.30, 3.31). This variant is characterised by the eruption of itchy vesicles, especially on the lateral margins of the fingers and toes, as well as the palms and soles.

Varicose eczema This subtype occurs in patients with longstanding varicose veins. The eczematous patches affect the lower leg and may or may not be associated with other skin disorders caused by varicose veins; for example, venous ulcers that occur in the region of the medial malleolus, pigmentation and oedema.

Psoriasis

The lesions are well-defined, slightly raised and erythematous. In the chronic phase, silvery scales cover the surface. The lesions vary in size from small (guttate)

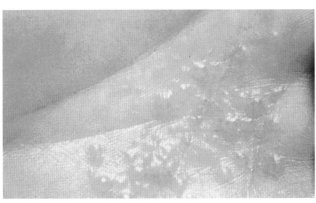

Fig. 3.30 Typical itchy vesicles of pompholyx.

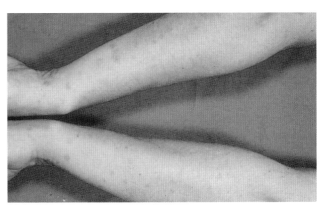

Fig. 3.33 Acute guttate psoriasis.

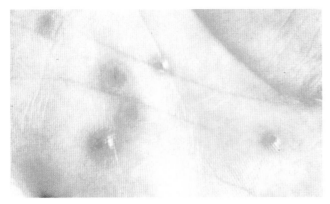

Fig. 3.31 Pompholyx: pruritic vesicles on the hand.

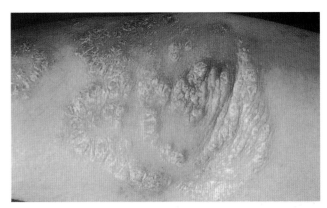

Fig. 3.34 Psoriatic plaque covered with a silvery scale.

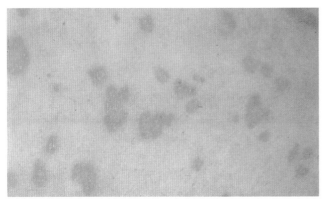

Fig. 3.32 Guttate (teardrop) psoriasis.

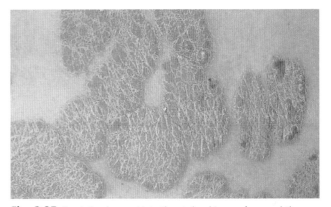

Fig. 3.35 Psoriatic plaque. Note the scaly, shiny surface and the sharp border.

(Figs 3.32, 3.33) to large plaques (Figs 3.34, 3.35). These guttate (1–3 cm) lesions are widely distributed over the body and may either resolve or persist as chronic psoriasis. Guttate psoriasis may follow streptococcal pharyngitis.

Chronic psoriasis The plaques of chronic psoriasis have a predilection for the scalp, elbows, knees, perineum, umbilicus and submammary skin. The lesions are usually symmetrical. A characteristic feature of psoriasis is the development of new psoriatic lesions where the skin is traumatised (the Koebner phenomenon). If you gently scratch the surface of a psoriatic plaque, tiny bleeding points appear.

Pustular psoriasis Pustular psoriasis is a variant, usually confined to the palms (Fig. 3.36) and soles, although some are occasionally more diffuse. The pustules, 2–5 mm in diameter, are yellow (Fig. 3.37). On the palms and soles they become pigmented and hyperkeratotic. Rarely, psoriasis may be so extensive that most of the skin is involved and exfoliation occurs.

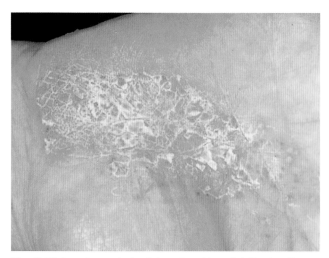

Fig. 3.36 Pustular psoriasis of the palm with well-defined scaling and erythema.

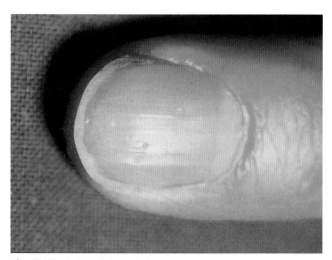

Fig. 3.38 Pitting of the nails in psoriasis.

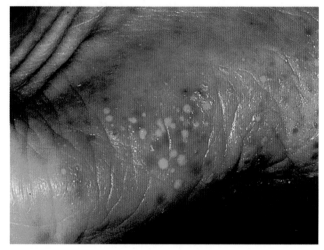

Fig. 3.37 Pustular psoriasis of the foot. The yellow pustules turn brown.

Fig. 3.39 Pityriasis rosea: the pink papules become oval macules.

Psoriatic arthropathy In psoriatic arthropathy, the distal interphalangeal joints are affected. Large joints may also be affected, either singly or symmetrically. Rarely, patients may have sacroiliitis or even spinal ankylosis. The nails may be involved even in the absence of skin disease. The typical features include pinpoint pitting of the nail (Fig. 3.38) and onycholysis (lifting of the distal nail from the nail bed). Unlike fungal nail lesions, nail psoriasis is symmetrical. Severe nail dystrophy may occur.

Pityriasis rosea

This is a common skin disorder in the younger patient. A single patch rash occurs days or even weeks before the more general eruption. This 'herald patch' may be confused with ringworm. The full blown rash affects the upper arms, trunk and upper thighs ('shirt and shorts' distribution). Pink papules evolve into 1–3 cm itchy oval macules (Fig. 3.39) that scale near the edge, giving a

characteristic appearance (Figs 3.40, 3.41). The rash resolves spontaneously within approximately 6 weeks.

Lichen planus

This is another itchy rash that can usually be diagnosed at the bedside by its typical appearance (Fig. 3.42). Occasionally, a lichenoid rash may be associated with systemic disorders (e.g. primary biliary cirrhosis, chronic graft versus host disease) or drugs (e.g. penicillamine and gold) but most commonly there is no associated disease.

The rash affects both the skin and mucous membranes. It has a predilection for the volar (front) aspect of the forearm and wrists, the dorsal (back) surface of the hands, the shins, ankles and lower back region. The rash is symmetrical and characterised by small, shiny, purple or violaceous papules which have a polygonal rather than rounded outline. A network of white lines on the surface of the papules is termed Wickham's striae (best seen after

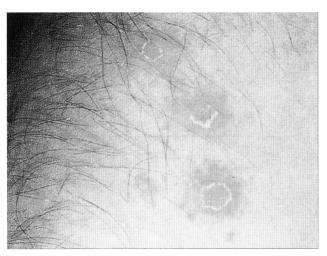

Fig. 3.40 In pityriasis rosea, the typical lesions are ovoid macules with scaling.

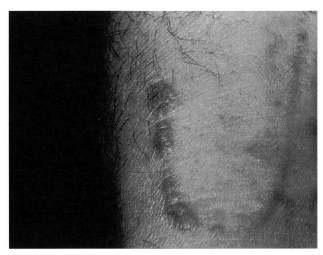

Fig. 3.43 Lichen planus: linear lesion of the Koebner syndrome.

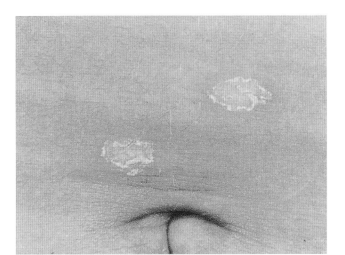

Fig. 3.41 Pityriasis rosea with obvious scaling.

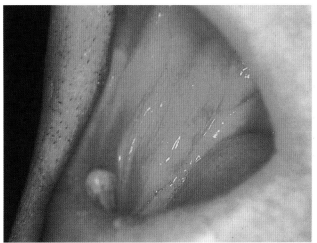

Fig. 3.44 Buccal involvement in lichen planus.

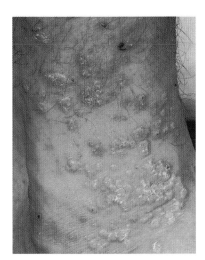

Fig. 3.42 Polygonal papules in lichen planus.

coating the lesion with mineral oil). As the papules resolve, the affected skin becomes pigmented. Eruptions occur after trauma (Koebner phenomenon) (Fig. 3.43) and linear lesions are tell-tale signs occurring in scratched areas. The buccal mucous membrane is commonly involved (Fig. 3.44). Use a spatula and light to inspect the mouth, looking for the lace-like network of white lines or spots. The scalp is usually, although not always, spared. The disease may affect the nails and penis.

Skin infections

BACTERIAL

Impetigo

This is a highly contagious skin lesion caused by β-haemolytic streptococci. The face is most commonly infected (Fig. 3.45). The lesions start as a papular eruption around the mouth and nose that then evolves into a vesicular eruption and spreads locally. The lesion breaks

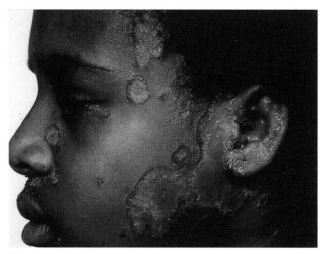

Fig. 3.45 Facial impetigo with crusting of the lesion.

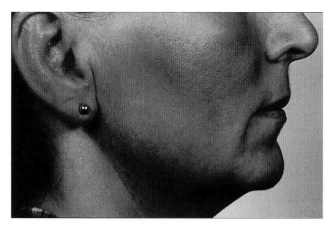

Fig. 3.46 Erysipelas. Note the erythema and oedema.

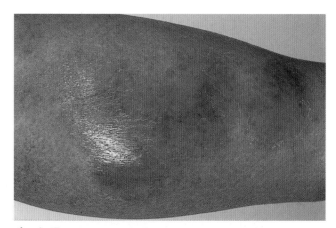

Fig. 3.47 Erythema and oedema associated with cellulitis.

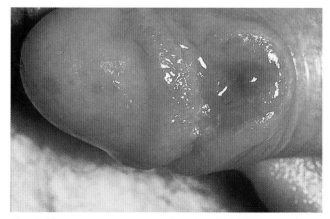

Fig. 3.48 Primary chancre in syphilis.

down to leave a typical honey-coloured crust. Secondary infection with *Staphylococcus aureus* is common.

Furuncle (boil)

A furuncle is an infection of a hair follicle, caused by *S. aureus*, that spreads locally into the surrounding tissue. A head of pus may be obvious at its apex. Furuncles usually affect adolescents. A local collection of furuncles is called a carbuncle. A stye (or hordeolum) is a small furuncle affecting an eyelash.

Erysipelas and cellulitis

Infection of the superficial skin layers by *Streptococcus pyogenes* is termed erysipelas, whereas an infection of the deeper skin layers is called cellulitis. The lower limbs are most commonly affected. Erysipelas is characterised by the abrupt onset of a well-demarcated slightly raised and tender erythematous rash (Fig. 3.46). Left untreated, the margins of the lesion advance rapidly. The patient is usually pyrexial and toxic. The infection responds quickly to antibiotics. The margin of an area of cellulitis is less well defined than erysipelas; in addition, superficial bullae may develop in the centre of an affected area of skin (Fig. 3.47).

Syphilis

There are numerous skin manifestations of syphilis and you should always suspect this disease when confronted with an unexplained, non-itchy rash, especially when the patient is generally unwell or when there is a high risk of sexually transmitted disease. In primary syphilis, a painless ulcer with an indurated edge (primary chancre) (Figs 3.48, 3.49) appears at the site of infection (usually on the genitalia but occasionally on the lips or even fingers). Approximately 2 months after the appearance of the chancre, the secondary rash appears: a pink macular rash on the trunk (Fig. 3.50) that becomes papular, affecting the genital skin, palms and soles. In the anal and groin regions, the moistness may cause erosions (condylomata accuminata) (Fig. 3.51). Raised oval patches

occur in the mucous membrane of the mouth (snail-track ulcers). In the tertiary stage, granulomas form (gummas); these can be felt as skin nodules which are prone to degenerate and ulcerate.

VIRAL

Warts

Common warts caused by papilloma viruses are self-limiting and generally occur in the young patient. Warts usually occur on the fingers and hands as discrete papules

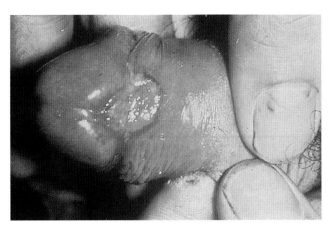

Fig. 3.49 Primary syphilitic chancre on the frenulum.

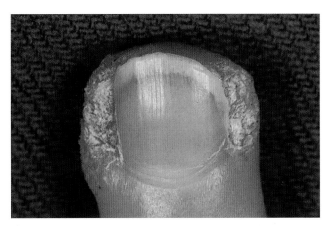

Fig. 3.52 Finger warts.

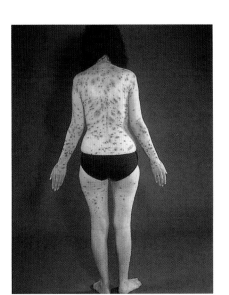

Fig. 3.50 The maculopapular rash of secondary syphilis.

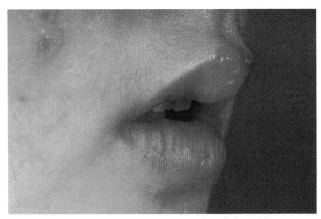

Fig. 3.53 'Fever blister' caused by herpes simplex.

with a typical irregular surface (Fig. 3.52). Plantar warts occur on the pressure-bearing areas of the feet and are consequently flattened rather than raised.

Molluscum contagiosum

This is a common infection caused by a member of the pox virus group. The lesions appear as flesh-coloured, dome-shaped papules varying in size from pinpoint to 1 cm in diameter. The most characteristic feature of the lesion is umbilication (a central depression of the surface). In children, the lesions are especially common on the face and trunk, whereas in adults, the genitalia may be affected. As the lesions resolve, an area of induration often develops in the surrounding skin.

Herpes simplex

There are two types of herpes simplex virus (HSV). Type 1 virus normally affects the mouth and lips (Fig. 3.53), whereas type 2 usually affects the genitals. Crossover infections do sometimes occur. The primary HSV infection presents with crops of painful superficial vesicles surrounded by an area of erythema. The vesicles erode superficially, then crust and finally heal without scarring. After the primary infection, the virus lies dormant in the dorsal root nerve ganglion, with recurrences occurring predictably in the same area as the initial infection.

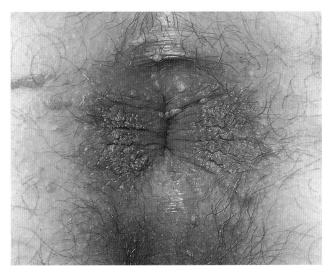

Fig. 3.51 Condylomata accuminata.

Reactivation is heralded by a tingling sensation in the skin which is followed within 1–2 days by the eruption of a crop of vesicles. Exacerbations may be precipitated by infection, stress, fever (hence the term fever blisters), abnormal exposure to sunlight, menstruation and trauma. Often, no obvious precipitating cause is discovered.

Herpes zoster (shingles)

After an attack of chicken pox, the varicella-zoster virus lies dormant in a dorsal root or cranial nerve ganglion. Reactivation of the virus causes a localised eruption called shingles. The cause of reactivation is often not apparent, although immunosuppression, lymphomas and ageing may be implicated.

The patient complains of pain or discomfort in a localised area of skin and, within a few days, a crop of vesicles appears in a characteristic dermatomal distribution (Fig. 3.54). Over 2–3 weeks, the vesicles evolve into pustules, scab, then heal. Often there is some residual scarring. In order of frequency, the thoracic, cervical, lumbar and sacral dermatomes are affected. If the ophthalmic branch of the trigeminal nerve is involved, there may be serious damage to the cornea. This is associated with a typical distribution of the vesicles on the tip and side of the nose. Involvement of the geniculate ganglion of the facial nerve causes a facial palsy with involvement of the outer ear (Ramsay Hunt syndrome). The most debilitating long-term effect of shingles, even when healing has occurred, is chronic pain and hyperaesthesia in the affected dermatome.

FUNGAL

Candida albicans

This is a common infection of the skin and mucous membranes. Oral candidosis tends to occur in immunosuppressed patients and diabetics, and after treatment with antibiotics. Candidosis is a major manifestation of AIDS. Look for candidosis in the mouth; the oral infection is characterised by white or off-white plaques that can be scraped off, leaving a raw red base. Other manifestations include angular stomatitis, vulval and vaginal infections and involvement of contact surfaces (e.g. the natal cleft, inner thighs, scrotum and inframammary fold – intertrigo).

Pityriasis versicolor (tinea versicolor)

This common condition of young adults is caused by *Malassezia furfur* and presents as small pigmented or hypopigmented macules on the upper trunk and arms. The macules tend to coalesce, resulting in lesions that vary in size and shape. Scales can be demonstrated by scraping or teasing the lesions with a scalpel blade. In sunburnt areas, the lesions appear to be hypopigmented in comparison to the surrounding skin.

Dermatophytes (tinea)

The dermatophytes inhabit the stratum corneum and the dead keratin of the nails and hair. Hair infection (tinea capitis) presents with localised patches of hair loss and skin inflammation. Skin infection (tinea corporis) affects the unhairy parts of the body. This presentation is often referred to as 'ringworm', because the lesion has an inflamed annular edge with a paler central area of healing (Fig. 3.55). Athlete's foot (tinea pedis) appears as a scaling erythematous rash between the toes. A nail infection (tinea unguium) is often asymmetrical and affects the toenails more often than the fingernails. The nail becomes yellow and thick; there is onycholysis and, at a later stage, the nail crumbles and breaks. If suspected, take nail clippings for mycology.

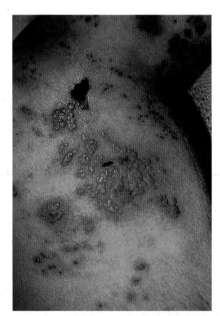

Fig. 3.54 Herpes zoster: note the haemorrhagic lesions (distribution of L2).

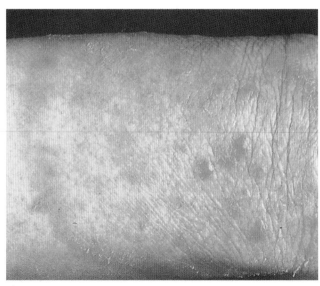

Fig. 3.55 Ringworm rash with inflamed periphery.

INFESTATIONS

Pediculosis

Infestation with lice causes skin irritation. Head lice infestation (pediculosis capitis) is common in children. The diagnosis is made by careful inspection of the hair for eggs (nits) which, unlike dandruff, cannot be shaken off the hair. Scratching may give rise to secondary inflammation and itching. Body lice infestation (pediculosis corporis) is rare and almost always occurs in malnutrition and when hygiene is poor. Infection of the pubic hair (pediculosis pubis) is caused by the crab louse and is usually sexually transmitted. Like other lice infections, the infestation causes intense pruritus and the nits (and lice) are seen with the naked eye.

Scabies

Consider scabies in any patient presenting with widespread pruritus. The mite (*Sarcoptes scabei*) burrows into the skin, where the female lays her eggs. The burrows can be seen on inspection; look for these along the sides of the fingers, the webs (Fig. 3.56) and the wrist. The burrows are linear and just palpable and the white dot of the mite can often be seen. The lesions may develop into inflamed papules and may affect the elbows, axillae and genitalia. Scratching causes secondary excoriation and infection.

BLISTERING LESIONS

Bullous pemphigoid

This disorder occurs most commonly in elderly people. The lesions are itchy and appear as tense, mainly symmetrical blisters overlying and surrounded by an area of erythema (Fig. 3.57). The blisters are initially small but enlarge to a considerable size over a few days (Fig. 3.58). Although truncal involvement also occurs, the blisters appear mainly on the limbs, especially along the inner aspects of the thighs and arms. The blisters become haemorrhagic and then degenerate, causing erosions that are susceptible to secondary infection (Fig. 3.59). Healing occurs without scarring.

Pemphigus

This autoimmune disorder occurs most commonly in middle-aged Ashkenazi Jews. The onset is usually insidious and the earliest lesions often start in the mouth or genital mucous membrane; however, patients usually present to the doctor once the skin is involved. Pemphigus is characterised by painful, flaccid blisters that rupture to reveal a raw base that heals slowly (Figs 3.60, 3.61). The skin adjacent to the bullous lesion slides over the underlying dermis (Nikolsky's sign). The umbilicus, trunk, intertrigenous areas and scalp are most commonly affected. The clinical diagnosis is confirmed by typical immunofluorescent staining, which shows immunoglobulin G (IgG) and complement deposition in the epidermis.

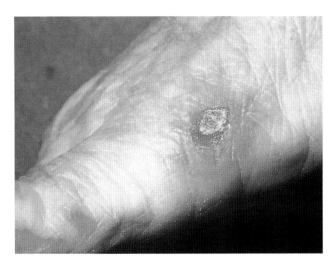

Fig. 3.57 Bullous pemphigoid with surrounding erythema.

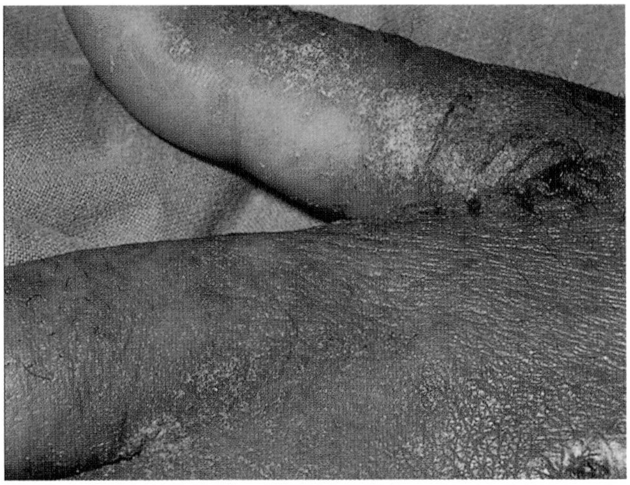

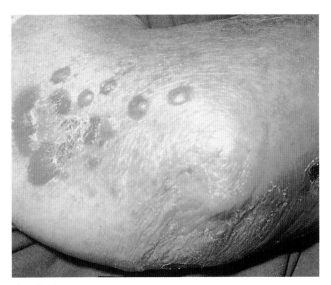

Fig. 3.56 Chronic scabies in the webs between fingers.

Fig. 3.58 Tense blisters of bullous pemphigoid.

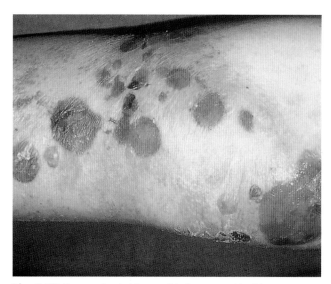

Fig. 3.59 Haemorrhagic blisters of bullous pemphigoid.

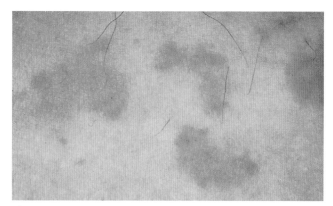

Fig. 3.62 The skin lesions of dermatitis herpetiformis.

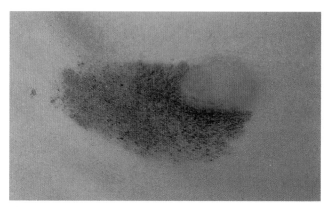

Fig. 3.63 Junctional naevus.

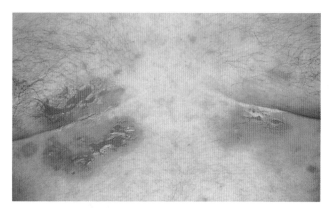

Fig. 3.60 Skin pemphigus.

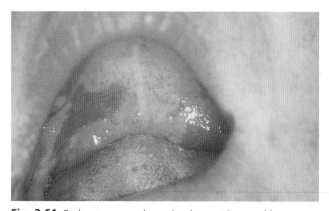

Fig. 3.61 Oral mucous membrane involvement in pemphigus.

Dermatitis herpetiformis

This disorder usually occurs in the third and fourth decades and is characterised by strikingly symmetrical groups of intensely itchy vesicles which most commonly erupt on the elbows, below the knees, buttocks, back and scalp (Fig. 3.62). Scratching causes local excoriation.

Healing leaves tell-tale areas of hyperpigmentation. The disorder is almost always associated with gluten-sensitive enteropathy (coeliac disease). Although almost all patients have villous atrophy, it is unusual for them to present with features of malabsorption.

Naevi

There are numerous skin blemishes collectively called naevi. Pigmented naevi cause the greatest concern because of the seriousness of malignant change. The junctional naevus is distinguished as a flat or slightly raised smooth lesion which has a uniform colour and varies in size up to about 1 cm (Fig. 3.63). A compound naevus is a raised, rounded, pigmented papular lesion from which hairs may project (Fig. 3.64). Dermal naevi are raised, flesh-coloured, dome-shaped lesions with a wrinkled surface, occurring most commonly on the face (Fig. 3.65).

Café-au-lait patches

These are flat, coffee-coloured patches (see Fig. 3.7), usually centimetres in size, which may occur as a benign blemish or a marker of neurofibromatosis (Von Recklinghausen's disease). The presence of five or more of these patches is a sure sign of the disorder. Neurofibromas appear as soft, sessile, pedunculated lesions or discrete subcutaneous nodules.

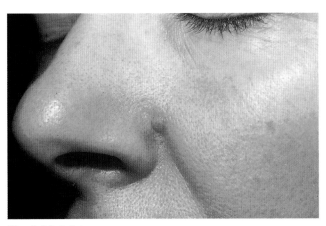

Fig. 3.64 Cellular naevus.

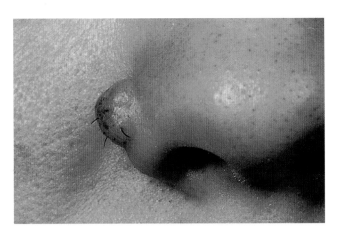

Fig. 3.65 Dermal naevus.

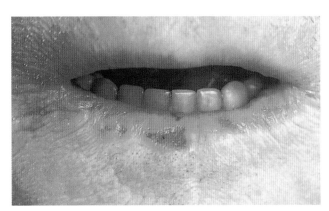

Fig. 3.66 Squamous cancer of the lip.

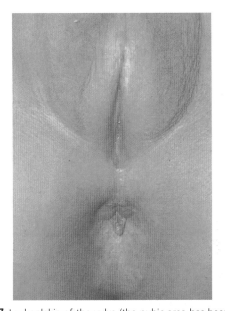

Fig. 3.67 Leukoplakia of the vulva (the pubic area has been shaved).

TUMOURS

Squamous cell carcinoma

There is usually a risk factor predisposing to this cancer. Consider excessive sun exposure, carcinomatous change in a chronic leg ulcer and areas of leukoplakia. The tumour presents as an ulcer or nodule with a firm indurated margin; the ulcer margin is often everted (Fig. 3.66). The cancer usually occurs in sun-exposed areas (face, back of the hands and forearm) or, in women, in an area of vulval leukoplakia (Fig. 3.67).

Basal cell carcinoma

This tumour most commonly affects the face and, like squamous carcinoma, sun exposure is an important predisposing factor. The 'rodent' ulcer starts as a small painless papule (Fig. 3.68) which ulcerates. The ulcer margin is well-defined and rolled at the edges. The tumour bleeds and scabs. Your index of suspicion must be aroused if any skin ulcer fails to heal.

Malignant melanoma

This is less common than squamous or basal cell carcinoma but is the most serious, because it spreads by the lymphatics and blood. Most lesions are not

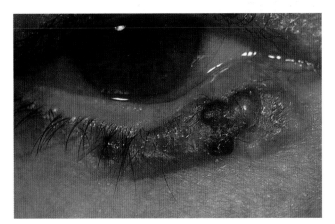

Fig. 3.68 Papular form of basal cell carcinoma.

associated with a pre-existing pigmented lesion but approximately one-third are associated with a junctional pigmented naevus. The tumour is usually pigmented and presents either as a nodule or a spreading area of pigmentation (Fig. 3.69). Consider the diagnosis if a

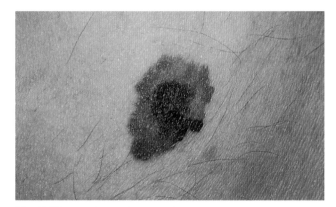

Fig. 3.69 Spreading malignant melanoma.

pigmented lesion is nodular, grows, darkens in colour, changes shape or bleeds. The back is a common site in men, whereas in women the legs are the most common site.

Red flag
Features suspicious of malignant melanoma

- Asymmetry with irregular border
- Irregular colorations
- Diameter usually > 0.5 cm
- Irregular elevation
- Loss of skin markings

Risk factors
Malignant melanoma

- New mole, change in pre-existing mole
- Prior melanoma or family history of melanoma
- Caucasian
- Oral psoralens and PUVA for psoriasis
- Immunosuppression
- Excessive sun exposure
- Red hair, blond hair, green or blue eyes

Kaposi's sarcoma

This tumour was once restricted to equatorial black Africans (Fig. 3.70) and elderly Ashkenazi Jews (Fig. 3.71). Immunosuppression is an important predisposing factor and the sarcoma occurs in transplant recipients on immunosuppressive drugs and is particularly associated with AIDS (Fig. 3.72). The Kaposi's lesion is characterised by red-blue nodules, especially affecting the lower legs but also involving the hands.

Skin manifestations of systemic disease

Many systemic disorders involve the skin and careful examination of the skin often helps in diagnosis.

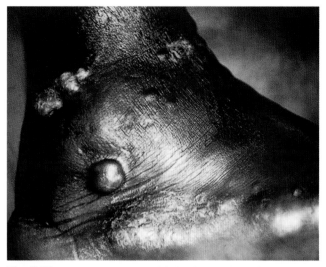

Fig. 3.70 Kaposi's sarcoma in a black African. The nodules are multiple and dark blue in colour.

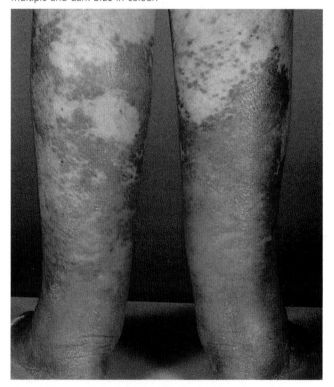

Fig. 3.71 Kaposi's sarcoma in an Ashkenazi Jew. The purple plaques particularly occur on the lower legs and feet.

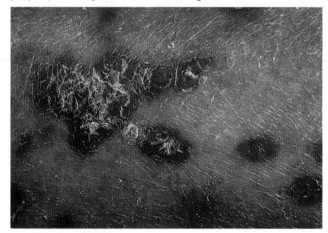

Fig. 3.72 Kaposi's sarcoma in an immunosuppressed AIDS patient.

Nail disorders

Examination of the nails can provide useful and often diagnostic physical signs. Patients often complain of cracking, ridging and brittleness of the nail. This may be caused by nail-biting, picking and poor nail care rather than disease. In addition, nails may have white spots which have no significance. First examine the nail face-on. Asymmetrical splinter-like lesions (splinter haemorrhages) may indicate microemboli from infected heart valves (subacute bacterial endocarditis) or vasculitis. Remember that manual labourers may have traumatic nail lesions that resemble splinter haemorrhages. Pitting of the nail occurs in psoriasis (Fig. 3.73) and may even occur in the absence of the typical skin rash. Premature lifting of the distal nail is called onycholysis (Fig. 3.74). This occurs in many chronic nail disorders and is also associated with hyperthyroidism (Plummer's nails). White nails with loss of the lunule (leukonychia) is typical of hypoalbuminaemia and severe chronic ill health (Fig. 3.75).

Acute severe illness may be associated with the later appearance of transverse depressions in the nail (Beau's lines) (Fig. 3.76) which grow out with normal nail growth on recovery. Infection of the skin adjacent to the nail is called paronychia and is characterised by pain, swelling, redness and tenderness of the skin at its interface with the nail (Fig. 3.77). Fungal infection of the nail causes opacification and distortion of the nail. Spooning of the nail (koilonychia) occurs in iron deficiency (Figs 3.78, 3.79).

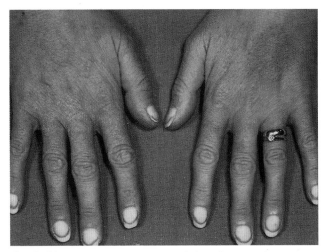

Fig. 3.75 Leukonychia in a patient with liver disease and hypoalbuminaemia.

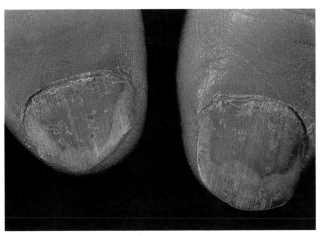

Fig. 3.73 Pitting and onycholysis of the nail caused by psoriasis.

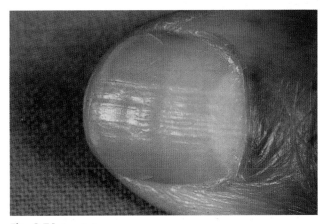

Fig. 3.76 Beau's lines.

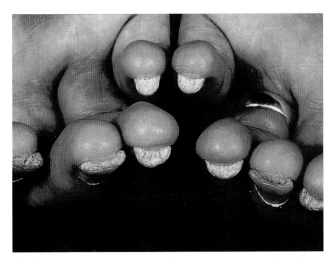

Fig. 3.74 Onycholysis caused by hyperkeratotic psoriasis beneath the nail.

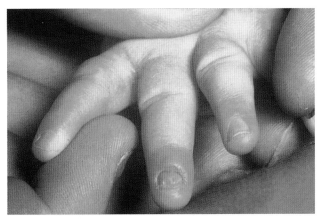

Fig. 3.77 Bacterial paronychia.

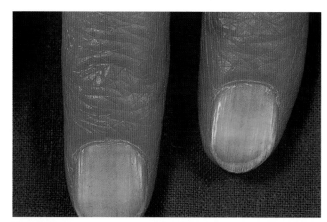

Fig. 3.78 Koilonychia with spooning of the nail in a patient with chronic iron deficiency anaemia.

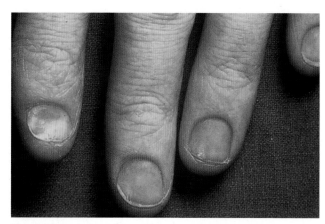

Fig. 3.79 Spooning of the nails.

Clubbing

floating nail base

increased angle (180°)

early clubbing

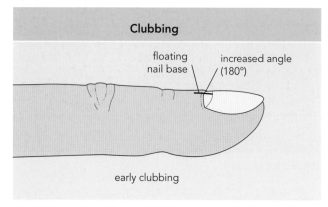

Fig. 3.80 Clubbing. The angle is increased and filled in and the nail base has a spongy consistency.

Always examine the lateral outline of the nails and fingertip to check for clubbing. The normal angle between the fingernail and nail base is 160° (Fig. 3.80) and the base is firm to palpation. Clubbing occurs when abnormal connective tissue and capillaries fill this angle. In early clubbing, the angle increases and if you press the nail base the nail appears to 'float'. In severe clubbing, such as occurs with lung cancer, the fingers may have a drumstick appearance and may be associated with wrist pain and tenderness due to periostitis (hypertrophic pulmonary osteoarthropathy).

Differential diagnosis

Finger clubbing

Lung disease
- Pyogenic (abscess, bronchiectasis, empyema)
- Bronchogenic carcinoma
- Fibrosing alveolitis

Heart disease
- Cyanotic congenital heart disease
- Subacute bacterial endocarditis

Gastrointestinal
- Cirrhosis
- Ulcerative colitis
- Crohn's disease

Idiopathic/congenital

Symptoms and signs

Skin manifestations of systemic disease

Disease	Skin findings
Sarcoidosis	Erythema nodosum, lupus pernio, nodules in scars
Systemic lupus erythematosus	Facial 'butterfly' rash (malar erythema over cheeks and bridging nose); occurs in 50% of patients on exposure to UV rays. Also alopecia areata and discoid lupus
Scleroderma	Thickened tight skin (especially fingers), skin telangiectasia, calcified skin nodules
Hyperlipidaemia	Xanthelasmata of eyelids, xanthomas of elbows, knuckles, buttock, soles and palms, and Achilles tendon
Diabetes mellitus	Necrobiosis lipoidica – symmetrical plaques on shins with atrophic, yellow appearance and waxy feel; cutaneous candida, ulcers on feet
Hyperthyroidism	Pretibial myxoedema – thickened skin on front of skin, clubbing
Cushing's syndrome	Purple striae, thin skin, easy bruising
Ulcerative colitis/Crohn's disease	Pyoderma gangrenosum – large ulcer
Dermatomyositis	Oedema and mauve discoloration of eyelid, erythema of the knuckles and other bony parts such as elbow and shoulder tip; photosensitive 'butterfly rash' on face
Cancer	Acanthosis nigricans – brown, velvet-like thickening of skin in axilla and groin; tylosis – thickening of palms/soles; ichthyosis – fish-skin appearance

Examination of elderly people

Skin changes in elderly people

- Skin becomes increasingly wrinkled with loss of elastic tissue and collagen
- Skin becomes fragile and even minor trauma can cause wounding and secondary infection
- Loss of spring makes it more difficult to use tissue turgor as a sign for assessing hydration
- Capillary fragility results in easy intradermal bleeding (senile purpura and ecchymosis)
- Warty pigmented lesions (senile keratosis) may become widespread and disfigure skin
- Sunburnt area increasingly predisposed to malignant change in the elderly (squamous and basal cell carcinomas)
- Pressure sores (decubitus ulcers) are a particularly serious complication of immobility; predisposing factors include capillary occlusion, friction and secondary infection
- Pressure sores most commonly develop over bony prominences, especially the heels and sacrum

Review

Skin examination

- Always expose the patient to allow examination of the whole skin organ
- Ensure good illumination (preferably natural light)
- Measure dimensions of skin lesions (especially helpful when assessing progression and regression)
- Attempt to transilluminate larger swellings (fluid-filled)
- Assess skin colour and variations
- Describe the primary morphology of a localised skin lesion
  - macule
  - patch
  - papule
  - plaque
  - wheal
  - vesicle
  - nodule
  - petechiae or ecchymosis
  - bulla
  - telangiectasia, spider naevus
- Describe the secondary characteristics
  - superficial erosion
  - ulceration
  - crusting
  - scaling
  - fissuring
  - lichenification
  - atrophy
  - excoriation
  - scarring or keloid
- Describe the distribution of a more widespread rash or colour change
- Assess the temperature of the affected area
- Perform a general examination, looking for evidence of systemic disease

4

Ear, nose and throat

Structure of the ear

A diagrammatic cross-section of the external, middle and inner parts of the ear is shown in Figure 4.1.

THE EXTERNAL EAR

The externally visible part of the external ear is the pinna (Fig. 4.2). This is a structure covered by skin with an internal structure of cartilage (which is absent in the lowest part, the tragus).

As well as the pinna, the external ear includes the external canal and peripheral surface of the tympanic membrane. The skin of the external canal contains normal epithelium with hair follicles and apocrine glands. It is the combination of desquamated skin and the ceruminous secretions of the apocrine glands that form wax. Wax is protective to the ear but over-accumulation or impaction reduces the conductive element of hearing. The external canal is straight in children (making the tympanic membrane easier to see) but in adulthood the canal passes through an angle of descent distal to the observer. The angle formed by the tympanic membrane and the external canal makes an acute-angled recess (the anterior recess) which can be difficult to visualise, and wax, discharge or a foreign body may be difficult to locate and remove. This difficulty may be compounded by the isthmus if it is narrow. The isthmus is the junction between the outer cartilaginous two-thirds of the external canal and the bony inner one-third.

The tympanic membrane (Fig. 4.3) is a translucent membrane visible at the inner extremity of the external canal. In its normal state the membrane appears grey and shiny and through it the handle of the malleus is visible with its inferior pole (the umbo) pointing posteriorly. The umbo can be seen fairly close to the centre of the tympanic membrane. Inferior to the umbo, an arc of light (the light reflex) reflects back to the observer. This arc is directed antero-inferiorly.

THE MIDDLE EAR

This extends from the inner surface of the tympanic membrane to the temporal bone and includes the air filled cavities containing the three ossicles (from proximal to distal to the observer these are the malleus, incus and stapes; see Fig. 4.4), the Eustachian tube and the mastoid air cells. The function of the middle ear is to magnify sound-waves sensed by the tympanic membrane and forms an important part of conductive hearing. This magnification of sound is done by the three ossicles, the last of which is the stapes whose foot-plate fits in the oval window which is connected to the cochlea of the inner ear. The function of the Eustachian tube is to aerate the middle ear so that the pressure in the middle ear is equal to the outside pressure (in the external canal) and thus allow the tympanic membrane to vibrate freely.

There are two important nerves that pass through the medial wall of the middle ear. These are the facial nerve and its off-shoot, the chorda tympani (concerned with taste from the tongue on the same side and with submandibular and sublingual salivary glands). The facial nerve passes in the bone above and behind the stapes footplate, whereas the chorda tympani emerges through the posterior wall of the middle ear and passes between the malleus and incus.

THE INNER EAR

The inner ear is that part of the auditory mechanism within the petrous temporal bone. The inner ear is called the labyrinth and is comprised of the cochlea, vestibule and semi-circular canals. The cochlea is the organ of hearing and the semicircular canals are the organ of balance. The sensorineural part of hearing is located here in the inner ear, whereas conductive hearing is managed by the external and middle parts of the ear. The *sensori-*

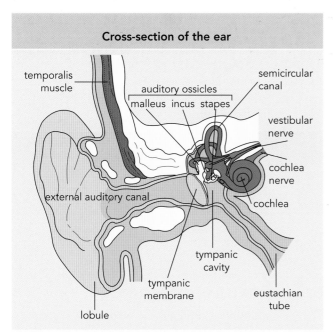

Fig. 4.1 Cross-section of the whole structure of the ear.

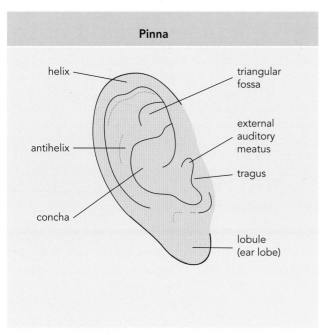

Fig. 4.2 The pinna.

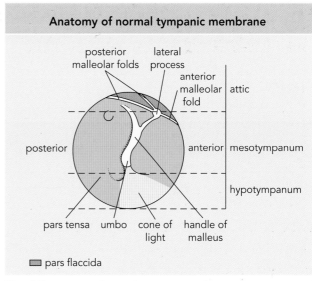

Fig. 4.3 Anatomy of normal tympanic membrane.

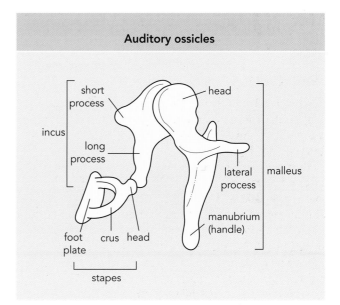

Fig. 4.4 The auditory ossicles.

part of hearing occurs within the cochlea, whereas the *neuro-* part occurs within the eighth (VIII) nerve and beyond.

The cochlea records the transmission of sound via hair cells which convert the signal received into electrical impulses. These are transmitted by the auditory (VIII) nerve to the cerebral cortex.

The semicircular canals or balance organ form the peripheral balance organ. There are three canals: the superior, lateral and posterior. The organ is neurologically connected to the eyes and cerebellum. The eyes, proprioception and cerebellum, together with the cerebral cortex, form the central balance control.

Symptoms of diseases of the ear

VISIBLE SYMPTOMS

Patients may present with symptoms of visible external abnormalities. The conditions that may be seen usually present because of concern about the cosmetic appearance of the ear.

Differential diagnosis

Cosmetic presentations

- Bat ears
- Preauricular sinus
- Accessory auricles
- Anotia and microtia
- Cauliflower ear (untreated haematoma)
- Chondrodermatitis nodularis helicis
- Basal cell carcinoma
- Squamous cell carcinoma

Questions to ask

Otalgia

- Where is the pain and does it radiate?
- How long has the pain been present?
- Is the pain constant or intermittent?
- Does anything provoke or relieve it?
- Is there any swelling, discharge, deafness or vertigo?
- Has anything been put in the ear?
- Is there a past history of ear problems?
- Is there a problem in other areas – teeth, pharynx, cervical spine?

PAIN IN THE EAR (OTALGIA)

Pain in the ear may arise from the ear itself (usually unilateral) but may arise from other sources. The cause can usually be determined on history and clinical examination. The possible causes of otalgia are summarised in the differential diagnosis box.

Differential diagnosis

Otalgia

Pinna	Perichondritis, cellulits
	Neoplasm (basal cell or squamous cell)
External canal	Furuncle, furunculosis
	Otitis externa
	Impacted wax
	Foreign body
	Herpes zoster (Ramsay Hunt syndrome)
	Neoplasm
Middle ear	Acute otitis media and its rare sequelae (mastoiditis, meningitis and cerebral abscess)
	Secretory otitis media (glue ear)
	Eustachian tube obstruction
	Barotraumas
	Neoplasm
Other sites	Teeth, tongue, pharynx (including tonsils and hypopharynx), sinuses, temporomandibular joint, cervical spine

To fully assess causes of otalgia it is necessary to exclude causes of referred pain. The clinician should directly question whether the patient has any problem with other structures such as teeth, the pharynx or cervical spine.

To assess aural causes of the symptom of otalgia, ask about any associated swelling, discharge, deafness, giddiness or vertigo. Any history of excessive contact with water such as by swimming, bathing or showering is relevant and it is wise to check that the patient has not been putting anything into the external canal (cottonwool buds, pins).

DISCHARGING EAR (OTORRHOEA)

The ear naturally discharges wax which is a mixture of skin debris and apocrine gland secretion.

Pathological discharge from the ear varies in nature from watery to foul-smelling or blood-stained. A green-coloured discharge often indicates pseudomonas infection, whereas a blackened discharge may indicate fungal infection.

With foul-smelling discharge, or with the presence of pseudomonas infection, middle ear disease (and therefore a perforated tympanic membrane) should be suspected. In the rare instance of a cerebrospinal fluid (CSF) leak, due to trauma or surgery, the discharge will be watery. A mucoid discharge is suggestive of middle ear disease. Purulent discharge is commonly from infection of the external canal.

A most common cause of a bloodstained discharge is infection, but the rare instance of a squamous cell carcinoma may present with this.

Discharge is often associated with otalgia and the timing of the two symptoms will often indicate the origin. Otalgia from middle ear disease is usually relieved when the tympanic membrane ruptures and discharges mucopus, whereas continuing pain associated with discharge usually indicates external ear inflammation.

Questions to ask

Otorrhoea

- How long has it been present?
- What is its relationship to pain?
- Has it occurred previously?
- What is its colour and consistency?
- Is it blood-stained?
- Is it offensive?

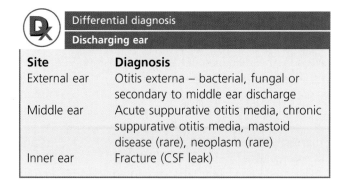

Differential diagnosis
Discharging ear

Site	Diagnosis
External ear	Otitis externa – bacterial, fungal or secondary to middle ear discharge
Middle ear	Acute suppurative otitis media, chronic suppurative otitis media, mastoid disease (rare), neoplasm (rare)
Inner ear	Fracture (CSF leak)

conduction and magnification of sound to the cochlea. For sound to be conducted, the external canal must be patent. It may be impeded by malformation, wax or discharge. The tympanic membrane should be intact and the middle ear aerated and free of discharge or adhesions. The ossicular chain in the middle ear must be intact and move freely. Testing of the integrity of middle ear function is explained in the section on examination of the ear (pages 90–92).

HEARING LOSS (DEAFNESS)

Hearing loss is recognised as being either conductive or sensorineural. It varies in degree from minor to profound and affects all age groups. Poor hearing is significant in infants because of the association with slow or abnormal development of speech. Assessment of hearing in infants and young children is difficult (see p. 92). The clinician should take careful note of parents' concerns. Hearing loss of old age is called presbyacusis. There are many causes of hearing loss.

Conductive deafness

Conductive deafness is the term used to indicate that hearing is being impaired by a malfunction in the

Sensorineural deafness

The sensory part of the ear is the cochlea, but for full function the neural element is required. This comprises the auditory nerve and cerebral cortex. To distinguish between the sensory and neural element can be difficult.

Hearing loss in the elderly (presbyacusis) is mainly due to degeneration of the cochlea. The cochlea may be damaged during life in other ways. This may be by infection, vascular ischaemia, noise, drugs, surgery, or Ménière's disease.

The red flag symptom to alert the clinician is unilateral deafness as this may indicate an acoustic neuroma. Early treatment of this space-occupying lesion lessens morbidity and mortality.

Differential diagnosis
Hearing loss

Age group	Causes	Type of loss
Infants	Congenital	Conductive or sensorineural
	Secretory otitis media (glue ear)	Conductive
Young children	Congenital	Conductive or sensorineural
	Secretory otitis media (glue ear)	Conductive
	Postinfective (meningitis, viral)	Sensorineural
Adolescents	Congenital	Conductive or sensorineural
	Malingering	—
	Postinfective (meningitis, viral)	Sensorineural
	Acoustic trauma or drugs	Sensorineural
20–40 years	Postinfective (meningitis, viral)	Sensorineural
	Acoustic trauma or drugs	Sensorineural
	Otosclerosis	Conductive
	Acoustic neuroma	Sensorineural
	Ménière's disease	Sensorineural
	Postoperative complications	Conductive or sensorineural
40–60 years	Acoustic trauma or drugs	Sensorineural
	Otosclerosis	Conductive
	Acoustic neuroma	Sensorineural
	Ménière's disease	Sensorineural
	Postoperative complications	Conductive or sensorineural
60+ years	Presbyacusis	Sensorineural
	Acoustic trauma or drugs	Sensorineural
	Acoustic neuroma	Sensorineural
	Postoperative complications	Conductive or sensorineural

TINNITUS

Tinnitus is the symptom of noise in the ears. It is difficult to investigate because it is a subjective symptom. It may be heard as a continuous, pulsatile or episodic sound. The sound may be difficult for the patient to describe but is often noted as whistling, buzzing or crackling. The sounds experienced are not complex auditory hallucinations as found in certain psychoses.

The most common cause of tinnitus is the onset of sensorineural deafness associated with degeneration of the cochlea. However, anything which interferes with the hearing mechanism (even wax) may produce tinnitus. All the possible causes of hearing loss should be considered when tinnitus is present. It is one of the triad of symptoms that are observed in Ménière's disease, the others being vertigo and loss of hearing. Tinnitus may arise from the Eustachian tube, which is also the site of the rare condition of palatal myoclonus.

In present day usage it is unusual to see tinnitus caused by drugs, but it may be seen in the treatment of rheumatic fever by high dose aspirin and is a recognised side-effect of aminoglycosides. High doses of nonsteroidal anti-inflammatory drugs may also induce tinnitus. This form of drug-induced tinnitus is usually reversible on stopping the medication.

A red flag sign is when the tinnitus is unilateral. As with unilateral deafness, an acoustic neuroma must be considered and investigated.

VERTIGO (DIZZINESS)

Vertigo is a symptom of imagined spinning or unsteadiness. The patient feels they or their surroundings are moving. This is true vertigo and is caused by inner ear, vestibular, dysfunction. Vertigo arising from the vestibular mechanism is known as peripheral vertigo.

Acute labyrinthine dysfunction

Acute labyrinthine dysfunction is the term used for severe episodic vertigo of sudden onset. Its cause includes diagnoses such as viral, idiopathic or vascular labyrinthitis. The disorder may last for days and may be prolonged in benign positional vertigo.

Benign positional vertigo

Benign positional vertigo is recognised by the short-lasting onset of vertigo with movement of the head. It may be one of the sequelae of acute labyrinthine dysfunction. Other causes are trauma or idiopathic.

Central causes of vertigo

Other manifestations of giddiness arise from different sites. The vestibular (inner ear) cause of vertigo is known as peripheral vertigo and that arising from other sites is termed central vertigo. Inputs from the eyes, proprioception, cerebellum, brainstem, cerebrum and reticular formation all have a function in balance. The loss of balance in central vertigo is not of the rotational type but is manifest by a feeling of unsteadiness and is not usually associated with nausea or vomiting. One possible cause of this is a hypotensive state, perhaps caused by drugs in the management of hypertension. Vertigo of vestibular (peripheral) origin is almost always accompanied by nausea and/or vomiting, whereas this is less common in central vertigo. Another distinguishing feature is that peripheral vertigo is usually intermittent and is not progressive. Giddiness of central origin is often constant and progressive.

The red flag sign in vertigo, requiring urgent investigation or referral, is the possibility of a transient ischaemic attack (TIA) or vertebrobasilar ischaemia. The other associated signs suggesting these conditions as a possible cause are raised blood pressure, dysarthria, visual disturbance, neck problems and loss of coordination.

Questions to ask
Vertigo

- How would you describe the giddiness?
- How long has it been present?
- Is it intermittent?
- How long does it last?
- What precipitates it (e.g. change of posture or head movement)?
- Are you on any medication (ototoxic or lowering blood pressure)?
- Do you have any nausea or vomiting?
- Have you ever had ear problems or surgery?
- Do you have any deafness or tinnitus?

Differential diagnosis
Central and peripheral vertigo

Diagnosis	Site
Acute labyrinthine dysfunction	Peripheral
Benign positional vertigo	Peripheral
Ménière's disease	Peripheral
Multiple sclerosis	Central
Transient ischaemic attack (TIA)	Central
Vertebrobasilar ischaemia	Central
Head injury	Central or peripheral

Examination of the ear

THE AUROSCOPE

Use the largest aural speculum that fits in the external canal comfortably. Hold the auroscope at its point of balance (centre of gravity). Balance it lightly in the hand. Do not grab it like a screwdriver! Use the same hand as the ear (left hand for left ear) (see Fig. 4.5). When inserting

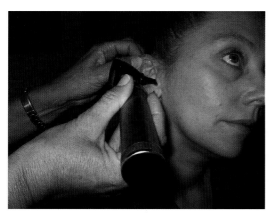

Fig. 4.5 How to hold the auroscope.

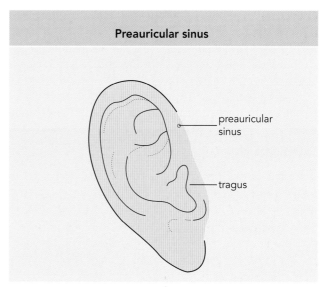

Fig. 4.6 Site of preauricular sinus.

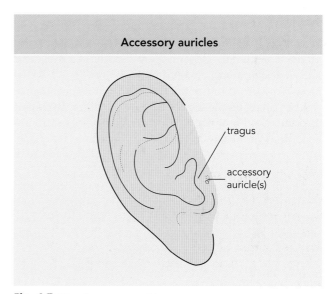

Fig. 4.7 Site of accessory auricles.

the auroscope retract the pinna posteriorly with the free hand (right hand for left ear). This opens the canal for easier inspection. Always examine the pinna before examining the external canal.

Do not rush to insert the auroscope and, when inserting it, look at the canal throughout its whole length. Observe for any anatomical abnormality and note the external appearance of any discharge or eczema. The appearance of discharge, if mucoid, may indicate middle ear disease rather than otitis externa, whereas evidence of eczematous skin in the pinna (or psoriasis) may indicate that otitis externa will be found in the canal.

Look also for scars of mastoid surgery (pre- or post-auricular) because passing the auroscope too hastily into the ear may result in a large posterior mastoid cavity being overlooked.

EXTERNAL EAR

Pinna

Minor congenital abnormalities Bat ears is the term given to ears which do not lie flat against the head but protrude outwards. They occur in about 2% of the population and if to be surgically corrected this is best left until after six years of age.

Pre-auricular sinus is a defect in embryological development and usually occurs antero-superiorly to the tragus (Fig. 4.6).

Accessory auricles occur anterior to the tragus (Fig. 4.7) and are another embryonic fault.

Gross congenital deformities are rare and include anotia (complete absence of the pinna). The conditions can occur with normal or abnormal development of the middle and inner ear.

Skin changes Eczema or psoriasis are common conditions which may involve the pinna and external canal. Like any skin condition, secondary infection is a possible complication and is more likely to occur in the external ear because of the accumulation of debris.

Infection/inflammation can be severe with pain, redness and swelling. The infection may be an extension of infection from the external canal but even if localised

to the pinna should be treated with systemic antibiotics. Infections of the pinna include cellulitis and perichondritis, where the underlying cartilage is infected.

Cauliflower ears are the result of previous untreated traumatic haematoma of the pinna. Early surgical treatment of the initial haematoma may prevent lasting deformity.

Chondrodermatitis nodularis helicis is a benign nodular condition usually of the helix of the ear. The aetiology is unknown but, as it occurs in later life, may be related to sun damage. It can only be differentiated from malignant conditions by biopsy.

Basal cell carcinomata and squamous cell carcinomata are tumours most commonly seen on the pinna and require appropriate surgical treatment.

Chondromata arise from cartilage, which forms the outer one-third of the canal. They may vary in size from being quite small to obstructing the whole canal.

They rarely need attention but may make it difficult to remove wax and observe the inner part of the canal and the tympanic membrane. To the inexperienced eye chondromata may appear alarming and arouse concern about malignancy. They are swellings that are covered by normal epithelium and vary greatly in size from minor swellings to those obstructing most of the external canal.

External canal

The diameter of the canal is very variable and even in some adults may be very narrow. In a child the canal is straight and the tympanic membrane is easily seen. In adults the distal part of the canal, close to the tympanic membrane, narrows (the isthmus) in its final third and deflects downwards. This results in a recess inferiorly with an acute angle being formed between canal and tympanic membrane. It is thus more difficult to see the whole tympanic membrane and debris or foreign bodies are more easily concealed from the clinician in the recess (see Fig. 4.1).

Wax Wax is the natural accumulation of skin debris and secreted oil from the apocrine glands of the external canal and unless causing symptoms does not need to be removed. Before full examination of the external canal can be complete, the ear should be cleaned of wax. Wax, impacted or otherwise, is one of the commonest conditions of the ear dealt with by the general physician. It may present with a difficulty in hearing or even with pain.

The production and accumulation of wax (rather than its natural expulsion) is dependent on occupational and genetic factors (gene on chromosome 16). The removal of impacted wax gives the greatest relief (in both hearing and discomfort) to an afflicted patient.

The most common method used to clear wax is by syringing or the now more acceptable irrigation (by an electrical pulsed pump). There are contraindications to syringing.

Review

Contraindications to syringing

- Previous ear surgery – mastoid, tympanoplasty, stapedectomy
- Previous otitis externa
- Perforation
- Tinnitus
- Labyrinthine disturbance

Water in the ears is a common trigger for otitis externa and it is important that the ears are fully cleaned if possible so that no water is trapped behind any remaining wax. The ears should be carefully dried after syringing and it is useful to have an operator trained in the use of

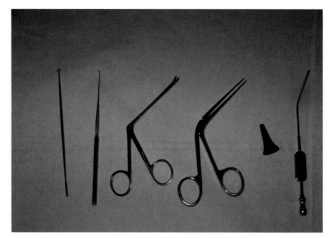

Fig. 4.8 Instruments useful in the removal of wax. From left to right: Jobson Horne probe, wax hook, crocodile forceps, aural forceps, aural speculum, aural sucker.

a Jobson Horne probe (tipped with cotton wool) to dry the outer part of the external canal. In addition to the Jobson Horne probe, useful instruments for removing wax include a wax hook, crocodile forceps and aural forceps (Fig. 4.8).

Water used to irrigate wax should be at 37°C (hand temperature). Variation in this temperature may stimulate the labyrinth, causing temporary giddiness.

The ENT specialist will have access to microsuction, which is light suction applied by an aural cannula under operating-microscope vision.

Whatever method is used to clean the external canal, this must be done before any external canal or middle ear disease can be diagnosed.

Otitis externa

Otitis externa is an infection of the external canal. Infections include furuncle or generalised furunculosis and otitis externa, bacterial or fungal. Otitis externa causes discharge, irritation and often pain. The colour of the discharge is discussed in the section on symptoms (see p. 83) but when observing the discharge the possible presence of the spores of a fungal growth should be noted.

Furunculosis

A single furuncle or generalised furunculosis of the external canal is usually painful and may be extremely so. Furuncles can be recognised as a small boil in the external canal. The lesion may be quite distal and it may be easily missed if the auroscope is inserted too deeply without observing the whole length of the canal. Furunculosis is recognised by the appearance of multiple boils or abscesses in the canal and is associated with severe pain and swelling of the external canal which may be completely occluded.

Myringitis bullosa

This is a manifestation of viral otitis externa where blisters are to be seen on the epithelial surface of the tympanic membrane.

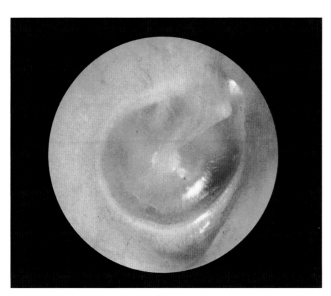

Fig. 4.9 Normal tympanic membrane.

THE MIDDLE EAR

Tympanic membrane

The whole circumference of the membrane should be visualised. In its normal state the membrane appears grey and shiny and through it the handle of the malleus is visible with its inferior pole (the umbo) pointing posteriorly. Inferior to the umbo, an arc of light reflects back to the observer. This arc is directed antero-inferiorly (Fig. 4.9).

Any vascular infiltration should be noted and this may occur either along the handle of the malleus or involve the tympanic membrane as a whole.

Superior to the handle of the malleus is the pars flaccida. This is the part of the tympanic membrane that is mobile and will move either by instigating a Valsalva manoeuvre or by using an auroscope with pneumatic attachment. Demonstration of the mobility of the pars flaccida will assure the clinician of aeration of the middle ear and therefore of patency of the Eustachian tube. The main area of the tympanic membrane is called the pars tensa and comprises the largest part of the membrane. It is in this part that a perforation may be noted. Here also chalk patches (tympanosclerosis) may be seen.

Acute otitis media

This is the most common middle ear infection and is particularly common in childhood. The presenting symptoms are fever and otalgia. In infancy, otalgia is recognised by the child being restless and crying. The onset is rapid and is usually associated with an upper respiratory tract virus infection.

On clinical examination of the ear, the tympanic membrane is inflamed and the epithelium of the membrane is often distorted ('pavement' epithelium) or bulging. The condition normally resolves with or without treatment.

Suppurative acute otitis media

Suppurative otitis media is one of the possible sequelae of acute otitis media. With this the tympanic membrane ruptures and releases the mucopus formed by the acute otitis media infection. Again this condition usually resolves spontaneously because of the release of the mucopus.

Chronic suppurative otitis media

This can be defined as a continuing discharging tympanic membrane perforation. The tympanic perforation of acute suppurative otitis media may remain, together with the discharge and become chronic. Referral to an ENT specialist is then indicated so that the possible extension of the infection into the mastoid and beyond (meninges and brain) can be assessed.

Acute mastoiditis, meningitis and cerebral abscess

Though rare, these are all possible sequelae of acute otitis media and should be considered when there is continuing fever, otorrhoea, otalgia and any suspicion of cerebral signs present. Acute mastoiditis may be detected by examination of the mastoid bone for swelling, redness or tenderness.

It should be noted that these conditions may progress very rapidly from an attack of acute otitis media.

Eustachian tube dysfunction

This may present with otalgia, reduced or distorted hearing, or with tinnitus. As the condition advances, vascular infiltration of the tympanic membrane along the handle of the malleus develops and the malleus becomes more prominent as the increasing negative pressure in the middle ear causes retraction of the tympanic membrane.

As a result of the negative pressure in the middle ear, and blockage of the Eustachian tube, the mobility of the pars flaccida is lost. This can be demonstrated by asking the patient to perform the Valsalva manoeuvre and observing for movement (or lack of) in the pars flaccida. This can be replicated by use of the puffer with a pneumatic auroscope. Graphical demonstration of Eustachian tube dysfunction can be obtained using tympanometry.

Tympanometry Tympanometry (Figs 4.10, 4.11) provides a good method for detecting middle ear effusion. A flat trace on the tympanogram indicates an immobile tympanic membrane suggestive of middle ear effusion.

Secretory otitis media (glue ear)

This is a condition of mucoid secretions in the middle ear which results primarily in reduction in hearing. It occurs as a result of poor aeration of the middle ear caused by Eustachian tube dysfunction. It is mainly a disease of children in whom adenoidal obstruction of the Eustachian tube is a prominent feature. However it can occur in adults whose nasal airway is compromised.

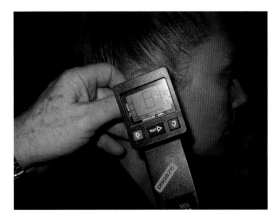

Fig. 4.10 Tympanometer in use.

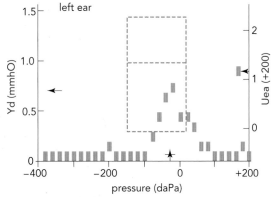

Fig. 4.11 Normal tympanogram showing tympanic membrane response to pressure.

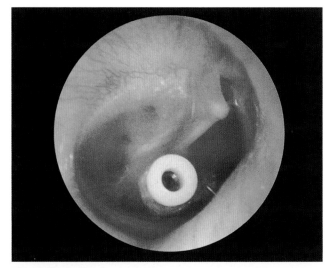

Fig. 4.12 Ventilation tube (grommet) in situ.

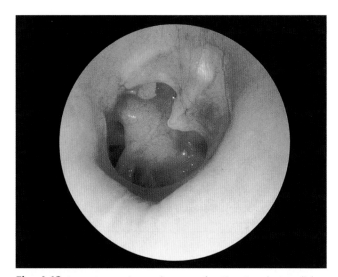

Fig. 4.13 Large tympanic membrane perforation. Incudostapedial joint just visible posterosuperiorly; round window visible posteriorly.

Clinical diagnosis is made in several ways. Bubbles of mucous may be seen on examination of the tympanic membrane. Otherwise all the clinical aspects of Eustachian tube dysfunction may be elicited (see above).

The importance of this condition is for children in whom speech, language or educational development may be delayed due to reduction in hearing. If there is evidence of such delay in development, or if there is a persistent (longer than three months) reduction of hearing, referral to an ENT specialist is advisable for consideration of grommet insertion (Fig. 4.12) and adenoidectomy.

Dry perforation

This may occur due to trauma or as a result of a previous middle ear infection and may be of varying size from very small to involving the vast majority of the tympanic membrane and exposing structures in the middle ear (Fig. 4.13).

THE INNER EAR

Information about inner ear disease is mainly obtained from the history of the condition that the patient gives, whether it is deafness, tinnitus or giddiness. The inner ear cannot be examined directly and information on its function is obtained by various methods and tests.

Deafness

Tuning fork tests Tuning forks are the first and an important tool to investigate deafness (Fig. 4.14). A tuning fork with a frequency of 256 Hz (C$_{256}$, middle C on the piano) can be used to undertake the Rinne and Weber tests (see below) with which it should be relatively easy for the clinician to differentiate conductive from sensorineural deafness.

It is also most helpful to have a high-tone tuning fork of about 4096 Hz. In deafness of old age (presbyacusis) it is the high tones that the patient first loses the ability to hear. Holding a sounding tuning fork of 4096 Hz a few centimetres away from the entrance of the external ear will ascertain whether there is a degree of high-tone hearing loss.

- *Weber test*. This test is performed by placing a tuning fork (C$_{256}$) on the midline of the skull, usually on the

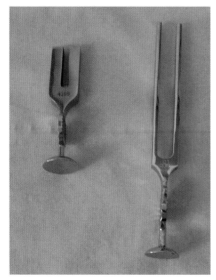

Fig. 4.14 Tuning forks: left, 4096 Hz; right, 256 Hz.

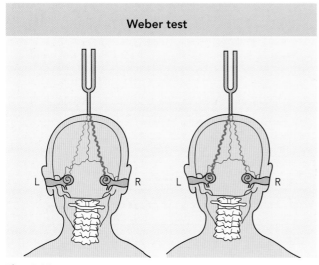

Fig. 4.15 Weber test.

forehead (Fig. 4.15). With normal hearing the sound of the tuning fork is heard centrally (equally in both ears). If it is referred to one side, that side either has a conductive deafness or has a better sensorineural hearing than the other side.

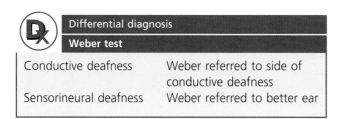

Differential diagnosis	
Weber test	
Conductive deafness	Weber referred to side of conductive deafness
Sensorineural deafness	Weber referred to better ear

- *Rinne test*. This test clarifies whether or not there is conductive deafness (Fig. 4.16). It tests the efficiency of the ossicular chain. In a normal ear the Rinne test will be positive. A tuning fork (C$_{256}$) is first placed on the

mastoid bone. It will be heard less well than if the tuning fork is placed close to the external canal. If it is heard louder on the mastoid bone, the test is negative and indicates that the ossicular chain is not magnifying the sound for some reason.

A false negative Rinne test may occur if the ear has a profound sensorineural deafness. With an ear conducting normally the test should be positive, but the bone conduction (the tuning fork placed on the mastoid bone) sound may be picked up by the opposite ear and therefore thought by the patient to be louder than air conduction; whereas such profound deafness in the tested ear negates the test for conduction (false negative Rinne). This finding will be supported by the fact that the Weber test will be referred to the other (less deaf) ear.

As already explained, in conductive deafness there is an interruption of sound, and/or sound magnification, in the external or middle ear. Sensorineural deafness indicates a problem with the cochlea or auditory nervous system.

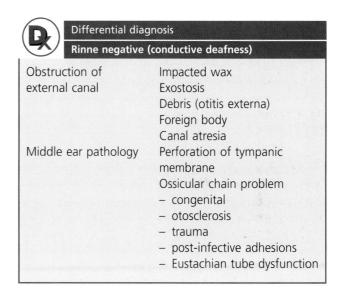

Differential diagnosis	
Rinne negative (conductive deafness)	
Obstruction of external canal	Impacted wax
	Exostosis
	Debris (otitis externa)
	Foreign body
	Canal atresia
Middle ear pathology	Perforation of tympanic membrane
	Ossicular chain problem
	– congenital
	– otosclerosis
	– trauma
	– post-infective adhesions
	– Eustachian tube dysfunction

Audiometry The definitive test for hearing acuity is by audiometry. There may be subjective errors in the tuning fork tests. There may also be subjective anomalies in audiometric testing but these are less likely. Audiometric testing shows in graphic form both bone and air conduction (Fig. 4.17).

The normal annotation used when producing an audiogram is as follows:

- X refers to air conduction in the left ear
- O refers to air conduction in the right ear
- ⊃ refers to bone conduction in the left ear
- ⊂ refers to bone conduction in the right ear

The horizontal axis indicates the frequency of the sound in Hz and the vertical axis indicates the hearing level in decibels (dB). Levels of hearing recorded between zero and 20 dB are considered to be within normal limits.

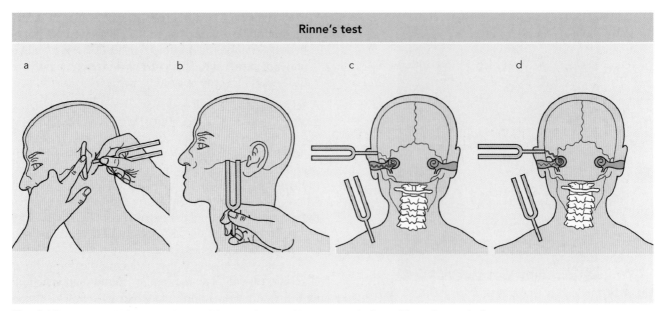

Fig. 4.16 Rinne test: (a) bone conduction, (b) air conduction, (c) perceptive deafness, (d) conductive deafness.

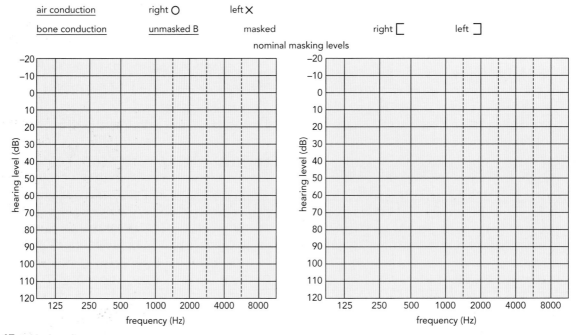

Fig. 4.17 A blank audiogram.

Oto-acoustic emissions test (to screen for deafness in infancy)

This is a screening test for neonates. It is non-invasive and relies on a sound transmitted to a baby's ear producing an auto-acoustic emission or echo. This echo can be measured by computer. A negative response may indicate infant hearing impairment, but the test can give false readings. The infant can then be referred for the more accurate auditory brain-stem response test.

Labyrinthine dysfunction

Nystagmus occurs with stimulation of the vestibular system. The direction of the nystagmus indicates the side affected. The direction of the fast element is away from the affected side, although the nystagmus is named to the side of the fast element. Thus nystagmus (fast) to the right indicates an affected left labyrinth.

The caloric test is carried out by irrigating the ear canal with cold or warm water. This induces nystagmus. Lack of response indicates no function in the labyrinth of the side tested. This finding may be indicative of Ménière's disease.

Benign positional vertigo

Hallpike (Dix–Hallpike) test This is a definitive test for benign positional vertigo. If vertigo is induced by the manoeuvre, the test is deemed positive. The manoeuvre is performed by sitting the patient on a couch with their legs extended. The clinician turns the head 45° to one side and lays the patient fully on their back and slightly extends the neck. The test is positive if nystagmus is provoked by this. The cause of the vertigo can then be established as peripheral (in the labyrinth) as opposed to central.

Red flag – urgent referral

The ear

- Sudden onset of unilateral deafness
- Unilateral deafness even if not of sudden onset
- Persistent unilateral tinnitus
- Unresolving ear discharge
- Acute and unremitting otalgia not responding to treatment
- Vertigo if TIA or vertebrobasilar ischaemia a possibility

The nose

Structure of the nose and sinuses

Diagrams of the nose and paranasal sinuses are shown in Figure 4.18.

EXTERNAL NOSE

The external appearance of the nose (before it may be distorted by injury or disease) is variable due to genetic factors. It is dependent on the shape of the cartilage and bone structure.

The external structure of the nose consists of skin overlying a bone and cartilaginous support. This skin continues into the anterior nares (the vestibule). The skin of the nose contains many sebaceous glands and within the vestibule the skin contains both hair and sebaceous cells. The proximal one-third of the nose is constructed of bone while the distal two-thirds is cartilage.

NASAL CAVITY

The interior structure is called the nasal cavity. After the vestibule, the surface is lined with ciliated columnar epithelium except in its upper part, which is lined with olfactory epithelium. The ciliated columnar epithelium lines the whole respiratory tract, indicating the importance of the nose in this system. The sinuses are also lined with ciliated columnar epithelium.

The central pillar at the entrance to the nose is the columella from which the nasal septum extends posteriorly. This is cartilaginous in its outer structure, becoming bony after about half its length. The bony part is formed by perpendicular plate of the ethmoid and inferiorly by the vomer, which is an extension of the maxillary crest. The septum is often not straight in its development.

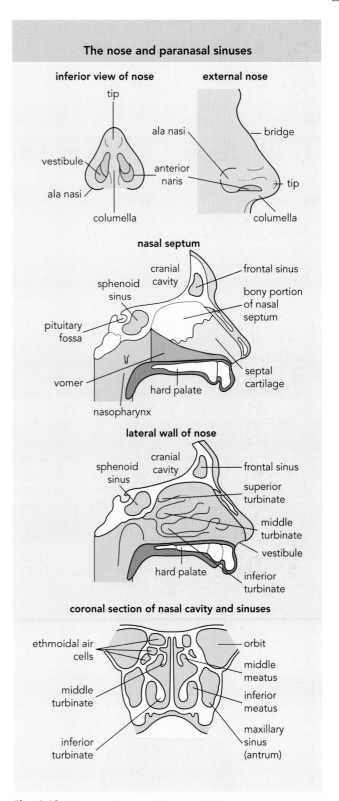

Fig. 4.18 Diagrams of nose and paranasal sinuses.

Turbinates extend from the lateral wall of the nasal cavity and act as air-warming processes. These are the inferior, middle and superior turbinates. The inferior turbinate is easily seen through the vestibule by elevating the tip of the nose. Drainage of the nasolacrimal duct occurs under the inferior turbinate; of the maxillary, anterior ethmoid and frontal sinuses from under the middle turbinate; of the posterior and sphenoidal sinuses from under the superior turbinate.

BLOOD SUPPLY

The blood supply of the nose is abundant and is derived from both internal and external carotid arteries. The lateral nose is supplied by the sphenopalatine artery and the anterior and posterior ethmoid arteries. The septum is supplied by these arteries. The anterior part of the septum also receives a supply from the superior labial artery and the posterior part from the greater palatine. The area of maximal confluence of these vessels is at Little's area, which is an area at the antero-inferior part of the nasal septum.

Venous drainage of the nose follows the arterial supply but is important in that they drain directly into the cavernous sinus. This is a route of potential infection into the cranium.

SINUSES

The sinuses – maxillary, ethmoidal, frontal and sphenoidal – are air-filled cavities (Fig. 4.19). All but the frontal sinuses are present at birth. All are represented bilaterally although the sphenoidal sinus is central with a separating septum. The importance of this sinus is that its posterior wall is the anterior wall of the pituitary fossa. The frontal sinuses border the orbit and anterior cranial fossa. The ethmoid sinuses are closely related to the orbit and the anterior cranial fossa and the maxillary sinuses are close to the orbit and teeth. Their drainage has been described in the section on the nasal cavity.

The function of the sinuses is unknown but they form part of the respiratory tract and are susceptible to infection.

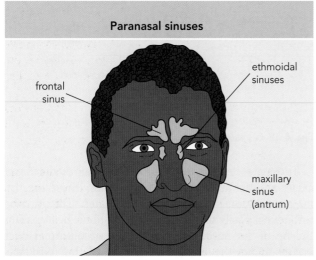

Paranasal sinuses

frontal sinus

ethmoidal sinuses

maxillary sinus (antrum)

Fig. 4.19 Topographical representation of the paranasal sinuses.

Symptoms of diseases of the nose and sinuses

ANOSMIA (COMPLETE LOSS OF SENSE OF SMELL)

Happily this is a fairly rare condition but it is very upsetting to those who suffer it. Hyposmia is when the sense of smell is partially lost and occurs more commonly than the complete anosmia. Dysosmia is an altered perception of smell and is usually a hallucination.

Risk factors
Disturbance of smell

- Nasal polyps or chronic sinus disease
- Viral upper respiratory tract infections
- Trauma or toxic chemicals
- Idiopathic
- CNS dysfunction (Alzheimer's)
- Hallucinogenic (epilepsy, schizophrenia)

EPISTAXIS (NOSE BLEED)

It is important to distinguish a frank blood loss from a bloody nasal discharge as the latter may have more serious implications.

Epistaxis usually occurs spontaneously or is caused by direct trauma. Associated conditions are vestibulitis or rhinitis, nose-picking or a foreign body. In the elderly, degenerative vascular disease or hypertension may be linked to the epistaxis, thus bleeding may be more severe in the elderly.

Bleeding is more common if there is an associated bleeding diathesis or if the patient is taking medication such as anticoagulants, aspirin or a nonsteroidal anti-inflammatory drug.

Questions to ask
Epistaxis

- How long and how severe is the bleeding?
- Which side did the bleeding start?
- Have you had nosebleeds before?
- Do you have hypertension?
- Are you on any medication? (specify these)
- Have you had nasal surgery in the recent past?
- Do you have a personal or family history of a bleeding disorder?

Emergency
Epistaxis

- Bleeding brisk and prolonged
- Ongoing (>30 minutes)
- Shortness of breath
- Clinically anaemic
- Shock (tachycardia, hypotension, sweating)

RUNNY NOSE (RHINORRHOEA)

The type of nasal discharge may suggest the diagnosis.

Rhinorrhoea may be intermittent, varying with the clock, or with contact with animals, dust, chemicals, certain foods or heat. It may also be intermittent and related to the season, typically in hay fever (seasonal allergic rhinitis). The differential diagnosis of these presentations is discussed in the examination of the nose section (p. 98).

Unilateral nasal discharge may signify a serious cause, whether it is an otherwise unrecognised foreign body in a child or neoplasm in an adult, and must always be thoroughly investigated.

Symptoms and signs	
Nasal discharge	
Type of discharge	**Potential causes**
Watery or mucous	Perennial allergic rhinitis
	Seasonal allergic rhinitis
	Vasomotor rhinitis
	Viral infection
Mucopurulent	Bacterial infection
	Foreign body
Serous	Cerebrospinal fluid leak
Bloody	Epistaxis
	Foreign body
	Trauma
	Neoplasia
	Bleeding diathesis

BLOCKED NOSE

This condition is often associated with rhinorrhoea and so taking the history is the same in both conditions.

As with unilateral nasal discharge, unilateral nasal obstruction may have a significant cause. The examiner must establish whether the nasal obstruction is a true obstruction or intermittent. If the obstruction is intermittent, and even varying from one side to the other, it is more likely to be caused by a physiological reaction rather than mechanical obstruction.

Mechanical nasal obstruction may be due to nasal septal, turbinate or other causes. Nasal septal distortion

occurs as a result of injury which may be of cartilage or fracture of the nasal bone. Abnormal development of the nasal septum may be congenital or due to a disease process such as collapse of the septum caused by cocaine or other chemicals. It may result from previous surgery.

The rare congenital obstruction of the nose seen in infants and young children is choanal atresia. The communication between the nose and pharynx may be absent in one or both nares.

Questions to ask
Rhinorrhoea and blocked nose

- What is the colour of any nasal discharge?
- Is the discharge from one nostril or both?
- Is any nasal obstruction one sided or both?
- Do you suffer from both nasal discharge and obstruction?
- Do the symptoms vary with the time of day or night, or with the time of year?
- Does anything aggravate your symptoms?
- Do you have any pets?
- Has any medication relieved your symptoms?
- Do you have any known allergies?
- Have you had any previous nasal surgery?

NASAL DEFORMITY

Deformity of the nose may be congenital or acquired. Patients will either present with a nose that has always dissatisfied them or with one that has become misshapen due to an injury or possibly due to a disease process.

When taking a history, the patient should be asked about any injury and the length of time the deformity has been present. Any other associated symptoms should be noted such as the presence of obstruction or discharge. The use of cocaine or contact with chemicals (such as chromium) should be noted.

PAINFUL NOSE AND FACE

Other than as a result of direct trauma or acute inflammation, it is unusual for nasal pain to be present as a symptom. If it is, care should be taken to establish the cause.

Facial pain may be caused by acute sinus infections but is often associated with causes other than the nose or sinuses. Sites to be considered in particular are the teeth and the trigeminal nerve.

Maxillary sinus pain is usually always associated with nasal obstruction or discharge and is typically worse on bending down. Frontal sinus pain is felt above the orbit and is usually accompanied by periorbital swelling. This condition requires urgent referral because of the closeness of the lateral sinus and it communication with the brain.

- Unilateral nasal discharge, especially if blood-stained (>2/52)
- Unilateral nasal obstruction (>2/52)
- Nasal pain with no obvious aetiology (>2/52)
- Unexplained facial pain (>2/52)
- Epistaxis, heavy and lasting longer than 30 minutes
- Periorbital swelling and pain

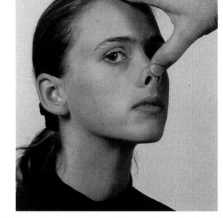

Fig. 4.20 Manual examination of the nasal vestibule and lower cavity.

Examination of the nose and sinuses

EXTERNAL APPEARANCE OF THE NOSE

The general appearance of the nasal structure and the skin overlying the nose should be observed. Any redness or abnormal swelling or shape should be noted. Swelling around the maxilla or orbit may indicate severe sinus infection but maxillary swelling may also highlight a dental abscess. The nose is not an uncommon site for skin tumours such as basal or squamous cell carcinomas.

SEBORRHOEIC DERMATITIS

This is a common skin condition often first seen at the side of the nose close to the alae. It is manifest by redness and scaling of the skin.

ACNE ROSACEA

While this skin condition is well recognised to be a redness of the skin seen in adults on various areas of the face, it may occur on the lower part of the nose.

RHINOPHYMA

This condition is thought to be an extension of acne rosacea. The excessive swelling and growth of the nose can be quite disfiguring. It is important to note that there is an increased incidence of skin neoplasia in this condition.

NASAL CAVITY

The nasal cavity can be visualised in a variety of ways and this depends on the equipment available to the clinician.

MANUAL EXAMINATION

In children and adolescents the nasal vestibule and lower cavity can be easily seen by elevating the tip of the nose (Fig. 4.20).

THUDICUM SPECULUM OR AUROSCOPE

This useful instrument allows a good view of the vestibule and lower part of the nasal cavity, while the clinician has one hand free to, for example, remove a foreign body. Figure 4.21 illustrates how to use the thudicum.

If a speculum is not available, an auroscope is a useful and simple alternative.

NASENDOSCOPE

A more complete view of the nasal cavity can be obtained with the use of a rigid (Fig. 4.22) or flexible (Fig. 4.23) nasendoscope. In particular the flexible nasendoscope allows a view of the whole cavity and can be advanced into the postnasal space, and beyond (Figs 4.24, 4.25).

DEFORMITIES OF THE NOSE

Genetic causes, injury or disease may result in structural deformities. Injury may result in fracture or dislocation of the nasal bone or cartilage. These may be visible from observing the external appearance or more usually from examining the nasal cavity.

The nasal structure may also be damaged by conditions which collapse the nasal bridge such as contact with various chemicals, notably cocaine. The structure may also be distorted by syphilis, tuberculosis or neoplasms within the cavity of the nose.

Most deformities of the nose involve the midline septum and such deformities are detected both externally and by examining the nasal septum.

The most common problem with the septum is deviation from the central position, often termed as deflection.

SEPTAL PERFORATION

The finding of a septal perforation should prompt the clinician to seek any possible pathology, although there

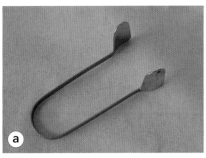

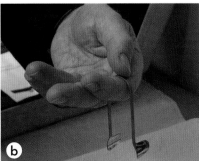

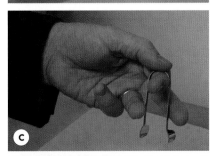

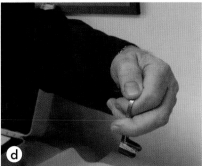

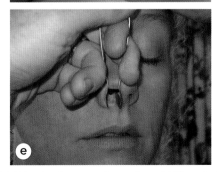

Fig. 4.21 (a) The thudicum nasal speculum. (b) Place thudicum on left index finger with the flanges pointing towards the wrist. (c) Rotate the hand so that the arms of the speculum are between the third and fourth fingers such that the flanges are protected from spreading too wide. (d) Flex the wrist and the speculum is ready for use. (e) Speculum in use.

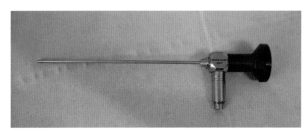

Fig. 4.22 Rigid endoscope.

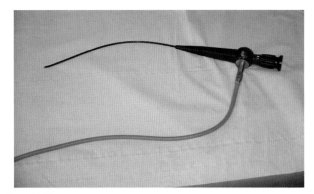

Fig. 4.23 Flexible endoscope.

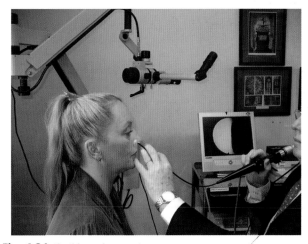

Fig. 4.24 Flexible endoscope in use.

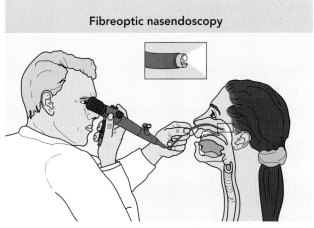

Fibreoptic nasendoscopy

Fig. 4.25 Fibreoptic examination of the postnasal space (transnasal).

may be none. Perforations usually occur low in the septum and should be visible to the nonspecialist by use of a thudicum speculum or auroscope.

Aetiology
Septal perforation

- Idiopathic
- Iatrogenic (previous cauterisation or surgery)
- Infection (tuberculosis, syphilis)
- Neoplastic (basal or squamous cell carcinoma, malignant granuloma)
- Chemicals (cocaine, chromic salts)

VESTIBULITIS

Inflammation and crusting in the area of the nasal vestibule indicates a bacterial infection. Such infection will cause dilatation of blood vessels, in particular in the plexus of Little's area which can result in epistaxes.

EPISTAXIS

The large majority of epistaxes come from Little's area on the nasal septum where there is a plexus of blood vessels. The clinician will be able to see dilated vessels in this area with simple instrumentation. Only by use of a nasendoscope will it be possible to detect bleeding points higher in the nose.

ALLERGIC RHINITIS

Allergic rhinitis may be seasonal (hay fever) or perennial. It can be recognised by observing the prominent inferior turbinates which will be swollen and oedematous. There will be a watery nasal discharge and sneezing may be a feature. Seasonal allergic rhinitis will be related to the seasons. Perennial allergic rhinitis will be related to dusts, cats, feathers or other allergens and will occur throughout the year.

VASOMOTOR RHINITIS (NONALLERGIC RHINITIS)

The signs on examination are similar to allergic rhinitis but it is not related to any allergy. Profuse watery nasal discharge is a feature, as is nasal obstruction. It is due to increased vascularity of the nasal mucosa. The difference from allergic rhinitis is that the turbinates may appear more reddened. The symptoms may be enhanced by a dry atmosphere, heat or hot foods, alcohol and certain chemicals.

RHINITIS MEDICAMENTOSA

The result of this condition is that by the misuse of nasal sympathomimetic sprays the mucosa behaves in a similar way to vasomotor rhinitis. Vascularity of the turbinates is increased causing turbinate swelling and watery nasal discharge.

ATROPHIC RHINITIS

The mucosa in this condition is very different to the other types of rhinitis. It is atrophied, dry and crusted. As a result, halitosis is often present.

SINUSES

Acute maxillary sinusitis

The diagnosis of acute sinusitis is usually made on the history of facial pain, blocked nose and purulent nasal discharge. It is usually associated with an upper respiratory tract infection and fever may be a feature. On examination the clinician may elicit maxillary tenderness. Diagnostically, however, mucopus should be observed coming from beneath the middle turbinate. A CT scan is the most helpful investigation to confirm the condition.

Acute frontal sinusitis

It is unusual for this condition to occur without associated maxillary sinusitis. Supraorbital tenderness, swelling and even redness may be observed. Again mucopus should be detected drained from under the middle turbinate.

Chronic sinusitis

The diagnosis of this condition is similar to acute sinusitis but the condition will have lasted longer and may be more associated with halitosis.

The throat

Structure of the throat

ORAL CAVITY

The structures within the oral cavity are the gums, teeth, tongue and tonsils (Fig. 4.26). The anterior border of the oral cavity is formed by the gums and its posterior boundary is the oropharynx. The surface of the cavity is lined by mucous membrane.

The salivary glands open into the oral cavity. The parotid glands open into the buccal mucosa at the level of upper second molar and the submandibular glands open into the floor of the mouth lateral to the frenulum of the tongue.

TEETH

There are 10 upper and 10 lower deciduous or milk teeth. In the adult there are 16 upper teeth and 16 lower teeth. Their average times of eruption are shown in Figures 4.27 and 4.28.

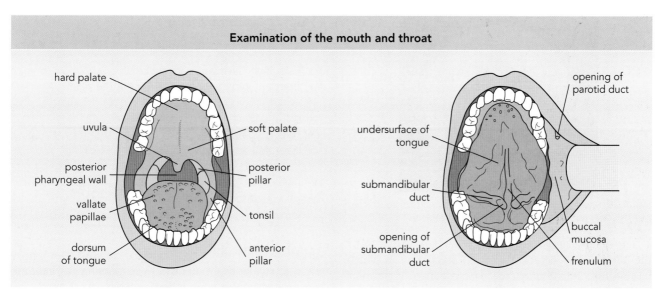

Fig. 4.26 Structure of the oral cavity.

Average eruption times of deciduous teeth

edcba | abcde
edcba | abcde

$\overline{a|a}$ 6 months

$\dfrac{d|d}{d|d}$ 14 months

$\dfrac{a|a}{}$ 7 months

$\dfrac{c|c}{c|c}$ 18 months

$\dfrac{b|b}{b|b}$ 8–9 months

$\dfrac{e|e}{e|e}$ 24 months

Fig. 4.27 Average eruption times of the deciduous teeth.

Average eruption times of permanent teeth

87654321 | 12345678
87654321 | 12345678

$\overline{1|1}$ 6 years

$\dfrac{4|4}{4|4}$ 10 years

$\dfrac{6|6}{6|6}$ 6 years

$\dfrac{53|53}{53|53}$ 11–13 years

$\dfrac{1|1}{}$ 7 years

$\dfrac{7|7}{7|7}$ 12 years

$\overline{2|2}$ 8 years

$\dfrac{8|8}{8|8}$ 18–25 years

$\dfrac{2|2}{}$ 9 years

Fig. 4.28 Average eruption times of the permanent teeth.

TONGUE

The tongue is a muscular organ whose ventral or under surface is mucous membrane. The dorsal or upper surface is of squamous epithelium in which are papillae containing taste buds. It has a rich blood and nerve supply. The anterior two-thirds of the tongue is divided from the posterior one-third by a V-shaped sulcus terminalis. In the posterior third of the tongue the papillae are particularly prominent.

The tongue has a central band of tissue tethering its ventral surface; this is called the frenulum.

TONSILS

The tonsils are lymphoid tissue that lie posterolaterally to the tongue between the anterior and posterior falces. The lymphoid tissue contains many mucus-secreting crypts which commonly contain harmless exudate, or food debris. Lymphoid tissue is also found in the nasopharynx (adenoids) and posterior to the tongue (lingual tonsil). All lymphoid tissue in the pharynx tends to regress with age.

PHARYNX AND LARYNX

The pharynx forms the space posterior to the oral cavity. It is anatomically divided into three parts.

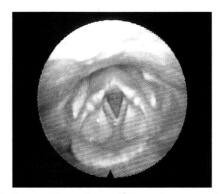

Fig. 4.29 Fibreoptic view of normal larynx, showing epiglottis, cords and arytenoid cartilages (courtesy of Wonersh Surgery).

The *nasopharynx* is the part of the pharynx that forms the postnasal space above the soft palate and in which, in children, lie the adenoids. The choanae of the nose form its anterior border.

The *oropharynx* is the posterior extension of the oral cavity.

The *hypopharynx,* or laryngopharynx, extends from the oropharynx to the cricoid cartilage which lies distal to the vocal cords. The internal structures to be observed here are the epiglottis and larynx. The main structures of the larynx are the vocal cords and their suspensory cartilages, the arytenoid cartilages. Above the cords is the ventricular sinus which is bordered proximally by mucous membrane folds (false chords). There is a recess posterior to the tongue but anterior to the epiglottis, the vallecula. The pyriform fossae are two recesses which lie either side of the larynx.

The larynx (Fig. 4.29) is enclosed in the thyroid cartilage (Adam's apple) and beneath (and above and connecting it to the cricoid cartilage) is the cricothyroid membrane (a site for tracheostomy).

Symptoms of diseases of the throat

BLOOD IN THE MOUTH

Patients may present with a history of finding blood in their mouth or throat. This should be distinguished from blood arising from vomiting (haematemesis) or coughing (haemoptysis).

The most common site for bleeding of the throat is from inflamed gums. Lesions from other sites in the oral cavity and pharynx where neoplasm might be concealed should be excluded.

SORE THROAT

Pain can arise from all the structures in the mouth and pharynx, from teeth to larynx. In the mouth the cause may be readily seen. It is important to establish the severity of the symptoms and if there is any associated fever. It is also important to establish the effect of the pain on swallowing solids and liquids.

Soreness in the throat may present as the feeling of a lump in the throat.

Questions to ask

Sore throat or mouth

- How long have you had the pain?
- Does anything aggravate or relieve the pain?
- Where do you feel the pain and does it radiate?
- Is the pain constant or does it vary?
- How is your swallowing?
- Have you any other symptoms?
- Have you been or are you presently taking any medication?
- Do you smoke or drink alcohol?

LUMP IN THE NECK

Thyroid swellings are dealt with in Chapter 2. There are other sites in the neck where swelling may arise. The clinician should establish the position of any mass and palpate the lumps presented (see 'Examination of the throat' p. 101). It is not uncommon in infections of the throat for the anterior cervical glands to be tender and enlarged. Posterior cervical gland enlargement (posterior to the sternomastoid muscle) may be of more sinister significance.

Neck lumps may be a sign of generalised disease and the possibility of other systems being involved must be considered.

Questions to ask

Lump in the neck

- How long has it been present?
- Has the lump changed in size?
- Is the lump painful?
- Do you have a cough?
- Have you any problem with your mouth or throat?
- Have you lost weight recently?
- How is your general health?
- Do you have any problem with sweating?
- Do you have any thyroid symptoms?

STRIDOR

Stridor is a harsh sound made on inspiration. It is associated with narrowing of the upper airway, usually of the glottic or vocal cord area. It should be distinguished from the expiratory wheeze of asthma. It is often associated with hoarseness and the age of the patient is relevant to the diagnosis.

HOARSE VOICE

Hoarseness is a term describing an altered voice. It may be extreme, in that there is little or no voice production. It is frequently associated with an upper respiratory tract infection and any symptoms of that should be elucidated.

The clinician should ascertain whether the voice has been overused (frequent singing or shouting) and obtain information about smoking and the use of alcohol.

Questions to ask

Hoarse voice

- How long have you been hoarse?
- Is it persistent or intermittent?
- Have you any other symptoms (cold or fever)?
- Have you been projecting your voice for any reason?
- Do you smoke or drink alcohol and how much?
- What is your job; do you work in dusty surroundings?

DYSPHAGIA

Difficulty on swallowing of oesophageal origin is dealt with in Chapter 7. It should be distinguished from oropharyngeal causes of pain or difficulty in swallowing. The anatomical level of discomfort and any associated symptoms should be ascertained when taking a history (see 'Questions to ask, sore throat or mouth' p. 100).

Examination of the throat

INSTRUMENTS

It would be unusual for a nonspecialist clinician to have access to fibreoptic equipment. Important requirements for a primary care physician are a good light source, tongue depressor and possibly an indirect laryngoscopy mirror (Figs 4.30–4.34).

BUCCAL MUCOSA

Ulceration

Ulceration is where there is loss of epithelium. There are many conditions that may cause ulceration of the buccal mucosa. Most causes are infective in origin but perhaps the most common are aphthous ulcers for which no cause

Differential diagnosis

Aphthous ulcers

- Viral (herpes simplex)
- Allergies to foodstuffs or certain chemicals found in toothpastes and mouthwashes
- Stress
- Medication such as nonsteroidal anti-inflammatory drugs, beta-blockers
- Medical conditions such as vitamin deficiencies, Crohn's disease, Behçet's syndrome, blood dyscrasias (agranulocytosis)
- Mechanical trauma

has been found. Associated factors in aphthous ulcer formation are listed in the 'differential diagnosis' box.

Other causes of buccal lesions are Vincent's angina (acute ulcerative stomatitis) and the more chronic infections of tuberculosis and syphilis.

Carcinoma in the mouth usually presents as an ulcer and may occur on any part of the mucosa or tongue. Kaposi sarcoma may involve the buccal mucosa and appear as small, firm, cytic-shaped, bluish lesions.

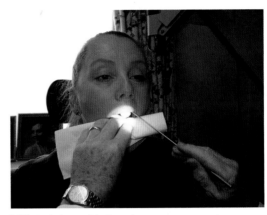

Fig. 4.30 Technique of indirect laryngoscopy.

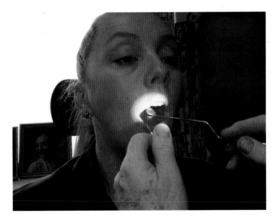

Fig. 4.31 Technique of examination of nasopharynx using postnasal mirror.

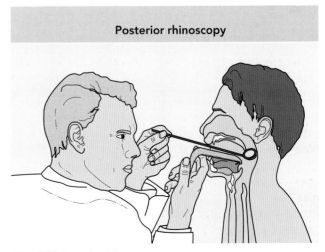

Posterior rhinoscopy

Fig. 4.32 Posterior rhinoscopy.

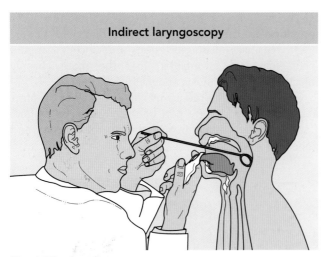

Indirect laryngoscopy

Fig. 4.33 Indirect laryngoscopy.

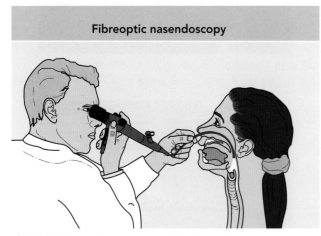

Fibreoptic nasendoscopy

Fig. 4.34 Fibreoptic examination of the larynx (transnasal).

White lesions

White lesions on the buccal mucosa are not uncommon in the oral cavity.

Candidiasis is the most common cause. This condition more commonly occurs in infants and frail elderly but also may be seen in those on antibiotic treatment or in immunocompromised patients.

Lichen planus and leucoplakia may be similar in appearance to candida and, if candida fails to respond to treatment, a biopsy may be necessary to distinguish these other two possibilities. All these lesions may present with some ulceration.

TONGUE

Geographical tongue

The tongue has various conditions of unknown aetiology and of no pathological importance. This condition can be recognised by random areas of desquamation which may concern the patient.

Hairy tongue

The tongue in this condition may be black in colour. It is caused by hypertrophy of filiform papillae and may be related to social factors such as smoking or drinking tea and coffee.

Fissured tongue

In this condition there is an exaggeration of fissures in the epithelium of the tongue. It may be a manifestation of iron-deficiency anaemia but is more often of genetic origin.

TONSILS AND OROPHARYNX

Pharyngitis

Inflammation of the pharynx without an associated tonsillitis is recognised by a redness and oedema of the soft palate and fauces. Its cause may be viral or bacterial and it is usually associated with fever and swelling of the anterior cervical glands.

Tonsillitis

When there is infection of the tonsils it is notoriously difficult for the clinician to determine whether the causative organism is viral or bacterial. Commonly tonsillar exudates are seen and every organism may produce these. Although exudates are commonly seen in infective mononucleosis (glandular fever) these can be seen in any inflammatory condition of the tonsil. The tonsils, as well as producing exudates, may enlarge with inflammation.

Unilateral enlargement of the tonsils

This is a significant finding and is a red flag indication for referral (see box).

If there is obvious redness, oedema and uvular displacement, a peritonsillar abscess (quinsy) should be suspected. Associated signs will be fever and anterior cervical gland enlargement.

Lymphoma of the tonsil may present in a similar fashion but usually without the signs of fever and inflammation.

Red flag – urgent referral

The throat

- Unilateral tonsillar enlargement
- Child with fever, cough, stridor and respiratory distress
- Child with fever, drooling and respiratory distress
- Airways obstruction in any age group
- Hoarseness lasting longer than 4 weeks

LARYNX

Infective causes involving the larynx may occur at any age but there are two conditions in children of particular importance.

Acute laryngotracheobronchitis (croup)

The usual organism causing this condition is the parainfluenza virus. It most commonly occurs in children under the age of 5 years and is of sudden onset. It is recognised by the presence of a barking cough, stridor (inspiratory wheeze), and hoarse voice. There will usually be fever present and symptoms are most prominent at night. The condition lasts about 48 hours.

Severe cases may cause acute respiratory distress (tachycardia, rapid respirations and possibly cyanosis) and require urgent admission to hospital.

Diagnosis of croup is mainly made on the symptoms alone.

Epiglottitis (supraglottitis)

This infection extends into a slightly older age group and the mean age is around 5 years old, and therefore older children may be affected. Again, onset is sudden and diagnosis is made mainly on the symptomatology. Cough in this condition is much less of a feature. Drooling of saliva is frequently present, as well as difficulty in swallowing and respiratory distress. As with any infection, fever may be present.

If this condition is suspected in a child, urgent admission is necessary as deterioration in the airway may be rapid.

Laryngitis

In the adult, laryngitis is usually diagnosed by its symptoms. Cough, throat discomfort and hoarseness of voice together with fever are the usual presenting symptoms. If the causative organism is bacterial, there will be an associated purulent sputum. Most cases however are viral.

Voice production, hoarseness or aphonia, may be due to misuse or overuse. There may also be symptoms in the larynx of pain or voice alteration caused by a psychological element (hysterical dysphonia and globus syndrome). These conditions can only be diagnosed in the absence of direct or indirect laryngoscopy by the history and lack of infective signs.

A patient in whom the hoarseness has lasted for longer than 4 weeks should be referred to a specialist for investigation.

Tumours of the larynx

Laryngeal carcinoma should be excluded in anyone with a persistent hoarse voice, which is the cardinal symptom of this condition. There may be an associated history of smoking or a family history of the disease.

Not all tumours of the larynx are malignant, however – singer's nodes and polyps are happily a more common finding. Vocal cord palsy may indicate a malignant bronchial tumour.

Examination of elderly people

The ear

- Wax removal may greatly help hearing
- Ear irrigation is perfectly acceptable as long as there are no contraindications
- Presbyacusis (sensorineural deafness of old age) may occur over 60 years of age; it is the most common cause of deafness in old age
- Presbyacusis is usually first recognised clinically by a high tone hearing loss
- Unilateral deafness may indicate significant pathology, so refer
- Unilateral tinnitus may indicate significant pathology, so refer
- Persisting unilateral otalgia may indicate significant pathology, so refer
- Persisting discharge from a perforated tympanic membrane may indicate significant pathology, so refer

The nose

- Epistaxis in the elderly is usually more difficult to control due to arteriosclerosis, so there should be a lower threshold for referral criteria
- Epistaxis in the elderly is more likely to be from higher in the nose than Little's area and will be more difficult for the primary care physician to control
- Incidence of carcinoma of the nose and sinuses increases with age

The throat

- Voice change occurs in the elderly due to loss of tissue elasticity
- The incidence of carcinoma of the larynx increases with age and so hoarseness lasting longer than 4 weeks should be referred to a specialist urgently
- Malignancies may cause hoarseness by involving the vocal cords directly or by recurrent laryngeal nerve palsy from a carcinoma in the hilum of the lung

A useful guide to a student of ear, nose and throat examination is to always take particular note of symptoms and signs that are unilateral.

The ears

- Always examine the pinna and entrance to the external canal before inserting the auroscope into the ear
- Irrigation of ears is a safe procedure except in defined circumstances
- The temperature of the water used should be 37°C otherwise the onset of a convection current in the labyrinth may result in temporary vertigo
- Water is a significant irritant of otitis externa and of the middle ear if there is a perforation and therefore irrigation should not be used in such circumstances
- Unilateral symptoms, such as sudden onset deafness or tinnitus, may be significant and should be referred – urgently in the case of sudden onset deafness
- Presbyacusis is signalled by an initial high tone hearing loss
- Continuing discharge from an ear should be referred to a specialist. If the discharge is from the external ear, aural toilet will speed resolution; if the discharge is from the middle ear specialist management is needed

The nose

- Look into the nose frequently. Use an auroscope if nasal speculae are not available. Get used to what is normal
- Nasal polypi are white and pearly and should not be confused with the appearance of a swollen inferior turbinate

- Rhinorrhoea and nasal obstruction are the most common symptoms of the nose presented to the clinician
- Allergic rhinitis is the most common reason for those symptoms
- Distinguishing allergic rhinitis from atrophic or vasomotor rhinitis is made on the history and findings in the nose
- Nasal fractures do not need correcting if there is no cosmetic deformity or if the nasal airway is unimpeded
- Unilateral nasal discharge in children may indicate a foreign body
- Unilateral nasal discharge in an adult may indicate neoplasm
- Uncontrolled epistaxis, lasting over 30 minutes, should be seen in a specialist clinic especially if the patient is elderly

The throat

- Unilateral tonsillar enlargement may be significant. Consider lymphoma or, if there is inflammation, peritonsillar abscess (quinsy)
- In children with stridor indicating acute laryngotracheitis and signs of respiratory distress admit to a specialist unit urgently
- In children with fever, drooling and respiratory distress suspect epiglottitis and admit to a specialist unit urgently
- Hoarse voice lasting more than 4 weeks should be referred for specialist examination to exclude malignancy

5

The respiratory system

Disease of the respiratory tract accounts for more consultations with general practitioners than any other of the body systems. It is also responsible for more new spells of inability to work and more days lost from work.

For example, asthma now affects approximately 10% of the population of many Western countries; lung cancer is the most common male cancer and in some places has already exceeded breast cancer as the most common female malignancy. Tuberculosis, for so long the staple of the respiratory physician is, after a long period of decline, increasing again. The respiratory complications of HIV infections have added to the burden. Increases in pollution, new industrial processes and the growing worldwide consumption of tobacco all have implications for the lungs. The average family practitioner, therefore, is likely to spend more of the working day examining the respiratory system than any other.

Respiratory disease is common in hospital practice. It accounts for approximately 4% of all hospital admissions and approximately 35% of all acute medical admissions. Surgeons and anaesthetists are very interested in ensuring an adequate respiratory system in any patient who needs a general anaesthetic.

Radiologists, pathologists and microbiologists are intimately involved in the diagnosis of lung conditions. Consequently, doctors in many branches of medicine spend a very substantial portion of their professional working life in the diagnosis and treatment of lung disease.

As with any other disease, a good history is the basis for a diagnosis of lung disease, particularly as examination may be normal even in advanced disease. A good history is aided by a knowledge of structure and function. Fortunately, two fairly straightforward techniques, radiography and spirometry (the analysis of the volume of expired air over time), illustrate normality and help the physician to understand the abnormal.

Structure and function

The respiratory tract extends from the nose to the alveoli and includes not only the air-conducting passages but the blood supply as well. The arrangement of the major airways is shown in Figure 5.1. An appreciation of this arrangement helps in the interpretation of radiographs (Fig. 5.2) and is essential for the bronchoscopist. More important for the examiner is the arrangement of the lobes of the lungs (Fig. 5.3). It will be seen that both lungs are divided into two and the right lung is divided again to form the middle lobe. The corresponding area on the left is the lingula, a division of the upper lobe. Figure 5.4 transposes this pattern on to a person, outlining the surface markings of the lungs. Examination of the front of the chest is largely that of the upper lobes, examination of the back the lower lobes. It will be seen how much more lung there is posteriorly than anteriorly, so it comes as no surprise that lung disease that primarily affects the bases is best detected posteriorly. Note how much lung is against the lateral chest wall. Students often examine a narrow strip of chest down the front and the back. Many signs are found laterally and in the axilla.

Computerised tomography (CT) adds an extra dimension to visualisation of the chest (Figs 5.5–5.10).

The fine detail of the airways is beautifully illustrated by wax injection models (Fig. 5.11). The same technique can be used to illustrate the intimate relationships between the supply of blood and air to the lungs (Fig. 5.12).

LUNG DEFENCE AND HISTOLOGY

The lung is exposed to 6 litres of potentially infected and irritant-laden air every minute. There are, therefore, numerous defence mechanisms to ensure survival. The nose humidifies, warms and filters the air and contains lymphocytes of the B series which secrete immunoglobulin

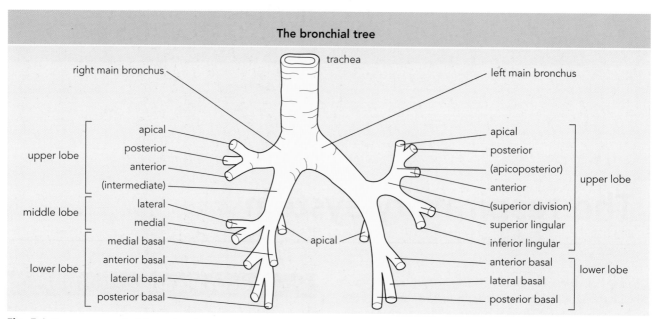

Fig. 5.1 The arrangement of the major airways.

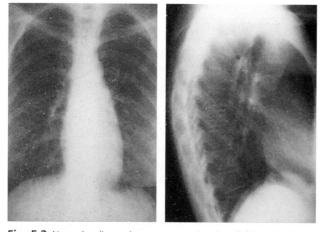

Fig. 5.2 Normal radiograph: posteroanterior view (left) and right lateral view (right).

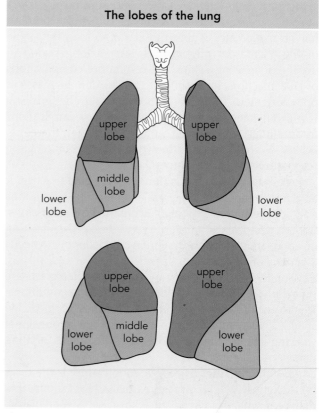

Fig. 5.3 Lobes of the lung: anterior view (upper) and lateral view (lower).

A. The epiglottis protects the larynx from inhalation of material from the gastrointestinal tract.

The cough reflex is both a protective and a clearing mechanism. Cough receptors are found in the pharynx, larynx and larger airways. A cough starts with a deep inspiration followed by expiration against a closed glottis. Glottal opening then allows a forceful jet of air to be expelled.

The main clearance mechanism is the remarkable mucociliary escalator. Bronchial secretions from bronchial glands and goblet cells, together with secretions from deeper in the lungs, form a sheet of fluid which is propelled upwards continuously by the beat of the cilia lining the bronchial epithelium (Figs 5.13, 5.14). This cilial action can fail either from the rare immotile cilia syndromes or commonly from cigarette smoke.

The chief defence of the alveoli is the alveolar macrophage (Fig. 5.15), which, in conjunction with complement and immunoglobulin, ingests foreign material that is then transported either up the airways or into the pulmonary lymphatics. T and B lymphocytes are

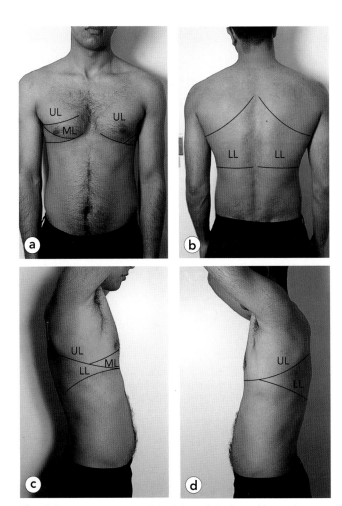

Fig. 5.4 Surface markings of the lobes of the lung: (a) anterior, (b) posterior, (c) right lateral and (d) left lateral (UL, upper lobe; ML, middle lobe; LL, lower lobe).

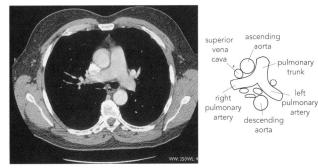

Fig. 5.7 CT scan at level of carina.

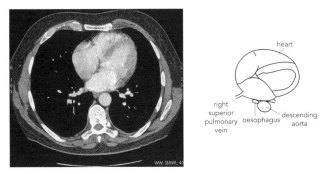

Fig. 5.8 CT scan at level of mid left atrium.

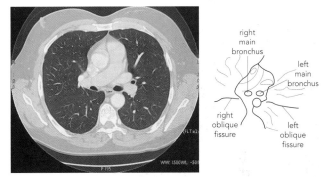

Fig. 5.9 CT scan – lung windows at level of carina.

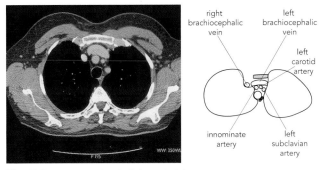

Fig. 5.5 CT scan at level of thoracic inlet.

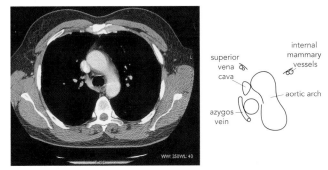

Fig. 5.6 CT scan at level of aortic arch.

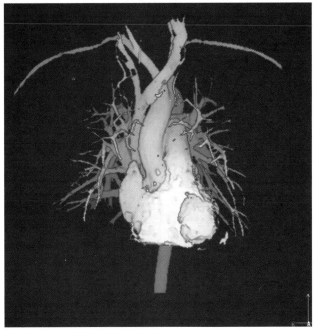

Fig. 5.10 Shaded surface display of reconstruction of dynamic magnetic resonance angiography of pulmonary and great vessels.

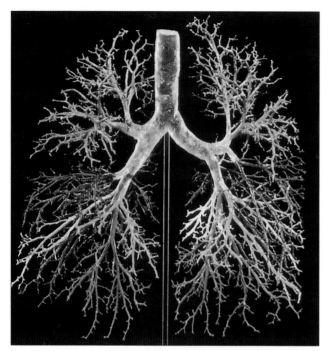

Fig. 5.11 A cast of the bronchial tree with the segments outlined in different colours.

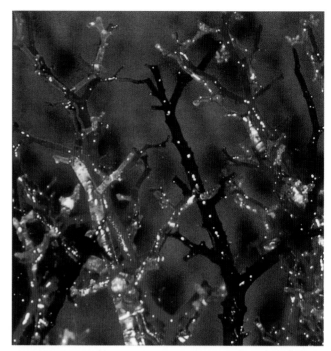

Fig. 5.12 Injection model showing bronchi (white), arteries (red but carrying deoxygenated blood) and veins (blue but carrying oxygenated blood).

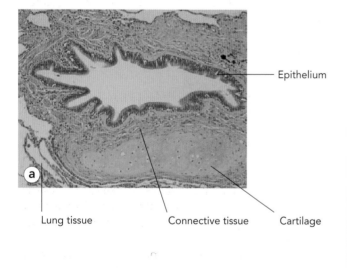

Epithelium

(a)

Lung tissue   Connective tissue   Cartilage

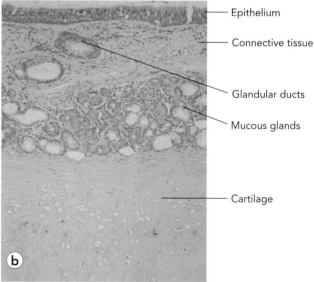

Epithelium

Connective tissue

Glandular ducts

Mucous glands

Cartilage

(b)

Fig. 5.13 (a) Low-power photomicrograph of a bronchus. (b) High-power photomicrograph of normal bronchial wall.

present throughout the lung substance and most of the immunoglobulin in the lung is made locally. The blood supplies neutrophils that pass into the lung structure in inflammation.

LUNG FUNCTION

The function of the lung is to oxygenate the blood and to remove carbon dioxide. To achieve this, ventilation of the lungs is performed by the respiratory muscles under the control of the respiratory centre in the brain. The rhythm of breathing depends on various inhibitory and excitatory mechanisms within the brainstem. These can be influenced voluntarily from higher centres and from the effect of chemoreceptors. The medullary or central chemoreceptors in the brainstem respond to changes in partial pressure of carbon dioxide in the blood ($P\text{CO}_2$). Chemoreceptors in the aortic and carotid body respond to low partial pressure of oxygen ($P\text{O}_2$) but only when this falls below 8 kPa. Thus, alteration in $P\text{CO}_2$ is the most important factor in respiratory control in health.

The sensitivity of the medullary chemoreceptor to $P\text{CO}_2$ can be reset either upwards in prolonged ventilatory failure or downwards, as when a patient is placed on a

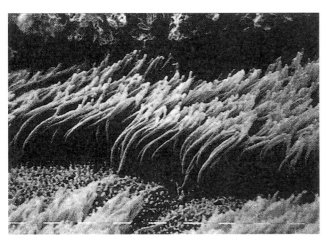

Fig. 5.14 Electron micrograph of bronchial cilia and the mucus sheet.

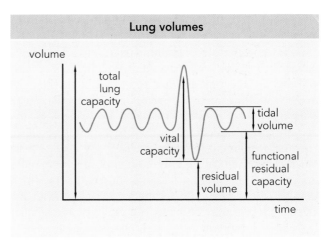

Lung volumes

Fig. 5.16 Subdivisions of lung volume.

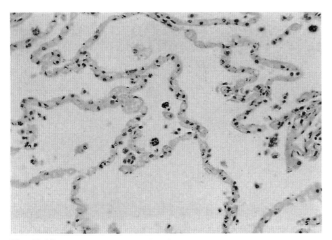

Fig. 5.15 Normal lung. Occasional pigment-containing macrophages are present within the alveolar spaces. Haematoxylin and eosin stain (× 25).

mechanical ventilator. The first situation is most commonly seen in chronic airflow limitation (chronic obstructive pulmonary disease) when patients may become dependent on hypoxic drive to maintain respiration. The injudicious administration of oxygen can then lead to ventilatory failure and death. In the second situation, 'weaning' a patient away from a ventilator is difficult because the medullary centre demands a low P_{CO_2} that cannot be maintained by the patient unaided.

Ventilation is largely performed by nerve impulses in the phrenic nerve acting to contract the diaphragm and expand the volume of the chest. Scalene and intercostal muscles act mainly by stabilising the chest wall. The result is to decrease the pressure in the pleura (already less than atmospheric). As the air inside the airways is at atmospheric pressure, the lungs must follow the chest wall through pleural apposition and expand, sucking in air. Expiration is largely a passive process: when the muscles relax the lung recoils under the influence of its own elasticity. Ventilation is, therefore, much more than just forcing air through tubes. Higher brain centres, the brainstem, spinal cord, peripheral nerves, intercostal

muscles, spine, ribs and diaphragm are all involved. Moreover, the lung tissue itself must overcome its own inertia and stiffness. Malfunction of any of these can lead to respiratory failure.

Diaphragm function is in two parts: contraction leads to descent of the diaphragm and the costal parts elevate the lower ribs. A common consequence of chronic airflow limitation and hyperinflation is a low flat diaphragm which may pull the ribs inwards rather than out.

ASSESSING RESPIRATORY FUNCTION

As the function of the lungs is to add oxygen to the blood and to remove carbon dioxide, it might be thought that measurement of the P_{O_2} and P_{CO_2} in the blood would be an adequate assessment of its efficiency. However, the lung has such an enormous reserve capacity that it can sustain considerable damage before blood gases are affected. There are, nonetheless, a number of other tests of lung function that are briefly described here. These are tests of static lung volumes, ventilation or dynamic lung volumes and gas exchange across the alveolar–capillary membrane.

Although some tests of pulmonary function are quite complex, most problems only need the simpler tests to diagnose. Spirometry and peak flow measurements can be made available in many primary care centres.

Static lung volumes

When attempting to take as deep an inspiration as possible we are eventually stopped partly by the resistance of the chest wall to further deformation and partly by the inability to stretch the lung tissues any further (Fig. 5.16). Total lung capacity (TLC) at one end is, therefore, largely influenced by this 'stretchability' or elasticity of the lung. The stiffer the lung, as in fibrosis or scarring, the less distensible it will be. Conversely, damage to the elastic tissue of the lung (e.g. emphysema) with destruction of the alveolar walls will make it more distensible, leading to an increase in TLC. TLC is also high is some patients with asthma and chronic obstructive bronchitis, probably because the lungs are overexpanded in an attempt to widen the airways.

As already indicated, breathing out from TLC is largely passive by progressive retraction of the lung; this process will end at functional residual capacity (FRC) when the tendency of the lung to contract is balanced by the thorax resisting further deformation. This point is also the end of normal expiration. Further expiration is an active process involving expiratory muscles. By using these muscles, more air can be forced out until, at least in older individuals, the limiting factor is closure of the small airways which have been getting smaller along with the alveoli. Beyond this the lungs can only become smaller by direct compression of gas (Boyle's law) by the expiratory muscles. At this point, the amount of air left in the lung is designated residual volume (RV).

In chronic bronchitis, the small airways are narrowed and inflamed; in emphysema, the elastic tissue supporting the small airways is lost and they collapse in expiration. Both mechanisms lead to an increase in RV. Conversely, if the lungs are stiffer (fibrosis), the increased tension in the lung tissue holds the airways open with closure occurring later in expiration, thus reducing the RV.

In summary, stiff lungs from fibrosis cause a low TLC and low RV, emphysema causes a high TLC and a high RV and chronic bronchitis causes a high RV. Vital capacity (VC) depends on the relative changes in RV and TLC but usually the overall effect in lung disease is a reduction.

Dynamic lung volumes

Assessment of airflow involves measuring the volume exhaled in unit time by use of a spirometric trace (Fig. 5.17). This is produced by a forced exhalation from TLC to RV. The conventional parameters derived from this trace are the forced vital capacity (FVC) and the forced expiratory volume in 1 second (FEV_1). FVC is the amount exhaled forcefully from a single deep inspiration, FEV_1 is the fraction of that volume exhaled in the first second. These are then expressed as a ratio of the FEV_1 over the FVC ($FEV_1\%$). This is normally approximately 75%, which indicates that a normal person can exhale forcibly three-quarters of their VC in 1 second. VC and FVC, one in slow expiration and the other in fast expiration, give similar results in normal individuals, although FVC is reduced in many disease states because of premature airway closure.

In diseases causing airways obstruction, the proportion of the VC that can be exhaled in 1 second is reduced and the $FEV_1\%$ falls. Conversely, in restrictive lung disease the airways are held open by the stiff lungs and the $FEV_1\%$ is normal, even increased. Nevertheless, the FVC will be reduced because the TLC is reduced. In restrictive lung disease, FEV_1 is reduced in proportion to FVC; in airways obstruction, it is reduced disproportionately.

Peak flow

The peak expiratory flow rate (PEFR) is the flow generated in the first 0.1 seconds of a forced expiration; the resulting

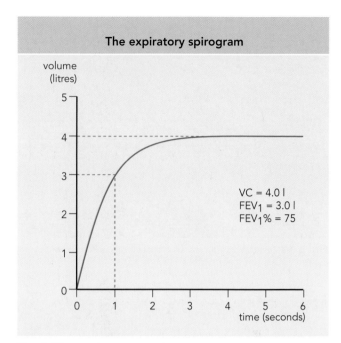

Fig. 5.17 Normal expiratory spirogram.

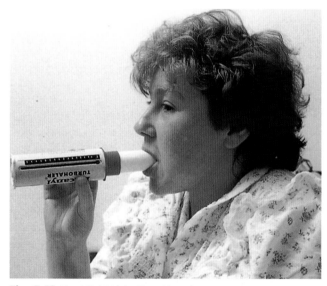

Fig. 5.18 The Mini-Wright Flow Meter in use.

figure is extrapolated over 1 minute. It can be measured easily by a variety of portable devices (Fig. 5.18) and serial recordings can be very useful in the diagnosis and monitoring of asthma (Fig. 5.19).

Gas exchange

The transfer factor (TF) is a measurement of gas transference across the alveolar–capillary membrane. For technical reasons carbon monoxide is used as the test gas but oxygen is affected in a similar way. TF is reduced when there is destruction of the alveolar–capillary bed, as in emphysema, and also when there is a barrier to diffusion. This may occur when the alveolar–capillary membrane is thickened or where there is lack of

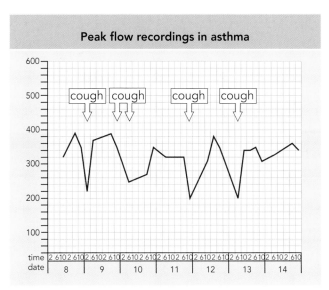

Fig. 5.19 Peak flow chart in a child with asthma whose main symptom was cough. The dips coincide with the symptoms.

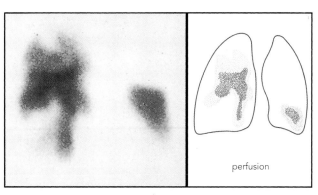

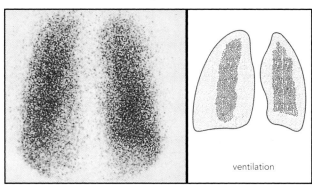

Fig. 5.20 Perfusion (upper) and ventilation (lower) scans in pulmonary emboli. Note the multiple perfusion defects but the normal ventilation pattern.

homogeneity in the distribution of blood and air at alveolar level. Both mechanisms are important in lung fibrosis.

The TF will naturally be reduced if the lungs are small or if one has been removed (pneumonectomy). The transfer coefficient (KCO or D_LCO divided by alveolar volume, calculated separately) is a more useful measurement because it reflects the true situation in the ventilated lung.

LUNG VOLUMES IN DISEASE

In summary, it is possible to distinguish two main patterns of abnormal lung function. An 'obstructive pattern' is seen in asthma, chronic obstructive bronchitis and emphysema. FVC, FEV_1 and FEV_1% are all reduced and RV increased; TLC is often reduced but high in emphysema. TF is low in emphysema but otherwise normal. A 'restrictive pattern' is seen in lung fibrosis, such as occurs in cryptogenic fibrosing alveolitis. TLC, VC, FEV_1, RV and TF are all reduced but FEV_1% is normal or high.

When other results do not give a clear pattern, RV can be very helpful, being high in airways obstruction and low in fibrosis.

DISTRIBUTION OF VENTILATION AND PERFUSION

Distribution of air within the lung is best assessed for clinical purposes by radioactive isotopes. The usual tracer gas is radioactive xenon. The measurement of radioactivity over the lung gives a measure of the distribution and also the rate at which gas enters and leaves various parts of the lung. Thus, it can be used to detect 'air trapping' or absence of ventilation. Perfusion of blood can be measured in a similar way, usually by microaggregates of albumin

labelled with technetium-99m, and injected into a peripheral vein. These microaggregates form small emboli within the lung and the radioactivity they give off is a measure of blood distribution. These tests are most useful in the diagnosis of pulmonary embolism when perfusion to an area of lung is reduced but ventilation is maintained (Fig. 5.20). If both ventilation and perfusion are reduced, then the defect probably lies within the airways and is a failure of ventilation with secondary changes in the blood supply.

BLOOD GASES

Blood gases can be measured directly by electrodes in blood obtained by arterial puncture. The results are expressed as partial pressure of gas in the plasma (P_{O_2} and P_{CO_2}). It is important to realise that this is not the same as the amount of gas carried by the blood. If all the red cells were removed, the P_{O_2} would be unchanged, yet the patient would be in a perilous state. The haemoglobin in the red cell packages and transports oxygen and carbon dioxide just as a subway train packages and transports passengers.

The relationship between P_{O_2} and saturation of the haemoglobin by oxygen (and hence the volume of oxygen carried) is given by the oxygen dissociation curve (Fig. 5.21). It will be seen that the P_{O_2} can drop significantly before there is a drop in the saturation, clearly a good thing in the early stages of lung disease. Nevertheless, it

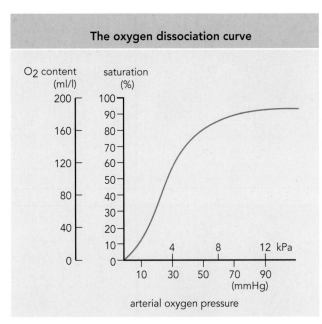

Fig. 5.21 Oxygen dissociation curve relating the partial pressure of oxygen in the blood to saturation of haemoglobin and amount of oxygen carried (assuming haemoglobin is normal).

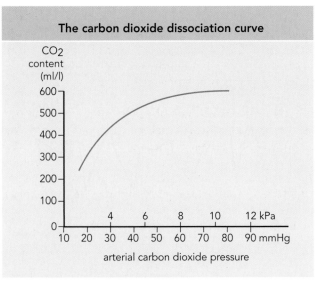

Fig. 5.22 Carbon dioxide dissociation curve relating partial pressure of gas in the blood to amount carried.

means that overventilation of the lung's good parts cannot fully compensate for underventilation of bad parts because the good parts on the flat part of the curve cannot increase the carriage of oxygen in the blood supplied to them beyond a certain maximum. Thus, when there is a shunt of blood from the right to the left heart, either directly through the heart or through unventilated lung, the total amount of oxygen carried is bound to be reduced and cannot be restored to normal either by increasing ventilation or administering oxygen.

The steep part of the curve indicates that a small increase in inspired oxygen gives a large increase in the amount of oxygen carried – clearly useful for oxygen therapy in sick patients. It also indicates how readily hypoxic tissues can remove large amounts of oxygen from the blood.

The dissociation curve for carbon dioxide is very different to that for oxygen; lowering the P_{CO_2} continuously lowers the saturation and hence the volume of gas carried (Fig. 5.22). This means that overventilation in one part of the lung can compensate for underventilation elsewhere. Arterial P_{CO_2} is a good measure of overall alveolar ventilation, being increased in alveolar hypoventilation (e.g. severe chronic airflow limitation) and decreased in alveolar hyperventilation (e.g. anxiety states, heart failure, pulmonary embolus, asthma), in which hypoxia and other factors stimulate an increase in ventilation.

The lungs help to regulate the acid–base balance by their ability to excrete or to retain carbon dioxide. In cases of metabolic acidosis (e.g. diabetic ketoacidosis, renal failure), the lungs can 'blow off' carbon dioxide to restore the pH towards normal. In cases of metabolic alkalosis (e.g. prolonged vomiting with loss of acid from the stomach), the retention of carbon dioxide again restores

the pH towards normal. Retention or secretion of carbon dioxide as a result of lung disease (respiratory acidosis and alkalosis) alters pH, which is then secondarily restored by excretion or retention of bicarbonate by the kidney. Thus, changes in arterial P_{CO_2} (whether primary or secondary) can be regarded as functions of the lung, and changes in bicarbonate (again, either primary or secondary) can be regarded as functions of the kidney.

Symptoms of respiratory disease

History-taking must follow the principles outlined earlier. Here, we are concerned with the analysis of the main symptoms of respiratory disease in turn. These are dyspnoea, cough, sputum, haemoptysis, pain and wheeze.

Questions to ask

Essential questions

- Do you get short of breath?
  - how much can you do?
- Do you have a cough?
  - do you cough anything up?
  - what colour is it?
  - is there any blood?
- Do you have any (chest) pain?
  - where is it?
  - does it hurt to breathe?
- Do you wheeze?
  - does it come and go or is it there all the time?

DYSPNOEA

Most lung diseases will cause dyspnoea or difficulty in breathing. Patients will express this in different ways as 'shortness of breath', 'shortwindedness', 'can't get my breath' or in terms of functional disability ('can't do the housework').

Some patients will talk about 'tightness'. It may not be immediately clear whether they are describing breathlessness or pain. If the complaint is really a pain then this may well be angina, which is in itself sometimes associated with breathlessness. If asked directly, patients can usually tell you whether their tightness means pain or breathlessness. Some patients with pleuritic pain complain of breathlessness, but what they really mean

Questions to ask

Dyspnoea

- Is the breathlessness recent or has it been present for some time?
- Is it constant or does it come and go?
- What can't you do because of the breathlessness?
- What makes the breathing worse?
- Does anything make it better?

Differential diagnosis

Some causes of breathlessness

Control and movement of the chest wall and pleura
- Hyperventilation syndrome
- Hypothalamic lesions
- Neuromuscular disease
- Kyphoscoliosis
- Ankylosing spondylitis
- Pleural effusion and thickening
- Bilateral diaphragm paralysis

Diseases of the lungs
- Airways disease
    - chronic bronchitis and emphysema
    - asthma
    - bronchiectasis
    - cystic fibrosis
- Parenchymal disease
    - pneumonia
    - cryptogenic fibrosing alveolitis
    - extrinsic allergic alveolitis
    - primary and secondary tumour
    - sarcoidosis
    - pneumothorax
    - pulmonary oedema
- Blood supply
    - pulmonary embolism
    - anaemia

Differential diagnosis

Duration of breathlessness

Immediate (minutes)
- Pulmonary embolism
- Pneumothorax
- Pulmonary oedema
- Asthma

Short (hours to days)
- Pulmonary oedema
- Pneumonia
- Asthma
- Pleural effusion
- Anaemia

Long (weeks to years)
- Chronic airflow limitation
- Cryptogenic fibrosing alveolitis
- Extrinsic allergic alveolitis
- Anaemia

is that they are unable to take a deep breath because of pain. It is of interest to consider why patients complain of breathlessness. Most normal people do not regard themselves as ill when they are short of breath, say when running for a bus. It seems probable that the sensations reported by patients are the same as the rest of us but they recognise that the work the lungs are being asked to do is disproportionate to the task the body is performing, that is, it feels inappropriate.

Causes of breathlessness

The causes of breathlessness may be listed as those to do with the control and movement of the chest wall, lung disease itself and problems with the blood and its supply to the lungs. The control of breathing can start with psychological factors in the brain, problems with the control centre in the medulla (rare) and the increased effort needed to overcome the effects of spinal cord disease (trauma or degeneration), neuropathies (e.g. Guillain–Barré syndrome), myopathies and chest wall problems (e.g. kyphoscoliosis, ankylosing spondylitis).

Lung diseases may require more work to overcome obstruction to airflow (e.g. chronic obstructive bronchitis, emphysema, asthma) or to stretch stiff lungs (e.g. pulmonary oedema, lung fibrosis).

Hypoxia needs to be severe to stimulate respiration but may be the mechanism in pneumonia, severe heart failure and other causes of pulmonary oedema. Pulmonary embolism leads to wasted ventilation in the affected area. Severe anaemia reduces the oxygen-carrying capacity of the blood.

J receptors are vagal nerve endings and are adjacent to pulmonary capillaries. Stimulation of these by pulmonary oedema, fibrosis and lung irritants is an additional mechanism causing breathlessness.

Duration of dyspnoea

The duration of dyspnoea may give a clue to the cause and can conveniently be divided into immediate (over minutes), short (hours to days) and long (weeks to years). There is some overlap but contrast, for example, the patient with a large pulmonary embolism who collapses in minutes in acute distress compared with the progressive relentless disability extending over a decade in the patient with smoking-related airflow limitation. Some patients find it difficult to remember duration accurately. Many report symptoms as lasting for only 'a few weeks' when they mean 'worse for a few weeks'. A question like 'When could you last run for a bus?' may reveal problems stretching back for years. A spouse is often more accurate in this respect than the patient.

Variability of dyspnoea

Questions about variability can be couched as 'Does it come and go or is it much the same?' or 'Do you have good days and bad days or is it much the same from one day to another?'. A reply suggesting variability is highly characteristic of variable airflow limitation, that is, asthma. If asthma is suspected, this can be followed-up by questions on aggravating factors. Follow this up with some more directed questions about particular factors. These are important not only as potentially preventable causes but because positive replies strengthen the diagnosis. The house dust mite is the most common allergen; patients will report worsening of symptoms on sweeping, dusting or making the beds. Exercise, at least in children, is a potent trigger of asthma but exercise will also make other forms of breathlessness worse. The difference is that in asthma the attack is caused by the exercise, may indeed follow it and may last for 30 min or more. In other causes of breathlessness, recovery starts as soon as exercise stops.

Asthma

Asthma due solely to emotional causes probably does not exist; nonetheless, most patients who have asthma are worse if emotionally upset. Patients may feel that admitting to stress is respectable when they would deny other emotions. Nocturnal asthma is very common. Few asthmatics smoke because they know it makes them worse. Ask what happens if they go into a smoky room. Many will say they are unable to do so because of the effects of the smoke. The response to household aerosol sprays can be helpful. Many breathless patients with a variety of illnesses will think it logical, rightly or wrongly, that 'dust' or 'fumes' will make them worse but only true asthmatics seem to notice a deterioration with the ubiquitous domestic spray can.

Questions to ask

Asthma

- Does anything make any difference to the asthma?
- What happens if you are worried or upset?
- Does your chest wake you at night?
- Does cigarette smoke make any difference?
- Do household sprays affect you?
- What happens when sweeping or dusting the house?
- Does exposure to cats or dogs make any difference?
- Have you lost time from work/school?

Symptoms and signs

Allergic and nonallergic factors in asthma

Allergic
- House dust mite
- Animals (especially cats)
- Pollens (especially grass)

Nonallergic
- Exercise
- Emotion
- Sleep
- Smoke
- Aerosol sprays
- Cold air
- Upper respiratory tract infections

Severity of dyspnoea

Severity can be assessed by rating scales, although it is much better to use some functional measure. Ask the patient in what way their breathlessness restricts their activities: can they go upstairs, go shopping, wash the car or do the garden? If they are troubled with stairs, how many flights can they manage? Do they stop half way up or at the top? Questions about gardening are useful, at least in the summer, as it is possible to grade activity from pulling out a few weeds to digging the potato patch. It is important to be certain that any restriction is caused by breathlessness and not some other disability (e.g. an arthritic hip or angina).

Orthopnoea and paroxysmal nocturnal dyspnoea

Orthopnoea and paroxysmal nocturnal dyspnoea need special consideration. Both are usually regarded as manifestations of left ventricular failure, yet this is an oversimplification. Orthopnoea is defined as breathlessness lying flat but relieved by sitting up. It is common in patients with severe fixed airways obstruction, as in some chronic bronchitics who may admit to not having slept flat for years. Normal people, when they lie flat, breathe more with the diaphragm and less with the chest wall. In patients with airways obstruction, the diaphragm is often flat and inefficient and may even draw the ribs inwards rather than out. Thus, when they lie down the diaphragm cannot provide the ventilation required.

The term paroxysmal nocturnal dyspnoea is self-explanatory and is a feature of pulmonary oedema from left ventricular failure. However, many asthmatics develop bronchoconstriction in the night and wake with wheeze and breathlessness very similar to the symptoms of left ventricular failure. In contrast, patients with severe fixed flow limitation usually sleep well even if they do have to be propped up.

The hyperventilation syndrome

The hyperventilation syndrome is more common than is generally realised but produces a distinct pattern of symptoms. It is usually associated with anxiety and patients overbreathe inappropriately. The initial complaint is often, although not always, of breathlessness. The hyperventilation is the response to this sensation. It may be described by the patient as a 'difficulty in breathing in' or an inability to 'fill the bottom of the lungs'. The hyperventilation induces a reduction in the $P\text{CO}_2$, creating a variety of other symptoms: paraesthesiae in the fingers, tingling around the lips, 'dizziness', 'lightheadedness' and sometimes frank tetany. Chest pain is the probable consequence of increased chest wall movement. The onset is often triggered by some life event; especially work related (e.g. redundancy or dismissal). The diagnosis can be confirmed by asking the patient to take 20 deep breaths, which will reproduce the symptoms.

Symptoms and signs

Features suggestive of the hyperventilation syndrome

- Breathlessness at rest
- Breathlessness as severe with mild exertion as with greater exertion
- Marked variability in breathlessness
- More difficulty breathing in than out
- Paraesthesiae of the fingers
- Numbness around the mouth
- 'Lightheadedness'
- Feelings of impending collapse or remoteness from surroundings
- Chest wall pain

Dyspnoea and hypoxia

Dyspnoea should be distinguished from tachypnoea (increased rate of breathing) and from hypoxia. It is a symptom, not a sign, and is not necessarily an indication of lung disease. Psychological factors, such as the hyperventilation syndrome, and acidosis from diabetic ketosis or renal failure may produce tachypnoea which may be felt as dyspnoea. Many patients think that if they are short of breath, they must be short of oxygen. This is sometimes the case but, as mentioned earlier, hypoxia only stimulates respiration when relatively severe. To illustrate the distinction between hypoxia and dyspnoea, consider that many patients with airflow limitation from chronic bronchitis have hypoxia severe enough to cause right-sided heart failure, yet they have relatively little dyspnoea (blue bloaters). In contrast, some patients with emphysema seem to need to keep their blood gases normal by a heroic effort of breathing (pink puffers); they are very dyspnoeic.

COUGH

Cough arises from the cough receptors in the pharynx, larynx and bronchi; it, therefore, results from irritation of these receptors from infection, inflammation, tumour or foreign body. Cough may be the only symptom in asthma, particularly childhood asthma. Cough in children occurring regularly after exercise or at night is virtually diagnostic of asthma. Many smokers regard cough as normal: 'only a smoker's cough' or may deny it completely despite having just coughed in front of the examiner. In these patients, a change in the character of the cough can be highly significant.

Patients can often localise cough to above the larynx ('a tickle in the throat') or below. Postnasal drip from rhinitis can cause the former and may be accompanied by sneezing and nasal blockage.

Laryngitis will cause both cough and a hoarse voice. Recurrent laryngeal nerve palsy causes a hoarse voice and an ineffective cough because the cord is immobile. The usual cause is involvement of the left recurrent laryngeal nerve by tumour in its course in the chest. Cough from tracheitis is usually dry and painful. Cough from further down the airways is often associated with sputum production (bronchitis, bronchiectasis or pneumonia). In the latter, associated pleurisy makes coughing very distressing and reduces its effectiveness. Other possibilities are carcinoma, lung fibrosis and increased bronchial responsiveness (this is an inflammatory condition of the airways, thought to be part of the mechanism underlying asthma and often made worse by the factors listed in the 'symptoms and signs' box on allergic and nonallergic factors in asthma). A cause of cough, which is often overlooked, is aspiration into the lungs from gastro-oesophageal reflux or a pharyngeal pouch. Cough will then follow meals or lying down. Prolonged coughing bouts can cause both unconsciousness from reduction of venous return from the brain (cough syncope) and also vomiting. Sometimes the history of cough is omitted, making diagnosis difficult!

SPUTUM

Patients may understand the term 'phlegm' better than sputum. It is the result of excessive bronchial secretion;

itself a manifestation of inflammation and infection. Like cough, smokers may not acknowledge its existence. Children usually swallow their sputum. It is essential to be certain that the complaint relates to the chest, because some patients have difficulty in distinguishing sputum production from gastrointestinal reflux, postnasal drip or saliva. Sometimes asking the patient to 'show me what you have to do to get phlegm up' can be helpful. If the patient denies sputum, a cough producing a rattle (a 'loose cough') suggests that it is present.

Sputum caused by chronic irritation is usually white or grey, particularly in smokers; if infected, it becomes yellow from the presence of leucocytes and this may turn to green by the action of the enzyme verdoperoxidase. Yellow or green sputum in asthma can be caused by the presence of eosinophils rather than infection. Questions on frequency are most useful in the diagnosis of chronic bronchitis, an epidemiological definition of this is 'sputum production on most days for three consecutive months for two successive years'. Sputum production is common in asthmatics and is occasionally the main complaint. The diagnosis of bronchiectasis is made on a story of daily sputum production stretching back to childhood.

Patients can often give an estimate of the amount of sputum they bring up each day, usually in terms of a cup or teaspoon and so on. Large amounts occur in bronchiectasis and lung abscess and in the rare bronchioloalveolar cell carcinoma.

Sticky 'rusty' sputum is characteristic of lobar pneumonia, and frothy sputum with streaks of blood is seen in pulmonary oedema.

Highly viscous sputum, sometimes with plugs, is characteristic of asthma and in some patients with chronic bronchitis. Small bronchial casts, like twigs, may be described by a patient with the condition of bronchopulmonary aspergillosis associated with asthma.

HAEMOPTYSIS

The coughing up of blood is often a sign of serious lung disease. Nevertheless, it is common in trivial respiratory infections. Like sputum production, it is essential to establish that it is coming from the lungs and not the nose or mouth or being vomited (haematemesis). Bleeding from the nose may run into the pharynx and be coughed out but usually the patient will also describe bleeding from the anterior nares. Bleeding in the mouth causes confusion, it is usually related to brushing the teeth (gingivitis).

The blood in haemoptysis is usually bright red at first, then followed by progressively smaller and darker amounts. This would be unusual in haematemesis.

Differential diagnosis
Haemoptysis

Common
- Infection including bronchiectasis
- Bronchial carcinoma
- Tuberculosis
- Pulmonary embolism and infarction
- No cause found

Uncommon
- Mitral stenosis and left ventricular failure
- Bronchial adenoma
- Idiopathic pulmonary haemosiderosis
- Anticoagulation and blood dyscrasias

Differential diagnosis
Pointers to the significance of an episode of haemoptysis

Probably serious
- Middle-aged or elderly
- Spontaneous
- Previous or current smoker
- Recurrent
- Large amount

Probably not serious
- Young
- Recent infection
- Never smoked
- Single episode
- Small amount – if single episode

Differential diagnosis
Sputum

White or grey
- Smoking
- Simple chronic bronchitis
- Asthma

Yellow or green
- Acute bronchitis
- Acute on chronic bronchitis
- Asthma
- Bronchiectasis
- Cystic fibrosis

Frothy, blood-streaked
- Pulmonary oedema

Questions to ask
Sputum

- What colour is the phlegm?
- How often do you bring it up?
- How much do you bring up?
- Do you have trouble getting it up?

All haemoptysis is potentially serious, although the most important cause is carcinoma of the bronchus. Repeated small haemoptyses every few days over a period of some weeks in a middle-aged smoker is virtually diagnostic of bronchial carcinoma.

Other serious causes are pulmonary embolism (sudden onset of pleuritic chest pain and dyspnoea followed by haemoptysis), tuberculosis (weight loss, fever, cough and sputum) and bronchiectasis (long history of sputum production and the haemoptysis associated with an exacerbation and increased sputum purulence). Blood-tinged sputum in pneumonia and pulmonary oedema has already been mentioned.

| **Risk factors** |
| **Pulmonary embolism** |

- Previous DVT or PE
- Surgery
- Immobility, especially stroke and heart failure
- Malignancy
- Pregnancy
- Leg trauma
- Haematological abnormalities

PAIN

The lungs and the visceral pleura are devoid of pain fibres, whereas the parietal pleura, chest wall and mediastinal structures are not. The characteristic 'pleuritic pain' is sharp, stabbing, worse on deep breathing and coughing and arises from either pleural inflammation or chest wall lesions. Pain from the pleura is caused by the two pleural surfaces rubbing together. The pain may interfere with breathing: 'I have to catch my breath'. Inflammation of the pleura occurs chiefly in pneumonia and pulmonary infarction from pulmonary emboli. Pneumothorax can produce acute transient pleuritic pain.

Most pains from the chest wall are caused by localised muscle strain or rib fractures (persistent cough can cause the latter). These pains are often worse on twisting or turning or rolling over in bed; an uncommon feature of other disease. Bornholm disease is thought to be a viral infection of the intercostal muscles and produces very severe pain. True pleuritic pain is often accompanied by a pleural rub; this is absent in chest wall pain but there may be striking local rib tenderness reproducing the symptoms. Unfortunately, this is not entirely reliable, for pleurisy can be associated with local tenderness. A particular type of chest wall pain is caused by swelling of one or more of the upper costal cartilages (Tietze's syndrome); however, this is rare and it is much more common to find tenderness without swelling. Severe constant pain not related to breathing but interfering

with sleep usually indicates malignant disease involving the chest wall. Moreover, spinal disease and herpes zoster may cause pain in a root distribution round the chest.

Pleural pain is usually localised accurately by the patient, yet if the pleura overlying the diaphragm is involved pain may be referred either to the abdomen from the costal part of the diaphragm or to the tip of the shoulder from the central part because the pain fibres run in the phrenic nerve (C3–5). Pain may subside when an effusion develops.

Although the lungs are insensitive to pain, the mediastinal structures are not. Cancer of the lung and other central lesions produce a dull, poorly localised pain – presumably from pressure on mediastinal structures.

A third type of pain is a central soreness over the trachea in acute tracheitis.

WHEEZE AND STRIDOR

Wheeze

Most patients will understand wheeze as a high-pitched whistling sound, although some require a demonstration by the doctor before they recognise it. It occurs in both inspiration and expiration but is always louder in the latter. Spouses sometimes pick this up better than patients, particularly if the wheeze is mainly at night. It implies airway narrowing and is, therefore, common in asthma and chronic obstructive bronchitis. In asthma, the wheeze is episodic and clearly associated with shortness of breath, fulfilling the definition of 'variable wheezy breathlessness'. Nevertheless, some asthmatics may have little wheeze and acute severe attacks can be associated with a 'silent chest'. In chronic obstructive bronchitis and emphysema, the associations are less clear-cut, with wheeze, shortness of breath, cough and sputum occurring in various proportions.

Stridor

Stridor is a harsh inspiratory and expiratory noise which can be imitated by adducting the vocal cords and breathing in and out. It is often more evident to the observer than the patient.

OTHER IMPORTANT POINTS IN THE HISTORY

Other body systems

The lungs do not exist in isolation from the rest of the body. Lung disease can affect other structures, and disease elsewhere can affect the lungs. The closest relationships are naturally with the heart. Lung disease can affect the right side of the heart (cor pulmonale). An early manifestation is peripheral oedema (ankle swelling), which is likely to be accompanied by a raised jugular venous pressure and an enlarged liver. Disease of the left heart causes pulmonary oedema (orthopnoea, paroxysmal nocturnal dyspnoea, cough and frothy sputum). Diseases of other systems that affect the lungs include rheumatoid arthritis, other connective tissue disease (scleroderma and dermatomyositis), immune deficiency syndromes (including AIDS) and renal failure. A variety of neuromuscular diseases and skeletal problems affect the mechanics of breathing.

Weight loss is an important manifestation of lung carcinoma, although by the time it occurs there are usually metastatic deposits in the liver. Less well known as a cause is chronic airflow limitation, presumably from the increased respiratory effort impairing appetite and diverting calories to the respiratory muscles. Chronic infection, particularly tuberculosis, causes weight loss. Gain in weight may be a cause of increased dyspnoea and sleep apnoea (see below). One cause is steroid therapy for lung disease (iatrogenic Cushing's syndrome).

Fever must be distinguished from feeling hot or sweating and generally implies infection, particularly pneumonia or tuberculosis. Less commonly, it is caused by malignancy or connective tissue disease affecting the lungs. If pulmonary embolism is suspected, pain or swelling in the legs suggests a deep venous thrombosis.

Sleep

Sleep disturbance may be caused by pain, breathlessness and cough from airways obstruction or from depression. In the sleep apnoea syndrome, patients are aroused repeatedly in the night from obstruction of the upper airways. The cause is not always clear but obesity is very common and hypertrophied tonsils often contribute. Sudden obstruction leads to greater and greater inspiratory efforts by the patient who, in a half-awake state, will thrash around and eventually overcome the obstruction to the accompaniment of loud snoring noises. This may be repeated many times during the night. Wives (the patients are usually men) will describe this in graphic detail! The poor quality of sleep leads to daytime somnolence and the carbon dioxide retention to morning headaches.

Many diseases of the respiratory system produce lasting disability and some are fatal. Therefore, depression and anxiety are to be expected and may influence the history.

Symptoms and signs

Clinical features suggesting the sleep apnoea syndrome

- Excessive daytime somnolence
- Intellectual deterioration and irritability
- Early morning headaches
- Snoring
- Restless nights
- Social deterioration (e.g. job, marriage, driving difficulties)

PREVIOUS DISEASE

A history of tuberculosis may explain abnormal shadowing on a chest radiograph. Current symptoms may be caused by relapse, especially if the patient was treated before the start of the antibiotic era (1950). Some operations for tuberculosis from those days (thoracoplasty and phrenic crush) produce lifelong chest or radiographic deformity. Bronchial damage from tuberculosis can lead to bronchiectasis.

BCG vaccination reduces the risk of tuberculosis but one degree of protection is disputed. In some areas in the UK it is performed at school at the age of 12 or 13 years. Babies born to immigrant mothers often receive it at birth. For children, tuberculin testing to assess sensitivity is performed first. A history of these procedures helps in the assessment of a possible case of tuberculosis.

A history of wheeze in childhood suggests asthma. This may have gone into remission and been forgotten only to occur in later life. Whooping cough or pneumonia in childhood may lead to bronchiectasis and patients may have been told by their parents that their problems started with such an episode.

Chest injuries, operations or pneumonia can all lead to permanent radiographic changes which otherwise would be very difficult to explain. Previous radiographs can be invaluable in these circumstances and may be available. 'Health checks' may have included chest radiography. Many patients will have had chest radiography before an operation.

SOCIAL HISTORY

Smoking

The importance of enquiry about smoking in lung disease can hardly be overemphasised (Figs 5.23, 5.24). Smoking is, for practical purposes, the cause of chronic bronchitis and carcinoma of the bronchus and neither diagnosis is likely to be correct in a lifelong nonsmoker. Patients seem to be generally accurate about their tobacco consumption contrasting sometimes with alcohol.

It is important not to appear censorious when enquiring about smoking. Tobacco is highly addictive and most patients would give up if only they could and are not being perverse when they continue despite evidence of lung damage. You should be aware that some patients claim to be nonsmokers when they only stopped last month, last week or even on the way to hospital! Ask nonsmokers: 'Have you smoked in the past?'. The risk of disease increases with the amount smoked. Cigarettes are the most dangerous; pipes and cigars are not free of risk. Risk declines steadily when smoking stops; it takes 10–20 years for the risk of lung cancer to equal that of lifelong nonsmokers.

Inhalation of another person's smoke at home or at work is increasingly recognised as a factor in lung disease. This is particularly true for asthma. Children in households with smokers have more respiratory infections.

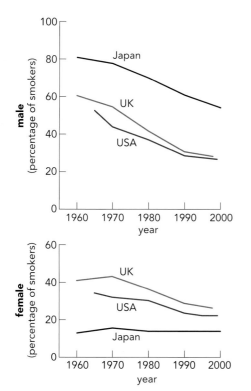

Fig. 5.23 Smoking trends in selected countries, based on data from the World Heath Organization.

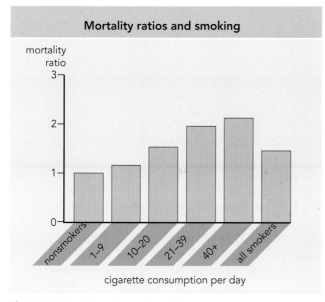

Fig. 5.24 Mortality ratios and smoking.

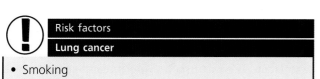

Risk factors

Lung cancer

- Smoking
- Atmospheric pollution
- Asbestos exposure
- Radon exposure (natural and occupational)
- Work in gas and coke industry

Pets and hobbies

For many asthmatics, cats and dogs are common sources of allergen. The allergen may remain in the house long after the offending animal has been banished.

Exposure to racing pigeons, budgerigars, parrots and other caged birds can cause extrinsic allergic alveolitis. The cause is protein material derived from feathers and droppings. Acute symptoms are usually seen in pigeon fanciers who, a few hours after cleaning out their birds, develop cough, breathlessness and 'flu-like' symptoms. Recovery takes place over the next day or two unless there is re-exposure. Chronic symptoms are seen in budgerigar owners, presumably because they are exposed continuously to low doses of antigen. Their complaint is of progressive breathlessness.

Parrots and related species transmit the infectious agent of psittacosis, a cause of pneumonia. You may need to extend your enquires beyond the home because patients may be exposed to birds belonging to friends and relations.

Occupation

The question 'What work do you do?' is more important for respiratory disease than for any other. The nature of the job and not just the title is important because the latter may convey no meaning to you at all. The question is important in two ways. Respiratory disease may affect a patient's ability to perform a job but may also be the result of the occupation. Any job involving exposure to noxious agents of a respirable size is potentially damaging; the most obvious example is pneumoconiosis in coal miners.

Risk factors

Some occupational causes of lung disease

Occupation	Agent	Disease
Mining	Coal dust	Pneumoconiosis
Quarrying	Silica dust	Silicosis
Foundry work	Silica dust	Silicosis
Asbestos (mining, heating, building, demolition, ship building)	Asbestos fibres	Asbestosis Mesothelioma Lung cancer
Farming	Actinomycetes	Alveolitis
Paint spraying	Isocyanates	Asthma
Plastics manufacture	Isocyanates	Asthma
Soldering	Colophony	Asthma

Enquiry may need to be searching and, if occupational lung disease is suspected, then a full list of all jobs performed will need to be constructed. For example, in the case of asbestos there can be an interval of 30 years between exposure, say in shipyard work, and the development of asbestosis or mesothelioma. Some will deny working with asbestos but nevertheless were exposed when others were performing lagging (putting asbestos on pipes) or stripping (taking it off). Other occupations in which exposure may not be obvious, although real nonetheless, are building and demolition work, electrical repair work, railway engineering and gas mask and cement manufacture. Environmental exposure, including that of wives of asbestos workers, seems important occasionally.

The easiest way to diagnose pneumoconiosis is to ask the patient. Miners in the UK undergo regular chest radiography while working. If significant pneumoconiosis is diagnosed the patient will be told.

Occupational asthma

The list of causes of occupational asthma grows longer yearly. A good screening question to any asthmatic is: 'Does your work make any difference to your symptoms?'. Follow this up with questions about improvement at weekends or on holiday. The latter is important because symptoms caused at work may not be manifest until the evening or night and sometimes changes take place over days or even weeks.

Common causes are isocyanates (paint hardeners and plastic manufacture) and colophony (soldering and electronics). The lack of an obvious culprit should not put you off the scent if the evidence is otherwise suggestive. Much detective work is necessary in individual cases.

Extrinsic allergic alveolitis

Extrinsic allergic alveolitis can be caused by occupation as well as by exposure to birds. The best example is farmer's lung: the agent is the microorganism thermophilic actinomycetes contaminating stored damp hay. The story is of shortness of breath, cough and chills a few hours after forking out fodder for cattle in the winter. Other occupations with similar risks are mushroom workers, sugar workers (bagassosis – mouldy sugar cane), maltworkers and woodworkers, although the antigens vary in each case.

FAMILY HISTORY

The most common lung disease with a genetic basis is asthma, although the development of the disease in an individual is much more complicated. A family history of asthma and the related conditions of hay fever or eczema are often found but these diseases are so prevalent that enquiry beyond the immediate family is of little value. Other diseases that run in the family include cystic fibrosis and α_1-antitrypsin deficiency, a rare cause of emphysema.

Tuberculosis is usually passed on within families. In the UK, tuberculosis is common in Asian and African migrants, particularly in their first 10 years in the country, and in individuals who have revisited the subcontinent. Most of the increased incidence of the disease seen in recent years has occurred in conditions of poverty.

Enquiry into sexual habits will be necessary if the illness could be a manifestation of AIDS, remembering that this is now becoming more common in the heterosexual population, especially in individuals who have travelled abroad, particularly to Africa and Asia.

DRUG HISTORY

The most useful questions are those concerning past treatment. Successful use of bronchodilators and corticoids in airways obstruction will indicate asthma. Aspirin and sometimes other nonsteroidal anti-inflammatory drugs and β-adrenergic receptor blockers can make asthma worse, and angiotensin-converting enzyme inhibitors cause chronic dry cough. Steroid therapy predisposes to infections, including tuberculosis.

PATIENT PERSPECTIVE

Many lung conditions are chronic and most of these are progressive. It is therefore particularly important to understand patients' reactions to the prospect of increasing disability and sometimes death. Ask about patients' hopes and fears for the future and how the disease is affecting their lives and that of their families.

General examination

Examination starts on first encounter. You should be able to continually pick up and store clues while talking and listening to the patient. As with all body systems, a good look at the patient as a whole will provide important evidence that will be missed in a rush to lay a stethoscope on the chest. Your findings should be divided into first impressions, then a more directed search for signs outside the chest likely to be helpful in lung disease and, finally, examination of the chest itself.

There are a number of circumstances when the examination may have to be focused on particular areas rather than attempting a comprehensive examination. This may be because the patient is too unwell or because the history only requires a specific confirmatory sign, say the presence or absence of wheeze. It may be difficult to undress some patients fully, particularly in primary care.

FIRST IMPRESSIONS

How breathless does the patient appear? Is it consistent with the story? If seen in the clinic or office, can the patient walk in comfortably and sit down or does the patient struggle to get in? Perhaps the patient is in a wheelchair; if so, is it because of breathing troubles or something else? Can the patient carry on a conversation with you or do they break up their sentences? How breathless is the patient when getting undressed? Details of breathing patterns are considered later but is the patient obviously distressed or quite comfortable? Is there stridor or wheeze? Is there cough, confirming or perhaps at variance with the history? Is there evidence of weight loss suggesting carcinoma or weight gain from steroid therapy?

Do not ignore clues around the patient. An air compressor by the bed will be used to deliver bronchodilator drugs. A packet of cigarettes in the pyjama jacket will have the opposite effect. In hospital you will be deprived of some of these features but not how the patient is positioned – does the patient have to sit up to breathe (confirming a history of orthopnoea)? Is the patient receiving oxygen?

After extracting as much information as you can, if it is feasible and appropriate position the patient comfortably on the bed or couch with enough pillows to support the chest at an angle of approximately 45° and begin the formal examination. This can conveniently start with the hands and a search for clubbing.

Clubbing

This refers to an increase in the soft tissues of the nail bed and the finger tip. The earliest stage is some softening of the nail bed which can be detected by rocking the nail from side to side on the nail bed (Fig. 5.25). This sign can be present to some extent in normal individuals but is exaggerated in the early stages of clubbing. Next, the soft tissue of the nail bed fills in the normal obtuse angle between the nail and the nail bed. This is usually approximately 160° but the area becomes flat, even convex in clubbing (Fig. 5.26). This is seen best by viewing

the nail from the side against a white background, say the bedsheets. Not surprisingly, there can be considerable disagreement about the presence or absence of clubbing in the early stages. When normal nails are placed 'back to back' there is usually a diamond-shaped area between them. This is obliterated early in clubbing (Fig. 5.27).

In the next stage, the normal longitudinal curvature of the nail increases. Some normal nails have a pronounced curve but in clubbing the increase in soft tissue in the nail beds needs to be present as well. In the final stage, the whole tip of the finger becomes rounded (a club) (Fig. 5.28). Clubbing less commonly affects the toes.

The pathogenesis of clubbing is unknown. There is increased vascularity and tissue fluid and this seems to be under neurogenic control because it can be abolished by vagotomy.

Clubbing is sometimes associated with hypertrophic pulmonary osteoarthropathy; this presents with pain in the joints – particularly the wrists, ankles and knees. The pain is not in the joint itself but over the shafts of the long bones adjacent to the joint. It is caused by subperiosteal new bone formation, which can be seen on a radiograph (Fig. 5.29). The condition is almost invariably associated with clubbing, although it can occur alone. Any cause of clubbing can also cause hypertrophic pulmonary osteoarthropathy; however, it is usually associated with a squamous carcinoma of the bronchus. The condition is often mistaken for arthritis, with consequent delay in diagnosis. Successful treatment

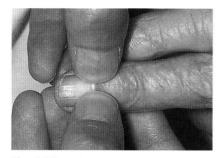

Fig. 5.25 Rocking the nail on the nail bed in clubbing.

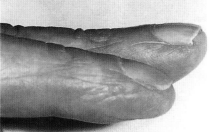

Fig. 5.26 Mild clubbing. The nail on the left shows obliteration of the angle at the nail fold compared with a normal nail on the right.

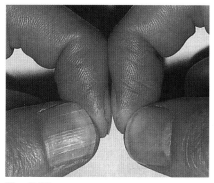

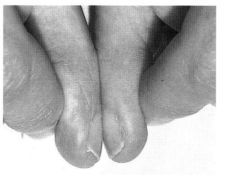

Fig. 5.27 Clubbing, showing how the diamond-shaped area formed between two normal nails (left) is obliterated (right).

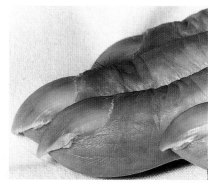

Fig. 5.28 Gross clubbing.

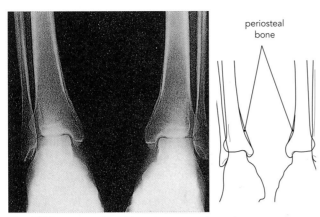

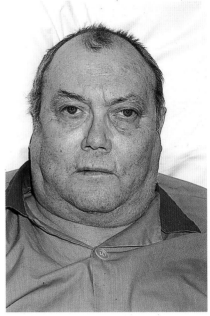

Fig. 5.29 Hypertrophic pulmonary osteoarthropathy.

periosteal bone

Differential diagnosis

Some common causes of clubbing

Pulmonary
- Bronchial carcinoma
- Chronic pulmonary sepsis
  - empyema
  - lung abscess
  - bronchiectasis
  - cystic fibrosis
- Cryptogenic fibrosing alveolitis
- Asbestosis

Cardiac
- Congenital cyanotic heart disease
- Bacterial endocarditis

Other
- Idiopathic/familial
- Cirrhosis
- Ulcerative colitis
- Coeliac disease
- Crohn's disease

Fig. 5.30 Cyanosis in a patient with chronic airflow limitation.

of the cause will relieve clubbing and the pain of hypertrophic pulmonary osteoarthropathy. While searching for clubbing, note any nicotine staining of the fingers.

Cyanosis

Cyanosis, a bluish tinge to the skin and mucous membranes, is seen when there is an increased amount of reduced haemoglobin in the blood (Fig. 5.30). Traditionally, it is thought to become visible when there is approximately 5 g/dl or more of reduced haemoglobin, corresponding to a saturation of approximately 85%; however, there is a good deal of interobserver variation. Severe anaemia and cyanosis cannot coexist otherwise most of the haemoglobin would be reduced. Conversely, in polycythaemia, in which there is an increase in red cell mass, there may be enough reduced haemoglobin to produce cyanosis, even though there is enough oxygenated haemoglobin to maintain a normal oxygen-carrying capacity.

Cyanosis can be divided into central and peripheral varieties. Central cyanosis is caused by disease of the heart or lungs and the blood leaving the left heart is blue. Peripheral cyanosis is caused by decreased circulation and increased extraction of oxygen in the peripheral tissues. Blood leaving the left heart is normal.

Central cyanosis Although the whole patient may appear cyanosed, the best place to look is the mucous membranes of the lips and tongue (Fig. 5.31). Good natural light is best. Any severe disease of the heart and lungs will cause central cyanosis but the most common causes are severe airflow limitation, left ventricular failure and pulmonary fibrosis.

Peripheral cyanosis Here, the peripheries, the fingers and the toes, are blue with normal mucous membranes. The usual cause is reduced circulation to the limbs, as seen in cold weather, Raynaud's phenomenon or peripheral vascular disease. The peripheries are also usually cold. There may be an element of peripheral cyanosis in heart failure when the perfusion of the extremities is reduced.

Cyanosis can rarely be caused by the abnormal pigments methaemoglobin and sulphaemoglobin. Arterial oxygen tension is normal.

Tremors and carbon dioxide retention

The most common tremor in patients with respiratory disease is a fine finger tremor from stimulation of β-receptors in skeletal muscle by bronchodilator

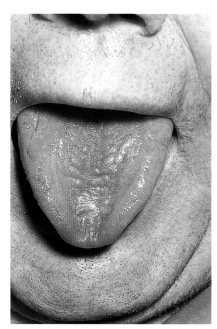

Fig. 5.31 Central cyanosis of the tongue.

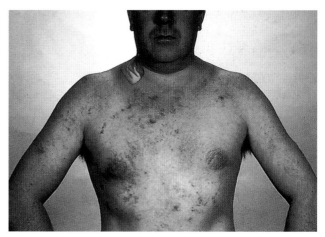

Fig. 5.32 Superior vena caval obstruction showing a swollen face and neck, dilated veins over the trunk and the site of a lymph node biopsy.

drugs. Carbon dioxide retention is seen in severe chronic airflow limitation. Clinically, it can be suspected by a flapping tremor (indistinguishable from that associated with hepatic failure), vasodilatation manifested by warm peripheries, bounding pulses, papilloedema and headache.

Pulse and blood pressure

Pulsus paradoxus is a drop in blood pressure on inspiration. A minor degree occurs normally. Major degrees occur in pericardial effusion and constrictive pericarditis but also in severe asthma. However, it probably adds nothing to other measures of severe asthma. For further discussion see Chapter 6.

Jugular venous pulse and cor pulmonale

The jugular venous pulse may be raised in cor pulmonale (right-sided heart failure due to lung disease). The common cause in the UK is chronic airflow limitation leading to hypoxia. The main mechanism is pulmonary vasoconstriction. Other signs are peripheral oedema (probably as much due to renal hypoxia as back pressure from the right heart), hepatomegaly and a left parasternal heave, indicating right ventricular hypertrophy. In severe cases, functional tricuspid regurgitation will lead to a pulsatile liver, large V waves in the jugular venous pulse and a systolic murmur in the tricuspid area (see Ch. 6). Sometimes overinflation of the lungs will displace the liver downwards and also obscure the cardiac signs, leaving the jugular venous pulse as the only sign.

Obstruction of the superior vena cava is a common presentation of carcinoma of the bronchus but can rarely be caused by lymphoma, benign tumours and mediastinal fibrosis. The tumour compresses the superior vena cava near the point where it enters the right atrium. The resulting high pressure in the superior vena cava causes distension of the neck, fullness and oedema of the face, dilated collateral veins over the upper chest (Fig. 5.32) and chemosis or oedema of the conjunctiva. The internal jugular vein is, of course, distended but may be difficult to see because it does not pulsate (the 'dog-in-the-night-time' syndrome). The external jugular vein should be visible. The patient may have noticed that shirt collars have become tighter.

Lymphadenopathy

Lymph nodes may enlarge either because of generalised disease (e.g. lymphoma) or from local disease spreading through the lymphatics to the nodes. Both may be important in respiratory disease. Palpation of lymph nodes is considered in Chapter 2, so here the examination of only those lymph nodes draining the chest is considered.

Lymphatics from the lungs drain centrally to the hilum then up the paratracheal chain to the supraclavicular (scalene) or cervical nodes. Chest wall lymphatics, especially from the breasts, drain to the axillae. Lung disease, therefore, rarely involves the axillary nodes. Examination of the cervical chain can be carried out by palpation from the front of the patient. Supraclavicular lymphadenopathy is best detected from behind the patient by placing your fingers either side of the neck behind the tendon of the sternomastoid muscle. It helps if the neck is bent slightly forward (Fig. 5.33). Cervical nodes can be palpated this way too.

It is sometimes difficult to examine in the supraclavicular area because lymph nodes may be only slightly enlarged. If palpable, the nodes are usually the site of disease. Careful comparisons should be made between the two sides. If lymph nodes are enlarged then biopsy or aspiration may be a simple way to confirm a diagnosis.

The respiratory system

Beware of performing a cervical node biopsy too readily. Throat cancer can involve these nodes and painstaking block dissection is the correct treatment.

Respiratory diseases that involve these nodes are carcinoma, tuberculosis and sarcoidosis. Nodes containing

> **Differential diagnosis**
>
> **Common respiratory causes of supraclavicular lymphadenopathy**
>
> - Lung cancer
> - Lymphoma
> - Tuberculosis
> - Sarcoidosis
> - HIV infection

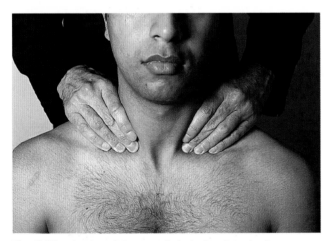

Fig. 5.33 Palpation of the supraclavicular lymph nodes from behind.

metastatic carcinoma are hard and fixed. Tuberculous nodes, common in Asian patients in the UK, are soft and matted and may have discharging sinuses. Healing and calcification leave small hard nodes.

Examination of the axillary nodes is shown in Figure 5.34. Abduct the patient's arm, place the fingers of your hand high up in the axilla, press the tips of the fingers against the chest wall, relax the patient's arm and draw your fingers downwards over the ribs to roll the nodes between your fingers and the ribs.

Skin

The early stages of sarcoidosis and primary tuberculosis are often accompanied by erythema nodosum (Fig. 5.35): painful red indurated areas usually on the shins; although occasionally more extensive, they fade through bruising. Severely affected patients may also have arthralgia. Sarcoidosis can also involve the skin, particularly old scars and tattoos, with nodules and plaques. Lupus pernio is a violaceous swelling of the nose from involvement by sarcoid granuloma.

Eyes

Horner's syndrome [miosis (contraction of the pupil), enophthalmos (backward displacement of the eyeball in the orbit), lack of sweating on the affected side of the face and ptosis (drooping of the upper eyelid; see also Chapter 11)] is usually due to involvement of the sympathetic chain on the posterior chest wall by a bronchial carcinoma.

Sarcoidosis and tuberculosis can cause iridocyclitis. Miliary tuberculosis can produce tubercles visible on the retina by ophthalmoscopy. Papilloedema can

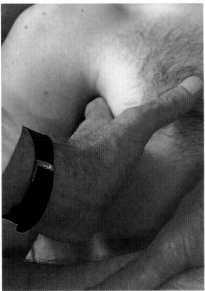

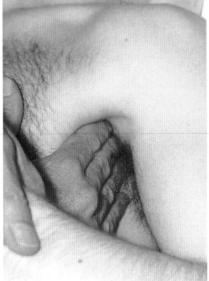

Fig. 5.34 Palpation of the axillary lymph nodes.

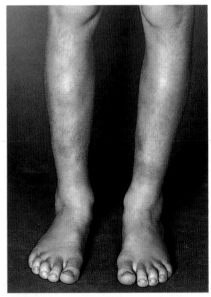

Fig. 5.35 Erythema nodosum, showing raised red lumps on the shins.

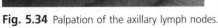

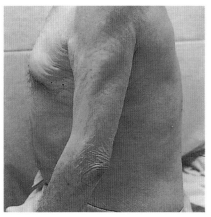

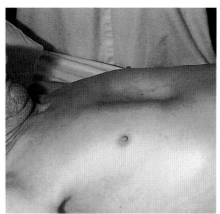

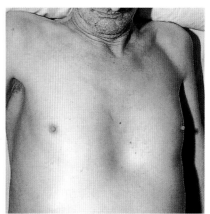

Fig. 5.36 'Barrel chest'. Note the increased anteroposterior diameter of the chest.

Fig. 5.37 Pectus excavatum, showing the depressed sternum.

 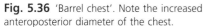

Differential diagnosis

Erythema nodosum

Infections
- Streptococci
- Tuberculosis
- Systemic fungal infections
- Leprosy

Others
- Sarcoidosis
- Ulcerative colitis
- Crohn's disease
- Sulphonamides
- Oral contraceptive pill and pregnancy

be caused by carbon dioxide retention and cerebral metastases.

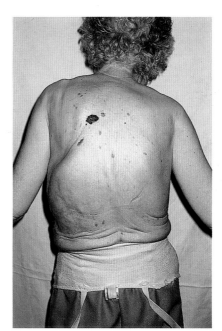

Fig. 5.38 Thoracoplasty with secondary changes in the spine.

Examination of the chest

You should follow the classical sequence of inspection, palpation, percussion and auscultation, not forgetting contemplation (Osler).

INSPECTION OF THE CHEST WALL

First look for any deformities of the chest wall. In 'barrel chest' the chest wall is held in hyperinflation (Fig. 5.36). In normal people the anteroposterior diameter of the chest is less than the lateral diameter but in hyperinflation the anteroposterior diameter may be greater than the lateral. The amount of trachea palpable above the suprasternal notch is reduced. The normal 'bucket handle' action of the ribs moving upwards and outwards, pivoting at the spinous processes and the costal cartilages, is converted into a 'pump handle' up-and-down motion.

Barrel chest is seen in states of chronic airflow limitation, with the degree of deformity correlating with its severity.

In pectus excavatum ('funnel chest'; Fig. 5.37), the sternum is depressed. The condition is benign and needs no treatment but can produce unusual chest radiographic appearances, with the heart apparently enlarged and displaced to the left. In pectus carinatum ('pigeon chest'), the sternum and costal cartilages project outwards. It may be secondary to severe childhood asthma.

Examine the chest wall for any operative scars or the changes of thoracoplasty. This was an operation performed in the 1940s and 1950s for tuberculosis and designed to reduce the volume of the chest. It can produce marked distortion of the chest wall, more clearly seen from the back (Fig. 5.38).

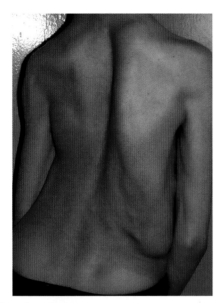

Fig. 5.39 Kyphoscoliosis.

| Emergency |
| **Signs of asthma in adults** |

Signs of acute severe asthma in adults
- Unable to complete sentences
- Pulse >110 beats/min
- Respirations >25 breaths/min
- Peak flow <50% predicted or best

Signs of life-threatening asthma in adults
- Silent chest
- Cyanosis
- Bradycardia
- Exhaustion
- Peak flow <33% predicted or best
- SpO_2 <92%, PaO2 <8 Kpa

Flattening of part of the chest can be due either to underlying lung disease (which usually has to be longstanding) or to scoliosis.

Kyphosis is forward curvature of the spine and scoliosis is a lateral curvature (Fig. 5.39). Both, but scoliosis in particular, can lead to respiratory failure.

Air in the subcutaneous tissue is termed surgical emphysema, although it is as commonly associated with a spontaneous pneumothorax as trauma to the chest. The tissues of the upper chest and neck are swollen, sometimes grossly so (Michelin man), although the condition is not dangerous in itself. The tissues have a characteristic crackling sensation on palpation. In pneumothorax, the air probably tracks from ruptured alveoli, through the root of the lungs to the mediastinum, thence up into the neck. On auscultation of the precordium, you may hear a curious extra sound in time with the heart (mediastinal crunch) but this can occur in pneumothorax without pneumomediastinum. Mediastinal air may be visible on a radiograph.

BREATHING PATTERNS

A good deal can be learnt from simple observation of the chest wall movements. Note rate, depth and regularity. Does the chest move equally on the two sides? Does breathing appear distressing? Is it noisy?

Counting the respiratory rate is often neglected and the precise rate is rarely of practical importance. However, changes can be of great help in the absence of other information. You should note an increase in rate or depth. An increase in rate may occur in any severe lung disease and in fever and sepsis. Patients with hyperventilation may breathe both faster and more deeply, although the increase can be subtle and easily missed. Patients with

acidosis from renal failure, diabetic ketoacidosis and aspirin overdosage will have deep sighing (Kussmaul) respirations as they try to excrete carbon dioxide. Acute massive pulmonary embolism gives a similar pattern.

Is the breathing regular? Cheyne–Stokes respiration is a waxing and waning of the respiratory depth over a minute or so from deep respirations to almost no breathing at all. It is thought to be caused by a failure of the central respiratory control to respond adequately to changes in carbon dioxide and is often seen in patients with terminal disease. Patients may seem unaware of the condition.

Is there any prolongation of expiration? The typical patient with airflow limitation has trouble breathing out. Inspiration may be brief, even hurried, but expiration is a prolonged laboured manoeuvre. Many of these patients breathe out through pursed lips as if they were whistling; this mechanism maintains a higher airway pressure and keeps open the distal airways to allow fuller although longer expiration.

Note if the chest expands unequally. If this is so and there is no structural abnormality of the chest or spine to account for it, then air is probably not entering the lung so well on the affected side. The difference has to be marked to be appreciated. The causes will be considered under palpation. It is possible to measure overall expansion with a tape-measure (the result is of little value and certainly no substitute for measures of lung volume). Breathing mainly from the diaphragm suggests chest wall problems (e.g. pleural pain, ankylosing spondylitis). Breathing mainly with the rib cage suggests diaphragm paralysis, peritonitis or abdominal distension. Normally, as the diaphragm descends in inspiration the anterior abdominal wall will move outwards. If it moves inwards (abdominal paradox) then the diaphragm is probably paralysed. Similarly, in tetraplegia, when the chest wall muscles are paralysed but phrenic nerve function preserved, descent of the diaphragm produces indrawing of the chest wall (chest wall paradox).

Is the patient distressed by breathing? Can the patient carry on a normal conversation or does he or she have to break up sentences, even perhaps to single words at a time? Patients with severe respiratory distress use their accessory muscles of respiration. They fix the position of the shoulder girdle by pressing the hands on the nearest fixed object and throw back their heads. This gives a purchase for accessory muscles of respiration, mainly the sternomastoids.

Does the patient breathe more comfortably in certain positions? Can the patient lie flat or does he or she have to be propped up? Patients with pulmonary oedema and severe airflow limitation will be unable to lie down for long but then most patients with breathing difficulty are more comfortable sitting up. Is breathing audible? Wheeze is a prolonged expiratory noise often audible to the patient as well as the doctor and implies airflow limitation. Stridor is a harsh inspiratory and expiratory noise and implies obstruction in the central airways. This may be at laryngeal level when the voice is usually hoarse but otherwise implies tracheal or major bronchial obstruction. In children, croup and foreign bodies are the usual causes; in adults, carcinoma or extrinsic compression.

'Pink puffers' and 'blue bloaters'

The terms 'pink puffers' and 'blue bloaters' are applied to the overall appearances of some patients with chronic airflow limitation. They describe polar groups and most patients are in between. 'Blue boaters' (Fig. 5.40) are cyanosed from hypoxia and bloated from right-sided heart failure. Further investigation shows features of chronic obstructive bronchitis. Cough and sputum are common but breathlessness less so. Carbon dioxide retention is a feature. 'Pink puffers' (Fig. 5.41) are not cyanosed and are thin. Investigation shows features associated with emphysema. Cough and sputum are less common, but the patients are breathless. Carbon dioxide levels in the blood are normal or low.

PALPATION

Trachea and mediastinum

Start palpation by feeling for the position of the trachea. Do this from the front by placing two fingers either side of the trachea and judging whether the distances between it and the sternomastoid tendons are equal on the two sides (Fig. 5.42). An alternative is to examine the patient from behind and hook your fingers round the tendons to meet the trachea. The trachea may be displaced by masses in the neck such as thyroid enlargement. Nonetheless, the trachea gives an indication about the position of the mediastinum, although often you will only be confident about tracheal displacement after you have seen the radiograph.

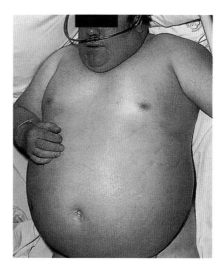
Fig. 5.40 A 'blue bloater' showing ascites from marked cor pulmonale.

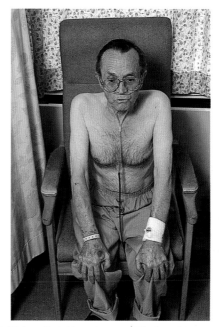
Fig. 5.41 'Pink puffer'. Note the pursed-lip breathing.

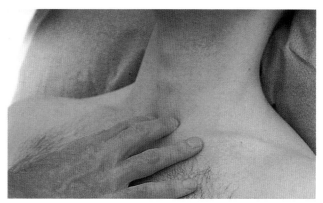
Fig. 5.42 Palpation of the trachea.

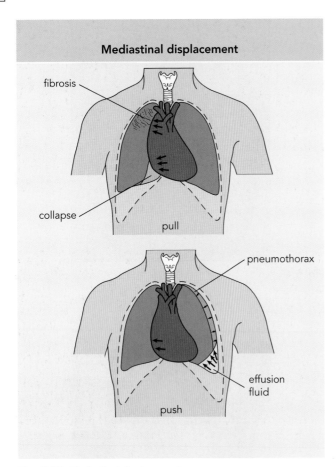

Mediastinal displacement

fibrosis

collapse

pull

pneumothorax

effusion fluid

push

Fig. 5.43 Mediastinal displacement.

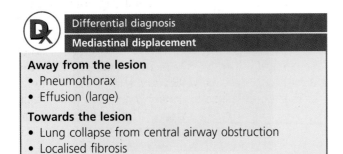

Differential diagnosis

Mediastinal displacement

Away from the lesion
- Pneumothorax
- Effusion (large)

Towards the lesion
- Lung collapse from central airway obstruction
- Localised fibrosis

The position of the apex beat also gives information about the position of the mediastinum so long as the heart is not enlarged. The trachea moves with the upper part of the mediastinum, the apex beat with the lower. The mediastinum may be pushed or pulled to either side. Large effusions push the position of the apex beat but very large effusions are needed to displace the trachea. Pneumothorax pushes the mediastinum even though the lung collapses. This is because the pressure in the pleural space (usually negative) approaches or even exceeds atmospheric pressure, that is, increases. Lung collapse and fibrosis pull the mediastinum (Fig. 5.43). Tumour, especially the pleural tumour mesothelioma, may 'fix' the mediastinum so that it cannot move despite these changes.

Chest wall

If the patient complains of chest pain, then you should gently palpate the chest for local tenderness. If present, this usually indicates disease of bones, muscles or cartilage. As indicated earlier, one variety is called Tietze's syndrome, in which there is pain and swelling of one or more of the upper costal cartilages, but much more commonly than this syndrome there is merely pain and tenderness of the cartilage but no swelling. Chest wall tenderness may also be present in pleurisy; point tenderness over a rib or cartilage is almost always due to benign local disease and the worried patient can be reassured.

A SYSTEMATIC APPROACH

From this point on, as with most parts of the physical examination, comparison is made between the two sides of the body as abnormality is likely to be confined to one side. Start from the front at the apex of the lung and work downwards, comparing each side immediately with the other. Remember that the heart will influence the result on the left. Do not forget the lateral sides and the axillae. Then sit the patient forwards and examine the back. Sometimes you will need an assistant to help a sick patient to lean forwards. When examining from the back, place the arms of the patient forwards in the lap. This will move the scapulae laterally and uncover more of the chest wall.

Vocal fremitus

This is performed by placing either the edge or the flat of your hand on the chest and asking the patient to say 'ninety-nine' or count 'one, two, three'. The vibrations produced by this manoeuvre are transmitted through the lung substance and are felt by the hand. The test is crude and the mechanism and the alterations in disease are the same as for vocal resonance.

Chest expansion

The purpose of this test is to determine if both sides of the chest move equally. Students often have difficulty with this examination. A good method is to put the fingers of both your hands as far round the chest as possible and then to bring the thumbs together in the midline but to keep the thumbs off the chest wall. The patient is then asked to take a deep breath in; the chest wall, by moving outwards, moves the fingers outwards and the thumbs are in turn distracted away from the midline (Fig. 5.44). The thumbs must be free: if they are also fixed to the chest wall they will not move. It is important to keep your fingers and thumbs in the same relationship to each other, for it is easy to move the thumb the way you think it ought to go. Examination can be performed on both the front and the back.

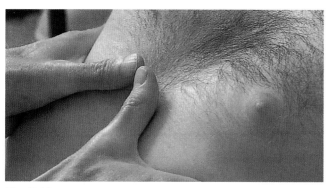 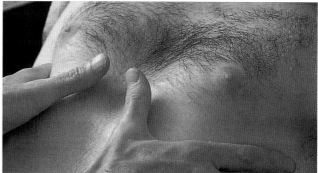

Fig. 5.44 Assessing chest expansion in expiration (left) and inspiration (right).

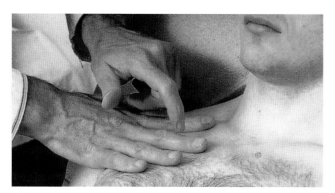

Fig. 5.45 Percussion over the anterior chest.

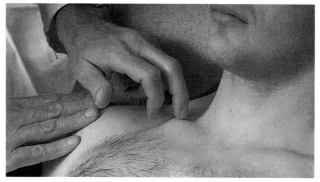

Fig. 5.46 Direct percussion of the clavicles for disease in the lung apices.

Expansion can be reduced on both sides equally. This is difficult to detect as there is no standard of comparison but is produced by severe airflow limitation, extensive generalised lung fibrosis and chest wall problems (e.g. ankylosing spondylitis).

Unilateral reduction implies that air cannot enter that side and is seen in pleural effusion, lung collapse, pneumothorax and pneumonia.

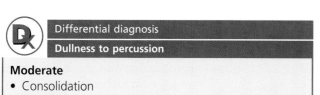

Differential diagnosis

Dullness to percussion

Moderate
- Consolidation
- Fibrosis
- Collapse

'Stony'
- Pleural fluid

PERCUSSION

The purpose of percussion is to detect the resonance or hollowness of the chest. Use both hands, placing the fingers of one hand on the chest with the fingers separated and strike one of them with the terminal phalanx of the middle finger of the other hand (Fig. 5.45); it must be removed again immediately, like the clapper inside a bell, otherwise the resultant sound will be damped. The striking movement should be a flick of the wrist and the striking finger should be at right angles to the other finger. As well as hearing the percussion note, vibrations will be felt by your hand on the chest wall. Again, each side is compared with the equivalent area on the other from top to bottom. Do not forget the sides.

The finger on the chest should be parallel to the expected line of dullness (e.g. in an effusion, parallel to the floor). This will then produce a clearly defined change in note from normal to dull; a finger straddling the demarcation will not do this. It should be placed in the intercostal spaces. Do not percuss more heavily than is necessary: it gives no more information and can be distressing to patients. The apex of the lung can be examined by tapping directly on the middle of the clavicle (Fig. 5.46). Remember that the lung extends much further down posteriorly than anteriorly (see Fig. 5.4).

The degree of resonance depends on the thickness of the chest wall and on the amount of air in the structures underlying it. The possibilities are increased resonance, dullness and 'stony dullness'. Obese patients and individuals with thick chest walls show less resonance, yet it is equal on the two sides. In contrast, patients with overinflated lungs, particularly those with emphysema, have increased resonance; however, it is generalised and without a reference point is difficult to grade. It might be thought that air in the pleural space (pneumothorax) would increase resonance but the difference is often insufficient to identify which is the affected side from percussion alone.

Resonance is decreased moderately in consolidation and fibrosis of the lung and markedly if there is fluid of any kind between the lung and the chest wall, that is, stony dullness. A collapsed lobe can compress to a very small volume and compensatory overinflation of the other lobe fills the space. The percussion note may then be normal. A whole lung cannot collapse completely (unless there is also a pneumothorax) so the chest will be dull. Percussion can also be used to determine movement of the diaphragm because the level of dullness will descend as the patient breathes in (tidal percussion). Dullness is to be expected over the liver, which anteriorly reaches as high as the sixth costal cartilage, and over the heart. Resonance in these areas, again a subjective finding, implies increased air in the lungs and is common in overinflation and emphysema. Bilateral basal dullness is more usually due to failure or inability to take a deep breath, to obesity or to abdominal distension than to bilateral pleural effusions. The right diaphragm is normally higher than the left so expect a slightly higher level of dullness.

AUSCULTATION

Many doctors prefer to use the diaphragm of the stethoscope for auscultation of the chest (Fig. 5.47). In thin bony chests, the bell may give a more airtight fit and is less likely to trap hairs underneath, which produce a crackling sound.

Ask the patient to take deep breaths through the mouth, then listen in sequence over the chest as before. Start at the apices and compare each side with the other. Some patients fail to understand the instruction to breathe through the mouth but the sounds are much clearer if

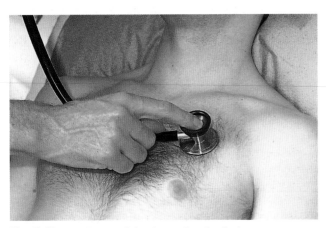

Fig. 5.47 Auscultation of the chest using the diaphragm.

they do. To help them you may have to press gently on the jaw to open it. Some take enormous slow deep breaths that, although otherwise satisfactory, do prolong the examination. A quick demonstration of what you want will resolve any problems.

The breath sounds are produced in the large airways, transmitted through the airways and then attenuated by the distal lung structure through which they pass. The sounds you hear at the lung surface are therefore different from the sounds heard over the trachea and are modified further if there is anything obstructing the airways, lung tissue, pleura or chest wall. When reporting on auscultatory changes, you must distinguish between the breath sounds and the added sounds. Breath sounds are termed either vesicular or bronchial and the added sounds are divided into crackles, wheezes and rubs.

Vesicular breath sounds

This is the sound heard over normal lungs; it has a rustling quality and is heard on inspiration and the first part of expiration (Fig. 5.48). Reduction in vesicular breath sounds can be expected with airways obstruction as in asthma, emphysema or tumour. The so-called 'silent chest' is a sign of severe asthma: so little air enters the lung that no sound is produced. The breath sounds can be strikingly reduced in emphysema, particularly over a bulla. Generalised reduction in breath sounds also occurs with a thick chest wall or obesity.

Anything interspersed between the lung and the chest wall (air, fluid or pleural thickening) will reduce the breath sounds; this is likely to be unilateral and therefore more easily detected.

Avoid the term 'diminished air entry' when you mean diminished breath sounds. The two are not necessarily synonymous.

Bronchial breathing

Bronchial breathing causes much confusion because the essential feature of bronchial breathing, the quality of the sound, is difficult or impossible to put into words. Traditionally, it is described by its timing as occurring in both inspiration and expiration with a gap in between (Fig. 5.49). In this way it is contrasted with vesicular breathing. These features are undoubtedly true but lead to the confusion in the mind of the student that if anything is heard in middle or late expiration it must be bronchial breathing. Many normal people and individuals with airways obstruction have a prolonged expiratory component to the breath sounds (this is sometimes designated 'bronchovesicular' but this term increases the confusion rather than diminishing it). It is best to forget about the timing and concentrate on the essential feature, the quality of the sound. It can be mimicked to some extent by listening over the trachea with the stethoscope, although a better imitation can be obtained by putting the tip of your tongue on the roof of your

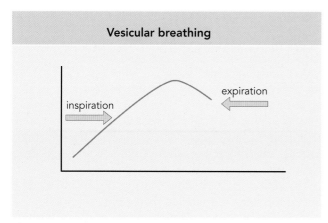

Fig. 5.48 Timing of vesicular breathing.

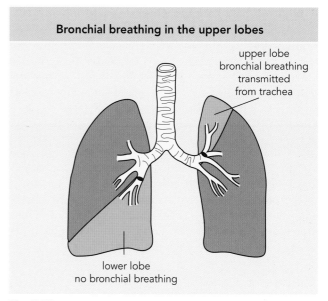

Fig. 5.50 Bronchial breathing may be heard over the upper lobes even if the bronchus is blocked.

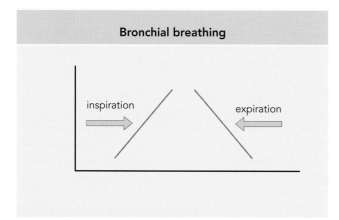

Fig. 5.49 Timing of bronchial breathing.

mouth and breathing in and out through the open mouth.

Bronchial breathing is heard when sound generated in the central airways is transmitted more or less unchanged through the lung substance. This occurs when the lung substance itself is solid, as in consolidation, but the air passages remain open. Sound is conducted normally to the small airways but then, instead of being modified by air in the alveoli, the solid lung conducts the sound better to the lung surface and, hence, to the stethoscope. If the central airways are obstructed by, say, a carcinoma, then no transmission of sound will take place and no bronchial breathing will occur even though the lung may be solid. An exception is seen in the upper lobes. Here, if the bronchi to either lobe are blocked, sounds from the central airways can still be transmitted directly from the trachea through the solid lung to the chest wall (Fig. 5.50).

The main cause of bronchial breathing is consolidation, particularly from pneumonia – so much so that in the minds of most clinicians the three terms are synonymous. Lung abscess, if near the chest wall, can cause bronchial breathing, probably because of the consolidation around it. Dense fibrosis is an occasional cause. Breath sounds

over an effusion will be diminished but bronchial breathing may be heard over its upper level, perhaps because the effusion compresses the lung.

Bronchial breathing is only heard over a collapsed lung if the airway is patent. This is rare as the collapse is usually caused by an obstructing carcinoma. Nevertheless, there is an exception with the upper lobes (see above).

Bronchial breathing has been divided into tubular, cavernous and amphoric but attempts to score points on ward rounds by using these terms are best left to others.

Vocal resonance

This is the auscultatory equivalent of vocal fremitus. Place the stethoscope on the chest and ask the patient to say 'ninety-nine'. Normally the sound produced is 'fuzzy' and seems to come from the chest piece of the stethoscope. The changes in disease should by now be predictable. The sound is increased in consolidation (better transmission through solid lung) and decreased if there is air, fluid or pleural thickening between the lung and the chest wall. The changes of vocal fremitus are the same. Both tests are of little value in themselves, yet a refinement of vocal resonance can be very useful. Sometimes the increased transmission of sound is so marked that even when the patient whispers, the sound is still heard clearly over the affected lung (whispering pectoriloquy). When this is well developed there is a striking difference between the normal side, where the sound appears to come from the end of the stethoscope, and the abnormal side, where the syllables are much clearer and seem as if they are being whispered into your ear.

Bronchial breathing and whispering pectoriloquy have the same mechanism so commonly occur together. Consequently, if you are in doubt about the presence of bronchial breathing then whispering pectoriloquy may confirm it. Like bronchial breathing, whispering pectoriloquy is characteristic of consolidation but can also occur with lung abscess and above an effusion.

Added sounds

There are three types of added sounds: wheezes, crackles and pleural rubs. Much confusion has been generated in the past by other terms such as rhonchi, which are equivalent to wheezes, and crepitations and rales, which are equivalent to crackles. Further subdivision is often attempted but is of very limited value.

Wheezes

These are prolonged musical sounds largely occurring on expiration, sometimes on inspiration, and are due to localised narrowing within the bronchial tree. They are caused by the vibration of the walls of a bronchus near to its point of closure. Most patients with wheeze have many, each coming from a single, narrowed area. As the lung gets smaller on expiration, so the airways get smaller too; each narrowed airway reaches a critical phase when it produces a wheeze then ceases to do so. Thus, during expiration, numerous narrowings produce numerous wheezes in sequence and together. A single wheeze can occur and may then suggest a single narrowing, often caused by a carcinoma or foreign body (fixed wheeze).

Wheezes are typical of airway narrowing from any cause. Asthma and chronic bronchitis are the most common and the narrowing is caused by a combination of smooth muscle contraction, inflammatory changes in the walls and increased bronchial secretions. Sometimes patients with these conditions have few or no wheezes. If so, ask the patient to take a deep breath and then to blow out hard. This may produce a marked wheeze. Occasionally, wheezing is heard in pulmonary oedema, presumably because of bronchial wall oedema.

The term bronchospasm suggests narrowing caused only by smooth muscle contraction and should be avoided as the bronchial narrowing is usually multifactorial.

Wheeze-like breath sounds can disappear in severe asthma and emphysema because of low rates of airflow. The amount of wheeze is not a good indicator of the degree of airways obstruction. Peak expiratory flow measurement is much better.

Stridor

Stridor may be heard better without a stethoscope by putting your ear close to the patient's mouth and asking the patient to breathe in and out. As indicated earlier, it is a sign of large airway narrowing in the larynx, trachea or main bronchi.

Crackles

In a sense the term crackles is self-explanatory. Problems arise because of various descriptions that are often added, such as coarse, medium, fine, wet or dry. These add little to our understanding; nonetheless, it is possible to distinguish two main types. The first occurs when there is fluid in the larger bronchi and a coarse bubbling sound can be heard that clears or alters as the secretions causing the sound are shifted on coughing or deep breathing.

The sound of other 'fine' crackles can be imitated by rolling the hairs of your temple together between your fingers. They occur in inspiration and are high-pitched, explosive sounds. The mechanism of their production is thought to be as follows. Many conditions lead to premature closure of the small airways at the end of expiration. During the succeeding inspiration, these units can only be reopened by overcoming the surface tension that keeps them closed. When they eventually 'pop open' crackles are produced. During inspiration, larger bronchi will open before smaller ones so crackles from chronic bronchitis and bronchiectasis tend to occur early. Conditions that largely involve the alveoli, such as left ventricular failure, fibrosis and pneumonia, tend to produce crackles later on inspiration. This distinction is of clinical value.

Differential diagnosis
Crackles
• Left ventricular failure
• Fibrosing alveolitis
• Extrinsic allergic alveolitis
• Pneumonia
• Bronchiectasis
• Chronic bronchitis
• Asbestosis

Note whether the crackles are localised. This would be expected in pneumonia and mild cases of bronchiectasis. Pulmonary oedema and fibrosing alveolitis typically affect both lung bases equally.

Normal people, especially smokers, may have a few basal crackles; these often clear with a few deep breaths.

Pleural rub

This is caused by the inflamed surfaces of the pleura rubbing together. The sound has been likened to new leather when it is bent or, more vividly, to the creaking noises made in a sailing ship heeling to the wind, which you may have experienced from films if not in reality. Some idea of the quality of the sound can be obtained by placing one hand over the ear and rubbing the back of

Red flag – urgent referral

Respiratory disease

- Haemoptysis. May be a symptom of cancer, although most are due to infection. Chest x-ray required.
- Persistent symptoms of chest infection. May be underlying cancer. Chest x-ray required.
- Right lower lobe collapse. Enquire about choking fit. May be foreign body.
- Absent breath sounds and wheeze in a breathless patient. Not necessarily a good sign. May imply severe asthma with little air movement.
- Equal inspiratory and expiratory wheeze may in fact be stridor from a central obstruction. If there is also a hoarse voice consider laryngeal carcinoma.
- In a patient with apparently mild COPD (chronic obstructive pulmonary disease) who develops oedema or excessive sleepiness consider type 2 respiratory failure.
- In a patient with a 'fat face' and full neck consider SVC (superior vena cava) obstruction and look for dilated veins over the chest wall.
- If clubbing develops in a patient with COPD this is likely to be due to a carcinoma.

Differential diagnosis

Some causes of pneumonia

- *Streptococcus pneumoniae*
- *Mycoplasma pneumoniae*
- *Haemophilus influenzae*
- Influenza virus
- *Legionella pneumophila*
- Psittacosis
- Q fever
- Chemical (for example, aspiration of vomit)
- Radiation

that hand with the fingers of the other. Pleural rubs are usually heard on both inspiration and expiration. At first you may think that you are moving the stethoscope on the chest. Sometimes coarse crackles can sound like rubs; a cough will shift the former. If there is any pain, ask the patient to point to the site of the pain, this often localises the rub too. Rubs are heard in all varieties of pleural inflammation, such as in pneumonia and pulmonary embolism. Any effusion will separate the pleura and the rub may well go but sometimes remain above the effusion.

Common patterns of abnormality

This section summarises what has been said before but from the perspective of the disease process. The diagnosis itself will need the integration of the history and any other information. The processes considered are consolidation, pleural fluid, pneumothorax, chronic airflow limitation, lung or lobar collapse and fibrosis. Not all the signs are present in every case and often there is more than one disease process at a time. The radiograph often illustrates the anatomical nature of the process, so examples are shown.

CONSOLIDATION

Consolidation is a confusing term as it means different things to different specialists. To a radiologist it means

an alveolar-filling process with no presumption about aetiology. To a pathologist it means a heavy airless lung and to a clinician it means bronchial breathing that is usually equated with pneumonia. To use pneumonia as an example, the affected lung or lobe is the same size or very slightly larger than normal lung. The alveoli are full of exudate, yet the air passages are open. The pleura are inflamed. The 'differential diagnosis' box lists some causes. Note that not all are infections.

Inspection of the chest may show diminished movement on the affected side, palpation shows no shift of the mediastinum but expansion is reduced, vocal fremitus may be increased, percussion note will be moderately impaired, breath sounds will be bronchial over the affected area with whispering pectoriloquy and there may be a pleural rub. Early and late in the disease process there may also be crackles and these may be the only auscultatory change in mild cases. In lobar pneumonia, the changes are localised to a lobe, which means that the signs are detected either anteriorly or posteriorly but not usually both. More widespread changes suggest 'bronchopneumonia', a complication of chronic bronchitis, or 'atypical pneumonia' caused by viruses, mycoplasma and other organisms. Radiology may show an 'air bronchogram' – air in the bronchi outlined by fluid in the alveoli (Fig. 5.51).

PLEURAL FLUID

Whether this be from an increase in pleural transudate, pleural exudate from inflammation, blood, pus or lymph, the signs are the same. A large amount of fluid is needed to displace the heart and an even larger amount, filling most of the hemithorax, to displace the trachea. The displacement is away from the fluid. Expansion is diminished on the affected side, vocal fremitus is reduced, percussion note is markedly reduced, 'stony dullness', and breath sounds are absent or markedly reduced. Bronchial breathing and a rub may be heard at the upper level of the effusion. An effusion, if large enough, is detected both anteriorly and posteriorly (Figs 5.52, 5.53).

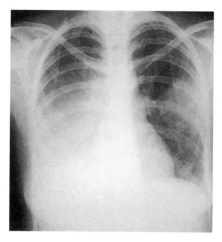 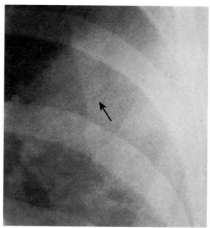

Mediastinum central
Expansion ↓
Percussion note ↓
Breath sounds bronchial
Whispering pectoriloquy
Crackles
Pleural rub

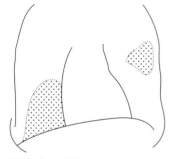

Fig. 5.51 Consolidation (unusual because it affects both lungs). Enlarged view showing air bronchogram (arrow).

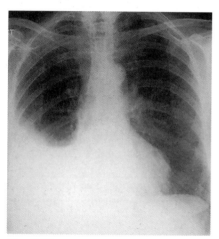 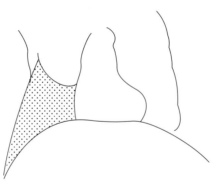

Mediastinum usually central
Expansion ↓
Percussion ↓
Breath sounds ↓
Sometimes bronchial breathing
   or a pleural rub at upper level

Fig. 5.52 Small effusion.

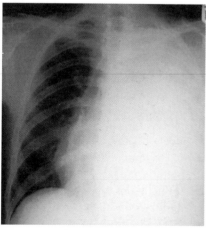 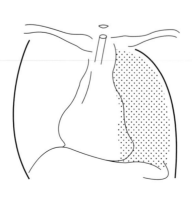

Mediastinum displaced
Expansion ↓
Percussion ↓
Breath sounds ↓

Fig. 5.53 Large effusion with mediastinal displacement.

Differential diagnosis
Some causes of pleural fluid

Transudates
- Congestive cardiac failure
- Cirrhosis
- Nephrotic syndrome

Exudates
- Tumours – primary, secondary and lymphomas
- Pneumonia
- Tuberculosis
- Rheumatoid arthritis and other connective tissue disorders
- Pulmonary embolism and infarction

Blood
- Trauma
- Pulmonary embolism
- Tumours

Pus
- Pneumonia
- Trauma

Lymph
- Tumours, especially lymphoma

Risk factors
Some causes of pneumothorax

- No cause found
- Apical blebs
- Chronic bronchitis and emphysema
- Staphylococcal pneumonia
- Asthma
- Tuberculosis
- Cystic fibrosis
- Trauma

there is also dullness to percussion. Vocal resonance is reduced and there are no added sounds (Fig. 5.54). Some causes of pneumothorax are given in the 'risk factors' box.

CHRONIC AIRFLOW LIMITATION

This term covers the entities of chronic obstructive bronchitis, emphysema and asthma, which are not always readily distinguishable from each other. There may be hyperinflation of the chest, pursed lip breathing and use of accessory muscles of respiration. Expansion may well be reduced but usually equally so. The mediastinum is not displaced. Vocal fremitus is normal, percussion is usually normal but there may be increased resonance and reduced hepatic and cardiac dullness. Breath sounds are vesicular and sometimes reduced, presumably from low flow rates; the added sounds are wheezes and often crackles. The radiograph is usually normal but sometimes shows overinflation with low flat diaphragms (Fig. 5.55).

LUNG AND LOBAR COLLAPSE

The usual cause is a central bronchial carcinoma, although a foreign body has the same effect. If the lung or lobe is not ventilated, the air within it is absorbed by the

PNEUMOTHORAX

The pressure in the pleural space is normally negative with respect to atmospheric pressure. In a pneumothorax, the affected side is at a higher pressure, that is, less negative. This pressure tends to displace the mediastinum to the opposite side, and if there is a flap valve effect producing a tension pneumothorax this can be extreme and dangerous. The affected side moves less well, vocal fremitus is reduced and the percussion note is normal. The expected increased resonance can be difficult to detect and it is the conjunction of diminished breath sounds with a normal percussion note that distinguishes it from other causes of diminished breath sounds when

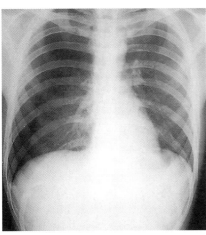

Fig. 5.54 Pneumothorax on right.

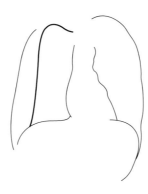

Mediastinum sometimes displaced
Expansion ↓
Percussion normal or ↑
Breath sounds ↓
No added sounds

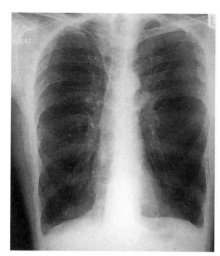

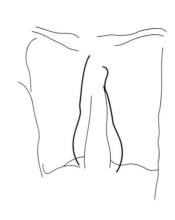

Hyperinflation
Mediastinum central
Hepatic and cardiac dullness ↓
Vesicular breath sounds
Wheezes and crackles
Radiograph often normal but
here shows overinflation
and low flat diaphragms

Fig. 5.55 Chronic airflow limitation.

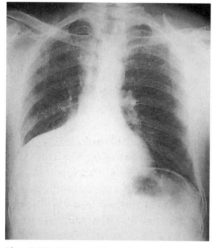

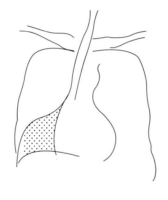

Mediastinum displaced
Expansion reduced
Percussion normal or ↓
Breath sounds vesicular
but ↓ or sometimes
bronchial

Fig. 5.56 Right middle and lower lobe collapse.

blood and the lung collapses. If the whole lung is involved, then the degree of collapse is limited by the capacity of the chest to shrink, but if a lobe is involved, then the other lobe can fill the space and the affected lung may come to occupy only a very small area. Lung collapse can also follow infection: tuberculosis and bronchiectasis are good examples. Here the airways remain open.

The findings on examination depend on whether the whole lung or only one lobe is involved. There is diminished movement on the affected side, with the mediastinum deviating to that side. The percussion note is markedly reduced if the whole lung is involved but can be difficult or impossible to detect if only a lobe is involved and has shrunk to a small space. Breath sounds are diminished but remain vesicular in lobar collapse and may be absent if the whole lung is involved. Vocal resonance is decreased. As already indicated, bronchial breathing, increased vocal resonance and whispering pectoriloquy can be heard in upper lobe collapse because

of direct transmission of sound from the trachea. Bronchial breathing is also heard in collapse of other lobes if (unusually) the airways remain patent (Fig. 5.56). Crackles and wheeze may be present if the cause is damage from an old infection.

LUNG FIBROSIS

This may be the end result of many lung conditions and minor degrees are undetectable clinically. Localised changes produce similar signs to lung collapse. Generalised disease is best illustrated by cryptogenic fibrosing alveolitis. The lungs are stiff, expansion may be reduced, but equally, and the mediastinum is central. Vocal fremitus is normal, percussion note is normal or slightly reduced, breath sounds are vesicular, although occasionally bronchial, yet there are marked crackles, initially confined to the bases but later extending up the chest (Fig. 5.57).

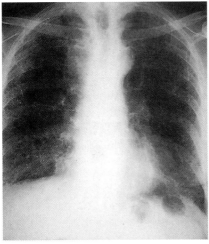

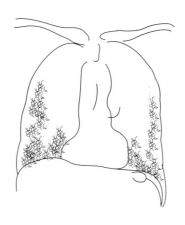

Mediastinum central
Expansion equally ↓
Percussion normal or ↓
Breath sounds vesicular
(occasionally bronchial)
Crackles

Fig. 5.57 Cryptogenic fibrosing alveolitis.

Emergency

Bedside assessment of acute respiratory failure

Bedside diagnosis of acute respiratory failure is difficult but:
- Look first for respiratory rate, cyanosis, respiratory distress, use of accessory respiratory muscles, ankle swelling
- Consider upper airways obstruction (e.g. anaphylactic shock, laryngeal tumour, foreign body, obstructive sleep apnoea)
  - look for swelling of lips and tongue, stridor, hoarse voice, snoring
- Consider central airways obstruction (e.g. tumour)
  - look for stridor, unilateral reduced breath sounds
- Consider generalised airway narrowing (e.g. asthma, COPD)
  - look for flapping tremor, wheeze, prolonged expiration, silent chest, perform PEF

- Consider parenchymal lung disease (e.g. pneumonia, pulmonary oedema, alveolitis)
  - look for crackles, bronchial breathing
- Consider pleural problems (e.g. effusion, pneumothorax)
  - look for displaced trachea, dullness with silence, resonance with silence
- Consider chest wall problems (e.g. ankylosing spondylosis, neurological disease)
  - look for scoliosis, upper limb weakness, poor chest wall movement, poor diaphragm movement, muscle fasciculations.

Further analysis depends crucially on vital capacity, chest radiograph, arterial blood gases, oxygen saturation

Respiratory examination

Examination of elderly people

- Be aware of multiple problems
- Occupational history still valid
  - mesothelioma occurs long after exposure
  - pneumoconiosis changes persist for life
- Not all breathless elderly patients have chronic obstructive pulmonary disease

- Respiratory and cardiac disease often coexist
- Right ventricular failure as a consequence of lung disease is difficult to distinguish from congestive cardiac failure
- Disability may be multifactorial

The respiratory system

1. While taking the history, watch for respiratory distress, particularly while talking. Note any clues from the patient's surroundings
2. Look at the hands for clubbing, cyanosis and evidence of carbon dioxide retention
3. Look at the mucous membranes for central cyanosis
4. Check the jugular venous pulse for evidence of cor pulmonale
5. Palpate for supraclavicular lymph nodes
6. Inspect the chest wall for deformities and inequalities
7. Note the pattern of breathing
8. Palpate the trachea for any displacement
9. Palpate the front of the chest for vocal fremitus and for right ventricular hypertrophy
10. Assess expansion of the chest from the front and note any inequalities
11. Percuss the front of the chest comparing one side with the other and noting any areas of dullness; include the axillae
12. Auscultate the chest similarly and decide on the presence and nature of the breath sounds
13. Test for vocal resonance and, where appropriate, whispering pectoriloquy
14. Note any added sounds
15. Repeat last six steps on the back of the chest
16. If appropriate, measure the peak flow rate

6

The heart and cardiovascular system

The cardiovascular system is fundamental to the functioning of almost every other organ system. Despite the availability of many sophisticated imaging techniques, which will be discussed later, the fundamental simplicity and accessibility of the structure and function of the heart and vascular system make its physical examination both important and extremely rewarding.

Structure and function

The adult heart (Fig. 6.1) consists of two pumps working in series. The 'right heart', comprising the right atrium, tricuspid valve, right ventricle, pulmonary valve and pulmonary artery, is a low pressure pump receiving blood

The chambers of the heart

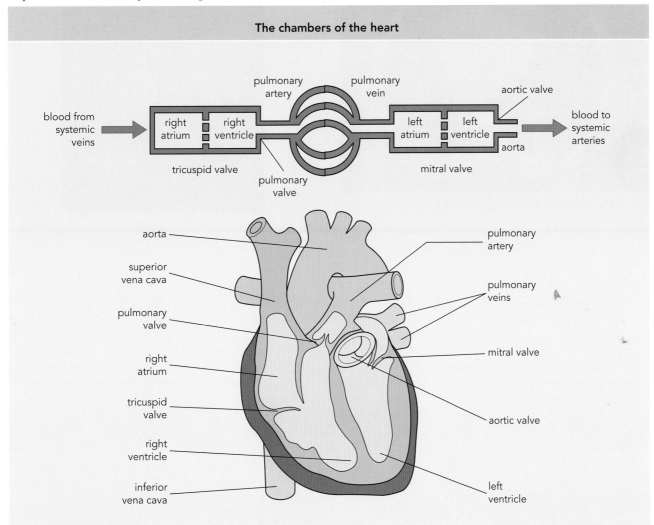

Fig. 6.1 Arrangement of the heart chambers as a flow diagram (above) and in their approximate anatomical positions (below).

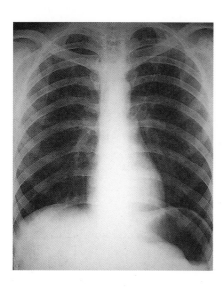

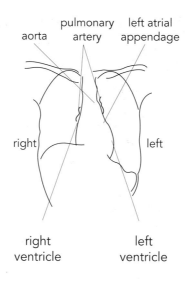

aorta   pulmonary
artery   left atrial
appendage

right   left

right
ventricle   left
ventricle

Fig. 6.2 Most of the anterior surface of the heart is formed by the right ventricle and pulmonary artery. The tip of the left ventricle and the left atrial appendage also appear on the left border of the heart.

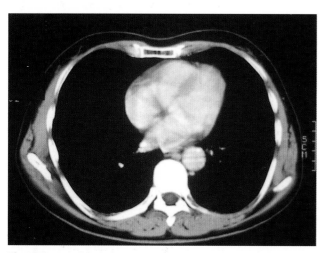

Fig. 6.3 Computerised tomography scan of the heart showing the position of the heart within the chest cavity. Viewed from below.

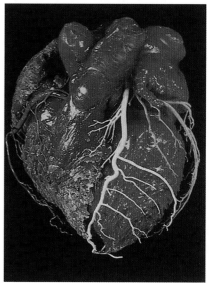

Fig. 6.4 A 'corrosion cast' of the chambers of the heart, made by filling the chambers with wax or plastic and dissolving away the muscle.

from the systemic veins and pumping it to the lungs. The left heart, comprising the left atrium, mitral valve, left ventricle, aortic valve and aorta, is a high pressure pump receiving blood from the lungs and pumping it round the body. In the early embryo, the heart forms as a simple tube down the midline of the body. As the embryo grows, the tube elongates more rapidly than the tissues around it and thus develops a loop and a twist. It also becomes divided into left and right chambers by the growth of a partition or septum down the middle.

In the ninth week of gestation, the fetal heart rotates in a clockwise direction until the right ventricle comes to rest anteriorly behind the sternum. Most of the left ventricle comes to lie posteriorly, apart from a small portion of left ventricular muscle which forms the left heart border when seen from the front and the extreme

tip or apex of the heart (Fig. 6.2). The way the heart is situated within the chest cavity is also well demonstrated on the computerised tomographic scan of the chest shown in Figure 6.3. Note that the heart lies obliquely in the chest and that its long axis, the planes of the interatrial and interventricular septum, and the planes of the various valves, are not aligned with any of the conventional anatomical planes. The chambers of the heart can be examined after death by injecting wax or plastic and dissolving away the muscle (Fig. 6.4). They can also be examined during life by injecting radio-opaque contrast medium through catheters placed in the various chambers of the heart and taking cine radiographs. By tilting the x-ray tube and image detector appropriately, it is possible to obtain detailed pictures of the full extent of the ventricular cavities (Fig. 6.5).

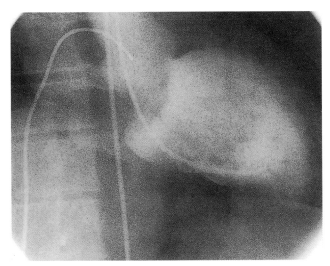

Fig. 6.5 Left ventricular cine-angiogram made by injecting radio-opaque contrast medium into the heart through a catheter passed via the femoral artery and aorta. The x-ray tube and image intensifier are tilted into the 'right anterior oblique' position to outline the full extent of the left ventricle.

HEART MUSCLE

Ventricles

Heart muscle or myocardium is a special type of muscle that is extremely resistant to fatigue. As a result of the higher pressures that it normally generates, the wall of the left ventricle is much thicker than the wall of the right ventricle. In a section taken through both ventricles, left ventricular myocardium, including the intraventricular septum, has a roughly circular outline with the right ventricle appearing to be wrapped around one side of it (Fig. 6.6). The muscle fibres of the heart are arranged in a complicated spiral arrangement so that when they contract (systole) not only is blood forced out of the ventricles but the heart also elongates and rotates on the fixed base provided by the attachment of the major blood vessels. It is this movement that is felt as the beating of the heart by a hand placed on the chest. The heart normally lies in its own serous cavity, the pericardium, which allows it to move without friction. Apart from moving with each heart beat, the position of the pericardium and the heart can be altered by the phase of respiration or by rolling from one side to the other.

Atria

The atria of the heart are also muscular but are much thinner walled than the ventricles (Fig. 6.7). They contract

Transverse ('short axis') view of the heart

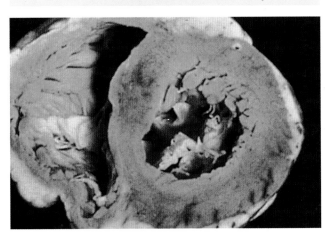

Fig. 6.6 'Short axis' view of the heart. In the short axis or transverse section, the thinner (low pressure) right ventricle is 'wrapped around' the left ventricle.

'Long axis' view of the heart

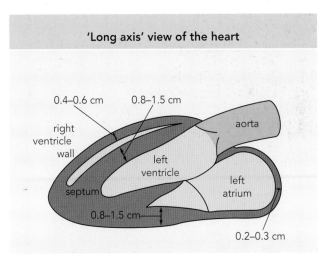

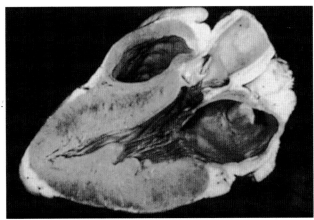

Fig. 6.7 Relative thickness of muscle in different parts of the heart.

a fraction of a second before the ventricles and, in doing so, they assist in the filling of the ventricles, particularly when there is a need for increased cardiac output. The atrial component of cardiac filling can contribute up to 30% of cardiac output. Patients in whom, as a result of disease, the atria are paralysed or are beating out of synchrony with the ventricles are usually comfortable at rest but may become short of breath on exercise.

CARDIAC HYPERTROPHY AND DILATATION

Like any muscle, cardiac muscle responds to an increased workload by growth. The heart responds in different ways to pressure load and volume load. Pressure load is caused by an increased resistance to ejection of blood from the heart. The response to pressure load is cardiac hypertrophy, initially without dilatation of the chamber involved. For example, in aortic stenosis, the left ventricular wall becomes excessively thickened but the left ventricular cavity remains of normal size. Eventually, when the pressure load is extreme or growth of the heart muscle has outstripped its blood supply, failure of the muscle occurs and the cavity begins to enlarge.

The heart responds to a volume load, for example, a leaking mitral or aortic valve, an arteriovenous fistula or left-to-right shunt, by both hypertrophy of the myocardium and dilatation of the chamber involved. This is to accompany the increased stroke volume that is required to deal with the volume load. The chest radiograph shows cardiac enlargement (Fig. 6.8) and this is also found on echocardiography. Ventricular hypertrophy produces characteristic electrocardiographic changes and it is possible to identify the cardiac chamber involved from the electrocardiographic appearances.

HEART VALVES

There are four heart valves. They fall anatomically and functionally into two groups: the inflow or atrioventricular valves and the outflow or 'semilunar' valves. The tricuspid and mitral valves separate right atrium and right ventricle and left atrium and left ventricle, respectively. Both develop from the endocardial cushions of the embryonic heart and are composed of thin flexible leaflets that are prevented from prolapsing back into the atrium when the ventricle contracts by being attached by chordae tendineae to specialised portions of ventricular muscle, the papillary muscles (Fig. 6.9). The hydrodynamic efficiency of the mitral and tricuspid valves is very high. Their pliable edges smooth out eddies and turbulence in blood flow and allow the rapid transfer of blood from atrium to ventricle with a very small pressure differential. The aortic and pulmonary valves develop from two spiral ridges that divide the single great vessel leaving the embryonic heart into aortic and pulmonary trunks. Each normally has three cusps whose arrangement reflects their embryonic origin (Fig. 6.10). As each cusp is shaped like a half moon, they are sometimes called the semilunar valves.

HEART SOUNDS

Closure of the heart valves at different stages of the cardiac cycle gives rise to sounds that are readily audible through a stethoscope. The sounds are normally described as 'lub-dup'. The first heart sound ('lub') is caused by the closure of the mitral and tricuspid valves, and the second heart sound, the rather higher pitched ('dup'), is caused by the closure of aortic and pulmonary valves. The relationship between the heart sound, the electrocardiogram and the arterial pulse wave is shown in Figure 6.11. In children or in young adults, the

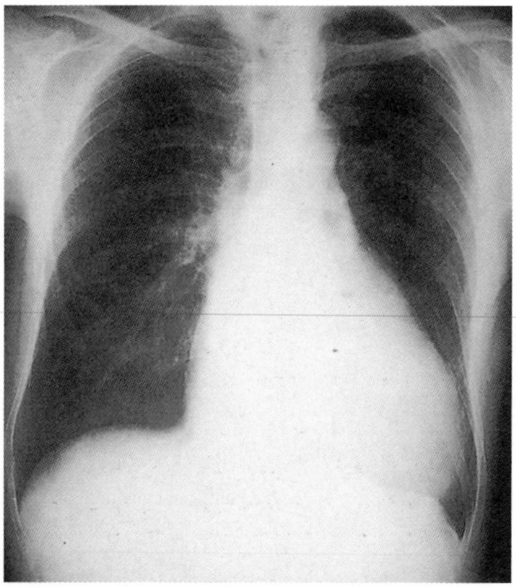

Fig. 6.8 Chest radiograph showing cardiac enlargement in response to a volume load chronic mitral regurgitation (compare with Fig. 6.2).

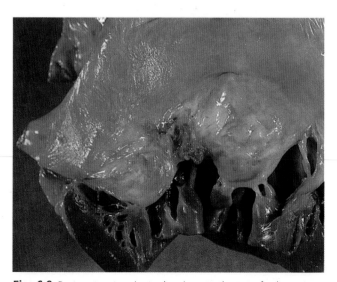

Fig. 6.9 Postmortem specimen showing attachment of valve cusps to papillary muscles by chordae tendineae.

Development of the aortic and pulmonary (semilunar) valves

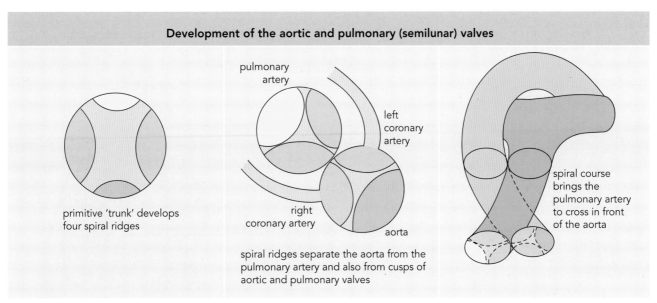

primitive 'trunk' develops
four spiral ridges

pulmonary
artery

left
coronary
artery

right
coronary artery

aorta

spiral ridges separate the aorta from the
pulmonary artery and also from cusps of
aortic and pulmonary valves

spiral course
brings the
pulmonary artery
to cross in front
of the aorta

Fig. 6.10 The common 'great vessel' of the fetal heart is divided into aorta and pulmonary artery by the growth of the spiral ridges.

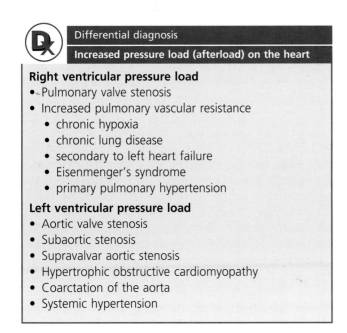

Differential diagnosis
Increased pressure load (afterload) on the heart

Right ventricular pressure load
- Pulmonary valve stenosis
- Increased pulmonary vascular resistance
  - chronic hypoxia
  - chronic lung disease
  - secondary to left heart failure
  - Eisenmenger's syndrome
  - primary pulmonary hypertension

Left ventricular pressure load
- Aortic valve stenosis
- Subaortic stenosis
- Supravalvar aortic stenosis
- Hypertrophic obstructive cardiomyopathy
- Coarctation of the aorta
- Systemic hypertension

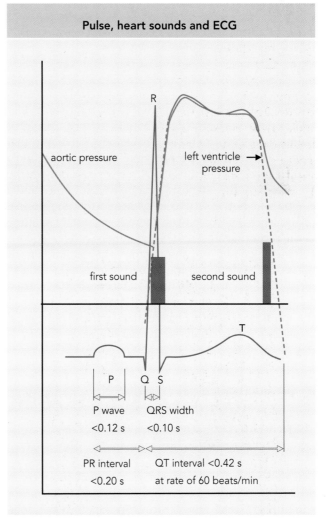

Pulse, heart sounds and ECG

R

aortic pressure

left ventricle
pressure

first sound

second sound

T

P   Q S

P wave   QRS width
<0.12 s   <0.10 s

PR interval   QT interval <0.42 s
<0.20 s   at rate of 60 beats/min

Fig. 6.11 Relationship between heart sounds, electrocardiogram and arterial pulse.

second heart sound splits into two components during inspiration ('lub da-dup') and comes together again in expiration. This physiological splitting of the second heart sound is the result of minor changes in the stroke volume of left and right ventricles during the normal respiratory cycle.

During inspiration, venous return to the right side of the heart is increased, thus increasing right ventricular stroke volume and delaying pulmonary valve closure. At the same time, pooling of blood in the pulmonary veins reduces filling of the left ventricle and makes aortic valve closure slightly earlier than in expiration. The split may

Splitting of the second heart sound

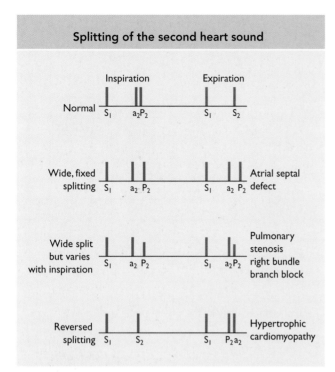

Fig. 6.12 Beat to beat variations in left and right ventricular stroke volume cause splitting of the second heart sound in phase with breathing. Splitting of the second sound with inspiration is normal. Other patterns may indicate cardiac abnormalities.

Electrical conduction in the heart

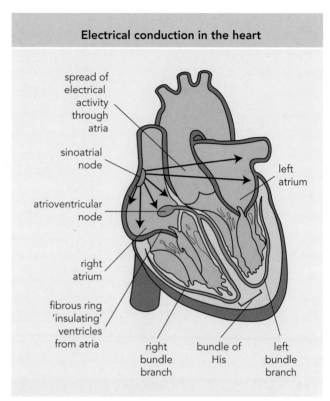

Fig. 6.13 Paths of the spread of electrical impulses in the heart (note that there are no specific electrical pathways in the atria).

be widened by other factors that delay right ventricular contraction, such as right bundle branch block or pulmonary valve stenosis. Conversely, anything that delays left ventricular contraction, such as left bundle branch block, hypertrophic obstructive cardiomyopathy or severe aortic stenosis, may so delay the aortic component of the second heart sound that the normal relationship is reversed and there is increasing splitting of the second heart sound on expiration with the sounds coming together on inspiration. This is known as paradoxical splitting of the second heart sound. Finally, in an atrial septal defect, there is a characteristically fixed splitting of the second heart sound because the hole in the intra-atrial septum means that left and right atrial pressure remains equal throughout the respiratory cycle (Fig. 6.12).

Electrical activity of the heart

The signal for contraction of each heart muscle cell is the electrical depolarisation of its membrane. The electrical signal is transmitted from cell to cell in an orderly way so that under normal circumstances the heart contracts in an orderly fashion. The physiological cardiac pacemaker comprises a small group of cells in the sinoatrial node situated close to where the right atrium joins the superior vena cava. Normally, these cells undergo cyclical repolarisation and depolarisation at a faster rate than

cells in other parts of the heart. The electrical impulse spreads out from the sinoatrial node (Fig. 6.13) through the cardiac muscle of the atria. The atria and the ventricles are separated by a fibrous ring of tissue to which the tricuspid and mitral valves are attached and which does not support conduction of the cardiac impulse. The only electrical pathway through this ring is through the atrioventricular node, a localised area of specialised conducting tissue lying between the tricuspid valve and the aorta. There is a delay of 0.12–0.20s while the impulse passes through the atrioventricular node, ensuring the correct delay between atrial and ventricular contraction. Once through the atrioventricular node, the electrical impulse is rapidly conducted to ventricular tissue through specialised conducting fibres which form the bundle of His and its branches.

ELECTROCARDIOGRAM

The electrocardiogram (ECG) is an electrical and structural map of the heart and is an invaluable aid to studying normal heart rhythm and its disturbances. It works by sensing and amplifying the very small electrical potential changes between different points on the surface of the body caused by the cyclical depolarisation and repolarisation of the heart cells. Electrical potentials are picked up by electrodes that are attached to the skin. The points at which the electrodes are attached and the conventional ways in which they are connected enable

The multilead ECG

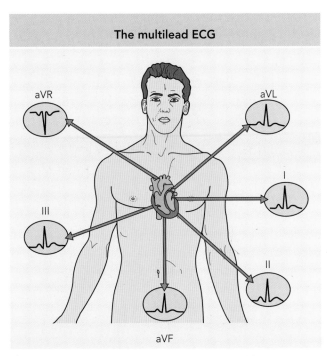

Fig. 6.14 How the ECG 'looks at' the heart from different directions (a concept due to Goldberger and Wilson).

The ECG 'complex'

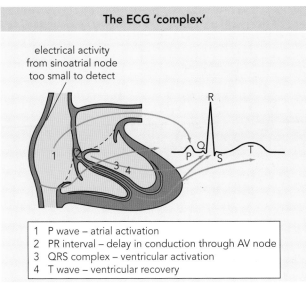

electrical activity from sinoatrial node too small to detect

1 P wave – atrial activation
2 PR interval – delay in conduction through AV node
3 QRS complex – ventricular activation
4 T wave – ventricular recovery

Fig. 6.15 Different parts of an ECG 'complex'.

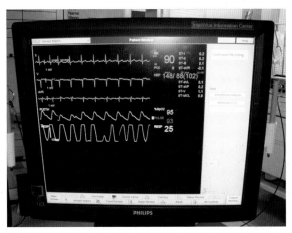

Fig. 6.16 ECG trace displayed on a monitor at the nursing station or bedside.

the ECG to 'look at' the heart from a sequence of different directions (Fig. 6.14). The cycle of electrical changes during a single heart beat is termed an ECG complex. Different parts of the ECG complex reflect the activation of different parts of the heart. The P wave signals atrial activity and the QRS complex indicates ventricular activity (Fig. 6.15).

In patients suspected of intermittent arrhythmias, the ECG may be displayed as a continuous monitor trace (Fig. 6.16). In patients outside hospital, the ECG can be recorded continuously digitally for periods of 24–48 h and then played back to analyse any rhythm disturbances. This process is called 'ambulatory ECG' or 'Holter monitoring'. The ECG can be used to detect hypertrophy of the different chambers of the heart (Fig. 6.17), abnormal rhythms and cardiac damage.

Cardiac arrhythmias

Abnormalities of heart rhythm can be divided into those in which the heart goes too slowly (bradycardia) and those in which the rate is abnormally rapid (tachycardia). Physiologically, heart rate can vary in a normal young adult from 40 beats/min during sleep to 180 beats/minute or more during vigorous exercise. The physiological control of heart rate is due to a balance between sympathetic nervous activity, which speeds the heart rate, and vagal activity, which slows it down.

There are two principal mechanisms of arrhythmia generation: automaticity and re-entry phenomena. The

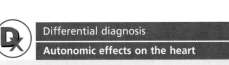

Differential diagnosis
Autonomic effects on the heart

Vagal tone (slows the heart)
- Increased in: children, athletes
- Stimulated by:
  - carotid baroreceptors, pain, trauma (via hypothalamus)
  - ventricular stretch receptors (fainting reflex)
- Excessive in:
  - malignant vasovagal syncope
  - carotid sinus syncope
- Blocked by: atropine

Sympathetic tone (speeds up the heart)
- Increased by: fear, pain, hypovolaemia, heart failure, physical activity
- Decreased: during sleep
- Blocked by: β-adrenoceptor blockers

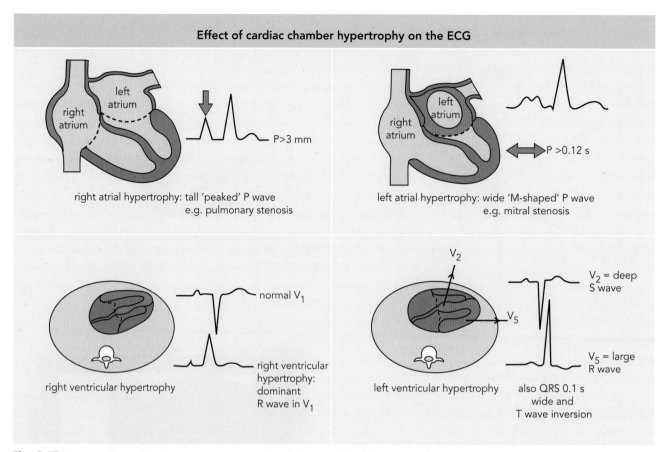

Fig. 6.17 Electrocardiographic changes can be used to identify hypertrophy of the cardiac chambers.

latter comprises 90% of arrhythmias. Automaticity implies normal conduction tissue or abnormal conduction (ectopic) tissue that is repetitively firing faster than usual. Re-entry phenomenon is described under tachycardia below.

BRADYCARDIA

Bradycardia may be caused by drugs, particularly β-adrenoceptor blocking drugs ('beta-blockers'); it may also be a physiological finding in fit young athletes with a high vagal tone. Extreme bradycardia may be caused by heart block with failure of conduction of the electrical impulse, most often as it passes through the atrioventricular node or bundle of His (Fig. 6.18).

TACHYCARDIA

Ectopic beats

As all heart muscle and not only the sinoatrial node exhibits the capacity for spontaneous depolarisation, it is not uncommon to find an 'ectopic focus' of electrical activity which can initiate extra beats out of time with the normal cardiac cycle. These extra beats or extrasystoles may be generated in the atrium or ventricle. In otherwise healthy people, extrasystoles are usually benign and harmless. Following myocardial

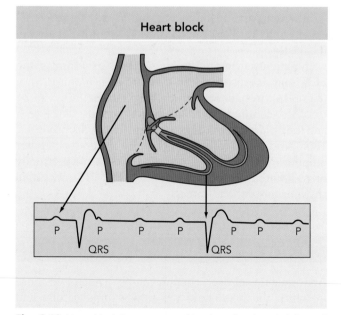

Fig. 6.18 Heart block is one cause of bradycardia; there is failure of conduction of the electrical impulses from atrium to ventricle.

infarction or during a viral infection of the heart, they may act as markers for metabolic damage and, consequently, excessive irritability of the heart muscle (Fig. 6.19).

Ventricular and atrial extrasystoles

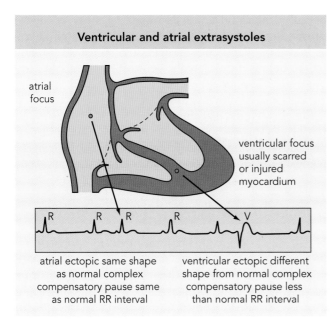

atrial focus

ventricular focus usually scarred or injured myocardium

atrial ectopic same shape as normal complex compensatory pause same as normal RR interval

ventricular ectopic different shape from normal complex compensatory pause less than normal RR interval

Fig. 6.19 Extrasystoles are caused by an ectopic focus of electrical activity.

Sustained tachycardia

A persistent tachycardia may be caused by several ectopic beats occurring in sequence (e.g. as the manifestation of a particularly irritable ectopic focus). This is called a 'focal tachycardia'.

A more common mechanism for sustained tachycardia is, however, the phenomenon of re-entry (Fig. 6.20). The basic principle of a re-entry tachycardia is that there are two alternative pathways for the conduction of the electrical impulse; these pathways differ both in their speed of conduction and their refractory period. Under normal conditions, the cardiac impulse will be conducted by both pathways but an exceptionally early beat may find one pathway still refractory to conduction and therefore the impulse will be conducted down the other one alone. However, by the time it reaches the end of this pathway, the other pathway will have recovered and be able to conduct the impulse in the reverse direction. This sets up the possibility of a 'circus movement' or oscillation and the re-entry circuit can act as a focus for

Re-entry tachycardia

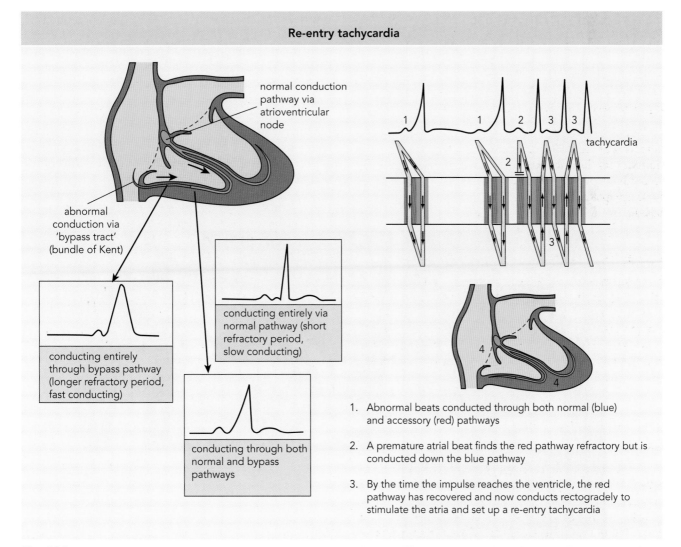

normal conduction pathway via atrioventricular node

abnormal conduction via 'bypass tract' (bundle of Kent)

conducting entirely through bypass pathway (longer refractory period, fast conducting)

conducting entirely via normal pathway (short refractory period, slow conducting)

conducting through both normal and bypass pathways

tachycardia

1. Abnormal beats conducted through both normal (blue) and accessory (red) pathways

2. A premature atrial beat finds the red pathway refractory but is conducted down the blue pathway

3. By the time the impulse reaches the ventricle, the red pathway has recovered and now conducts rectogradely to stimulate the atria and set up a re-entry tachycardia

Fig. 6.20 Mechanism of a re-entry tachycardia, based on the 'paradigm' of the Wolff–Parkinson–White syndrome. The left hand diagram shows the ECG pattern produced when conduction is all along the bypass pathway, when it is all along the normal pathway and when it is along both simultaneously.

generating a tachycardia. This tachycardia may continue until one of the pathways fatigues and cannot conduct fast enough to maintain the circuit or until the process is interrupted by an electrical stimulus which breaks the circuit and re-establishes normal conduction (Fig. 6.21).

Fibrillation

The most extreme form of arrhythmia occurs when the coordinated conduction of impulses between cells completely breaks down and individual cells contract haphazardly. This process is termed fibrillation. Atrial fibrillation is common but not particularly hazardous because the atrioventricular node acts as a 'filter', preventing the ventricles from being stimulated at too rapid a rate. Ventricular fibrillation is, however, rapidly lethal because the rapidly contracting ventricles are ineffective and unable to pump any blood into the circulation. The only treatment for ventricular fibrillation is to pass an artificial competing electric current through the heart. This technique is referred to as defibrillation and causes momentary extinction of all electrical activity, allowing the whole system to reset (Fig. 6.22).

Blood supply to the heart

Heart muscle needs a supply of blood to support both its basal metabolic needs and the increased oxygen requirements of exercise. The blood supply must be capable of increasing to meet the heart's demands during exercise because heart muscle, unlike skeletal muscle, can only work aerobically. The arterial blood supply to the heart is provided by the right and left coronary arteries. The right coronary artery supplies mainly the right ventricle and the inferior surface of the left ventricle. It divides at the end of its course into the posterolateral branch and the posterior descending branch, which supplies the posterior and lateral parts of the left ventricle The left coronary has a common trunk (the left main stem) which divides soon after its origin into the left anterior descending coronary artery, which supplies the interventricular septum, the anterior surface and the apex of the left ventricle, and the circumflex coronary artery, which supplies the lateral part of the left ventricle (Fig. 6.23).

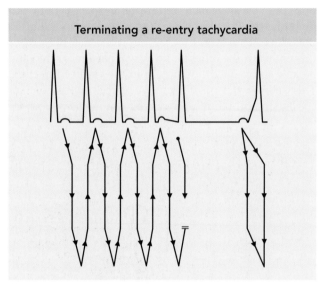

Terminating a re-entry tachycardia

Fig. 6.21 A critically timed extra stimulus can terminate a re-entry tachycardia by making both pathways refractory.

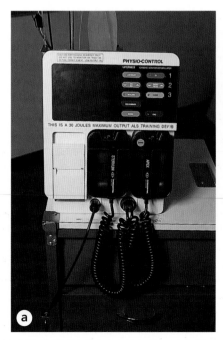

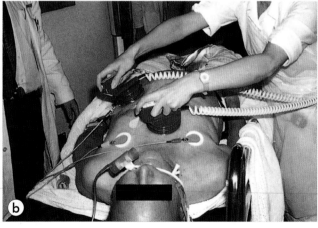

Fig. 6.22 A defibrillator (a). An electrical charge is built up within the machine and discharged through paddles applied to the patient's chest (b).

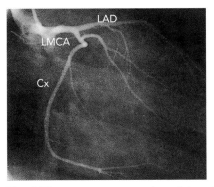
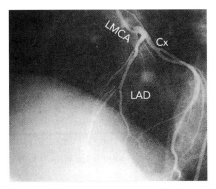
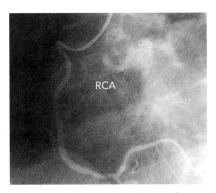

Fig. 6.23 Cine-angiograms to show (left and middle) the left coronary artery and (right) the right coronary artery (RCA) (Cx, left circumflex artery; LAD, left anterior descending artery; LMCA, left main coronary artery).

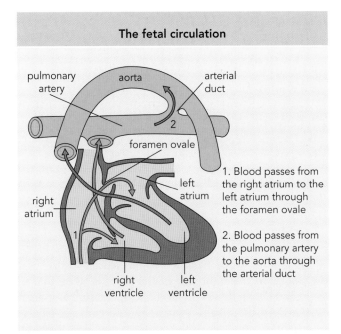

Fig. 6.24 In the fetal circulation, oxygenated blood from the umbilical vein bypasses the liver through the ductus venosus; a portion is shunted from the right to left atrium through the foramen ovale and a further portion passes through the arterial duct.

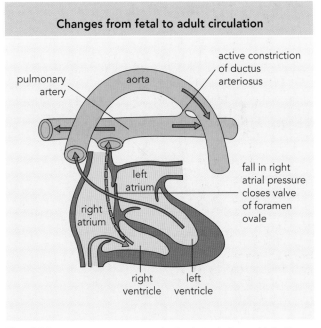

Fig. 6.25 Changes that occur in the fetal circulation at birth. The ductus arteriosus constricts and the fall in right arterial pressure as the lungs expand closes the foramen ovale.

In common with other arteries in the body, coronary arteries are prone to atheroma which predisposes to thrombosis and coronary artery occlusion. The clinical features of coronary thrombosis and the myocardial infarction are described later.

INTRACARDIAC SHUNTING

In the fetus, the placenta, rather than the lungs, participates in respiratory gas exchange and the unexpanded lungs offer a high resistance to blood flow. Both sides of the fetal heart work to pump a mixture of deoxygenated blood from the systemic veins and oxygenated blood from the placenta into the aorta and thus to the rest of the body. Blood entering in the right atrium may pass either through the tricuspid valve into the right ventricle or through a hole in the intra-atrial septum, the foramen ovale. Blood entering the right ventricle is pumped into the pulmonary artery, with only a small proportion of it entering the lungs. The remainder passes via the ductus arteriosus into the aorta (Fig. 6.24).

After birth, as the lungs inflate with air, intrapulmonary vascular resistance of the lungs rapidly falls. The subsequent fall in right atrial pressure and rise in left atrial pressure creates a pressure change which forces the valve-like foramen ovale to close and seals the interatrial septum. At the same time, the ductus arteriosus constricts and closes (Fig. 6.25). This separates the work of the right and left sides of the heart and causes them to work in series rather than in parallel. However, abnormalities in the process of transition from fetal to adult circulation, or

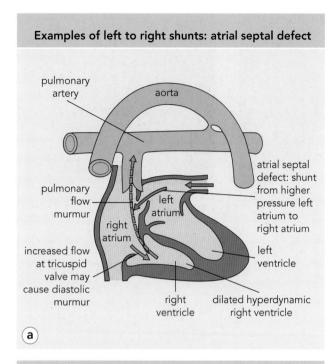

Examples of left to right shunts: atrial septal defect

pulmonary artery

aorta

pulmonary flow murmur

left atrium

right atrium

atrial septal defect: shunt from higher pressure left atrium to right atrium

increased flow at tricuspid valve may cause diastolic murmur

right ventricle

left ventricle

dilated hyperdynamic right ventricle

(a)

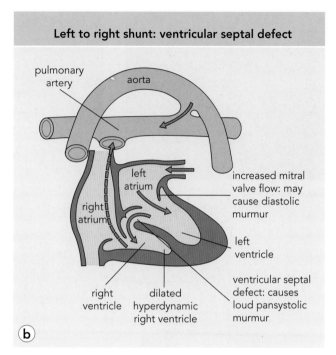

Left to right shunt: ventricular septal defect

pulmonary artery

aorta

left atrium

right atrium

increased mitral valve flow: may cause diastolic murmur

left ventricle

right ventricle

dilated hyperdynamic right ventricle

ventricular septal defect: causes loud pansystolic murmur

(b)

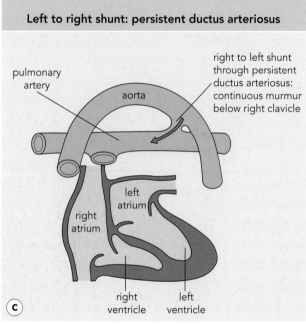

Left to right shunt: persistent ductus arteriosus

pulmonary artery

aorta

right to left shunt through persistent ductus arteriosus: continuous murmur below right clavicle

left atrium

right atrium

right ventricle

left ventricle

(c)

Fig. 6.26 (a) Left to right shunt atrial septal defect. Blood passes from the left to right atrium. The overall result is an increase in pulmonary blood flow. (b) Left to right shunt: ventricular septal defect. Blood passes from the high pressure left ventricle to the lower pressure right ventricle. (c) Left to right shunt: persistent ductus arteriosus. Blood passes from the high pressure aorta to the lower pressure pulmonary artery.

the heart has to cope with the extra load of blood shunted from the left. A two-to-one shunt means that the output at the right side of the heart is twice that of the left side of the heart and the increased workload on the right side of the heart may lead to heart failure. Alternatively, the excessively high blood flow through the lungs may lead to irreversible damage to the pulmonary vasculature and the development of pulmonary hypertension. Examples of left to right shunts are shown in Figure 6.26.

Right to left shunt

If a septal defect or persistent ductus arteriosus is combined with a further lesion that raises the pressure on the right side of the heart then, instead of blood flowing from the left-sided chamber to the right-sided chamber, it will flow in the opposite direction, from the right side of the heart to the left. The most common example of congenital heart disease causing a right to left shunt is Fallot's tetralogy (Fig. 6.27) which is physiologically equivalent to a ventricular septal defect plus pulmonary valve stenosis. A right to left shunt can occur when pulmonary vascular damage occurs in a patient with a severe left to right shunt. The resistance of the pulmonary arteries rises, resulting in increased pressure on the right side of the heart and a reversal of the shunt. This is called Eisenmenger's syndrome (Fig. 6.28).

anatomical defects in the partitions or 'septa' dividing the right and left sides of the heart, may lead to short-circuits or 'shunts'.

Left to right shunt

A congenital or acquired defect in the interatrial septum, interventricular septum or failure of closure of the ductus arteriosus will produce a left to right shunt. Blood follows the path of least resistance from the high pressure left-sided chamber to the lower pressure right-sided chamber. The result is that, instead of matching left and the right sided cardiac outputs, the right side of

Fallot's tetralogy

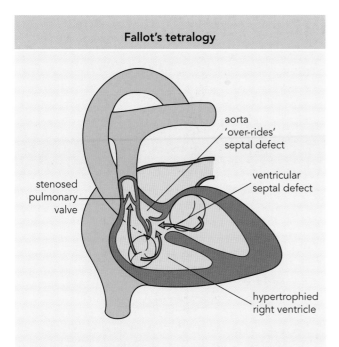

Fig. 6.27 Fallot's tetralogy is the most common 'congenital' cause of a right to left shunt. (The 'tetralogy' comprises pulmonary stenosis, ventricular septal defect, over-riding aorta and right ventricular hypertrophy.) (Note that cyanosis sometimes develops several weeks after birth because dynamic hypertrophy of muscle in the right ventricular outflow tract worsens the obstruction.)

Eisenmenger's syndrome

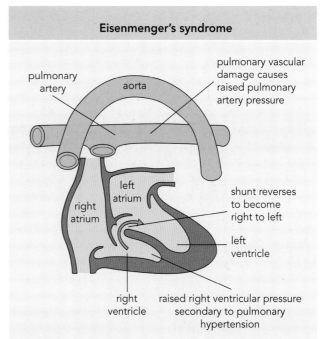

Fig. 6.28 Eisenmenger's syndrome is caused by a secondary rise in pulmonary vascular resistance as a consequence of pulmonary damage from increased blood flow initially due to a left to right shunt. (In some children, the pulmonary vasculature may never develop normally in the presence of such a shunt.)

The striking clinical feature about patients with right to left shunts is central cyanosis due to the admixture of desaturated venous blood with saturated blood coming from the pulmonary vein. It differs from cyanosis caused by lung disease or pulmonary oedema as it is not corrected by administering supplemental oxygen.

In patients with right to left shunts clinical signs of long-term adaptation to chronic reduction in systemic arterial oxygen saturation include finger clubbing (Fig. 6.29), polycythaemia and acne (particularly in adolescent children).

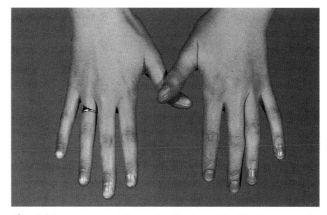

Fig. 6.29 Cyanosis and finger clubbing in a girl with Eisenmenger's syndrome.

Differential diagnosis
Factors that affect the shape of the pulse

- Velocity of cardiac ejection
- Stroke volume (decreased with tachycardia, heart failure or hypovolaemia)
- Peripheral resistance (low peripheral resistance leads to 'collapsing' pulse)
- Left ventricular outflow obstruction ('slow rising' pulse in aortic stenosis)
- Elasticity of peripheral vessels (inelastic vessels, e.g. in elderly people, may 'sharpen' pulse waves)
- Reflection of pulse waves from the periphery

The arterial system

The arterial system distributes oxygenated blood from the heart to the tissues and organs of the body. At the points where arteries pass close to the body surface or can be compressed against the bony skeleton, they can be felt as 'pulses' (Fig. 6.30). During each cardiac cycle, the left ventricle ejects blood into the aorta and initiates a pulse wave that is transmitted to the periphery. It is important to remember that the pulse wave travels to the periphery much more rapidly than the actual flow of blood.

The arterial pulses

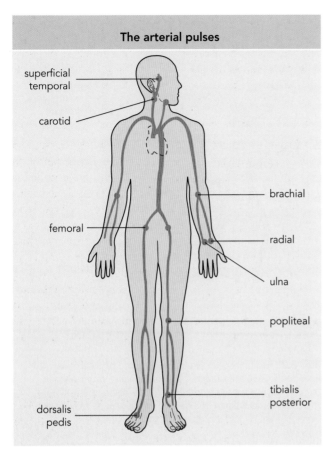

Fig. 6.30 Some of the points at which arterial pulsation can be felt. (Note the similarity to first-aiders' 'pressure points'.)

The pulse wave

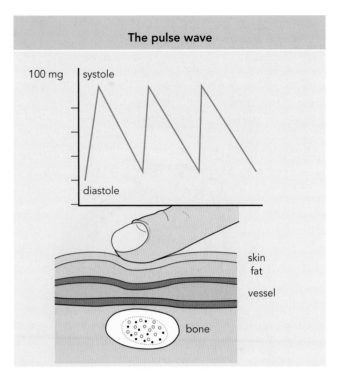

Fig. 6.31 Relationship between the pulse and the arterial waveform.

An intra-arterial recording of pressure against time indicates the shape of the pulse wave, which approximates to that which would be felt by a finger placed on the arterial wall (Fig. 6.31). The shape of the arterial pulse wave depends on many factors (see 'differential diagnosis' box).

The venous system

The most important mechanism allowing individual organs to adjust their blood supply according to metabolic need is by decreasing or increasing the arteriolar resistance to inflow (i.e. very small arteries 200–300 mm in diameter). Thus, food ingestion considerably reduces gut vascular resistance and increases gut blood flow. Similarly, exercising skeletal muscle strikingly reduces its vascular resistance, thereby increasing local blood flow. Alteration of blood flow to the skin is one of the important mechanisms controlling heat loss or conservation. The arteriolar resistance in the skin and the gut is under autonomic sympathetic nervous system control; sympathetic nervous system stimulation causes arteriolar constriction resulting in a rise in blood pressure. The most important blood vessels contributing to control of peripheral vascular resistance are the small muscular arteries and arterioles; larger blood vessels such as the femoral, carotid or radial arteries are conduits and play little or no role in the control of blood pressure.

The major veins of the body are shown in Figure 6.32. Systemic veins collect blood from the tissues and return it to the right atrium of the heart. The venous return from the gut is specialised because it flows into the hepatic portal vein and first enters the liver before flowing out through the hepatic veins into the inferior vena cava. The venous system operates at a much lower pressure than the arterial system. Veins draining the chest and abdomen drain passively into the vena cava, either directly or via the azygos vein. In the upright position, venous drainage from the head and neck is assisted by gravity. Passive venous drainage alone is inadequate for the limbs and, in particular, the lower limbs. Here, the venous system is divided into superficial and deep veins (Fig. 6.33) separated by one-way valves. Contraction of the arm and leg muscles during normal activities massage the deep veins and this pumping action actively propels blood back towards the heart. The one-way valve system between the deep and superficial venous systems of the lower limb ensures unidirectional blood flow.

Clinical history

A carefully taken history sets the scene for the subsequent physical examination. Particular symptoms that need to

Venous drainage

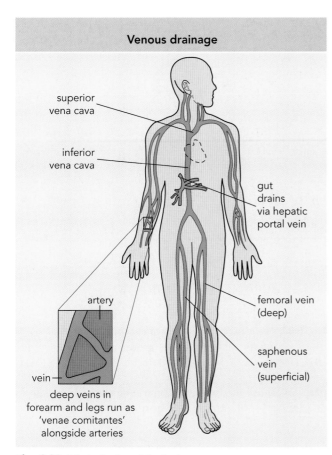

superior
vena cava

inferior
vena cava

gut
drains
via hepatic
portal vein

femoral vein
(deep)

saphenous
vein
(superficial)

artery

vein

deep veins in
forearm and legs run as
'venae comitantes'
alongside arteries

Fig. 6.32 Principal veins of the body.

Veins in the leg

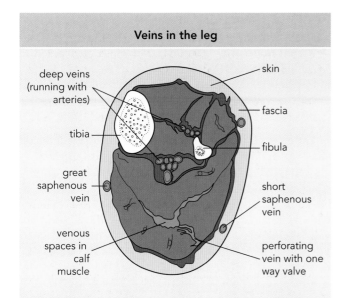

deep veins
(running with
arteries)

skin

fascia

tibia

fibula

great
saphenous
vein

short
saphenous
vein

venous
spaces in
calf
muscle

perforating
vein with one
way valve

Fig. 6.33 Veins in the leg form a 'muscle pump' in conjunction with the calf muscles. Muscle contraction forces blood from superficial to deep veins, and from periphery to centre.

be enquired of in the cardiovascular history include breathlessness, chest pain, palpitation, syncope and claudication. The presence or absence of these symptoms provides clues to the likely findings anticipated on physical examination.

BREATHLESSNESS

Patients with heart disease characteristically experience breathlessness during physical exertion (exertional dyspnoea) and sometimes when lying flat (known as positional dyspnoea or orthopnoea). There is evidence that orthopnoea is caused by stimulation of fine nerve endings in the lungs as a result of increased pulmonary capillary pressure, caused by redistribution of fluid between peripheral tissues and the lungs when the patient lies flat. Sometimes, the patient wakes extremely breathless from sleep and has to sit up gasping for breath, a symptom known as paroxysmal nocturnal dyspnoea. In extreme forms, this may be accompanied by a cough productive of white frothy sputum indicative of pulmonary oedema.

> **?** Questions to ask
>
> **Breathlessness**
>
> - Do you ever feel short of breath?
> - Does this happen on exertion?
> - How much can you do before getting breathless?
> - Do you ever wake up gasping for breath?
> - If so, do you have to sit up or get out of bed?
> - How many pillows do you sleep on?
> - Do you cough or wheeze when you are short of breath?

The mechanism of exercise-associated dyspnoea is controversial. It may be partly due to the same mechanism as orthopnoea, with increased venous return from exercising muscles raising left atrial pressure. However, in exercising patients, the sensation of breathlessness does not always correlate well with directly measured left atrial pressure. Other factors such as reduced arterial blood oxygen saturation and alteration of muscle function in chronic heart failure have also been invoked as mechanisms contributing to the sensation of breathlessness.

A commonly used classification of exercise tolerance in heart failure is that proposed by the New York Heart Association (NYHA). This is commonly used in clinical trials and has been shown to correlate with prognosis. For practical purposes, when taking the history, it is helpful to record the symptoms verbatim. Reflecting the patient's description of symptoms over time can be particularly useful in assessing progress. Left ventricular failure may present with associated wheezing. However, cardiac asthma should always be distinguished from obstructive airways disease; both history and examination should be helpful in distinguishing heart failure from asthma.

Symptoms and signs	
New York Heart Association classification of heart failure	
Grade I	No symptoms at rest, dyspnoea only on vigorous exertion
Grade II	No symptoms at rest, dyspnoea on moderate exertion
Grade III	May be mild symptoms at rest, dyspnoea on mild exertion, severe dyspnoea on moderate exertion
Grade IV	Significant dyspnoea at rest, severe dyspnoea even on very mild exertion. Patient often bed bound

It can sometimes be difficult to decide whether dyspnoea is caused by heart disease or lung disease. Paroxysmal nocturnal dyspnoea or orthopnoea points more to left ventricular failure, whereas wheezing or productive cough accompanying dyspnoea and risk features for lung disease would favour a pulmonary cause.

Differential diagnosis	
Dyspnoea	

- Heart failure
- Ischaemic heart disease (atypical or 'silent' angina)
- Pulmonary embolism
- Lung disease
- Severe anaemia

Anxiety should always be considered in the differential diagnosis of breathlessness. The pattern described by the patient is different; they might describe the sensation of suddenly feeling the need to take a deep breath unrelated to physical exertion, excessive sighing or a feeling of air hunger.

CHEST PAIN

Chest pain caused by myocardial ischaemia

Angina pectoris is the most common presenting cardiac chest pain. The characteristic features of anginal

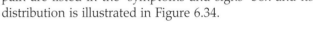

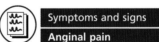

Fig. 6.34 Characteristic distribution of anginal pain.

pain are listed in the 'symptoms and signs' box and its distribution is illustrated in Figure 6.34.

Symptoms and signs	
Anginal pain	

- Brought on by physical or emotional exertion
- Relieved by rest
- Usually crushing, squeezing or constricting in nature
- Usually retrosternal (Fig. 6.34)
- Often worse after food or in cold winds
- Often relieved by nitrates

The characteristic feature of angina is exercise-induced chest pain that remits soon after the exertion is discontinued. It is usually described as a crushing, squeezing or constricting pain (the Greek word from which it is derived means 'choking'). Most patients with angina have stenosis of one or more coronary arteries and the retrosternal pain is precipitated when physical or emotional exertion increases the metabolic demand. The discomfort and pain are caused by an imbalance between myocardial blood supply and the metabolic demand resulting in anaerobic metabolism. Less often, angina may be a symptom of aortic stenosis, hypertrophic cardiomyopathy and other rare causes such as syndrome X (angina with normal coronary arteries) and Prinzmetal's angina (due to coronary spasm).

Pain similar in nature to angina but occurring at rest may be caused by the acute coronary syndrome, otherwise

Questions to ask

Angina

- Do you get pain in your chest on exertion (e.g. climbing stairs)?
- Whereabouts in the chest do you feel the pain?
- Is it worse in cold weather?
- Is it worse if you exercise after a big meal?
- Is it bad enough to stop you from exercising?
- Does it go away when you rest?
- Do you ever get similar pain if you get excited or upset?

Differential diagnosis

Chest pain on exertion

- Angina caused by coronary atheroma
- Aortic stenosis
- Hypertrophic cardiomyopathy
- 'Syndrome X' (anginal syndrome with normal coronary arteries)

known as unstable angina or myocardial infarction. The pain of myocardial infarction is severe, persistent and often accompanied by autonomic symptoms including nausea, vomiting and sweating (diaphoresis). Some patients describe a feeling of impending death.

Differential diagnosis

Chest pain at rest

- Myocardial infarction
- Unstable angina
- Dissecting aortic aneurysm
- Prinzmetal's angina (due to coronary spasm)
- Oesophageal pain
- Pericarditis
- Pleuritic pain
- Musculoskeletal pain
- Herpes zoster (shingles)

Red flag – urgent referral

Chest pain

- Chest pain at rest lasting >15–20 min
- Recent onset crescendo angina symptoms
- Unresponsive to GTN (glyceryl trinitrate)
- Associated autonomic symptoms (nausea, vomiting, sweating)

Pericarditis

Pericarditis is an inflammation of the pericardium, the serous sac surrounding the heart. It may be a complication following myocardial infarction or may result from a viral or bacterial infection or uraemia. The patient usually complains of pain that is perceived as a constant retrosternal soreness and which is often aggravated by deep breathing. The pain of pericarditis is characteristically aggravated by change in posture (e.g. turning over in bed) rather than physical exertion and sometimes radiates to the left shoulder tip.

Musculoskeletal chest pain

Pain arising in the chest wall or thoracic spine is often mistaken for cardiac pain. Characteristically, it is described as an aching pain, the onset of which may relate to a postural movement and the pain is usually present at rest. Costochondritis, or Tietze syndrome, should also be considered in patients presenting with chest pain. The anterior chest pain is usually present at rest and associated with localised tenderness over the costal cartilages and costochondral joints. This syndrome is due to local inflammation which may be viral in origin or occur spontaneously. A variant of musculoskeletal pain is the precordial catch syndrome, in which the patient describes a sudden, sharp needle-like jabbing pain in the precordium. The pain is short-lasting but may recur. The cause is unknown and the symptom runs a benign course.

Dissecting aortic aneurysm

Dissecting aneurysm of the thoracic aorta is a rare cause of chest pain which has a characteristic presentation. The pain is usually described at the outset as a 'tearing' sensation. It is often felt between the shoulder blades or in the mid-back and is usually severe, persistent and readily mistaken for the pain of myocardial infarction.

Other chest pains

Other chest pains that may masquerade as cardiac pain include the pain of pleurisy, acute pneumothorax or herpes zoster (shingles).

PALPITATION

Palpitation is defined as abnormal awareness of the heart beat. This may be perceived with exercise, when it is quite normal, or when there is an irregularity of the heart beat. It may be helpful to ask the patient to tap out the heart rhythm on the table. Ask about the duration of the palpitations and whether they end abruptly. In patients with extrasystoles, it is often not the extra beat itself that the patient perceives, but rather the following beat, which is characterised by a longer than usual pause and an excessively forceful beat. The patient may describe a jumping sensation or the feeling that the heart is about to stop. Ask about precipitating factors such as exercise, emotion or foods, in particular tea, coffee, alcohol and chocolates. You should also ask carefully about any medication, particularly over-the-counter decongestants and 'cold cures' which often contain sympathomimetic drugs.

Ectopic beats are often more apparent when the background heart rate is slow (e.g. when the patient lies down to rest). Paroxysmal tachycardias are often precipitated by exercise or by particular movements such as stooping down to open a drawer or reaching to remove an item from a high shelf.

Questions to ask
Palpitation

- Please tap out on the table the rate at which you think your heart goes during an attack
- Is the heart beat regular or irregular?
- Is there anything that sets an attack off?
- Can you do anything to stop an attack?
- What do you do when you have an attack?
- Are there any foods that seem to make symptoms worse?
- What medicines are you taking?

Differential diagnosis
Palpitation

- Extrasystoles
- Paroxysmal atrial fibrillation
- Paroxysmal supraventricular tachycardia
- Thyrotoxicosis
- Perimenopausal

The need to treat an arrhythmia is usually dictated by its haemodynamic effects. Enquire whether the arrhythmia is simply a transient inconvenience or whether the patient has to stop their activity and perhaps even lie down. Cardiac arrhythmias may cause loss of consciousness (cardiac syncope).

Many patients with paroxysmal tachycardia learn to use a modified Valsalva manoeuvre to terminate an attack. This might be achieved by forcibly exhaling with the nose and the mouth held shut or even by head immersion in cold water. Some patients with tachycardia describe a period of excessive urination following the palpitation. This is due to the release of atrial natriuretic hormone (ANP) during the tachycardia.

SYNCOPE (FAINTING, BLACKOUTS)

Syncope is defined as loss of consciousness resulting from a transient failure of blood supply to the brain. The presentation is readily confused with certain forms of epilepsy. Key features in the history that distinguish cardiogenic syncope from epilepsy includes lack of warning or aura, colour change (patients look pale during the event and flushed upon recovery due to hyperaemia) and rapid recovery. Remember that generalised convulsions can also occur following cerebral anoxia if the blood supply to the brain is interrupted for long enough. Common causes of syncope include simple fainting (vasovagal syncope), its variants such as micturition and cough syncope, postural hypotension, vertebrobasilar insufficiency and cardiac arrhythmias, particularly intermittent heart block.

Simple fainting is caused by a vagally mediated bradycardia combined with sudden reflex vasodilatation. It is usually caused by a combination of diminished venous return (e.g. standing still on a hot parade ground), coupled with increased sympathic drive caused by excitement, fear or disgust. *Malignant vasovagal syncope* is a rare disorder characterised by an exaggerated tendency to faint, resulting in recurrent episodes of unexpected syncope. *Micturition syncope* characteristically occurs at night in middle-aged or elderly men with a degree of prostatic obstruction, in whom the fall in venous return is caused by straining to empty the bladder accompanied by the sympathic stimulation of the consequences of not doing so. *Cough syncope* is an exaggerated vagal response to violent coughing and, uncommonly, is a cause of syncope in patients with chronic lung disease.

The Stokes–Adams attack is a term used by some physicians to describe cardiogenic syncope. It was originally defined as syncope due to cortical hypoperfusion caused by transient asystole or a ventricular tachyarrhythmia.

Differential diagnosis	
Stokes–Adams versus epilepsy	
Stokes–Adams	**Epilepsy**
No aura or warning	Aura often present
Transient loss of consciousness	Prolonged loss of consciousness
Pale during attack	Tonic/clonic phases
Rapid recovery	Prolonged recovery/drowsy
Hot flush on recovery	No hot flush on recovery

In fainting, loss of consciousness is seldom abrupt. The patient appears pale both before and immediately afterwards and both consciousness and motor power are rapidly restored by elevating the legs. In contrast, syncope caused by heart block is sudden, unheralded and complete and is usually witnessed as a drop attack. The patient looks pale while collapsed and recovery, which is often equally sudden, may be heralded by a pink flush. Vertebrobasilar insufficiency is common in elderly patients. There is often restricted neck movement and active or passive movements of the neck may precipitate symptoms. Postural hypotension is more common in elderly patients and may be exacerbated by antihypertensive medication, particularly diuretics. Important clinical questions in taking the history are highlighted in the 'questions to ask' box.

> **Questions to ask**
>
> **Syncope**
>
> (Wherever possible history should be taken from a family member or observer as well as the patient.)
> - What were the exact circumstances of the blackout?
> - Did you have any warning of the attack?
> - How quickly did you recover?
> - Did you go pale or red during or after the attack?
> - Are you taking any medication?

> **Red flag – urgent referral**
>
> **Syncope**
>
> - Complete loss of consciousness
> - Associated injury
> - Recurrent syncope
> - Known aortic stenosis
> - Family history of premature sudden cardiac death <40 years of age

CLAUDICATION

Intermittent claudication is the term given to a condition where the patient experiences pain in one or both legs on walking and which eases when the patient rests. Just as angina is the usual initial symptom of atheromatous disease of the coronary arteries, so intermittent claudication is usually the earliest symptom of narrowing of the arteries supplying the legs. The pain is usually described as 'aching' felt in the calf, thigh or buttocks. Intermittent claudication is more common in men and most common in smokers.

Occupation and family history

The family history is important in evaluating patients with heart disease as many cardiac diseases have an underlying genetic predisposition (e.g. towards hyperlipidaemia). The relevance of a positive family history of coronary heart disease applies to first degree relatives only. Sometimes it is more helpful to ask whether specific family members are still alive or about the circumstances of their death because the significance of this may not be apparent to the patient. For example, early death from stroke may indicate a family susceptibility to hypertension. The significance of cardiac disease may be very relevant to the patient's occupation; an example would be an airline pilot or heavy goods vehicle driver where clinical coronary artery disease or arrhythmias might be incompatible with safety at work.

HABITS

Do not forget to enquire specifically about cigarette smoking, alcohol intake and any medication the patient may be taking.

> **Questions to ask**
>
> **Family history**
>
> - Is there any heart disease in the family?
> - Are your parents still alive?
> - Did they live to a good age?
> - Do you know what they died from?
> - Have you any brothers or sisters?
> - Do any of them have a heart problem?

Clinical examination of the cardiovascular system

There are three interlinking facets to the cardiovascular examination. First, the examination routine should ensure that the cardiovascular system is examined smoothly and efficiently and in appropriate detail. Second, the examination should aim to build on the clinical clues derived from the history. Third, the discovery of an unexpected sign, such as a heart murmur or anaemia, might alter the interpretation of the history and the differential diagnosis.

GENERAL OBSERVATION

The position of the patient on the examination couch is important. The patient should lie comfortably at 45°, with the head supported and the body exposed to the waist. Prior to starting the formal examination, spend a few moments observing the patient as important signs can be elicited from inspection alone. Is the patient comfortable at rest or distressed? Is the patient able to lie flat? Is the patient breathless or cyanosed and, if cyanosed, is this peripheral or central cyanosis? (See 'symptoms and signs' box.)

Blood appears bluish or purplish when there is more than 5 g of reduced haemoglobin in the circulation. In peripheral cyanosis, the prolonged capillary circulation

Symptoms and signs

General observation

- Tachypnoea at rest
- Central or peripheral cyanosis
- Mitral facies
- Scars (sternotomy, lateral thoracotomy, closed mitral valvotomy, saphenous vein graft harvest)
- Dentition (as a possible source of bacterial endocarditis)
- Xanthelasma
- Corneal arcus
- Anaemia

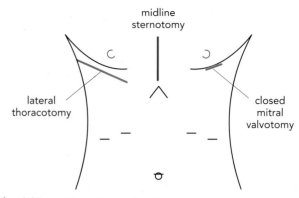

Fig. 6.35 Location of surgical incisions.

time caused by peripheral vasoconstriction results in excessive haemoglobin desaturation whilst the normal circulation time in the warm tongue and oral mucous membranes does not predispose to excessive deoxygenation. Central cyanosis indicates the presence of more than 5 g of reduced haemoglobin throughout the circulation and is indicative of anatomical or functional shunting of venous blood into the arterial circulation.

Is there evidence of previous cardiac surgical scars? The commonest cardiac scar is a mid-line sternotomy scar; also, check the legs for scars from veins stripped for use as bypass grafts. A lateral thoracotomy scar is often used in thoracic surgery. A small scar in the subclavicular region is a tell-tale site for a permanent pacemaker and a small scar under the left breast may indicate a previous closed mitral valvotomy (Fig. 6.35). Patients with mitral stenosis sometimes have a pink flushed colouration of the face, the so-called 'mitral facies'.

Symptoms and signs

Cyanosis

Peripheral cyanosis
- Cold fingers and toes
- Not dyspnoeic or tachypnoeic
- Peripheral vasoconstriction
- Bluish or purple discoloration of fingers and toes
- Normal pink coloured tongue

Central cyanosis
- Dyspnoea and tachypnoea
- Polycythaemia (secondary)
- Bluish or purple discolouration of the fingers and toes
- Similar discoloration of the tongue and oral mucous membranes
- Deoxygenated Hb level >5 g/dl

THE HANDS IN HEART DISEASE

Hand temperature gives a guide to the extent of peripheral vasodilatation. Patients in heart failure are usually vasoconstricted and their hands feel cold and sometimes sweaty from increased sympathetic drive. The fingernails may reveal splinter haemorrhages (Fig. 6.36) suggestive of subacute infective endocarditis. Finger clubbing is a sign of endocarditis and is a classical sign of cyanotic congenital heart disease.

Differential diagnosis

Cyanosis

Peripheral cyanosis
- Cold ambient temperature
- Shock with vasoconstriction
- Raynaud's phenomenon
- Beta-blocker drugs

Central cyanosis
- Severe chronic obstructive pulmonary disease
- Severe pulmonary infection
- Severe pulmonary embolism
- Congenital right to left shunt

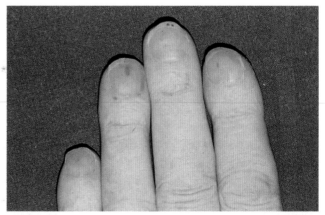

Fig. 6.36 Splinter haemorrhage in the ring finger of a man with infective endocarditis. There is an older, fading 'splinter' under the nail of the index finger. Splinter haemorrhages are often smaller and darker than this.

PALPATING THE PERIPHERAL PULSES

The radial pulse

The right radial pulse is usually best felt with the fingers of the examiner's left hand (Fig. 6.37) and is used to assess heart rate and rhythm. As the radial pulse is distant from the heart, it is an unsatisfactory landmark from which to attempt to assess pulse character. If there is suspicion of an abnormality in the aortic arch or the brachial artery on either side, it may be helpful to feel both radial pulses and simultaneously compare their volume and timing. In patients with suspected coarctation of the aorta, it is helpful simultaneously to feel the radial and the femoral pulse. In the presence of coarctation not only is the volume of the femoral pulse diminished but it is also appreciably delayed compared with the radial pulse (Fig. 6.38). As the blood flow leaving the aorta meets the restriction of a coarctation, there is dilatation of proximal collaterals and blood flows through intercostal

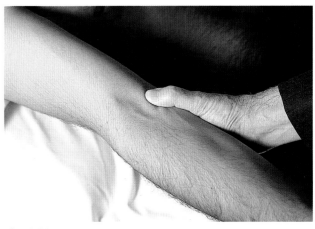

Fig. 6.39 Using the thumb to assess the character of the brachial pulse. The artery lies just medial to the tendinous insertion of the biceps muscle and deep to the fascial insertion of this muscle. It was called the 'grâce à dieu' (thanks be to God) fascia by medieval barber surgeons because it saved them from fatally damaging the artery when blood letting at the elbow!

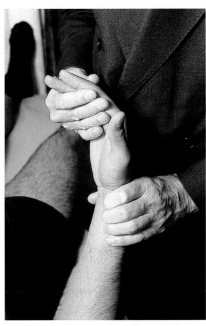

Fig. 6.37 Feeling the right radial pulse.

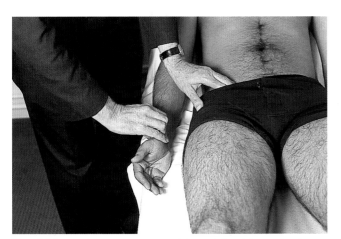

Fig. 6.38 Simultaneous palpation of the radial and femoral pulses: a delayed femoral pulse is a feature of aortic coarctation.

Pulse character		
Name	**Feels like**	**Associated with**
Normal	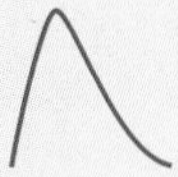	—
Slow rising	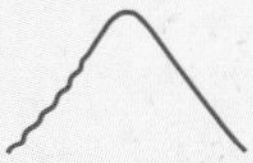	Aortic stenosis
Bisferiens ('two peaks')	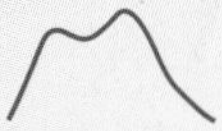	Mild aortic stenosis plus reflux
Collapsing	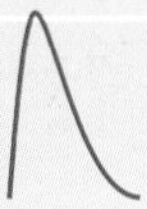	Aortic reflux Persistent ductus arteriosus
No pulse		Occluded bronchial or axillary artery

Fig. 6.40 Different pulse waveforms are associated with different cardiac or vascular abnormalities.

collaterals to rejoin the aorta distally. The extended route of the collateral circulation is the reason for radial femoral delay.

The brachial pulse

The right brachial pulse is best palpated using the thumb of the right hand, applied to the front of the elbow just medial to the biceps tendon with the fingers cupped round the back of the elbow (Fig. 6.39). The use of the thumb for feeling the pulse is helpful as it is the character of the pulse rather than rate or rhythm which is important at this point (Fig. 6.40).

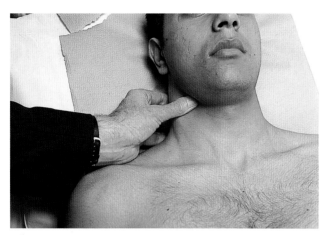

Fig. 6.41 Palpation of the carotid artery using the thumb.

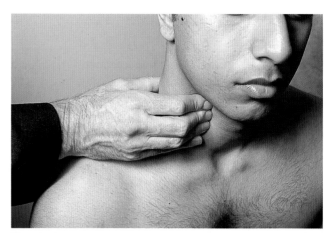

Fig. 6.42 Palpation of the carotid artery by different means.

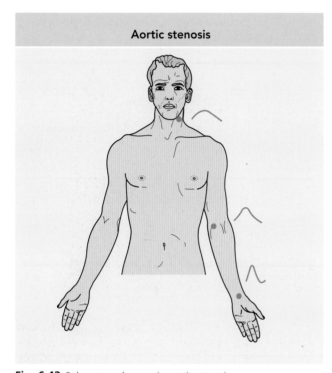

Fig. 6.43 Pulse wave changes in aortic stenosis.

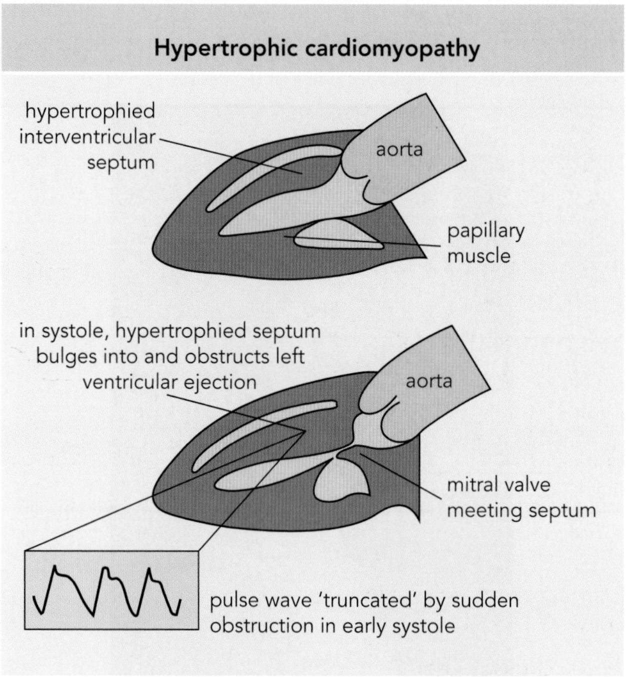

Hypertrophic cardiomyopathy

hypertrophied interventricular septum

aorta

papillary muscle

in systole, hypertrophied septum bulges into and obstructs left ventricular ejection

aorta

mitral valve meeting septum

pulse wave 'truncated' by sudden obstruction in early systole

Fig. 6.44 Hypertrophic cardiomyopathy. A 'jerky' carotid pulse may result from dynamic left ventricular outflow obstruction.

The carotid pulse

The carotid pulse is even closer to the heart than the brachial pulse and therefore even better for assessing pulse character as a reflection left ventricular mechanics. The best way to feel the patient's right carotid artery is to locate the tip of the left thumb against the patient's larynx and then gently but firmly press directly backwards so that the carotid artery is felt against the precervical muscles (Fig. 6.41). Alternatively, the carotid pulse can be felt from behind by curling the fingers around the side of the neck (Fig. 6.42). In severe aortic stenosis, there is characteristically a slow rising carotid pulse, usually called a 'plateau' pulse. If the carotid pulse is difficult to feel in a patient whose radial and brachial pulses are easily felt,

the cause may be aortic stenosis because the pulse form becomes more 'normal' the nearer the periphery it is felt (Fig. 6.43). Another sign best appreciated at the carotid is the jerky pulse of hypertrophic cardiomyopathy. This starts normally and then suddenly peters out as the contracting left ventricular outflow tract obstructs ejection (Fig. 6.44).

The femoral pulse

The femoral pulse is almost as valuable as the carotid pulse in assessing cardiac performance. It is more likely to be weak or absent in patients with disease of the aorta or iliac arteries. It is best examined with the patient exposed and lying flat with the thumb or finger placed directly above the superior pubic ramus and midway

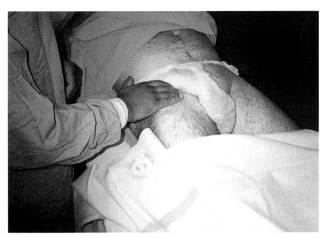

Fig. 6.45 Palpation of the femoral artery.

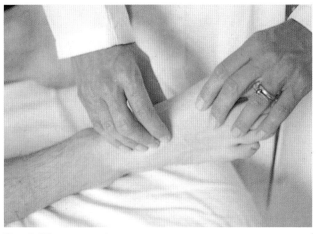

Fig. 6.47 Palpation of the dorsalis pedis pulse.

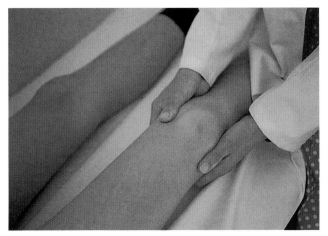

Fig. 6.46 Palpation of the popliteal artery.

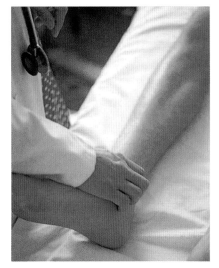

Fig. 6.48 Palpation of the tibialis posterior pulse.

between the pubic tubercle and anterior superior iliac spine (Fig. 6.45).

The popliteal pulse

Assessment of the popliteal and foot pulses is important in the examination of patients suspected of having peripheral arterial disease (see p. 178).

The popliteal pulse lies deep within the popliteal fossa but is readily felt by compressing the artery against the posterior surface of the distal end of the femur. The patient lies flat with the knee slightly flexed. The fingers of one hand are used to press the tips of the fingers of the other hand into the popliteal fossa to feel the popliteal artery against the back of the knee joint (Fig. 6.46). Palpating the popliteal artery is routinely used to evaluate arterial flow in patients with symptoms of intermittent claudication.

The dorsalis pedis and tibialis posterior pulses

Like the popliteals, these peripheral pulses are examined to assess the adequacy of the peripheral arterial tree in suspected peripheral vascular disease. The dorsalis pedis pulse is felt with the fingers aligned along the dorsum of

the foot lateral to the extensor hallucis longus tendon (Fig. 6.47); the tibialis posterior pulse is felt with the fingers cupped round the ankle just posterior to the medial malleolus (Fig. 6.48).

MEASURING BLOOD PRESSURE

The most convenient way of measuring blood pressure is with a stethoscope and sphygmomanometer. To measure the blood pressure reliably, all clothing must be removed from the arm and the sphygmomanometer cuff smoothly applied (Fig. 6.49). The patient's arm should be supported at heart level by an arm rest or by the examiner. For accurate measurement, pressure in the cuff should be reduced slowly, ideally at about 1 mmHg/s. Mercury manometers must be upright and not tilted. Aneroid manometers invariably become inaccurate with time and should be regularly recalibrated. Most practitioners now use automated devices as standard. This includes an electronic monitor with a pressure sensor, a digital display and an upper arm cuff that is inflated by an electrically driven pump.

It is good practice to check the systolic pressure roughly by palpation of the radial artery before applying the stethoscope. As the pressure in the sphygmomanometer cuff increases above the brachial artery systolic pressure, the artery is compressed and the radial pulse becomes impalpable. As the pressure in the cuff is gradually lowered, a pressure is reached where the blood is able to force its way past the obstruction created by the inflated cuff. Initially, this creates the sound of turbulent flow that can be heard with a stethoscope placed over the brachial artery at the elbow. These sounds are called the Korotkoff sounds after the Russian physician who first described them. The generation of the Korotkoff sounds is shown diagrammatically in Figure 6.50. As pressure in the cuff is lowered, the first appearance of the sound (phase 1) corresponds to the systolic blood pressure. The Korotkoff sounds then become louder and more ringing in character due to further increased turbulence (phase 2/3) before becoming muffled (phase 4). Finally, at the point where the flow again becomes linear, rather than turbulent, the audible sounds disappear altogether. Although the point of muffling of the sounds (phase 4) corresponds most closely to the diastolic pressure, as measured by an indwelling arterial cannula, the point of disappearance of the Korotkoff sounds (phase 5) is now used to define diastolic pressure for clinical and epidemiological purposes. This is because phase 5 readings are more reproducible amongst different observers.

Most people consciously or unconsciously round off the blood pressure reading to the nearest 5–10 mmHg, but this should be avoided. The most accurate method for assessing blood pressure is to use a random zero sphygmomanometer in which the operator presses levers to indicate when he or she thinks systolic and diastolic pressures have been reached and then opens the back of the instrument to read the results off a concealed scale.

Important points about the measurement of blood pressure are summarised in the 'symptoms and signs' box.

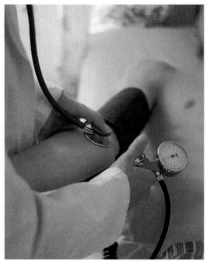

Fig. 6.49 Measuring blood pressure using a sphygmomanometer and stethoscope. The sphygmomanometer cuff is smoothly applied around the unclothed upper arm and the examiner supports the patient's arm at 'heart height'.

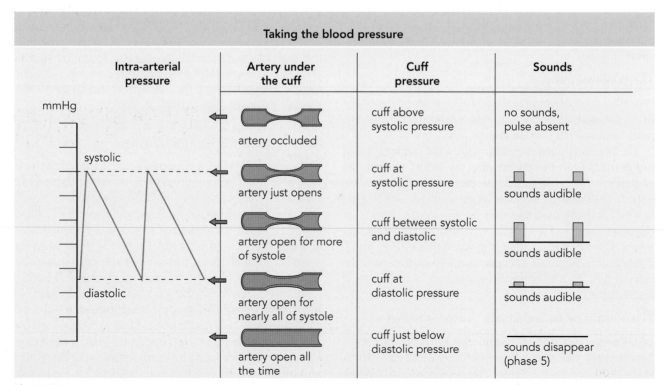

Fig. 6.50 The relationship between cuff pressure, Korotkoff sounds and arterial pressure.

Symptoms and signs

Important points about measuring blood pressure

- Remove all clothing from arm
- Support arm comfortably at heart level
- Use correct size of cuff: wide cuff for obese arms, paediatric cuff for children
- Check systolic pressure by palpitation
- Release pressure no faster than 1 mmHg/second
- Take phase 5 (disappearance of sounds) as diastolic pressure

Patients with very high blood pressure often have other evidence of hypertensive disease. End-organ damage includes retinal changes, left ventricular hypertrophy and proteinuria due to hypertensive renal damage. In the absence of end-organ signs, it is important not to make a final diagnosis of hypertension based on a single blood pressure recording. Repeated blood pressure measurements will nearly always show some tendency to regress towards normal. Some patients have high blood pressure when measured in a hospital clinic, yet measurement in their own home or by continuous blood pressure monitoring reveals a more normal pattern. This is sometimes referred to as 'white coat hypertension'. Use of a 24-hour ambulatory blood pressure monitor is employed to distinguish artefactual from true essential hypertension.

Differential diagnosis

Systemic hypertension

Primary:	'Essential' hypertension
Secondary:	Aortic coarctation
Hormonal:	Congenital
	– adrenal hyperplasia
	– 11-hydroxylase deficiency
	Acquired
	– phaeochromocytoma
	– Conn's syndrome
	– Cushing's syndrome
Renal:	Polycystic kidneys
	Renal artery stenosis
	Acute glomerulonephritis
	Chronic renal disease
Drug-related:	Steroids
	Contraceptive pill
	Non-steroidal anti-inflammatory drugs
	Ciclosporin

The definition of what constitutes high blood pressure has long been a subject for controversy. In any given population, the distribution of systolic and diastolic blood pressures is continuous. In Western populations, there is a tendency for both systolic and diastolic pressures to increase with age, although this does not necessarily apply to other populations, particularly peoples in whom there is a low salt intake. Most authorities accept a blood pressure of over 140/90 mmHg on repeated measurement as defining a hypertensive population. In the diabetic population the corresponding level defining hypertension is a reading consistently greater than 130/80 mmHg. A diastolic pressure of greater than 120 mmHg and evidence of end-organ damage would define patients with severe hypertension. Accelerated phase or malignant hypertension is a rare form of severe uncontrolled blood pressure associated with retinal haemorrhages and requires immediate hospital admission.

Red flag – urgent referral

Hypertension

- Severe hypertension (BP >200/120 mmHg)
- Retinal haemorrhages and cottonwool spots
- Proteinuria
- Left ventricular hypertrophy on ECG
- Headache

The converse of hypertension is hypotension or low blood pressure. Although a systolic blood pressure of less than 100 mmHg is part of the definition of shock, hypotension is usually characterised by its consequences such as impaired cerebral or renal function rather than by an arbitrary pressure level. Postural hypotension, which most commonly presents as dizziness, is precipitated by changing posture from a recumbent or sitting position to a standing position. The diagnosis is made by measuring the blood pressure with the patient lying supine at rest and then re-measuring the systolic and blood pressure 2 minutes after changing the position to standing.

Differential diagnosis

Hypotension

Impaired cardiac output
- Myocardial infarction
- Pericardial tamponade
- Massive pulmonary embolism
- Acute valve incompetence

Hypovolaemia
- Haemorrhage
- Diabetic pre-coma
- Dehydration from diarrhoea or vomiting

Excessive vasodilatation
- Anaphylaxis
- Gram-negative septicaemia
- Drugs
- Autonomic failure

Emergency

Severe hypotension (shock)

Emergency medical assessment of the patient with severe hypotension (shock):

History (from patient, relatives or attendants)

- Has there been any trauma, haemorrhage or substance abuse?
- Has onset been sudden or gradual (over hours or days, e.g. diabetic ketoacidosis, dysentery)?
- Has there been any pain (i) in the chest (myocardial infarction, dissecting aneurysm) or (ii) elsewhere (e.g. headache in meningococcal septicaemia)?
- Is there any other relevant history (e.g. bed rest, airline travel in massive pulmonary embolism)?

Clinical examination

- Before starting the examination, check that the patient's airway is safe and, if possible, attach an ECG monitor
- Check whether the patient is more comfortable sitting up (think of pulmonary oedema) or lying flat (think of hypovolaemia or pulmonary embolism)
- Remove external clothes and conduct a quick but thorough examination for signs of trauma or haemorrhage if appropriate. Usually the skin in shock is pale and cold but if it is warm or red think of septicaemia or allergy
- Assess the pulse. Normally it would be fast (100–120 beats/min) in shock, if very slow think of heart block, if more rapid consider an arrhythmia
- Quickly assess the major pulses (carotid, femorals). If asymmetrical, think of dissecting aortic aneurysm
- Try and assess the jugular venous pressure. A very high jugular venous pressure suggests pulmonary embolism or cardiac tamponade
- Check that the trachea is central and that air entry can be heard on both sides of the chest (if not, think of tension pneumothorax). If there are widespread crackles in the lungs, think of pulmonary oedema
- Listen to the front of the chest for murmurs or abnormal heart sounds (often very difficult if the heart rate is rapid)
- Gently palpate the abdomen for tenderness or pulsation (think of ruptured aortic aneurysm)
- If appropriate consider rectal or vaginal examination for hidden haemorrhage

Investigation

- As soon as possible record an ECG (diagnosis of myocardial infarction, arrhythmia, pulmonary embolism) and take a chest radiograph (and if appropriate other radiographs, e.g. in the case of trauma). Consider emergency echocardiography if diagnosis is still in doubt

Examination of the jugular venous pulse

Evaluation of the jugular venous pulse is a key clinical sign used to assess the performance of the 'input' side of the heart. The internal jugular vein is in direct communication with the superior vena cava and the right atrium. The normal pressure in the right atrium is equivalent to that exerted by a 10–12 cm column of blood. Therefore, when standing or sitting upright the internal jugular vein is collapsed, when lying flat it is completely filled by a gravitational effect. If the patient lies supine at approximately 45°, the point at which jugular venous pulsation becomes visible is usually just above the clavicle; this is the position usually chosen for examination of the jugular venous pulse (Fig. 6.51). To examine the pulse, the patient rests the head comfortably against a pillow, with the neck slightly flexed and looking straight ahead. It is important not to tense the sternomastoid muscles because the internal jugular vein lies directly beneath this muscle. Reliable ways of telling the jugular venous pulse from the carotid arterial pulse are listed in the 'differential diagnosis' box.

Differential diagnosis

Distinction between jugular venous and carotid pulses

Venous
- Most rapid movement inward
- Two peaks per cycle (in sinus rhythm)
- Affected by compressing abdomen
- May displace earlobes (if venous pressure raised)

Arterial
- Most rapid movement outward
- One peak per cycle
- Not affected by compressing abdomen
- Never displaces earlobes

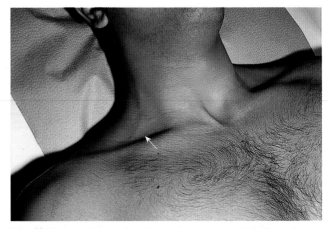

Fig. 6.51 Assessing the jugular venous pressure. With the patient lying supine at 45°, jugular pulsation is normally just visible above the clavicle.

Measuring the height of the jugular venous pulse

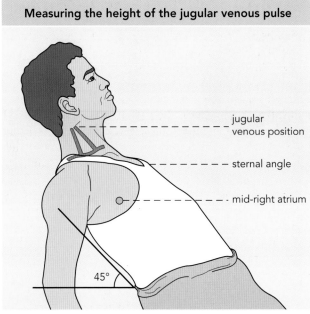

jugular
venous position

sternal angle

mid-right atrium

45°

Fig. 6.52 Relationship of the jugular venous pulsation, right atrium and manubriosternal angle.

It is sometimes said that jugular venous pulsation can be obliterated by gentle finger pressure and that the jugular pulse is never palpable. Whilst generally true, both statements are refuted in patients with severe tricuspid regurgitation where the venous pulse can be palpated.

Once the jugular venous pulse has been identified, both its mean height above right atrial level and the waveform are assessed. As it is not possible to see or feel the right atrium, it is usual to express the height of jugular venous pulsation by its height above the manubriosternal angle (Fig. 6.52). A normal jugular venous pressure is conventionally reported if less than 4 cm above the manubriosternal angle.

The waveform of the normal jugular venous pressure is biphasic with an 'a' wave and a 'v' wave (Fig. 6.53). Changes in the waveform reflect changes in right atrial pressure. The 'a' wave is a reflection of the pressure caused by atrial contraction and is therefore absent in atrial fibrillation. The 'v' wave is due to atrial filling against the closed atrioventricular valve and therefore occurs immediately after the first heart sound. Distinguishing 'a' from 'v' waves is best made by timing with the aortic pulse pressure because the 'a' wave is not synchronous with the arterial pulse pressure whereas the 'v' wave is synchronous.

In patients with a very high jugular venous pressure, such as occurs in pericardial tamponade or constrictive pericarditis, the internal jugular vein may be completely filled with the patient positioned at 45°. In the setting, it is necessary to sit the patient bolt upright to visualise the apex of the pulsation. As a quick rule of thumb, the jugular venous pressure must be raised if jugular venous pulsation is visible above the clavicle with the patient

Venous pressure waveforms

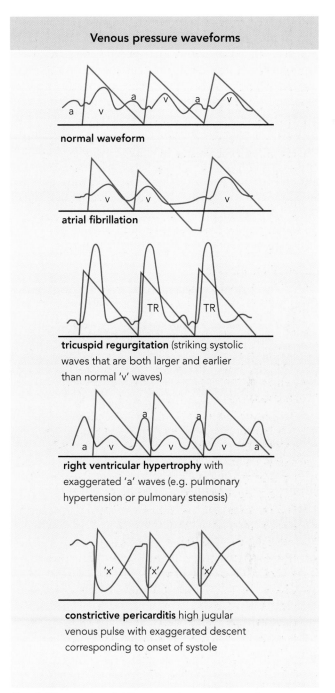

normal waveform

atrial fibrillation

tricuspid regurgitation (striking systolic waves that are both larger and earlier than normal 'v' waves)

right ventricular hypertrophy with exaggerated 'a' waves (e.g. pulmonary hypertension or pulmonary stenosis)

constrictive pericarditis high jugular venous pulse with exaggerated descent corresponding to onset of systole

Fig. 6.53 Examples of different jugular pressure waveforms.

sitting bolt upright. Even sitting the patient upright may fail to expose a very high venous pressure. When this is suspected, a rough estimate can be made by raising the patient's outstretched hand to a horizontal position at the level of the sternomanubrial angle and then slowly raising the hand and watching carefully for the point at which the veins on the back of the hand collapse. At this point, the difference in height between the hand and the right atrium or sternal angle is a crude reflection of right atrial pressure.

By far the most common cause of a raised jugular venous pressure is congestive heart failure, in which the raised venous pressure reflects right ventricular failure and a raised right atrial pressure. Examples of different jugular pressure waveforms are shown in Figure 6.53. In practice, the waveform that accompanies tricuspid regurgitation is the most common and most important abnormality of wave pattern. Free retrograde flow of blood from the right ventricle into the right atrium and jugular vein causes the characteristic large 'CV' wave that may even be palpable and provides a clue to the likelihood of discovering tricuspid regurgitation on direct examination and auscultation of the heart. Circumstances where the atrium contracts against a closed tricuspid valve give rise to a 'cannon' 'a' wave. This occurs in complete heart block and ventricular tachycardia. A raised but non-pulsatile jugular venous pressure should raise the suspicion of superior vena cava obstruction.

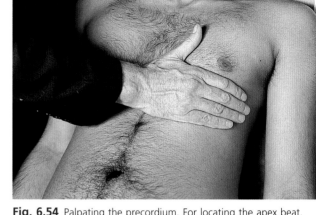

Fig. 6.54 Palpating the precordium. For locating the apex beat, the patient should lie flat on the back but to assess the quality of the impulses the patient should be rolled onto the left side.

Differential diagnosis

Causes and characteristics of raised jugular venous pressure

Common
- Congestive heart failure
- Tricuspid regurgitation
- Normal wave pattern usually preserved
- Large 'V' waves

Less common
- Pericardial tamponade
- Massive pulmonary embolism
- Iatrogenic fluid overload

Rare
- Superior vena cava obstruction
- Constrictive pericarditis
- Tricuspid stenosis

Palpation of the precordium

Palpate the precordium by laying the flat of the hand with outstretched fingers on the chest wall to the left of the sternum (Fig. 6.54). The first manoeuvre is to locate the apex beat, which coincides with the tip of the left ventricle. The apex beat is the furthest outward and downward point at which cardiac pulsation is palpable. With the patient lying supine at 45°, the normal adult apex beat lies in the fifth or sixth left intercostal space, extending no further than the midclavicular line. Remember that the heart has some mobility within the thorax, so if you roll the patient onto, for example, the left side, the apex beat will displace further outwards. There are circumstances where the apex beat is difficult to palpate. This occurs in markedly obese patients and patients with chronic airways disease and hyperinflated chests such as occurs in emphysema. In this setting, you might need to roll the patient onto the left side in order to feel the apex beat – and even then the pulsation might be undetectable.

Types of apex beat

Normal

'Sustained' or 'heaving' apex beat of left ventricular hypertrophy, often associated with a double impulse from concomitant left atrial hypertrophy

atrial component

'Tapping' apex in mitral stenosis

Diffuse or dyskinetic apex beat after anterior myocardial infarction

Fig. 6.55 Types of apical impulse.

In addition to demarcating the position of the apex beat, it is important to evaluate the quality of the impulse (Fig. 6.55). The quality of the normal apex beat and the range of abnormality is learnt by experience. A thrusting, forceful or heaving apex beat, palpated within the midclavicular line, indicates a hypertrophic myocardial response to increased left ventricular workload. This is characteristic of the myocardial response to hypertension and aortic stenosis prior to the development of cardiac

Differential diagnosis

Left ventricular hypertrophy

- Hypertension
- Aortic stenosis
- Hypertrophic cardiomyopathy

decompensation. Displacement of the apex beat lateral to the midclavicular line indicates left ventricular dilatation. A diffuse, displaced, poorly localised apex beat is indicative of more profound damage to the ventricular muscle. This occurs in extensive myocardial infarction, as a result of cardiomyopathy and in particular, in patients with severe aortic incompetence. This diffuse impulse can often be seen on inspection of the precordium. Another characteristic sign that can be detected on pulsation is the tapping apex beat of mitral stenosis. This is partly caused by left atrial enlargement causing displacement of the left ventricle nearer to the examining hand and, partly, due to a loud first heart sound which becomes both palpable and audible if the valve cusps are still pliable. Right ventricular hypertrophy or dilatation is felt as a parasternal heave close to the left sternal border. This is felt by

positioning the thenar eminence of the flat of your hand just to the left of the lower half of the sternum.

While palpating the heart, the examining hand will occasionally detect a vibration or 'thrill'. Thrills are 'palpable murmurs' and are always accompanied by an easily heard murmur on auscultation. A diastolic thrill, which conveys a sensation akin to that felt when stroking a purring cat, can occasionally be felt in patients with mitral stenosis. Systolic thrills may accompany aortic stenosis, ventricular septal defect or mitral regurgitation.

Auscultation of the heart

The stethoscope was originally introduced into medical practice by the French physician Laennec at the beginning of the nineteenth century. In its original form it consisted of a wooden cylinder with a small hole drilled from end to end. In addition to introducing a decorous distance between the head of the physician and the chest of the patient, the stethoscope has two principal functions. First, it transmits sounds from the patient's chest and, second, it selectively emphasises sounds of certain frequencies, enabling the examiner to interpret the

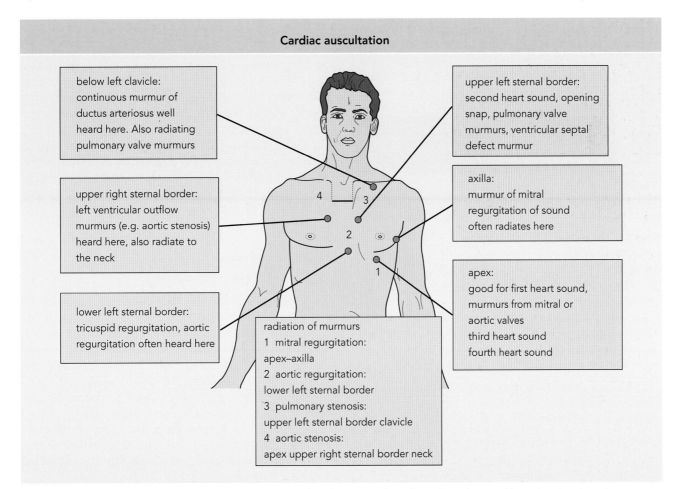

Cardiac auscultation

below left clavicle: continuous murmur of ductus arteriosus well heard here. Also radiating pulmonary valve murmurs

upper left sternal border: second heart sound, opening snap, pulmonary valve murmurs, ventricular septal defect murmur

upper right sternal border: left ventricular outflow murmurs (e.g. aortic stenosis) heard here, also radiate to the neck

axilla: murmur of mitral regurgitation of sound often radiates here

lower left sternal border: tricuspid regurgitation, aortic regurgitation often heard here

apex: good for first heart sound, murmurs from mitral or aortic valves third heart sound fourth heart sound

radiation of murmurs
1 mitral regurgitation: apex–axilla
2 aortic regurgitation: lower left sternal border
3 pulmonary stenosis: upper left sternal border clavicle
4 aortic stenosis: apex upper right sternal border neck

Fig. 6.56 Cardiac auscultation; the best sites for hearing sounds and murmurs depend on where the sound is produced and to where turbulent blood flows radiate.

auditory information. Indiscriminate amplification of the sound coming from the chest, as would be produced by a sensitive high fidelity microphone, actually produces a signal that is very hard for the human ear to interpret. The ear pieces of the stethoscope should be angled forwards to match the direction of the examiner's external auditory meati. They should fit snugly but comfortably and the tubing should not be too long. The bell and diaphragm selectively emphasise sounds of different frequencies. The bell is more efficient for listening to low-pitched sounds such as the mid-diastolic murmur of mitral stenosis or the third heart sound of cardiac failure. In contrast, the diaphragm filters out low-pitched sounds and, therefore, emphasises high-pitched ones. The diaphragm is best for analysing the second heart sound, ejection murmurs, ejection and mid-systolic clicks and the soft but high-pitched early diastolic murmur of aortic regurgitation.

When auscultating the heart, you should listen at the apex (known as the mitral area), the tricuspid area (between the apex and the sternum) and the aortic and pulmonary areas which are located respectively in the second intercostal space to the right and left of the sternum (Fig. 6.56). If an abnormal heart is heard, the stethoscope can be moved around until the abnormality is heard most clearly. Relate the auscultatory findings to the cardiac cycle by simultaneously palpating the carotid artery while listening to the heart (Fig. 6.57). A useful technique is to listen sequentially to the heart sounds. Initially, focus on auscultating the first heart sound in the mitral and tricuspid areas. Follow this with a similar focus

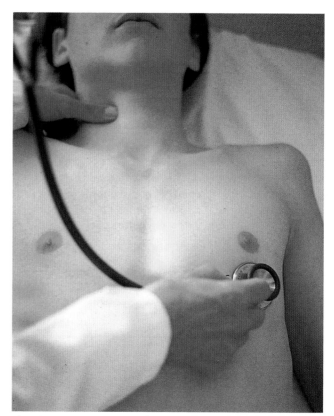

Fig. 6.57 Simultaneously listening to the heart sounds and timing them against the carotid pulse.

on the pulmonary and aortic components of the second heart sounds. Once the first and second heart sounds have been assessed, listen systematically for a third or fourth heart sound, systolic and diastolic murmurs and, where appropriate, ejection clicks. On discovering a systolic or diastolic murmur, determine whether there is radiation of the sound. The pansystolic ejection murmur of mitral incompetence typically radiates towards the axilla whilst the ejection systolic murmur of aortic stenosis characteristically radiates to the carotids.

HEART SOUNDS

First and second heart sounds

The mechanics of the first and second heart sounds and the mechanism and physiology of splitting the second heart sound have already been described. The first heart sound can be easily identified with both the bell and diaphragm but the diaphragm is more efficient for auscultating and analysing the second heart sound, with the stethoscope usually best placed at the midleft sternal edge. It is usual to record the heart sounds in a shorthand notation which is derived from the recording made by phonocardiography (Fig. 6.58). Factors causing a change in the intensity of the heart sounds are summarised in the 'differential diagnosis' box.

The most common causes of a loud first heart sound include any cause of increased cardiac output and mitral

Differential diagnosis

Factors that might influence the intensity of the heart sounds

Loud first sound
- Hyperdynamic circulation (fever, exercise)
- Mitral stenosis
- Atrial myxoma (rare)

Soft first sound
- Low cardiac output (rest, heart failure)
- Tachycardia
- Severe mitral regurgitation

Variable intensity of first sound
- Atrial fibrillation
- Complete heart block
- Ventricular tachycardia

Loud aortic component of second sound
- Systemic hypertension
- Dilated aortic root

Soft aortic component of second sound
- Calcific aortic stenosis

Loud pulmonary component of second sound
- Pulmonary hypertension

Shorthand notation for heart sounds

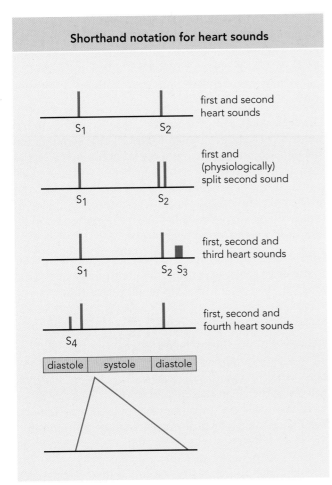

Fig. 6.58 Shorthand notation (derived from phonocardiography) for recording the heart sounds.

The fourth heart sound

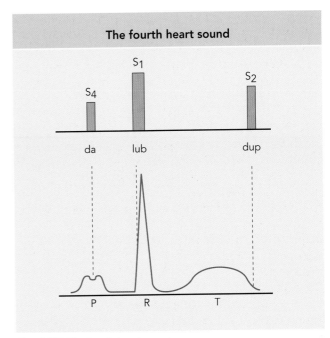

Fig. 6.59 The fourth heart sound.

stenosis (with pliable valve cusps). The most common causes of an abnormally quiet first heart sound are reduced cardiac output, severe mitral valve incompetence and the acoustic effect of a thick chest wall or hyperinflated lungs. The second heart sound is usually softer in the second left interspace than the equivalent right interspace, reflecting the lower closing pressure of the pulmonary compared to the aortic valve. A louder than expected ringing second heart sound may be auscultated in systemic hypertension or, occasionally, pulmonary hypertension.

Third and fourth heart sounds

These are additional heart sounds that convey important haemodynamic information. The third heart sound is a low-pitched, thudding sound that occurs in early diastole and coincides with the end of the rapid phase of ventricular filling. It is important to recognise that a third heart sound may be either physiological or pathological. A physiological third heart sound occurs in young fit adults in circumstances of increased cardiac output (e.g. in athletes, in the presence of a fever or during pregnancy). In this setting, the discovery of a third heart sound is of no pathological significance. A pathological third

heart sound usually indicates severe impairment of left ventricular function and in particular, occurs with left ventricular dilatation. Consequently, a third heart sound might be anticipated in patients with dilated cardiomyopathy, following acute myocardial infarction or in acute massive pulmonary embolism, when the third heart sound originates from the right ventricle and is consequently best heard during inspiration. A pathological third heart sound is usually accompanied by a tachycardia and, because the phenomenon occurs in the presence of left ventricular dilatation, the first sound is usually soft because of failure to generate sufficient power to cause full closure of the mitral valve. The cadence of first, second and third heart sounds is usually described by the sound 'da-da-boom' and the timing is likened to the sound of 'Kentucky'. The combined sound pattern of first, second and third sound has been described by the term 'gallop rhythm'.

A fourth heart sound is an additional heart sound occurring late in diastole. This sound coincides with atrial contraction and reflects the contraction of the left atrium against a raised left ventricular end diastolic pressure. Consequently, a fourth heart sound can be anticipated in patients with left ventricular hypertrophy such as occurs in systemic hypertension. A fourth heart sound is also often heard in the early phase following acute myocardial infarction when the left ventricle is 'stunned', less compliant and consequently develops a raised end-diastolic pressure. A fourth sound sounds a little like 'da-lub-dup' and timed like 'Tennessee' (Fig. 6.59).

Other extra heart sounds

Ejection clicks This is a high-pitched ringing sound that usually follows very shortly after the first heart sound

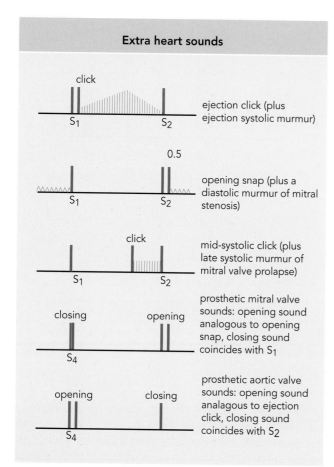

Extra heart sounds

click

S$_1$ S$_2$ — ejection click (plus ejection systolic murmur)

0.5

S$_1$ S$_2$ — opening snap (plus a diastolic murmur of mitral stenosis)

click

S$_1$ S$_2$ — mid-systolic click (plus late systolic murmur of mitral valve prolapse)

closing   opening

S$_4$ — prosthetic mitral valve sounds: opening sound analogous to opening snap, closing sound coincides with S$_1$

opening   closing

S$_4$ — prosthetic aortic valve sounds: opening sound analogous to ejection click, closing sound coincides with S$_2$

Fig. 6.60 Extra heart sounds.

(Fig. 6.60). An ejection click is a feature of aortic or pulmonary valve stenosis, where it is probably generated by the sudden opening of the deformed valve. Sometimes, patients with a dilated pulmonary artery or ascending aorta may have an ejection click without a stenotic valve.

Opening snap This is a diastolic sound heard in mitral stenosis caused by the snappy opening of a stenosed but still pliable mitral valve under the influence of the higher than normal left atrial pressure. A fibrosed and nonpliable mitral valve will generate only a soft opening snap or no snap at all. The opening snap is best heard to the left of the sternum and sounds rather like the second component of a widely split second heart sound.

Mid-systolic clicks These are most often associated with mitral valve prolapse and are caused by the tensing of the long and redundant chordae tendineae of these valves. The clicks may or may not be associated with a late systolic murmur (Figs 6.61, 6.62).

Sounds from artificial heart valves The ball, disc or poppet in an artificial heart valve usually makes a noise both when it opens and closes. The closing sound is usually louder than the opening sound. Thus, an aortic prosthesis will have a soft opening click just after the first heart sound and a loud closing click which contributes to the second heart sound. Conversely, a mitral valve will give a soft opening click in a similar position to the opening snap of mitral stenosis and a loud closing click which contributes to the first heart sound.

Murmurs

Murmurs are musical sounds caused by turbulent flow occurring at specific points in the cardiac cycle. The

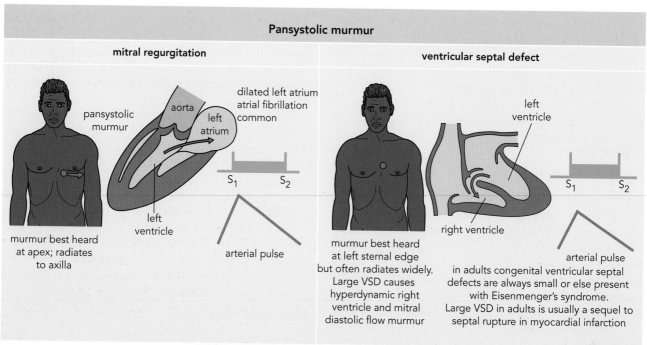

Fig. 6.61 Pansystolic (holosystolic) murmurs: mitral regurgitation (left), ventricular septal defect (right).

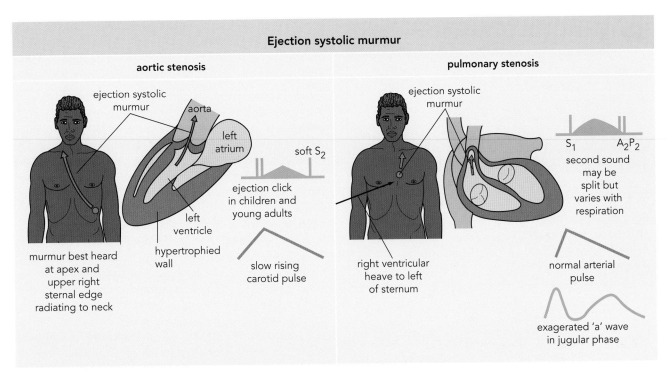

Ejection systolic murmur

aortic stenosis

ejection systolic murmur · aorta · left atrium · left ventricle · hypertrophied wall · soft S₂ · ejection click in children and young adults · slow rising carotid pulse

murmur best heard at apex and upper right sternal edge radiating to neck

pulmonary stenosis

ejection systolic murmur · right ventricular heave to left of sternum · S_1 · A_2P_2 · second sound may be split but varies with respiration · normal arterial pulse · exaggerated 'a' wave in jugular phase

Fig. 6.62 Ejection systolic murmurs: aortic stenosis and pulmonary stenosis.

important points in analysing a murmur include its timing in the cardiac cycle, what it sounds like, where it is best heard, where it radiates to and what happens during manoeuvres like deep breathing.

Symptoms and signs
Grading the intensity of murmurs

Grade 1 – just audible with a good stethoscope in a quiet room
Grade 2 – quiet but readily audible with a stethoscope
Grade 3 – easily heard with a stethoscope
Grade 4 – a loud, obvious murmur
Grade 5 – very loud, heard not only over the precordium but elsewhere in the body

Systolic murmurs Systolic murmurs result from one of three causes: leakage of blood through a structure that is normally closed during systole (e.g. mitral or tricuspid valves or the interventricular septum), blood flow through a valve normally open in systole but which has become abnormally narrowed (e.g. aortic or pulmonary stenosis), or increased blood flow through a normal valve (a flow murmur).

Murmurs that are due to leakage of blood through an incompetent mitral or tricuspid valve or a ventricular septal defect are usually of similar intensity throughout the length of systole and are termed pansystolic or holosystolic murmurs (Fig. 6.61). Occasionally, a valve is competent at the onset of systole but starts to leak halfway through. This occurs in mitral valve prolapse and results in a murmur that starts in mid or late systole and is termed a mid-systolic or late systolic murmur.

Differential diagnosis
Sites of radiation of murmurs

Cause	'Primary' site	Radiation
Tricuspid regurgitation	Lower left sternal edge	Lower right sternal edge, liver
Pulmonary stenosis	Upper left sternal edge	Towards left clavicle, beneath left scapula
Mitral regurgitation	Apex	Left axilla, beneath left scapula
Aortic regurgitation	Left sternal edge	Down left sternal edge towards apex
Aortic stenosis	Apex	Towards upper right sternal edge, over carotids
Ventricular septal defect	Left sternal edge	All over pericardium
Mitral stenosis	Apex	Does not radiate

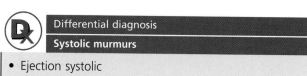

Differential diagnosis

Systolic murmurs

- Ejection systolic
- Innocent systolic murmur
- Aortic stenosis
- Pulmonary stenosis
- Hypertrophic cardiomyopathy
- Flow murmurs
  - atrial septal defect
  - fever
  - athlete's heart

Pansystolic murmurs

- Tricuspid regurgitation
- Mitral regurgitation
- Ventricular septal defect

Murmurs caused by blood flow through a narrowed aortic or pulmonary valve or due to increased blood flow through a normal calibre aortic or pulmonary valve tend to initiate quietly at the beginning of systole, rise to a crescendo in midsystole and then quieten again towards the end of systole. These diamond-shaped murmurs are called ejection systolic murmurs (Fig. 6.62).

Innocent murmurs Innocent murmurs are murmurs not associated with any cardiac structural abnormality nor with any haemodynamic disturbance. They occur commonly in children and young adults and have the

following characteristics: always systolic and quiet; usually best heard at the left sternal edge; not associated with ventricular hypertrophy; associated with normal heart sounds, pulses, chest radiology and electrocardiography.

Diastolic murmurs Diastolic murmurs can be divided into early and mid-diastolic murmurs. An early diastolic murmur is characteristic of aortic and pulmonary valve incompetence. Its cadence is maximal at the onset of diastole when aortic or pulmonary pressure is highest and the murmur rapidly becomes quieter as pressure in the aortic or pulmonary artery falls (decrescendo) (Fig. 6.63). The sound of an aortic diastolic murmur has aptly been described as like a whispered letter 'r'.

A mid-diastolic murmur is usually caused by blood flow through a narrowed mitral valve (or, rarely, the tricuspid valve). Occasionally, a similar murmur is generated when there is increased blood flow through one of these valves. Characteristically, this occurs in children with atrial septal defect where the tricuspid valve is anatomically normal but where increased flow derived from the shunt creates turbulence. The characteristic murmur of mitral stenosis is a low-pitched, rumbling murmur heard during diastole (Fig. 6.64). Sometimes, in patients in sinus rhythm, the murmur intensifies just prior to the onset of systole. This phenomenon is caused by atrial contraction increasing the blood flow through the narrowed valve and is termed 'presystolic accentuation'. Sometimes patients with aortic regurgitation have a mid-diastolic murmur known as an Austin Flint murmur. As a result of the aortic valvular incompetence, a regurgitant jet of blood creates a vibration of the anterior leaflet of

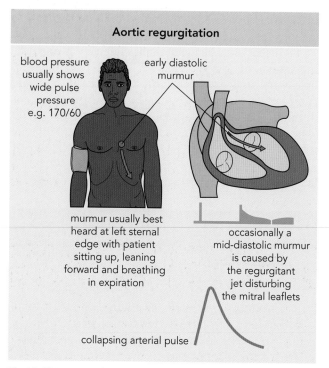

Fig. 6.63 Aortic regurgitation as an example of an early diastolic murmur.

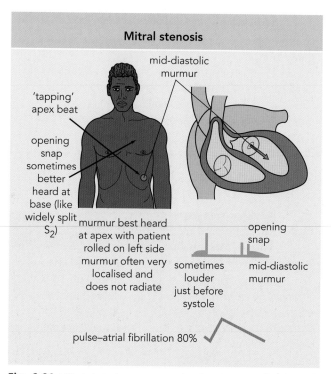

Fig. 6.64 Mitral stenosis as an example of a mid-diastolic murmur.

the mitral valve and also causes mild functional mitral narrowing, both of which contribute to this functional murmur.

Murmurs are usually most obvious over the site of the causative lesion and there may be radiation in the direction of the turbulent bloodstream that generates the sound. It is sometimes possible to intensify the murmur by positioning the patient appropriately. The murmur of mitral stenosis is best heard when the patient is rolled onto the left side and the stethoscope bell applied to the cardiac apex (Fig. 6.65). The murmur of aortic regurgitation is more intense and best heard if the patient is asked to sit up, lean forward and breathe out fully while the stethoscope is applied at the left side of the lower part of the sternum (Fig. 6.66).

The behaviour of murmurs during the respiratory cycle provides further clues to their origin and nature. Murmurs arising from the right side of the heart, such as pulmonary stenosis flow murmurs or tricuspid regurgitation pansystolic murmurs, tend to get louder during inspiration and quieter during expiration. Conversely, murmurs arising on the left side of the heart tend to sound quieter during inspiration and appear louder in expiration. Asking the patient to perform a Valsalva manoeuvre by forcibly expiring against a closed glottis makes most murmurs quieter, as cardiac output is diminished. However, the ejection murmur of hypertrophic obstructive cardiomyopathy arising from obstruction the left ventricular outlet tract tends to intensify as the degree of obstruction increases. The mid-diastolic murmur of mitral stenosis is often easier to hear if the patient is made to exercise before listening for it.

Differential diagnosis

Behaviour of murmurs in respiration

Louder immediately on inspiration
- Pulmonary stenosis
- Pulmonary valve flow murmurs

Quieter immediately on inspiration (may become louder later)
- Mitral regurgitation
- Aortic stenosis

Louder during Valsalva manoeuvre
- Hypertrophic obstructive cardiomyopathy
- The murmur of mitral prolapse may become louder or softer during inspiration

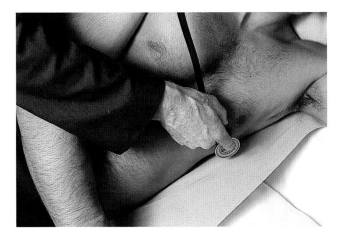

Fig. 6.65 Mitral diastolic murmurs are best heard using the bell, with the patient rolled onto the left side.

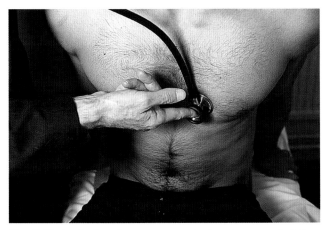

Fig. 6.66 Aortic diastolic murmurs may be heard more easily if the patient sits up, leans forward and holds the breath in expiration.

Cardiovascular system and chest examination

The most important pulmonary sign in patients with cardiac disease is the presence of crackles at the lung bases. These occur during inspiration and are an early sign of pulmonary oedema. Crackles are believed to be derived from the sound of collapsed alveoli snapping open. In mild heart failure, crackles are confined to the lower zones posteriorly but in severe failure they may be heard throughout the chest. Patients with severe heart failure and peripheral oedema may also develop pleural effusions. Examination of the chest is discussed in detail in Chapter 5.

Cardiovascular system and abdominal examination

In patients with cardiovascular disease, the abdominal examination (see Ch. 7) can add useful information. For example, in patients with biventricular or right ventricular failure and raised right atrial pressure, congestion caused by impaired hepatic venous outflow might cause liver enlargement. The patient may complain of right upper quadrant pain and the hepatomegaly is smooth and tender. In patients with significant tricuspid incompetence, the enlarged liver may also be pulsatile, reflecting the transmitted impulse from the right ventricle. The abdominal examination might also reveal an abdominal aortic aneurysm and, in patients with systemic hypertension, a renal artery bruit or the presence of enlarged kidneys might implicate this organ in the aetiology of the raised blood pressure. The presence of a renal artery bruit can be sought by applying the diaphragm of the stethoscope to a point 2.5 cm lateral and superior to the umbilicus on either side. The most common cause of probable large kidneys is polycystic disease of the kidney which inevitably results in hypertension and chronic renal failure. Ascites occurs rarely in very severe heart failure as a result of generalised fluid retention and the effect of impaired hepatic venous outflow on hepatic and splanchnic haemodynamics.

Rarely, splenomegaly may be apparent in patients with severe congestive heart failure. This is due to passive congestion. The presence of an enlarged spleen in patients with cardiac disease should also alert to the possibility of subacute bacterial endocarditis where splenomegaly develops as part of the immune response in this disease.

Aneurysm of the abdominal aorta is common, particularly in men over the age of 60 years. It is important to detect because early elective surgery carries a much lower mortality than emergency surgery. On examination, the characteristic finding is pulsation at about the level of the umbilicus. It is often possible to feel the normal aorta at this level, particularly in thin patients. If the abdominal aorta is aneurysmal, the aorta feels wider than normal (Fig. 6.67) and there may be an associated aortic bruit.

Abdominal ultrasound examination provides an accurate method for confirming the diagnosis of aortic aneurysm and of measuring its size.

Peripheral vascular system

Because blood flow to the skin determines the skin temperature, temperature change is a common sign of peripheral vascular disease. In the lower limbs, it is often possible to determine the level where the skin temperature changes from warm to cold and this should be documented. Trophic skin changes also occur as a result of arterial insufficiency and this is characterised by thin, smooth and hairless skin which is easily traumatised. Examination of the femoral, popliteal, posterior tibial and dorsalis pedis pulses helps determine whether vascular disease is due to large or small vessel disease. Look for varicose veins, the characteristic mottled discoloration caused by postphlebitic changes, and the presence of varicose ulcers, which localise to the medial aspect of the lower limb and are relatively painless.

OEDEMA

Oedema reflects the abnormal accumulation of fluid in the interstitial space. Fluid in the interstitial space is normally in dynamic equilibrium with plasma, so that the amount of fluid escaping from and re-entering the capillary network and lymphatic system is normally finely balanced (Fig. 6.68). The oedema of heart failure is largely the result of increased venous pressure creating increased end capillary pressure, but factors such as a slightly reduced plasma albumin concentration and abnormal capillary permeability may also play a role.

The oedema of heart failure can be divided into pulmonary oedema and peripheral oedema. Peripheral

Abdominal aortic aneurysms

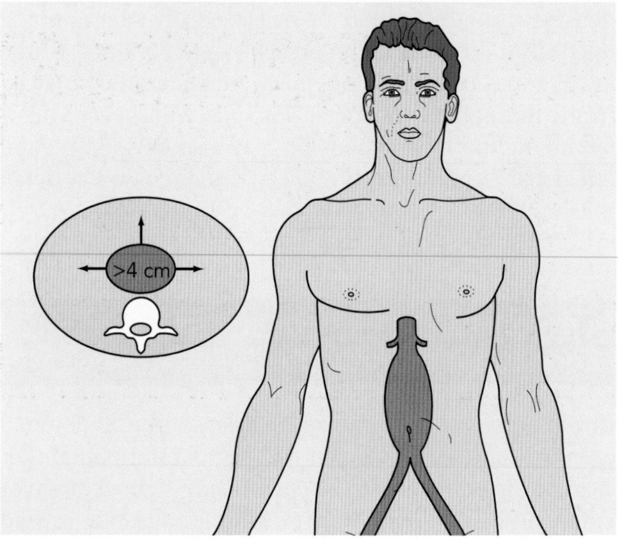

Fig. 6.67 Abdominal aortic aneurysm is felt as an 'expansile swelling' in the abdomen.

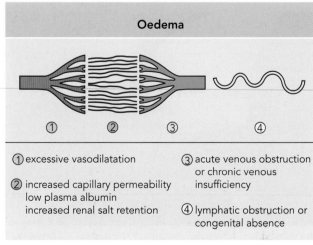

Oedema

① excessive vasodilatation

② increased capillary permeability low plasma albumin increased renal salt retention

③ acute venous obstruction or chronic venous insufficiency

④ lymphatic obstruction or congenital absence

Fig. 6.68 The factors contributing to oedema formation.

oedema is the characteristic feature of right-sided heart failure or biventricular congestive cardiac failure. Peripheral oedema characteristically accumulates at the lowest gravitational parts of the body and is known as 'dependent oedema'. Consequently, when patients are ambulant, the oedema tends to accumulate in the feet and ankles. In the recumbent position, there is redistribution of fluid with less pedal oedema and an increase in interstitial fluid in the back, especially the presacral region – where it is termed 'sacral oedema'. The more severe the oedema the further up the leg it tends to extend. In severe and untreated cardiac failure, the oedema may extend to involve the thigh, the scrotum and the lower part of the abdominal wall. This phenomenon is known as anasarca. Severe oedema is frequently accompanied by increased transudation of fluid into the serous cavities and may cause ascites and pleural effusions. It is virtually unknown for cardiac oedema to involve the facial tissues.

Clinically, peripheral oedema is detected by swelling that can be displaced by firm finger pressure which leaves a pitted impression when the finger is removed. This is known as 'pitting oedema'. The main differential diagnosis of cardiac oedema is stasis oedema, which occurs in elderly or immobile patients. This is caused by lack of muscle pump activity, in addition to chronic damage to venous valves and possibly a degree of lymphatic obstruction. The distinction is best made by looking for other signs of cardiac failure. In a patient who has a normal jugular venous pressure, peripheral oedema is seldom the result of heart failure.

HEART FAILURE

Heart failure refers to the inability to generate a cardiac output adequate to satisfy the body's needs. The European Society of Cardiology (2001) definition broadly encompasses the different facets of the clinical syndrome including symptoms of exercise intolerance, signs of fluid retention and response to therapy, accompanied by objective evidence of cardiac dysfunction at rest. Heart failure can be subdivided into acute and chronic heart failure and also into left-sided, right-sided or mixed heart failure, depending on the cause.

Acute heart failure

One of the most common manifestations of acute heart failure is tachycardia and a low systemic blood pressure – although sometimes intense peripheral vasoconstriction supports a normal or even increased blood pressure despite a very much reduced cardiac output. Acute left heart failure is accompanied by pulmonary oedema, tachycardia and a third heart sound. Pulmonary oedema is caused by a rise in pulmonary venous pressure to a point where there is net movement of fluid into the interstitial, and ultimately, alveolar spaces of the lungs. The patient becomes extremely breathless, develops a

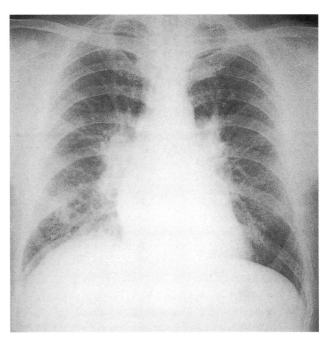
Fig. 6.69 Chest radiograph of acute left heart failure caused by mitral stenosis. (Note that left heart failure does not equate with left ventricular failure: the left ventricle in mitral stenosis is fine!)

cough and in severe left ventricular failure may even produce frothy pink-stained sputum. The characteristic clinical sign of pulmonary oedema is the presence of widespread crepitations or crackling sounds, usually best heard at the base of the lungs. The chest radiograph shows white fluffy shadows in both lungs (Fig. 6.69). In severe disease, both lung fields become almost opaque. With acute right-sided heart failure, such as occurs as a consequence of acute massive pulmonary embolism, there is no pulmonary oedema but the jugular venous pressure is markedly elevated and blood pressure is very low.

Symptoms and signs
Acute heart failure

- Acute dyspnoea (pulmonary oedema)
- Hypotension (may be marked by general vasoconstriction)
- Cold clammy skin (peripheral vasoconstriction)
- Anxiety
- Confusion (impaired cerebral blood flow, hypoxaemia)
- Oliguria

Chronic heart failure

In chronic heart failure, the body invokes physiological responses to compensate for the cardiac insufficiency. In

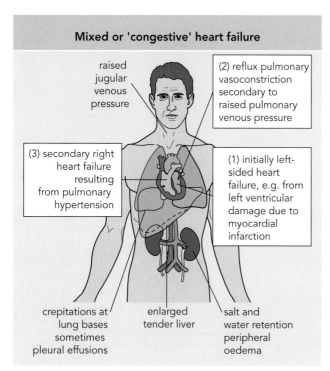

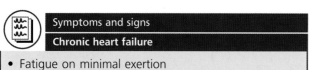

Mixed or 'congestive' heart failure

raised jugular venous pressure

(2) reflux pulmonary vasoconstriction secondary to raised pulmonary venous pressure

(3) secondary right heart failure resulting from pulmonary hypertension

(1) initially left-sided heart failure, e.g. from left ventricular damage due to myocardial infarction

crepitations at lung bases sometimes pleural effusions

enlarged tender liver

salt and water retention peripheral oedema

Fig. 6.70 Mixed or 'congestive' heart failure starts as left heart failure, but secondary pulmonary vasoconstriction then causes right heart failure.

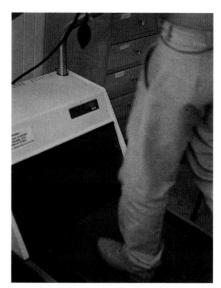

Fig. 6.71 Treadmill exercise testing is best used to confirm a clinical diagnosis of angina and to get an objective estimate of exercise tolerance.

Symptoms and signs

Chronic heart failure

- Fatigue on minimal exertion
- Exertional dyspnoea
- Peripheral oedema
- Abdominal discomfort (from hepatic distension)
- Nocturia (reversal of diurnal rhythm)
- Weight loss and cachexia

---

chronic left heart failure, there is often a reflex elevation of pulmonary vascular resistance, protecting the patient from pulmonary oedema but at the cost of generating secondary right heart failure. This combination is sometimes called mixed, biventricular or congestive heart failure (Fig. 6.70).

Another important compensatory mechanism is fluid retention mediated by the renin–angiotensin system which increases renal salt and water reabsorption. This has the effect of increasing cardiac filling pressure (manifested by a raised jugular venous pressure) at the cost of increased oedema.

CORONARY ARTERY DISEASE

Angina

Coronary artery disease is the most common form of heart disease in the Western world. It has three principal manifestations: angina, the acute coronary syndrome (myocardial infarction) and chronic heart failure. The characteristic features of angina have already been described in the section on taking a cardiac history.

Physical examination of the angina patient is frequently normal. Nonetheless, the examiner should seek signs of hyperlipidaemia, such as corneal arcus, tendon xanthomata and xanthelasma. Because the resting ECG is frequently entirely normal in patients with angina, confirmation of myocardial ischaemia is usually made by ECG exercise testing (Fig. 6.71). Other tests used commonly for the diagnosis of coronary artery disease include myocardial perfusion scanning (Fig. 6.72) and coronary arteriography (Fig. 6.73).

Risk factors

Coronary artery disease

Inherited
- Familial hyperlipidaemia
- High lipoprotein a (e.g. Indo origin)
- Others*

Acquired
- Smoking
- Acquired hyperlipidaemia
- Diabetes
- Hypertension
- Physical inactivity

---

*This includes many common polymorphisms with small (but cumulative) effects and some rare polymorphisms (e.g. pseudoxanthoma elasticum) with large effects.

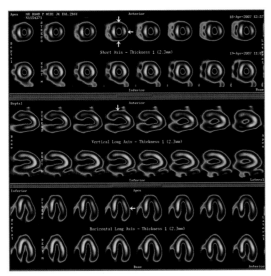

Fig. 6.72 Myocardial perfusion scan showing evidence of anterior reversible ischaemia.

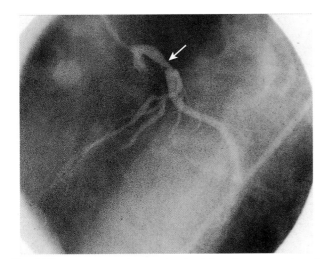

Fig. 6.73 Coronary arteriogram showing left main coronary stenosis (arrow).

ECG in myocardial infarction

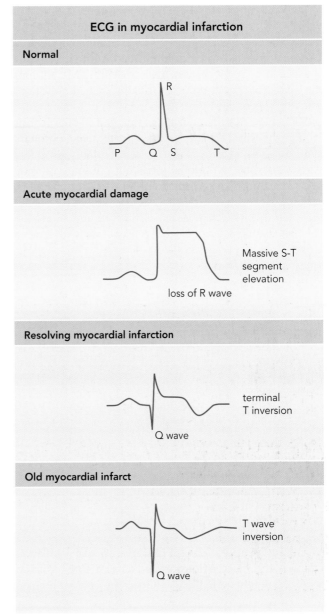

Fig. 6.74 ECG showing features of acute myocardial infarction.

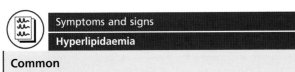

Symptoms and signs
Hyperlipidaemia

Common
- Corneal arcus (nonspecific in patients over 50 years old)
- Xanthelasma (nonspecific in patients over 50 years old)
- Tendon xanthomas (mainly in familial hypercholesterolaemia)

Less common
- Palmar xanthomas
- Eruptive xanthomas
- Ejection systolic murmur (familial hypercholesterolaemia)
- Lipaemia retinalis

Acute coronary syndrome

Acute coronary syndromes are nearly always caused by coronary thrombosis. The coronary thrombosis occurs at the site of disruption of an atheromatous plaque triggered by inflammation. Three distinct clinical syndromes are currently recognised including unstable angina, non-ST segment elevation myocardial infarction (NSTEMI) and ST segment elevation myocardial infarction (STEMI). However, the clinical presentation is identical. STEMI is associated with typical electrocardiographic changes of ST elevation and Q wave formation due to transmural myocardial ischaemia (Fig. 6.74) and is always associated with myocardial necrosis confirmed by a rise in plasma level of cardiac enzymes including creatine kinase or troponin.

Unstable angina and NSTEMI are associated with a variety of electrocardiographic changes including a normal ECG, T wave inversion or ST segment depression. Unstable angina can be distinguished from NSTEMI by the absence of myocardial necrosis. NSTEMI patients have a rise in cardiac enzymes (but without ST elevation) due to sub-endocardial ischaemia. The patient may previously have suffered from angina, but frequently this is not the case. The hallmark of an acute coronary syndrome is angina pain at rest, often associated with autonomic symptoms including nausea, vomiting and sweating. In a small proportion of patients, particularly elderly people and individuals with diabetes mellitus, myocardial ischaemia and infarction can be painless and might present with dyspnoea alone.

Symptoms and signs
Acute myocardial infarction

Symptoms
- Severe pain
- Pain persists despite rest

Physical signs
- Signs of sympathetic activation (pallor, sweating)
- Narrow pulse pressure
- May be extrasystoles
- May be added (third) heart sound

An early complication of STEMI is ventricular fibrillation which is the most serious of cardiac arrhythmias, often requiring urgent defibrillation. Late complications include other cardiac arrhythmias such as ventricular tachycardia, atrial fibrillation or bradycardia, cardiac failure, cardiac rupture (myomalacia), severe mitral valve regurgitation and, occasionally, the development of ventricular septal defect or mild mitral regurgitation due to papillary muscle fibrosis. These complications are now less common since the advent of prompt reperfusion therapy.

Chronic heart failure due to ischaemic heart disease has the clinical features of any other form of chronic heart failure and diagnosis can usually be made on the basis of the history of effort dyspnoea and orthopnoea.

Peripheral vascular disease

Peripheral vascular disease refers to disease of both the peripheral arterial and venous systems. Peripheral arterial disease results mainly from acute or chronic impairment of peripheral blood supply to a limb. This may result from atheromatous narrowing of the artery,

from thrombosis or much more rarely from embolism from the heart.

Acute arterial obstruction presents with a cold, white, painful, pulseless limb. The site of obstruction is usually obvious from examining the pulses but confirmation by vascular imaging is generally necessary, especially prior to planned surgery. Check all the pulses of the unaffected limbs, as there might be some clinical evidence of more diffuse or chronic peripheral vascular disease. This might manifest as reduced pulse volumes or absent pulses where a collateral circulation maintains function and tissue viability. Embolism to multiple sites may be the first clue to a cardiac disease such as atrial myxoma.

Chronic arterial insufficiency occurs most commonly in the lower limb and usually presents as intermittent claudication. The patient is aware of exercise-induced pain in the leg, thigh or buttock. Characteristically the pain relieves rapidly on stopping to rest. Examination of the leg reveals weak or absent foot, knee and sometimes femoral pulses. There may be a murmur or bruit over the femoral artery because of turbulence caused by upstream narrowing in the internal or external iliac arteries. As the disease progresses, the time to claudication reduces until finally the patient experiences rest pain. Pain is often worse at night. Patients with severe chronic arterial insufficiency in the leg often gain partial relief by hanging the leg over the side of the bed outside the bedclothes. Paradoxically, this often makes perfusion of the foot worse. Chronically ischaemic skin tends to become discoloured and shiny, and hair is lost from the foot. Infection, is often initiated by a minor injury such as that occurring during toenail clipping and infection characteristically spreads rapidly. Eventually, gangrene may affect the toes and foot (Fig. 6.75).

Patients with diabetes mellitus are particularly susceptible to peripheral arterial disease. As diabetes affects both large and small blood vessels as well as the intercellular tissue matrix, peripheral tissue damage tends to be disproportionately more severe than would be expected from the clinical assessment of the large vessels. The damage potential is further aggravated when there

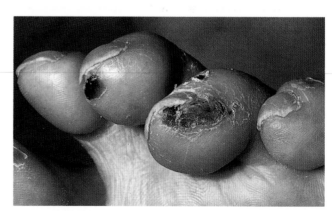

Fig. 6.75 Gangrene of toes in peripheral vascular disease.

is also accompanying diabetic sensory neuropathy, and indeed, diabetic patients may sustain injuries giving rise to infection without noticing much discomfort until the infection is well established.

The main aids to clinical diagnosis of peripheral arterial disease are Doppler ultrasound examination, which evaluates both vessel diameter and blood flow, and either contrast or magnetic resonance angiography.

DISEASES OF THE PERIPHERAL VEINS

The principal diseases of the peripheral veins are varicose veins, thrombophlebitis and deep venous thrombosis.

Varicose veins

Varicose veins are readily apparent as excessively dilated superficial leg veins. In adopting an upright posture, the human species has a special adaptation to ensure adequate venous drainage from the legs towards the heart. A system of one way valves in the venous system of the lower limbs ensures flow toward the heart orchestrated by the pump action of the lower limb muscles. Varicose veins usually result from defects in the valvular system that normally directs the venous blood flow from the legs via the deep veins against the force of gravity. The two major causes of varicose veins are defective valves in the 'perforating veins' which connect the deep and superficial venous systems in the calf, and defective valves in the upper part of the long saphenous vein where it joins the femoral vein at the thigh. Commonly, the problem is initiated by incompetent valves in the perforating veins and saphenofemoral incompetence is secondary to the resulting dilatation of the superficial venous system.

Risk factors

Varicose veins

- Obesity
- Stasis from sitting or standing (position)
- Pregnancy
- Pelvic venous obstruction
- Damage to deep veins from thrombosis
- Trauma to short or long saphenous vein
- Hereditary

Varicose veins are always most apparent when the patient is standing upright and the dilated veins empty completely when the legs are raised above heart level. By elevating the legs to empty the veins and then watching them refill as the leg is lowered, it is often possible to localise the sites of incompetent perforating veins and control them by local finger pressure. If the saphenofemoral junction is incompetent, it may be necessary first to

prevent blood flowing back from the femoral vein by tying a tourniquet around the upper thigh. Identification of the site of perforating veins is an important step in treating varicose veins by injecting a sclerosant solution around incompetent perforators. Very advanced varicose veins may require ligation and stripping of the long (and sometimes the short) saphenous vein. The importance of the long saphenous vein as a source of vascular tissue in coronary bypass surgery makes it important to preserve this vessel if possible.

Chronic venous insufficiency

Failure or inadequacy of the 'muscle pump' mechanism may also lead to chronic oedema of the legs and feet. This is more common in elderly, obese and sedentary patients and tends to become self-perpetuating because the legs are often painful and underused. The oedema is often relatively firm or 'brawny' and pits only reluctantly on pressure. The oedema is readily distinguished from heart failure because the jugular venous pressure is normal. Sometimes chronic venous insufficiency is associated with obstruction of the inferior vena cava but in this setting there are usually grossly distended collateral veins visible on the abdominal wall.

Varicose ulceration and eczema

Chronic venous insufficiency results in a rise in tissue pressure affecting skin and subcutaneous tissue attrition. This may lead to skin necrosis and ulceration, most commonly at the ankle just above the medial malleoli. The skin is often dusky and indurated. Scarring as part of the healing process tends to impair the microcirculation further and the condition may become self-perpetuating (Fig. 6.76).

Thrombophlebitis

Superficial thrombophlebitis refers to inflammation and thrombosis of a superficial vein. This commonly results either from local trauma or from an intravenous infusion but may occur spontaneously. There is local pain, redness and tenderness over the course of the vein. The condition is usually benign and self-limiting but septic thrombophlebitis from a drip site infection can lead to septicaemia.

Deep vein thrombosis

Thrombosis of the deep veins in the calf or pelvis usually occurs as a result of a combination of intravascular stasis and damage of the endothelial lining. Inactivity is the major predisposing factor and it is well known that bed rest, hospitalisation and long haul flights place individuals at particular risk. Until measures were taken to prevent inactivity by encouraging early mobilisation and using low dosage low molecular weight heparin, deep venous thrombosis was a common and potentially fatal complication of major surgery. Deep vein thrombosis

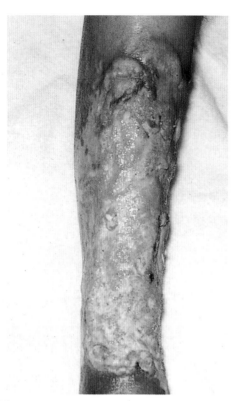

Fig. 6.76 Severe varicose ulceration of the leg.

may also occur in the absence of any obvious predisposing factor. On more extensive investigation, these patients may have abnormalities of the blood clotting and fibrinolytic systems (thrombophilia) and should be further investigated. Hereditary causes of thrombophilia include the Factor V Leiden, prothrombin gene mutation, Protein C and S deficiency, anti-phospholipid antibody syndrome and anti-thrombin III deficiency.

The characteristic clinical features of deep vein thrombosis in the leg are pain, swelling and occasionally redness. The pain is a deep aching pain which is worse on activity but persists at rest. Often, the pain is absent despite the presence of extensive venous thrombosis. Leg swelling can be assessed clinically by comparison of calf diameters at a fixed point below the patella. There is often dilatation of the superficial veins and warm skin resulting from diversion of blood flow from the deep to the superficial veins. Pain in the calf can sometimes be produced by dorsiflexing the foot (Homan's sign) but this sign is most often absent in patients with deep venous thrombosis. If pain and swelling are mainly below the knee, it is likely that the thrombosis is in the calf veins. If the swelling and tenderness extends to the thigh or the groin, then the thrombosis may involve the femoral or iliac veins: this is potentially more serious because thromboembolism from these sites is frequently massive.

The main differential diagnosis of deep vein thrombosis of the legs is spontaneous rupture of the gastrocnemius muscle and rupture of a Baker's cyst in the popliteal fossa.

The diagnosis of deep vein thrombosis needs to be confirmed by either Doppler ultrasound scanning or venography. It is important to remember that deep vein thrombosis, particularly in elderly people, may be accompanied by very few clinical signs and often goes unnoticed until it presents as pulmonary embolism.

Differential diagnosis
Deep vein thrombosis

Pain and swelling in the leg may be caused by:
- deep vein thrombosis
- ruptured head of gastrocnemius muscle
- ruptured osteoarthritic cyst (Baker's cyst) or knee joint
- anterior compartment syndrome (skin splints)

Pulmonary embolism is the most important complication of deep venous thrombosis. If extensive thrombosis occurs in the deep veins of the lower limb, a distal fragment may become detached and travel through the great veins to the heart, where it may either lodge in the right ventricle or in the pulmonary artery. Clinically, pulmonary embolism may present as a pulmonary infarct, acute massive pulmonary embolus and a more chronic pulmonary thromboembolic disease.

Acute pulmonary infarction

This is usually the consequence of a relatively small pulmonary embolus lodging in a branch of the pulmonary artery. As a result of vasospasm and reduced air entry, a wedge-shaped section of the lung downstream of the block becomes necrotic. This, in turn, causes inflammation of the pleura straddling the infarct and this results in the characteristic presentation with sudden onset pleuritic pain. The patient may complain of dyspnoea and tachypnoea might be evident on examination. There is seldom hypotension. A further clue to the diagnosis is profound arterial hypoxaemia with normal partial pressure of carbon dioxide. The chest radiograph may show a wedge-shaped opacity with its base along the pleural edge. The diagnosis is supported by an isotopic ventilation and perfusion lung scan which often shows other perfusion defects.

Acute massive pulmonary embolism

This occurs most commonly in postoperative patients. The patient suddenly becomes extremely breathless, profoundly hypotensive and may not be able to sit upright. There is often an accompanying urge to evacuate the bowels. The jugular veins are markedly distended and the liver may also be enlarged by congestion. Heart sounds are usually quiet because of the reduced cardiac output and there might be a third sound best heard to the left of the sternum. The chest radiograph is usually unhelpful but the ECG shows a characteristic pattern of acute right ventricular strain (S-wave in standard lead I, Q waves in standard lead III associated with an inverted T wave). Echocardiography shows a dilated, poorly contracting right ventricle and a small underfilled left ventricle. Definitive diagnosis is by isotopic ventilation perfusion scanning and/or CT pulmonary angiography.

Chronic pulmonary thromboembolic disease

Chronic thromboembolic disease results from the showering of multiple small pulmonary emboli over a period of time. The clinical features are those of chronic pulmonary hypertension (see below). The diagnosis should be suspected in patients who develop chronic pulmonary symptoms or right-sided heart failure against a background of chronic or recurrent deep vein thrombosis or evidence of thrombophilia.

PULMONARY HYPERTENSION

Pulmonary hypertension is defined by a mean pulmonary arterial pressure >25 mmHg and can be caused by obstruction or increased vascular tone at any point in the pulmonary vascular tree. In order to better understand pulmonary hypertension, it is useful to divide causes into those predominantly precapillary, capillary or postcapillary. Precapillary pulmonary hypertension is due to pathology involving the pulmonary arteries and arterioles including chronic pulmonary thromboembolic disease, primary pulmonary hypertension and pulmonary vasculitis. Capillary pulmonary hypertension occurs in conditions associated with parenchymal lung disease including cystic fibrosis and other chronic lung diseases such as chronic obstructive pulmonary disease. Postcapillary pulmonary hypertension is caused by left heart failure due to primary left ventricular myocardial dysfunction or ventricular failure secondary to aortic and/or mitral valve disease. Symptoms may be insidious, beginning with exertional dyspnoea which becomes progressively more severe. Rarely, chest pain occurs, which is sometimes called right ventricular angina. Progressive right heart failure supervenes and this is detected by the signs of right heart failure and fluid overload (see 'symptoms and signs' box).

Symptoms and signs
Pulmonary hypertension

- Loud pulmonary component of the second sound
- Parasternal (right ventricular) heave
- Dominant a wave in jugular venous pressure
- Tricuspid regurgitation
- Pulmonary regurgitation
- Signs of right heart failure (pedal oedema, ascites, pleural effusion)

INFECTIVE ENDOCARDITIS

Infection of the endocardium of the heart is known as infective endocarditis. There are three principal clinical types of endocarditis: acute, subacute, and postoperative endocarditis.

Acute endocarditis

Acute endocarditis is the result of endocardial infection occurring in a normal or abnormal heart with a virulent organism such as *Staphylococcus aureus* or *Streptococcus pneumoniae*. The infection usually involves one of the heart valves but may involve the endocardium adjacent to a defect such as a ventricular septal defect. The infection may destroy valve tissue, or result in abscess formation or the formation of large vegetations composed of an aggregation of bacteria, platelets and thrombin. The patient is usually seriously ill with a fever and profound systemic symptoms. One of the characteristic clinical findings is rapidly developing or changing cardiac murmurs, indicative of the destructive underlying process. Other signs include finger clubbing and splinter haemorrhages. The cardiac vegetations are a potential source of septic systemic emboli that may be carried through the circulation to reach distant parts of the body.

Subacute endocarditis

Subacute endocarditis may result from a more indolent intercurrent infection of an already diseased heart valve or septal defect. The time course of the illness is much more insidious than acute endocarditis. The most common organism associated with subacute endocarditis is *Streptococcus viridans*. Another cause of subacute endocarditis is partial treatment of acute endocarditis with inadequate doses of antibiotics.

Patients present with fatigue and tiredness, depression, unexplained fever, and symptoms related to the progressive valve destruction or systemic emboli. There is nearly always a heart murmur and the combination of fever and a heart murmur should always raise the suspicion of endocarditis. Like acute endocarditis, the murmurs may change but this usually occurs over a time course of days or weeks rather than hours. Finger clubbing and splinter haemorrhages are common cardinal physical signs. In untreated cases there may be anaemia and pigmentation of the skin. There is often splenomegaly, reflecting of the involvement of the immune system in this subacute infection. Other signs include localised subconjunctival haemorrhages, tender swellings in the finger pulps (Osler's nodes), painless macules on the palms and soles (Janeway lesions) and haemorrhagic spots in the retina characterised by an area of central pallor (Roth spots). Many of the systemic features of subacute endocarditis are due to immune complex deposition and systemic vasculitis.

Postoperative endocarditis

Postoperative endocarditis most commonly follows open heart surgery and may involve artificial heart valves or other implanted material. The most common organism is a coagulase-negative staphylococcus. The clinical features may resemble those of acute or subacute endocarditis.

MYOCARDITIS

Myocarditis is an inflammatory infection of heart muscle, usually resulting from a virus infection. Clinically, myocarditis usually presents with heart failure or an arrhythmia. There is often cardiac dilatation, a third heart sound and there may be a pansystolic apical murmur arising from 'functional' mitral incompetence caused by dilatation of the ventricle and consequent stretching of the chordae tendinae and papillary muscles.

CARDIOMYOPATHY

Cardiomyopathy is a general term meaning 'heart muscle disease'. Clinically, cardiomyopathy can be classified into hypertrophic, dilated and restrictive types.

Hypertrophic cardiomyopathy

Hypertrophic cardiomyopathy is characterised by abnormal cardiac muscle hypertrophy in the absence of a stimulus such as hypertension. The hypertrophy may be 'asymmetrical', that is, it specifically affects the interventricular septum, which bulges into the left ventricular outflow tract and causes obstruction to blood flow during ventricular systole. This variant, called hypertrophic obstructive cardiomyopathy (HOCM), has been associated with sudden death, often occurring during sport or exercise. The clinical features of hypertrophic obstructive cardiomyopathy are summarised in Figure 6.77.

Dilated cardiomyopathy

Dilated cardiomyopathy is characterised by a global impairment of left ventricular function, leading to progressive dilatation of the ventricles. Most commonly, the cause is unknown and this is termed idiopathic dilated cardiomyopathy. Similar pathology can occur in alcoholic patients and patients with systemic diseases such as sarcoidosis, haemochromatosis, thyrotoxicosis and myocarditis; a very rare form occurs in pregnancy (peripartum cardiomyopathy). Dilated cardiomyopathy has been associated with certain drugs, especially anthracyclines used in chemotherapy. The clinical presentation is dominated by symptoms and signs of biventricular heart failure. The apex beat is displaced laterally, indicating left ventricular dilatation, and invariably there is a gallop rhythm (third and fourth heart sounds). There may be mitral or tricuspid regurgitation caused by stretching of the chordae tendinae and papillary muscles attached to the dilated utricular wall.

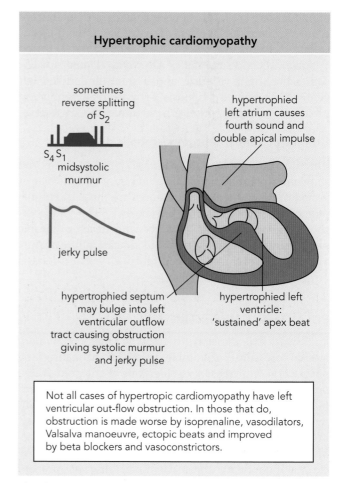

Hypertrophic cardiomyopathy

sometimes reverse splitting of S_2

S_4 S_1 midsystolic murmur

jerky pulse

hypertrophied left atrium causes fourth sound and double apical impulse

hypertrophied septum may bulge into left ventricular outflow tract causing obstruction giving systolic murmur and jerky pulse

hypertrophied left ventricle: 'sustained' apex beat

Not all cases of hypertropic cardiomyopathy have left ventricular out-flow obstruction. In those that do, obstruction is made worse by isoprenaline, vasodilators, Valsalva manoeuvre, ectopic beats and improved by beta blockers and vasoconstrictors.

Fig. 6.77 Findings in hypertrophic cardiomyopathy.

Restrictive cardiomyopathy

This is a rare condition in Western countries. The clinical presentation mimics constrictive pericarditis and the differential is readily made by echocardiography. Causes of restrictive cardiomyopathy include systemic amyloidosis and eosinophilic heart disease.

ACUTE RHEUMATIC FEVER

Acute rheumatic fever is caused by a throat infection with certain strains of beta-haemolytic streptococci. Many of the features are a consequence of an autoimmune response to this organism. Whilst rheumatic fever is now uncommon in Western countries, the condition remains prevalent in the developing world. The long-term consequences of the acute infection and the immunological response remains an important cause of chronic valvular heart disease. Clinically, acute rheumatic fever presents in children or young adults either with pharyngitis, an acute, migratory polyarthritis or with Sydenham's chorea. Other features include an erythematous non-itchy skin rash called erythema marginatum which is fleeting, variable and has a serpiginous margin and subcutaneous rheumatic nodules which are pathognomonic and located on the extensor surfaces of the knees and elbows.

Cardiac involvement is caused by a pancarditis affecting the endocardium, myocardium and pericardium. Endocardial involvement is usually signalled by the development of a pansystolic murmur caused by regurgitation of blood through an incompetent oedematous mitral valve. Another important murmur is a soft mid-diastolic murmur resembling the murmur of mitral stenosis and caused by oedema of the mitral valve and platelet vegetations. Listening at different times of the day, this murmur varies in intensity and is called a Carey Coombs murmur. Its presence has prognostic significance as in these patients the acute valvulitis invariably progresses to a fibrotic mitral stenosis. Myocarditis usually manifests as prolongation of the PR interval of the ECG.

Symptoms and signs

Criteria for the diagnosis of rheumatic fever

Major criteria
- Carditis
- Polyarthritis
- Subcutaneous rheumatic nodules
- Sydenham's chorea
- Erythema marginata

Minor criteria
- Prolonged PR interval
- Recent history of a throat infection
- Serological evidence of recent streptococcal infection
- Arthralgia
- Raised ESR

Diagnosis requires the presence of either two major criteria or one major criterion and two minor criteria.

PERICARDIAL DISEASE

The heart normally contracts within a smooth, closely fitting serous cavity – the pericardium. The principal pericardial diseases are acute pericarditis, pericardial effusion and chronic constrictive pericarditis.

Acute pericarditis

The symptoms of acute pericarditis have already been discussed under chest pain. The most characteristic physical sign on examination is the pericardial rub. This is often mistaken for a murmur but usually has a distinct scratchy quality that sounds like two leather surfaces being rubbed together. In sinus rhythm, the rub is rhythmic and occurs in the presystolic, systolic and diastolic phases of cardiac contraction. Pericardial rubs may be best heard with the patient sitting up, leaning forward and holding their breath in deep expiration (similar to the position for hearing aortic diastolic murmurs). The pericardial rub is usually evanescent and

usually varies in intensity when listened to interpretively over a period of a few hours. Patients with acute pericarditis are often pyrexial and may feel systemically unwell.

Pericardial effusion

Normally, there is only just sufficient fluid in the pericardial cavity to lubricate the visceral and parietal pericardial surfaces during cardiac movement. Excessive accumulation of pericardial fluid is called a pericardial effusion.

Differential diagnosis

Pericardial effusion

Infection
- Viral pericarditis
- Bacterial pericarditis (streptococcus)
- Tuberculous pericarditis

Myocardial infarction
- Peri-infarct pericarditis
- Cardiac rupture
- Dressler's syndrome

Malignant pericarditis
- Secondary (common) or primary (rare) tumours
- Leukaemia

Autoallergic
- Acute rheumatic fever
- Rheumatoid arthritis

Other
- Myxoedema
- Trauma (stab wounds)
- After cardiac surgery

The clinical features of a pericardial effusion depend both on the amount of fluid and the speed with which it accumulates. A large amount of fluid or the very rapid accumulation of fluid causes compression of the heart, particularly the right ventricle, causing a substantial reduction in cardiac output. This is termed 'cardiac tamponade' and is a medical emergency. The patient is often very ill, hypotensive and peripherally vasoconstricted. There may be pulsus paradoxus which is a variation in pulse volume with respiration (Fig. 6.78). The jugular venous pressure (JVP) is very high but this may be difficult to see because the patient may be too hypotensive to sit upright. Whereas normally the upper level of the JVP falls during inspiration as blood is sucked into the chest and returned to the right heart, in pericardial tamponade, the upper level rises paradoxically due to obstructed passage of the increased venous inflow occurring in inspiration. Even a small amount of fluid, acuminating rapidly, can cause cardiac tamponade. In this setting, the usual signs of a pericardial effusion, including increased area of dullness to percussion in the front of the chest and an

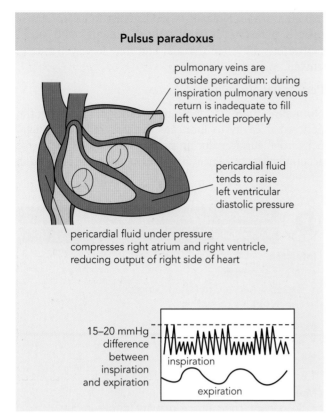

Pulsus paradoxus

pulmonary veins are outside pericardium: during inspiration pulmonary venous return is inadequate to fill left ventricle properly

pericardial fluid tends to raise left ventricular diastolic pressure

pericardial fluid under pressure compresses right atrium and right ventricle, reducing output of right side of heart

15–20 mmHg difference between inspiration and expiration

inspiration

expiration

Fig. 6.78 Pulses paradoxus, or the apparent diminution of the pulse on inspiration, is a feature of pericardial tamponade.

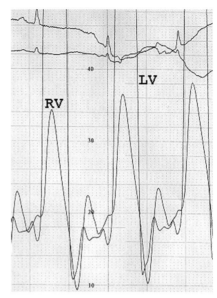

RV

LV

Fig. 6.79 Characteristic diastolic equalisation of right and left ventricular pressures leading to 'dip and plateau' appearance.

enlarged globular cardiac shadow on a chest radiograph, are unreliable in diagnosing cardiac tamponade. Bedside echocardiography is the best way of confirming the diagnosis of a pericardial effusion and, if necessary, this can be followed by pericardiocentesis.

Red flag – urgent referral

Cardiac tamponade

Causes
- Any cause of pericardial effusion (see 'pericardial effusion differential diagnosis' box)
- Pneumonia
- Trauma

Clinical presentation
- Hypotension
- Oliguria
- Raised jugular venous pulse
- Paradoxical pulse

Diagnosis
- Chest radiograph: enlarged heart shadow
- ECG: small voltages, 'electrical alternans'
- Echo: effusion with collapse of right ventricle

Treatment
- Pericardiocentesis
- Surgical drainage

If pericardial fluid accumulates slowly over days or weeks, this is often accommodated by stretching of the pericardium rather than cardiac tamponade. A chronic pericardial effusion may be detected accidentally or, more commonly, it presents as chronic right-sided cardiac failure, with marked peripheral oedema and, sometimes, ascites. Breathlessness is conspicuously absent despite the signs of right heart failure. The jugular venous pressure is usually markedly elevated and there is paradoxical movement with respiration. There is often an enlarged area of dullness on percussion to the left of the sternum. Depending on the volume of effusion there may or may not be a pericardial rub. In the presence of a large effusion, the apex beat will be impalpable and the heart sounds soft or virtually inaudible. There may be a pulsus paradoxus, but this is often less prominent than in acute cardiac tamponade. Chest radiography shows cardiac enlargement and echocardiography is the simplest investigation to confirm the diagnosis.

Chronic constrictive pericarditis

Chronic inflammation of the pericardium may lead to a thickened fibrotic pericardial membrane that constricts and compresses the heart. Worldwide, tuberculous pericarditis remains the most common cause, although it may also follow acute viral pericarditis, cardiac surgery or chest wall or lung radiation.

The clinical features of chronic constrictive pericarditis are similar to those of chronic pericardial effusion. There are readily visible signs of right-sided heart failure, often with severe and widespread oedema. Abdominal distension is common and due to ascites. The jugular venous pressure is elevated and often has a characteristic waveform, with a very rapid dip in the pulse as the tricuspid valve opens, followed by an equally abrupt termination as filling of the ventricle is curtailed. In longstanding severe constrictive pericarditis, the pericardium may become adherent to the ribcage and the examiner can feel a tugging on the posterior ribs in time with the heart beat (pericardial rub). Diagnosis is made by echocardiography or at cardiac catheterisation. There is a characteristic 'dip and plateau' or 'square root' sign in the pressure curves of the right and left ventricles and equalisation of pressure in the range of 5 mmHg or less (Fig. 6.79).

Examination of elderly people

Cardiovascular examination

- General approach and techniques unaltered
- Some stress tests may be impractical but there are alternatives
- Likely to be multisystem disease
- Common problems are hypertension, ischaemic heart disease and peripheral vascular disease
- Ischaemic heart disease may be asymptomatic
- Acute myocardial infarction may be 'silent'
- Ankle swelling usually a clue to venous insufficiency not heart failure
- Aortic stenosis is common and difficult to diagnose but worth treating if severe

- Cardiac arrhythmias are common and do not generally require investigation unless symptomatic
- Causes of dizziness or transient loss of consciousness include postural hypotension (often drug induced), vertebrobasilar insufficiency, arrhythmias (especially bradycardia)
- Multiple drug therapy may be the cause of the problem – nonsteroidals cause fluid retention and hypertension

Review

Framework for the routine examination of the cardiovascular system

1. Observe the patient. Are they comfortable at rest? Watch for features of breathlessness or cyanosis. Look out for any cardiac scars that may be relevant.
2. Take the patient's hand and assess warmth, sweating and peripheral cyanosis; examine the nails for clubbing or splinter haemorrhages.
3. Palpate the radial pulse and assess the rate and rhythm.
4. Locate and palpate the brachial pulse and assess its character. Measure the blood pressure. If there is any suspicion of a problem with the aortic arch, compare pulses in both arms.
5. Palpate the carotid pulse and assess its volume and character.
6. With the patient lying supine at 45°, assess the height of the jugular venous pressure and the jugular venous pulse waveform.
7. Take an opportunity for a closer look at the face, the conjunctivae, the tongue and the inside of the mouth.
8. With the patient's chest exposed, inspect the precordium and assess the breathing pattern and the presence of any abnormal pulsation.

9. Palpate the precordium, locate the apex beat and assess its character. Assess the feel of the rest of the precordium and the presence of any abnormal vibrations or thrills.
10. Listen with the stethoscope and assess heart sounds and murmurs systematically in the four valve areas: mitral, tricuspid, pulmonary and aortic. If appropriate, listen over the carotid artery for radiating murmurs or bruits.
11. Percuss and auscultate the chest both front and back looking for pleural effusions. Listen for crepitations at the lung bases.
12. Lie the patient flat and palpate the abdomen, feeling in particular for the liver and any dilatation of the abdominal aorta.
13. Assess the femoral pulses and the popliteal and foot pulses. Look for ankle or sacral oedema.
14. If appropriate, assess the patient's exercise tolerance by taking the patient for a short walk.
15. Test the urine.

The abdomen

The abdominal examination follows that of the heart and lungs. Diseases of the abdominal organs may already be apparent from the general examination: for example, you may have noticed jaundice when examining the skin and eyes and in patients with obstructive jaundice, scratch marks may be apparent. You may have been aware of abnormal weight loss, signs of malnutrition or anaemia. Underlying iron deficiency may be revealed by a smooth, atrophic tongue and by cracks at the angles of the mouth (cheilosis), which may also suggest a vitamin B group deficiency.

Structure and function

The symptoms and signs of abdominal disease reflect disorder in the anatomy and physiology of the major abdominal organs. These organs are packed neatly into the abdominal cavity (Fig. 7.1) The liver, gallbladder and spleen lie protected under cover of the lower thoracic ribs, whereas the stomach, 6 m of small intestine and 1.5 m of large bowel cover and cushion the pancreas, kidneys and ureters. The urinary bladder, and in women the ovaries and adnexae, lie hidden deep in the protective wall of the pelvis.

GASTROINTESTINAL TRACT

Mouth and oesophagus

Digestion begins in the mouth where food is chewed and moistened with saliva. The salivary fluid is a cocktail of enzymes, including amylase and lingual lipase and bicarbonate and lysozyme. Saliva is secreted by the parotid, submandibular and sublingual glands, with a small contribution from the labial glands on the inner aspects of the lips.

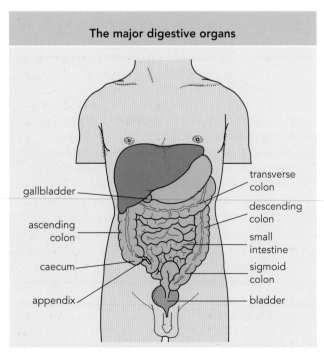

The major digestive organs

gallbladder

ascending colon

caecum

appendix

transverse colon

descending colon

small intestine

sigmoid colon

bladder

Fig. 7.1 The anatomical relationships of the major digestive organs.

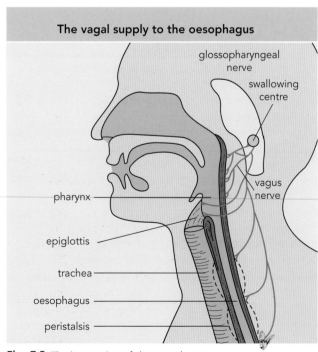

The vagal supply to the oesophagus

glossopharyngeal nerve

swallowing centre

pharynx

epiglottis

trachea

oesophagus

peristalsis

vagus nerve

Fig. 7.2 The innervation of the oesophagus.

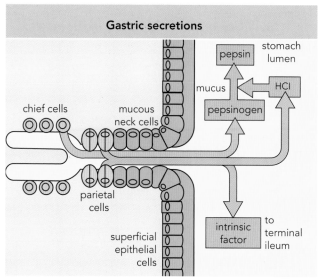

Fig. 7.3 Cells found in the mucosa of the stomach body are responsible for the principal gastric secretions.

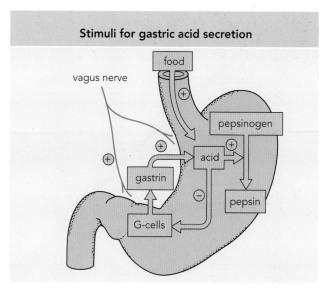

Fig. 7.4 The control of gastric acid secretion by food, vagal stimulation and gastrin. Pepsinogen is activated to pepsin at low pH.

Swallowing is controlled by a medullary centre in the brainstem which relays to and from the pharynx and oesophagus via the glossopharyngeal and vagus nerves (Fig. 7.2). There is also an intrinsic innervation within the smooth muscle of the oesophagus. There are three phases to the swallowing reflex: oral, pharyngeal and oesophageal. During the oral phase, the tongue presses the bolus up against the hard palate and drives the food into the pharynx. In the pharyngeal phase, the respiratory tract closes off, the upper pharyngeal sphincter (cricopharyngeus) relaxes and the upper, middle and lower pharyngeal constrictors propel the food into the oesophagus. In the oesophageal phase, a powerful peristaltic wave propels the bolus towards the stomach. The lower oesophageal sphincter has intrinsic tone that prevents regurgitation of the gastric contents: it relaxes in advance of the peristaltic wave and remains relaxed for a few seconds after the wave has passed.

Difficulty swallowing (dysphagia) may be caused by damage to the neural control, abnormalities of the oesophageal muscle or obstruction of the lumen.

Stomach

The churning action of the antrum continues the mixing process started in the mouth and prepares food for its journey into the duodenum. The parietal cells in the body of the stomach (Fig. 7.3) secrete hydrochloric acid, which sterilises the meal, and intrinsic factor, which is necessary for the absorption of vitamin B_{12} in the terminal ileum. The chief cells secrete pepsinogen which is converted to the proteolytic enzyme pepsin by the low pH of the stomach lumen. The secretion of acid is stimulated by the vagus nerve, distension of the stomach with food and the secretion of the hormone gastrin from the G-cells of the gastric antrum (Fig. 7.4). A mucous layer coats the

stomach mucosa, protecting it from self-inflicted injury by acid and pepsin.

Regurgitation of gastric contents into the oesophagus is prevented by an antireflux mechanism at the gastro-oesophageal junction. This includes the intrinsic tone of the lower oesophageal sphincter, the flap-valve effect of the angle of His and the squeezing effect of intra-abdominal pressure on the small segment of oesophagus that protrudes through the diaphragm into the abdomen (Fig. 7.5). If one or more of these antireflux mechanisms breaks down, gastric contents may regurgitate into the lower oesophagus, damaging the mucosa and causing heartburn.

Small intestine

The small intestine comprises the duodenum, the jejunum and the ileum. It fills most of the anterior abdomen and is framed by the ascending, transverse and descending colon. Blood is supplied by the superior mesenteric vessels (Fig. 7.6). The principal role of the small intestine is digestion and absorption, which is achieved by a combination of macroscopic and microscopic folds creating a vast absorptive area (Fig. 7.7).

Most of the enzymes necessary for the digestion of fat, protein and carbohydrate are present in the duodenum. Enterocytes develop in the base of the crypts of Lieberkuhn and migrate to the tip of the finger-shaped villi (Fig. 7.8). Both the enterocyte's capacity to produce specialised digestive enzymes on the brush border membrane and its absorptive properties develop progressively as the cell migrates towards the villous tip, at which point these functions are maximally developed.

Carbohydrate digestion is initiated by salivary and pancreatic amylase. Enzymes, such as lactase and sucrase, on the brush border membranes of the enterocytes, complete the digestion of complex polysaccharides and

The antireflux mechanism

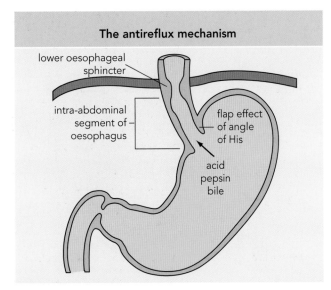

Fig. 7.5 The antireflux mechanism comprises the intrinsic tone of the lower oesophageal sphincter, the acute angle formed at the oesophagogastric junction (angle of His) and the pressure on the intra-abdominal oesophagus.

Blood supply to the intestine

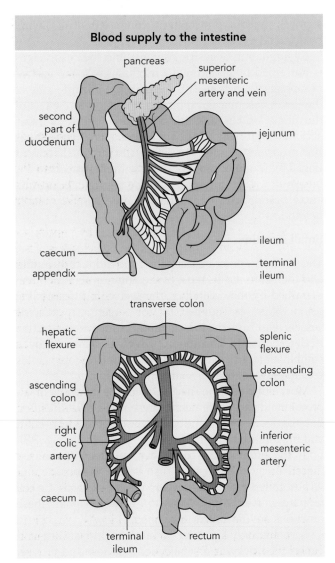

Fig. 7.6 The blood supply of the small intestine, colon, sigmoid and rectum.

The fold forming the surface of the bowel

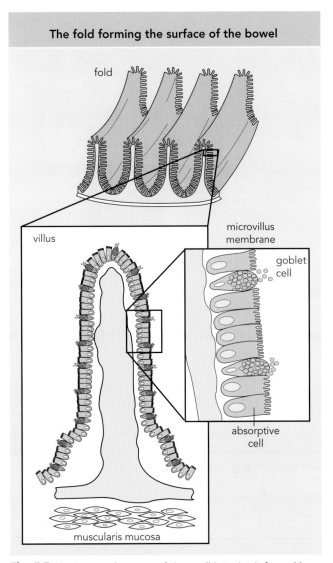

Fig. 7.7 The large surface area of the small intestine is formed by the duodenal folds, the villi and the microvillus membrane of the enterocyte.

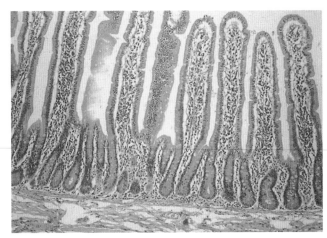

Fig. 7.8 Duodenal enterocytes develop in the crypts and migrate towards the villus tip.

Digestion of carbohydrate, fat and protein

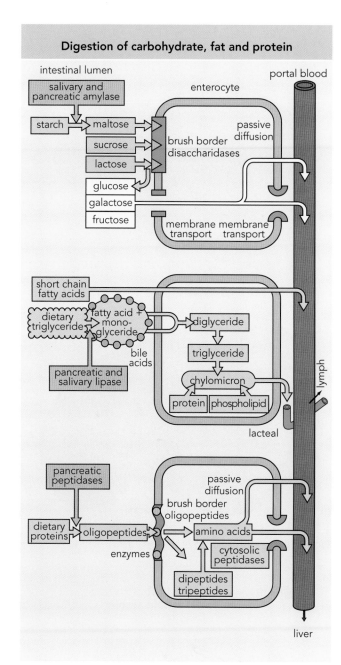

Fig. 7.9 Digestion in the small intestine. Digestion of complex carbohydrates occurs in the lumen and at the brush border membrane. Monosaccharides can then be absorbed through the brush border membrane into the portal circulation. Fat digestion occurs in the lumen and triglyceride is reconstituted in the enterocyte before absorption. Proteins are digested in the lumen and at the brush border membrane. Amino acids are then absorbed into the enterocyte and portal circulation.

Table 7.1 Principal effects of gastrointestinal hormones

Hormone	Function
Gastrin	Stimulates gastric acid secretion
Cholecystokinin	Stimulates gallbladder contraction and pancreatic enzyme secretion
Secretin	Stimulates secretion of pancreatic fluid and bicarbonate
Gastric inhibitory polypeptide	Potentiates the insulin response to glucose
Enteroglucagon	Trophic to small intestine
Vasoactive intestinal polypeptide (VIP)	Secretin-like effect on pancreas Affects intestinal motility and mesenteric blood flow
Motilin	Stimulates intestinal motility between meals
Somatostatin	Inhibits secretion of gastrin, other gut hormones and pepsin Stimulates gastric mucus production
Insulin	Lowers blood glucose Stimulates glycogen synthesis Stimulates protein and fat anabolism
Pancreatic glucagon	Promotes glucogenolysis, lipolysis, gluconeogenesis Slows intestinal motility
Pancreatic polypeptide	Inhibits pancreatic secretion Relaxes the gallbladder
Ghrelin	Stimulates appetite

disaccharides to monosaccharides, which are then transported through the enterocyte by specialised transporters on the brush border and basolateral membranes (Fig. 7.9). Pancreatic lipase hydrolyses triglycerides to fatty acids and monoglycerides. These products are emulsified by bile acids which help form micelles. The micelles are then taken up at the brush border membrane and diffuse passively into the enterocyte, where the triglyceride is reconstituted (Fig. 7.9). These triglycerides, as well as absorbed cholesterol, are formed into fat aggregates (chylomicrons) that are absorbed into the lymphatics and discharged into the circulation through the thoracic duct. The fat-soluble vitamins A, D, K and E are absorbed in a similar manner to other lipids.

Proteolysis is initiated in the stomach by pepsin, yet the bulk of protein digestion is mediated by trypsin and other pancreatic peptidases in the small intestine (Fig. 7.9). The action of these enzymes produces small peptides with 4–6 amino acids that undergo further processing to amino acids, dipeptides and tripeptides by oligopeptidases on the enterocyte brush border membrane. These are absorbed into the enterocytes where the final digestion to single amino acids occurs. The amino acids are transported to the liver by the portal blood.

The addition of pancreatic juice and bile, which are secreted through the ampulla of Vater, modifies and enriches the chyme (semi-liquid food) entering the duodenum from the stomach.

Absorption of nutrients occurs in the jejunum and ileum, along with the production and secretion of a range of hormones. The terminal ileum absorbs vitamin B_{12} and bile acids.

The small intestine has a considerable functional reserve and only fails when there is less than 100 cm of bowel following surgical resection.

Table 7.1 lists the principal effects of gastrointestinal hormones.

Colon

The ileum enters the caecum through the ileocaecal valve, which prevents reflux of colonic contents into the small intestine. Whereas the small intestine is relatively microbe free, the colon is heavily colonised by bacteria. Approximately 1.5 litres of ileal fluid empties into the caecum each day. Most of this effluent is reabsorbed as it passes through the ascending, transverse and descending colon. The colon concentrates the ileal outflow so that the daily stool output on a Western diet averages 200 g; 75% of stool weight is water and the remainder is unabsorbed food and bacteria. The colonic mucosa is rich in glands producing mucus, which provides constant lubrication for the passage of faeces and protects the mucosa from bacterial enzymes. The rectum is the storage organ for stool.

Infection or inflammation of the colonic mucosa may provoke fluid and electrolyte secretion and interfere with absorption, causing diarrhoea and dehydration. Diarrhoea may also occur in small bowel disease when the volume of ileal effluent exceeds the colon's absorptive capacity.

Liver

The liver is the largest intra-abdominal organ. The falciform ligament divides the liver into a large right lobe and a smaller left lobe (Fig. 7.10). Two smaller lobes, the anterior quadrate and posterior caudate, are squeezed between the left and right lobes on the visceral surface of the liver.

The liver is the focal point of intermediary metabolism and energy production and it lies in a strategic position between the gut and the systemic organs. The products of digestion are absorbed into the mesenteric veins which drain into the portal vein and ultimately into the hepatic sinusoids (Fig. 7.11). Specialised macrophages (Kupffer cells) straddle the sinusoids and mount an almost impenetrable defence against unwanted microbes or matter that has escaped the first line of defence in the bowel. Nutrient-rich plasma filters through the small holes (fenestrae) in the endothelial cells lining the sinusoids and passes into the space of Disse, which lies between the endothelial cells and hepatocytes (Fig. 7.12). The plasma filtrate bathes these highly adaptable cells, which are enriched with a range of enzymes able to metabolise the wide variety of incoming digestion products. Three hepatic veins collect the sinusoidal outflow and deliver it into the inferior vena cava.

Hepatocytes perform a remarkable array of synthetic and catabolic functions, with many clinical features of liver disease resulting from derangement of these processes. They convert glucose to glycogen (which can be stored and later reconverted, on demand, to glucose), synthesise a range of proteins (including albumin and the clotting factors), degrade protein to amino acids, synthesise urea from ammonia, and manufacture cholesterol and bile acids. The lateral borders of hepatocytes are modified to form bile canaliculi which

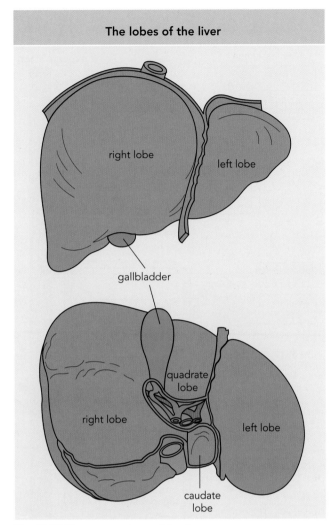

The lobes of the liver

Fig. 7.10 The gross anatomy of the liver.

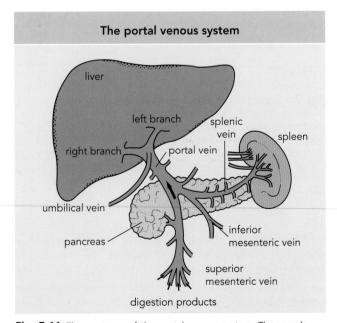

The portal venous system

Fig. 7.11 The anatomy of the portal venous system. The vessels drain into the liver sinusoids carrying nutrients from the intestine, pancreatic hormones from the islets of Langerhans and antibodies from the spleen.

Microanatomy of the liver

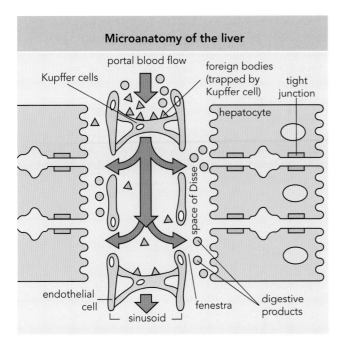

Fig. 7.12 Microanatomy of the liver sinusoids, the space of Disse and hepatocytes. Tight junctions adjacent to the bile canaliculi bind the hepatocytes together.

interconnect and eventually converge as the left and right main hepatic ducts at the liver hilum. The liver cells secrete bile into the canaliculi. Bile is a fluid comprising bile salts, cholesterol and bilirubin. Bilirubin is a pigment derived from haemoglobin released from dead erythrocytes. It cannot be excreted in bile until it has been rendered water-soluble by conjugation with glucuronic acid in the liver (Fig. 7.13).

The liver is an important storage site for iron and vitamins and plays a central role in the hydroxylation of vitamin D. Other functions include the conjugation and excretion of steroid hormones, the detoxification of drugs and the conversion of fat-soluble waste products to water-soluble substances for excretion by the kidneys.

Gallbladder

The gallbladder is a pear-shaped organ with a fundus, a body and a neck that narrows to give rise to the cystic duct. It lies protected beneath the lower surface of the liver in the gallbladder fossa that separates the right and quadrate lobes. The gallbladder concentrates and stores bile and, under the influence of cholecystokinin, it pumps the bile through the cystic duct into the common bile duct and through the ampulla of Vater into the duodenum, where it blends with the other products of digestion (Fig. 7.14).

Pancreas

The pancreas is an elongated retroperitoneal organ that lies in the transpyloric plane with its head end tucked into the C-shaped loop of the duodenum and its tail end abutting the spleen (Fig. 7.15). Its posterior position places the organ well out of reach of the examining

Bilirubin metabolism

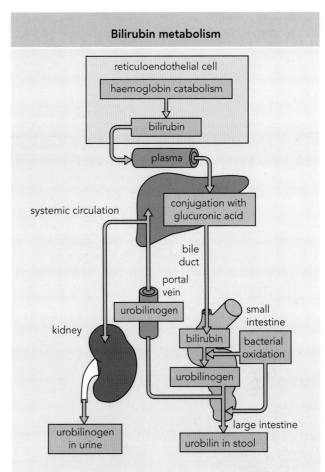

Fig. 7.13 Bilirubin is a product of haemoglobin catabolism.

Anatomy of the pancreatic and bile ducts

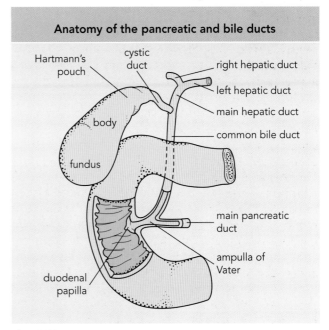

Fig. 7.14 The gallbladder and related ducts. Bile and pancreatic juice both enter the duodenum through the ampulla of Vater.

hand and diagnosis of pancreatic diseases is largely dependent on the use of special imaging techniques such as CT scanning, magnetic resonance cholangiopancreatography (MRCP) and endoscopic retrograde cholangiopancreatography (ERCP) (Fig. 7.16).

The pancreas has mixed exocrine and endocrine functions. The duct cells secrete bicarbonate which protects the duodenum from gastric acid and ensures an optimum pH for digestive enzyme activity. The exocrine acinar cells secrete lipase, phospholipase, amylase and peptidases (trypsinogen, chymotrypsinogen, elastase and carboxypeptidase). All the pancreatic enzymes are secreted in an inactive precursor form and are only cleaved to their active forms in the duodenum by enterokinase, which is fixed on the enterocyte brush border membranes. The hormone cholecystokinin mediates pancreatic enzyme secretion, whereas secretin

promotes the secretion of fluid and bicarbonate from duct cells. The mucosa of the duodenum synthesises both these hormones. The endocrine secretion of the pancreas arises from the islets of Langerhans, which secrete insulin, glucagon, somatostatin and pancreatic polypeptide into the pancreatic and portal veins.

Blockage of the main pancreatic duct by a carcinoma, or diffuse damage caused by pancreatitis, may cause maldigestion of protein, fat and carbohydrate. Patients with pancreatic exocrine failure pass pale, fatty stools that are difficult to flush (steatorrhoea).

Spleen

The spleen is a highly modified lymphoid organ which also regulates the destruction of red blood cells. Reticuloendothelial cells populate the bulk of the spleen, forming the white pulp. These cells provide an important line of defence and the organ is a major site of antibody production. The remainder of the spleen, the red pulp, consists of capillaries and venous sinuses that act as a sump for the storage of red blood cells, white blood cells and platelets. When the spleen enlarges, excessive pooling of these cells may occur, causing a fall in the peripheral blood count. The splenic venous outflow drains into the portal vein, adding a rich supply of antibodies to the portal blood entering the liver.

Kidneys

The kidneys control fluid electrolyte balance and produce the hormones erythropoietin and renin. Each kidney contains approximately 1.2 million nephrons. The structural and functional arrangement of a typical nephron is shown in Figure 7.17.

The capillary loops of the glomerulus form between the afferent and efferent arterioles supplying each glomerulus; the capillary tuft is embedded in the mesangium, which consists of a matrix and specialised mesangial cells. The basement membrane of the capillary tuft impinges on the epithelium of Bowman's capsule via foot processes (podocytes) that arise from the visceral

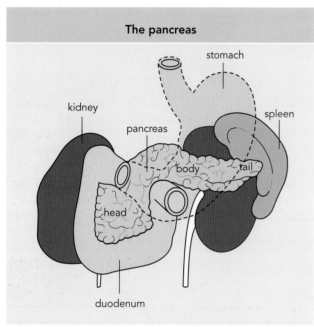

The pancreas

stomach

kidney

pancreas

spleen

body

tail

head

duodenum

Fig. 7.15 The anatomical relationships of the pancreas.

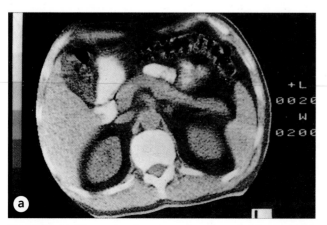

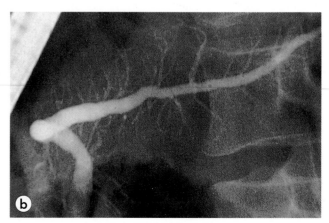

Fig. 7.16 (a) CT scan showing a normal pancreas and the surrounding structures; (b) the pancreatic duct visualised after ERCP injection of radio-opaque contrast medium through the ampulla of Vater.

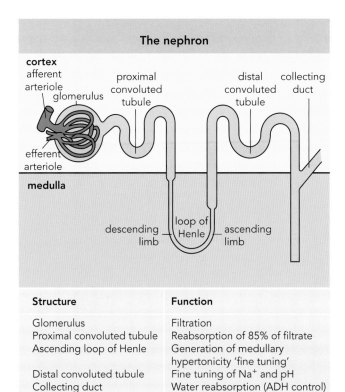

The nephron

Fig. 7.17 The structure and function of a typical nephron.

Structure	Function
Glomerulus	Filtration
Proximal convoluted tubule	Reabsorption of 85% of filtrate
Ascending loop of Henle	Generation of medullary hypertonicity 'fine tuning'
Distal convoluted tubule	Fine tuning of Na$^+$ and pH
Collecting duct	Water reabsorption (ADH control)

cells. This complex anatomical relationship allows a protein-free fluid to filter under pressure from the blood into the proximal convoluted tubule, where specialised epithelium allows the reabsorption of sodium, water, bicarbonate, glucose and amino acids into the efferent arteriole. Approximately two-thirds of the glomerular filtrate is reabsorbed in the proximal convoluted tubule.

The fluid entering the descending limb of the loop of Henle is isosmotic. The proximal and distal limbs of this loop are highly differentiated in their ability to secrete water, chloride and sodium and this, together with the spatial orientation of the loop, is responsible for the progressive increase in the sodium chloride concentration gradient between the cortex and medulla. This medullary hyperosmolality is vital for the further reabsorption of water. The thin descending limb of the loop of Henle is permeable to the outflow of water but not to that of sodium and chloride, so as the filtrate approaches the hairpin bend in the loop it becomes hypertonic. The thick ascending limb of the loop is impermeable to the efflux of water, yet permeable to the efflux of sodium which follows the active secretion of chloride ions. In the ascending limb, the tubular fluid becomes hypotonic while medullary interstitium becomes hypertonic. More sodium is reabsorbed from the distal convoluted tubule in exchange for potassium under the modulating influence of aldosterone.

The final composition of urine is determined by the collecting ducts that course through the medulla. The collecting ducts are normally impermeable to water but they are rendered permeable by the action of antidiuretic hormone (ADH), which is secreted by the pituitary. This allows water to be reabsorbed passively down the osmotic gradient that exists between the duct lumen and interstitial fluid. The permeability of the collecting duct is modified in response to body water requirements and is important for the fine tuning of fluid balance. Failure to produce ADH or insensitivity of the renal tubule to ADH causes inappropriate loss of water through the kidneys and excess urine secretion (polyuria), a syndrome known as diabetes insipidus. Sodium is also actively reabsorbed in the collecting tubules under the influence of aldosterone.

Symptoms of abdominal disorders

GASTROINTESTINAL DISEASES

The principal symptoms of gastrointestinal disease include dysphagia, heartburn, abdominal pain, loss of appetite, nausea and vomiting, weight loss, constipation or diarrhoea and rectal bleeding.

Dysphagia

Difficulty in swallowing is the principal symptom of oesophageal disease. Patients can usually indicate the level of obstruction but this does not always correspond to the actual level. Determine whether the dysphagia developed suddenly or gradually over weeks or months. Enquire whether the symptom is constant or intermittent and whether the dysphagia occurs with both solids and liquids. Associated symptoms such as weight loss and

Differential diagnosis

Dysphagia

- Benign oesophageal stricture
- Carcinoma of the oesophagus
- Oesophageal motor disorders
- Systemic sclerosis
- Old age (presbyoesophagus)
- Bulbar and pseudobulbar palsy

Questions to ask

Dysphagia

- At what level does food stick?
- Has the symptom developed over weeks, months or longer?
- Is the dysphagia intermittent or progressive?
- Are both food and drink equally difficult to swallow?
- Is there a history of reflux symptoms?
- Has there been weight loss?

pain or cough with swallowing may help you construct a differential diagnosis.

The more common causes of dysphagia include oesophageal cancer, benign stricture caused by longstanding acid reflux, and motility disorders including achalasia of the cardia (where there is increased tone in the lower oesophageal sphincter and failure of oesophageal peristalsis). The history may indicate the underlying cause, although special tests such as barium swallow, oesophagoscopy and manometry are required to make a definitive diagnosis.

Dysphagia caused by a carcinoma usually progresses rapidly over 6–10 weeks and is worse for solids than liquids. Profound weight loss results from reduced food intake and the wasting effect of the cancer.

Patients with a benign 'peptic' stricture often have a long history of heartburn, a slower rate of progression and less marked weight loss. In dysmotility syndromes the dysphagia often varies in intensity and is not accompanied by profound weight loss. Solids and fluids may be equally difficult to swallow. When dysphagia is caused by disease of the swallowing centre in the brainstem (e.g. pseudobulbar palsy) or damage to the vagus nerve (e.g. bulbar palsy caused by polio), the symptom is accompanied by coughing and spluttering as food spills into the larynx and trachea.

Heartburn

Malfunction of the antireflux mechanism of the gastro-oesophageal junction allows gastric acid, pepsin and bile to reflux into the oesophagus, causing damage to the mucosa, muscle spasm and pain felt behind the sternum. Most people have experienced heartburn: the pain is a scalding or burning sensation that wells up behind the sternum and radiates towards the throat. An acid or bitter taste may develop in the mouth and reflex salivation may cause it to fill with saliva (water brash). The patient's description is often accompanied by a hand gesture that illustrates the upward radiation of the pain behind the sternum. Heartburn is rapidly relieved by antacids. Retrosternal chest pain caused by reflux or oesophageal spasm may closely mimic the pain of myocardial ischaemia.

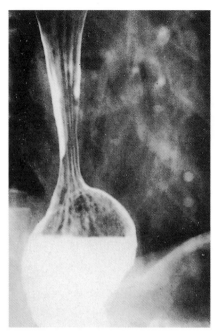

Fig. 7.18 Barium meal showing a sliding hiatus hernia with the gastro-oesophageal junction and a segment of stomach prolapsing into the chest.

A common cause of heartburn is a hiatus hernia, in which the oesophagogastric junction prolapses into the chest through the oesophageal hiatus (Fig. 7.18). The heartburn is often provoked by postures which raise intra-abdominal pressure, such as stooping, bending or lying down. The diagnosis may be suspected in overweight patients but confirmation relies on visualising the hernia, either by barium meal or endoscopy, and assessing the response to treatment with antacids.

Heartburn may result from a particular diet and lifestyle: chocolate, alcohol consumption and cigarette smoking relax the lower oesophageal sphincter, allowing reflux to occur. It is a common symptom in the later months of pregnancy. This is due both to the increase in intra-abdominal pressure and the loss of sphincter tone caused by high oestrogen levels.

Differential diagnosis

Distinguishing clinical features of reflux and myocardial ischaemic pain

	Position	Character	Associated features	Aggravating factors	Relieving factors
Reflux	Radiates towards the chest from the epigastrium	Burning, scalding	Water brash	Bending, lying down, eating	Antacids
Myocardial ischaemia	Radiates across the chest, into the jaw and down the left arm	Gripping vice-like pressure	Nausea, shortness of breath	Exercise	Ceasing exercise, nitrates

Pain on swallowing (odynophagia)

Chest pain caused by swallowing has a deep 'boring' quality which differs from heartburn, although both may occur together. The symptoms suggest deep inflammation or ulceration of the oesophageal wall or intense spasm of the oesophagus; it may be provoked by obstruction or an intrinsic motor disorder causing abnormal, intense and uncoordinated contraction ('nutcracker' oesophagus).

Loss of appetite (anorexia)

Loss of appetite is a nonspecific symptom that commonly accompanies both acute and chronic ill health; return of appetite usually heralds recovery. Prolonged or unexplained anorexia, especially when accompanied by weight loss, should alert you to a serious underlying disease. Anorexia may be a prominent feature of digestive diseases, failure of the major organs (kidneys, liver, heart and lungs) and generalised debilitating illnesses (e.g. cancer, tuberculosis).

Profound anorexia occurs in anorexia nervosa, a psychiatric disorder occurring mainly in young women. Anorexia in these patients results in marked weight loss, malnutrition and cessation of menstruation (amenorrhoea). Suspect anorexia nervosa in teenagers and young adults, otherwise healthy, who present with an eating disorder associated with depression, vomiting or purgative abuse.

Weight loss

Weight loss is an important but rather unspecific symptom of gastrointestinal and other diseases. Enquire about appetite, eating habits and average daily diet. When eating causes pain (as in gastric ulceration, mesenteric angina or pancreatitis), the inclination to eat is suppressed. Weight loss may be caused by inappropriate wastage of calories due to steatorrhoea, thyrotoxicosis or diabetes mellitus. Marked weight loss accompanies serious diseases such as chronic pancreatitis, advanced malignancy, chronic infections and failure of the major organs.

Questions to ask

Weight loss

- Is your appetite normal, increased or decreased?
- Over what time span has the weight been lost?
- Do you enjoy your meals?
- Describe your usual breakfast, lunch and supper
- Is the weight loss associated with nausea, vomiting or abdominal pain?
- Are your motions normal in colour and consistency?
- Has there been a fever?
- Do you pass excessive volumes of urine?
- Have you noticed a recent change in weather tolerance?

Dyspepsia and indigestion

Most people have experienced 'indigestion' or 'dyspepsia'. Patients and doctors use these terms rather loosely and interchangeably to describe a range of subjective abdominal symptoms. This term applies to a sensation of pain, discomfort or fullness in the epigastrium, often accompanied by belching, nausea and early satiety. Dyspepsia should focus your attention on foregut disorders.

Differential diagnosis

Dyspepsia

- Nonulcer dyspepsia
- Peptic ulcer disease
- Gastritis
- Gallstones
- Chronic pancreatitis

Risk factors

Dyspepsia

- Cigarette smoking
- Alcohol
- Aspirin
- Nonsteroidal anti-inflammatory drugs (NSAIDs)
- Corticosteroids and NSAIDs
- Oral bisphosphonates
- *Helicobacter pylori* infection

Red flag – urgent referral

Dyspepsia

- Weight loss
- Vomiting
- Haematemesis or melaena
- Dysphagia
- Anaemia

Nausea

Nausea describes the sensation experienced before vomiting, although it often occurs without vomiting. Nausea may last hours or days, usually comes in waves and is often associated with belching. It may be relieved by vomiting. The symptom may be provoked by unpleasant sights, smells and tastes or by abnormal stimulation of the inner ear labyrinths (motion sickness). Nausea may be accompanied by other complaints such as abdominal pain and diarrhoea (Fig. 7.19). It is a

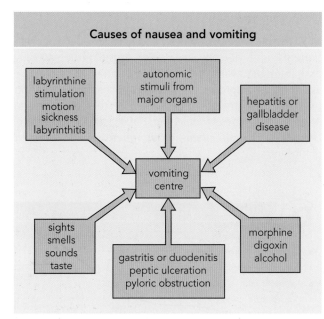

Fig. 7.19 The causes of nausea and vomiting.

Differential diagnosis

Gastrointestinal bleeding

Cause	Frequency (%)
Gastric ulcer	30
Duodenal ulcer	21
Gastritis or erosions	9
Oesophagitis or oesophageal ulcer	8
Duodenitis	4
Varices	3
Tumours	2
Mallory–Weiss tear	1
Others	22

Emergency

Assessment of patient presenting with haematemesis and melena

- Pulse rate (consider whether on beta-blockers)
- Respiratory rate
- Recumbent blood pressure
- Evidence of postural hypotension and reduced capillary filling time
- Hydration (dry tongue, sunken eyes, reduced skin turgor)
- Pallor (caused by shock and peripheral vasoconstriction or anaemia)
- Urine output
- Stigmata of liver disease (flap, jaundice, spider naevi)

Questions to ask

Vomiting

- Is the vomiting worse in the mornings?
- Does the vomiting occur in relation to meals?
- Is there associated abdominal pain?
- Is the vomit blood- or bile-stained?
- Is there recognisable food or 'coffee-grounds' in the vomit?
- What drugs are being taken?

characteristic of the prodromal phase of viral hepatitis and often accompanies biliary diseases (e.g. cholecystitis). Drugs causing gastric irritation (e.g. nonsteroidal analgesics) or those stimulating the vomiting centre (e.g. digoxin, morphine and anticancer drugs) cause nausea. Early morning nausea commonly occurs during the first trimester of pregnancy.

Vomiting and haematemesis

A wave of nausea usually heralds vomiting and the causes of nausea and vomiting are similar. Vomiting may occur in diseases of the gastrointestinal and biliary tracts, as well as in a variety of systemic and metabolic disorders. It may also be the presenting symptom of psychological disorders such as anorexia nervosa, bulimia and fear. Suspect an iatrogenic cause in patients taking digoxin or morphine and in individuals undergoing cancer treatment with cytotoxic drugs. Try to establish whether the vomit is bile-stained because this indicates patency between the stomach and duodenum. The presence of undigested food and a lack of bile suggest pyloric obstruction. Early morning nausea and vomiting are characteristic of early pregnancy and alcoholism.

Vomiting blood (haematemesis) indicates bleeding from the oesophagus, stomach or duodenum. If the bleeding is brisk the vomit may be heavily bloodstained but if bleeding is slower or vomiting delayed, gastric acid reacts with haemoglobin, turning it a dark brown or 'coffee-ground' colour. The patient's history often yields clues to the cause of haematemesis. If the bleeding is preceded by repeated bouts of retching or vomiting, consider as the cause a Mallory–Weiss tear which results from mechanical disruption of the mucosa at the gastro-oesophageal junction. Enquire about ingestion of alcohol or other gastric irritants (e.g. aspirin). If there is evidence of coincident liver disease, consider oesophageal varices to be the cause of bleeding. Weight loss may suggest bleeding from a gastric cancer, and a history of epigastric pain or heartburn suggests bleeding from a peptic ulcer or ulcerated oesophagus.

Abdominal pain

Pain is an important symptom of abdominal disease that may present in various forms, ranging from a

Diagnostic features of abdominal pain

Disorder	Localisation	Character	Aggravating factors	Relieving factors	Visceral symptoms	Major physical signs	Diagnostic test
Acute pancreatitis	Epigastric and left hypo-chondrium radiating to back	Severe, constant pain		May improve when sitting forward	Nausea, vomiting	Tachycardia, shock, tender upper abdomen with guarding. Bruising in flanks	Raised serum and urinary amylase
Acute cholecystitis/ biliary colic	Right hypo-chondrium/ epigastrium radiating to right scapula and shoulder	Initially colicky, becomes continuous. Patient writhes	Palpation over the gallbladder bed (below 10th rib in right upper quadrant)		Nausea, vomiting, may have fever and rigors	Tender right hypochondrium, positive Murphy's sign, may be jaundiced	Biliary tract ultrasound, ERCP
Renal colic (ureteric stones)	Loin pain radiating to groin, and in males the scrotum	Very intense colicky pain. Patient writhes			Nausea, vomiting, frequency	Microscopic or obvious haematuria	Abdominal radiograph (90% stones visible), ultrasound intra-venous urogram
Intestinal obstruction	Large bowel: lower abdomen Small intestine: periumbilical	Colic	Food, drink		Large bowel: constipation, vomiting occurs later Small intestine: vomiting, constipation occurs later	Abdominal distension, empty rectum	Radiograph of abdomen shows air–fluid levels in bowel
Acute appendicitis	Initially, periumbilical pain, later localises to right iliac fossa	Initially dull, later intense	Movement, hip extension	Lying still	Nausea, anorexia, vomiting	Fever, tenderness and guarding in the right iliac fossa	Laparoscopy
Perforated peptic ulcer	Sudden onset of epigastric pain. May radiate to the shoulder and extend to whole abdomen	Severe, persistent	Movement	Lying still	Nausea, vomiting	Fever, tachycardia, hypotension, shock, rigid abdomen with rebound tenderness	Chest radiograph reveals air under the diaphragm
Ruptured ectopic pregnancy	Lower abdomen	Sudden onset, severe pain	Movement	Lying still		Tachycardia, hypotension, shock. Lower abdominal tenderness may become generalised. Guarding and rebound tenderness, tender cervix	Positive pregnancy test, anaemia, ultrasound
Ruptured aortic aneurysm	Pain radiating to the back	Moderately severe			Nausea, sweating	Pulsatile tender mass, hypo-tension, shock, oliguria/aneuria	Abdominal radiograph (calcification), ultrasound angiography

Fig. 7.20 The characteristics of abdominal pain which may help in making a differential diagnosis.

dull ache to cramp, colic and peritonitis. A differential diagnosis can often be constructed from the position, character and timing, the aggravating and relieving factors and other distinctive or associated features (Fig. 7.20). When taking a history of abdominal pain, aim to distinguish between visceral, parietal and referred pain.

Visceral pain is caused by stretching or inflammation of a hollow muscular organ (gut, gallbladder, bile duct,

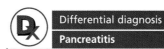

Differential diagnosis

Pancreatitis

- Idiopathic
- Toxic (alcohol, drugs)
- Common bile duct stone
- Abdominal trauma
- Mumps

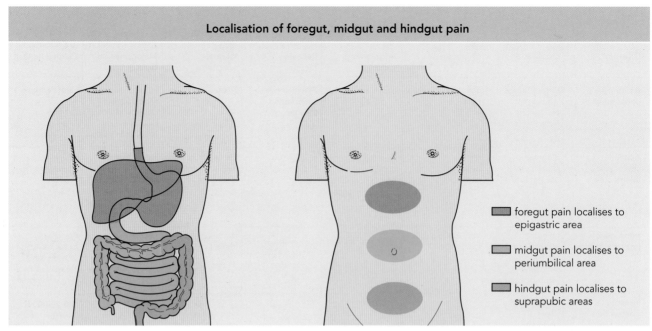

Localisation of foregut, midgut and hindgut pain

foregut pain localises to epigastric area

midgut pain localises to periumbilical area

hindgut pain localises to suprapubic areas

Fig. 7.21 Perception of visceral pain is localised to the epigastric, umbilical or suprapubic region according to the embryological origin of the diseased organ.

ureters, uterus). It is often described as a 'dull ache' or a 'gnawing' or 'cramping' sensation that is perceived near the midline, irrespective of the location of the organ. The pain can usually be localised to the epigastric, periumbilical or suprapubic areas, depending on whether the affected organ is derived from the embryological foregut, midgut or hindgut (Fig. 7.21). Pain arising from foregut is felt in the epigastrium; midgut pain is perceived around the umbilicus; pain arising from the hindgut is felt in the suprapubic area. Visceral pain may also radiate to specific sites and this helps to establish its origin (Fig. 7.22). It is commonly accompanied by nonspecific, 'visceral' symptoms (e.g. anorexia, nausea, pallor, sweating).

Colic is a characteristic manifestation of visceral pain and is caused by concerted and excessive smooth muscle contraction. It signifies obstruction of a hollow, muscular organ, such as the intestine, gallbladder, bile duct or ureter, and consists of recurring bouts of intense, cramping, visceral pain which build to a crescendo and then fade away. When the smaller organs such as the gallbladder, bile duct or ureters are acutely obstructed by a stone, the cyclical nature of colic soon gives way to a continuous visceral pain caused by the inflammatory effect of the impacted stone or secondary infection. Movement does not aggravate visceral pain, so the patient may writhe or double-up in response to it.

Unlike the visceral peritoneum, the parietal peritoneum is innervated by pain-sensitive fibres. Therefore, pain arising from the parietal peritoneum is well localised to the area immediately overlying the area of inflammation or irritation. Parietal pain is aggravated by stretching or moving the peritoneal membrane; the patient lies as still

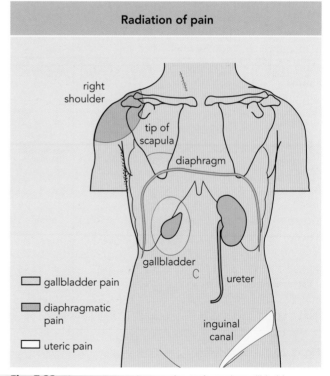

Radiation of pain

right shoulder

tip of scapula

diaphragm

gallbladder

ureter

inguinal canal

gallbladder pain

diaphragmatic pain

uteric pain

Fig. 7.22 Characteristic radiation of pain from the gallbladder, diaphragm and ureters. The pain is not always felt in the organ concerned.

as possible. Palpation over the area is extremely painful, with the overlying muscles contracting to protect the peritoneum (guarding). When the pressure of the examining hand is suddenly released, the pain is further aggravated and the patient winces. This sign is known as 'rebound tenderness'.

Questions to ask

Abdominal pain

- Describe the position, character and radiation of the pain
- Has the pain been present for hours, days, weeks, months or years?
- Is the pain constant or intermittent?
- Have you noticed specific aggravating or relieving factors?
- Is the pain affected by eating or defecation?
- Does the pain awake you from sleep?
- Is there associated nausea or vomiting?
- Has there been associated weight loss?
- Is there a history of ulcerogenic drugs?
- Has there been a change in bowel habit?

Abdominal pain may progress from a visceral sensation to a parietal pain. Acute appendicitis provides an excellent example of this transition. When this midgut structure becomes inflamed and obstructed, a dull pain localises to the periumbilical area and the patient may feel nauseous and sweaty. As the inflammation advances through the visceral covering to the parietal peritoneum, the pain appears to shift to the right iliac fossa where it localises over McBurney's point. The character of the pain also changes from dull to sharp. The area overlying the appendix is very tender and palpation causes reflex guarding and rebound tenderness.

Mesenteric angina

When the mesenteric arteries are stenosed by atherosclerosis the blood supply to the bowel may be impaired. The collateral supply to the bowel is well developed and the pain of bowel ischaemia usually becomes apparent only on eating, when the metabolic demands of digestion and absorption require an increase in the blood supply. Patients complain of a severe visceral periumbilical pain occurring soon after meals (mesenteric angina). The pain causes anorexia, which, together with damage to the bowel mucosa, results in considerable weight loss.

Wind

Most gas in the gastrointestinal tract is swallowed, with a smaller contribution arising from fermentation of cellulose in the colon. Small, imperceptible amounts of gas constantly escape from the bowel via the mouth and anus. Excessive belching (flatulence) or the passage of wind through the anus (flatus) are common symptoms that cause considerable distress. These symptoms are rather unspecific and occur in both functional and organic disorders of the gastrointestinal tract. Flatulence is usually caused by excessive air swallowing (aerophagy) and often

occurs with a hiatus hernia, peptic ulceration and chronic gallbladder disease. The symptom may be accompanied by a feeling of abdominal distension. Intestinal gas is produced by fermentation of certain foods, especially legumes, in the colon and your history should seek to identify a possible dietary cause of excessive flatus and flatulence.

CHANGE IN BOWEL HABIT

Constipation

Most people on a Western diet expect bowel actions once or twice daily. Consequently, constipation usually implies failure to produce a stool over 24 h. However, normal expectations vary between individuals and cultures; some healthy individuals evacuate every other day or even only three times a week, whereas others, particularly people on high roughage diets, expect up to three bulky bowel actions daily. Constipation is described more precisely as a disorder of bowel habit characterised by straining and the infrequent passage of small, hard stools. Constipated patients often complain that they are left dissatisfied, with a sense of incomplete evacuation (tenesmus). Patients with troublesome constipation often seek medicinal relief and a history of laxative use may be a helpful guide to the severity of the condition.

When constipation has troubled a patient for years or even decades, the cause is likely to be functional rather than obstructive and it may be attributed to diet, lifestyle or psychological make-up. Lack of exercise, inadequate fibre intake, irritable bowel syndrome and depression may all cause constipation.

When constipation presents as a recent change, and especially if it is associated with colic, suspect an organic cause such as malignancy or stricture formation. Enquire about constipating drugs (e.g. codeine-containing analgesics, aluminium-containing antacids) and about rectal bleeding, an alarm symptom that raises the suspicion of cancer. Consider hypothyroidism or electrolyte abnormalities. Anal pain caused by a fissure

Differential diagnosis

Constipation

- Low-residue diet
- Motility disorder (irritable bowel syndrome)
- Physical immobility
- Drugs (especially opiates and antidepressants)
- Depression and dementia
- Organic disease
  - colon cancer
  - diverticular stricture
  - Crohn's stricture
  - hypothyroidism
  - electrolyte imbalance

Questions to ask

Constipation

- What is the normal stool frequency?
- Do you strain at stool?
- How long have you been constipated?
- Is there associated abdominal pain, distension, nausea or vomiting?
- Are the stools large or small and pellet-shaped?
- Have you noticed intercurrent diarrhoea (spurious diarrhoea)?
- Are any constipating drugs, such as codeine or other opiates, being used?

Questions to ask

Diarrhoea

- What is the normal stool frequency?
- How many stools daily?
- How long have you had diarrhoea?
- Are you awoken from sleep to open the bowels?
- What is the colour and consistency of stools?
- Are blood and mucus present?
- Any travel abroad or contact with diarrhoea?
- Is there associated nausea, vomiting, weight loss or pain?
- Any purgative abuse?
- Any antibiotics?

or a thrombosed pile may cause profound constipation because of the patient's fear of pain at stool.

Constipation caused by chronic partial obstruction may be punctuated by periods of loose or watery stool. This 'spurious diarrhoea' occurs in elderly patients with faecal impaction and also when colon cancer causes a partial obstruction. The proximal bowel dilates and fills with liquid, which then seeps around the obstruction, presenting as liquid diarrhoea.

Differential diagnosis

Steatorrhoea

- Chronic pancreatitis
- Gluten enteropathy
- Small bowel bacterial overgrowth
- Blind loops
- Short bowel syndrome

Diarrhoea

The usual stool weight is 200–300 g/day. Diarrhoea implies increased stool volume and frequency and a change in consistency from formed to semiformed, semiliquid or liquid. Always enquire about the presence of blood and mucus and establish whether or not there is accompanying pain or colic. There is a wide differential diagnosis and the history may give some leads. Functional diarrhoea caused by anxiety, stress or the irritable bowel syndrome does not wake the patient from sleep, nor is it associated with rectal bleeding. Recent travel abroad, eating out or an outbreak among people living in close proximity suggests an infective cause.

Enquire about colour; in fat malabsorption, the stool is pale, malodorous, poorly formed and difficult to flush. Blood and mucus mixed in the stool suggest an infective colitis or inflammatory bowel disease. When a cause is not readily apparent, consider laxative abuse and recent broad-spectrum antibiotic treatment, both of which may precipitate diarrhoea. Thyrotoxicosis may present with increased stool frequency and weight loss.

Rectal bleeding

Rectal bleeding is a symptom common to several disorders (Fig. 7.23) and the history is not of much diagnostic value. Bright-red rectal bleeding usually arises from the sigmoid colon or rectum and more proximal colonic bleeding is often a darker red or maroon colour. The blood usually coats the stool, although in haemorrhoidal bleeding the blood may be most noticeable on the toilet paper. Colon cancer and polyps often present with intermittent rectal bleeding, whereas patients with inflammatory bowel disease pass blood, often mixed with mucus, with each stool. Torrential haemorrhage may occur from diverticular disease and marked bleeding may occur in mesenteric vascular disease when the ischaemic colonic mucosa ulcerates and bleeds. Microscopic blood loss (occult

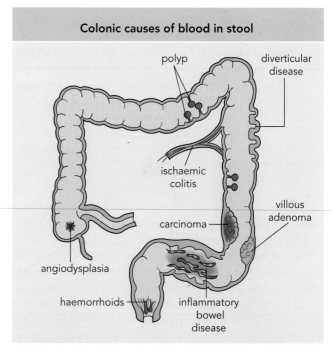

Colonic causes of blood in stool

Fig. 7.23 Potential causes of bright-red or maroon-coloured rectal bleeding.

bleeding) usually presents with symptoms of anaemia. Always consider a diagnosis of gastric, caecal or colon cancer in older patients with unexplained iron deficiency anaemia. Haemorrhoids are common, so always consider other causes of bleeding in patients aged 45 and over.

Questions to ask

Gastrointestinal bleeding

- Is there a past history of abdominal pain or other gastrointestinal symptoms?
- Is there a history of chronic alcoholism or excessive intake?
- Is there a past history of haematemesis, melaena or anaemia?
- Are any nonsteroidals, steroids or proprietary medicines being taken?
- Was the bleeding preceded by intense retching?
- Has there been ingestion of iron or bismuth that may stain the stools?

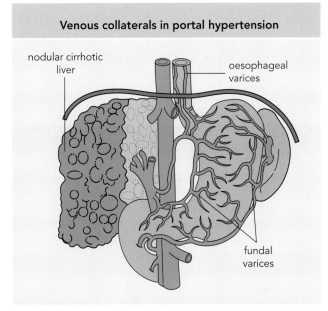

Venous collaterals in portal hypertension

nodular cirrhotic liver

oesophageal varices

fundal varices

Fig. 7.24 Cirrhosis of the liver. When portal pressure rises, collateral veins open and blood bypasses the liver through dilated fundal and oesophageal varices that eventually drain into the azygos vein and superior vena cava.

The passage of sticky, black stools with the colour and consistency of tar (melaena) usually indicates bleeding from the oesophagus, stomach or duodenum. The characteristic appearance and smell is attributed to the denaturing effect of gastric acid and enzymes on blood. Treatment with iron and certain drugs (e.g. bismuth-containing preparations) also blackens the stool and this cause must be distinguished from melaena.

LIVER DISEASE

The background symptoms of liver disease may reflect damage to the parenchymal liver cells (hepatocellular disease) or obstruction of the biliary tree (intrahepatic or extrahepatic cholestasis). Patients may also complain of symptoms related to the development of portal hypertension. Liver cell damage and obstruction of the bile duct both have numerous clinical consequences, the most striking of which are jaundice, pale stools and darkening of the urine. When sufficient hepatocyte damage occurs, the patient becomes jaundiced because bilirubin excretion fails and the pigment deposits in tissues. When hepatocytes are damaged or dead, enzymes leak into the blood, where they can be measured. The high plasma activity of these enzymes is the basis of biochemical tests for liver damage.

In cirrhosis, liver architecture is severely disturbed, with regenerating nodules distorting and compressing the sinusoids and intrahepatic portal venous radicals. In addition, collagen is deposited between the sinusoidal lining cells and the hepatocytes, causing gradual obliteration of the space of Disse. Blood flow through the liver is partially obstructed and pressure rises in the portal vein. Resistance to blood flow through the liver encourages

diversion of portal blood through collaterals (Fig. 7.24). A collateral circulation is established through the veins of the oesophagus. At endoscopy these abnormally dilated oesophageal veins are seen as tortuous, dilated veins (varices). Oesophageal varices are prone to rupture and may cause torrential haemorrhage.

Gut bacteria metabolise unabsorbed protein, releasing potentially neurotoxic breakdown products into the portal blood. The liver normally detoxifies these gut-derived products but in patients with portal hypertension, portal blood bypasses the liver (portosystemic shunting), and the brain is exposed to gut-derived products which depress brain function, causing a characteristic neurological syndrome known as hepatic encephalopathy.

A further clinical consequence of portal hypertension is fluid retention in the abdominal cavity (ascites). The combination of high portal pressure and low serum albumin allows fluid to escape and to accumulate in the abdominal cavity.

Risk factors

Factors predisposing to hepatitis B

- Intravenous drug abuse
- Exposure to contaminated blood or blood products
- Reuse of hypodermic needles, ritual scarification
- Unprotected sex
- Needle-stick injury from infected individual
- Vertical transmission from mother to newborn
- Horizontal transmission between children at play, toothbrushes, razors

Liver cell damage

The earliest symptoms of liver damage are not very specific and include malaise, fatigue, anorexia and nausea. Viral hepatitis is preceded by prodromes such as fatigue, nausea and a profound distaste for alcohol and cigarettes. Before the onset of jaundice the patient may notice darkening of the urine and lightening of stool colour. This is caused by failure of the liver cells to excrete conjugated bilirubin.

Enquire about the principal causes of liver damage. Calculate the number of units (or grams) of alcohol consumed in a week as this provides a good guide to the risk of liver damage (see Ch. 1). Ask about any foreign travel, intravenous drug abuse or exposure to blood products, and establish the patient's sexual orientation. Enquire about drugs that may cause liver damage and ask about a family history of liver disease.

The principal complications of chronic liver cell damage are jaundice, cirrhosis and portal hypertension. The patient may notice increasing girth and weight gain. This is caused by the accumulation of ascites. If encephalopathy occurs, the sleep pattern may be reversed and the patient may undergo a change in personality.

BILIARY OBSTRUCTION

The principal symptom is itching (pruritus) and this may occur long before the patient becomes jaundiced. The cause of pruritus is unknown, although the deposition of bile acids in the skin has been suggested. As with viral hepatitis, lightening of the stools and darkening of the urine often precedes jaundice. The history may not help distinguish between the different causes of intrahepatic and extrahepatic obstruction. Severe epigastric and right hypochondrial pain accompanied by fever and jaundice suggests impaction of a gallstone in the common bile

Questions to ask

Jaundice

- Have you travelled to areas where hepatitis A is endemic?
- Is there a history of alcohol or intravenous drug abuse?
- Have you ever had a blood transfusion?
- Have you had contact with jaundiced patients?
- Have you experienced skin itching?
- What medication has been used recently (including nonprescription drugs)?
- Have you had occupational contact with hepatotoxins?
- Is there pain and weight loss?
- What colour are the stools and urine?
- Is there a family history of liver disease?

duct, whereas 'painless' jaundice suggests either a more chronic obstruction of the common bile duct (e.g. cancer of either the bile duct or head of the pancreas) or damage to the intrahepatic biliary tree (e.g. primary biliary cirrhosis, sclerosing cholangitis, drugs). Impaired bile flow into the duodenum causes fat malabsorption and steatorrhoea; marked weight loss may occur.

PANCREATIC DISEASE

Acute pancreatitis presents with the onset of upper abdominal pain that is most prominent in the epigastrium and left upper quadrant. The pain may radiate through to the back, with its intensity varying from mild to severe. It is persistent and often lasts a few days before abating. The pain is commonly accompanied by nausea and vomiting; some relief may be obtained by sitting forward. Ask about alcohol intake and drugs (e.g. azathioprine, furosemide, corticoids) and consider underlying gallstones, which may precipitate acute pancreatitis.

Recurrent attacks of acute pancreatitis may result in chronic pancreatitis. This is often characterised by persistent, severe upper abdominal pain that may radiate circumferentially to the back. Progressive loss of exocrine function eventually leads to steatorrhoea and weight loss. Endocrine failure with diabetes is a late manifestation. Occasionally, chronic pancreatitis develops insidiously and presents with weight loss and steatorrhoea. Progressive fibrosis may occlude the lower bile duct causing jaundice.

KIDNEY AND BLADDER DISEASE

The principal symptoms of diseases affecting the kidneys, ureters and bladder are pain and an alteration in the volume and frequency of bladder emptying.

Frequency and urgency

Frequency refers to the desire to pass urine more often than normal, although there is not necessarily an increase in the volume of voided urine. Urgency may accompany

Differential diagnosis

Jaundice

Prehepatic or unconjugated hyperbilirubinaemia
- Haemolytic anaemias
- Gilbert's syndrome

Hepatocellular disease
- Viral hepatitis (types A, B, C, D and E)
- Alcoholic hepatitis
- Autoimmune hepatitis (lupoid)
- Drug hepatitis (halothane, paracetamol)
- Decompensated cirrhosis

Intrahepatic cholestasis
- Drugs (phenothiazines)
- Primary biliary cirrhosis
- Primary sclerosing cholangitis

Extrahepatic cholestasis
- Bile duct stricture (benign and malignant)
- Common duct stone
- Cancer of the head of the pancreas

frequency (i.e. a strong urge to urinate even though only small amounts of urine are present in the bladder).

Nocturia

It is unusual to be woken from sleep to pass urine (nocturia) but this may occur in patients with daytime frequency or individuals producing excessive quantities of urine (polyuria). Incomplete bladder voiding caused by prostatism often presents with nocturia.

Incontinence

Incontinence is an involuntary leakage of urine. If the symptom is provoked by increased intra-abdominal pressure (coughing, sneezing or laughing), it is referred to as 'stress incontinence'.

Diseases causing excessive bladder filling (e.g. bladder outlet obstruction or damage to the nervous supply of the bladder) may cause 'overflow incontinence' which reflects spill-over from an overfilled, hypotonic bladder.

Symptoms and signs
Some renal symptoms and their causes

Frequency
- Irritable bladder
  - infection, inflammation, chemical irritation
- Reduced compliance
  - fibrosis, tumour infiltration
- Bladder outlet obstruction
  - in prostatism, detrusor failure may limit the volume voided

Polyuria
- Ingestion of large volumes of water, beverages or alcohol
- Chronic renal failure (loss of concentrating power)
- Diabetes mellitus (osmotic effect of glucose in urine)
- Diabetes insipidus (caused by a lack of ADH or tubules insensitive to circulating ADH)
- Diuretic treatment

Dysuria
- Bacterial infection of the bladder (cystitis)
- Inflammation of the urethra (urethritis)
- Infection or inflammation of the prostate (prostatitis)

Incontinence
- Sphincter damage or weakness after childbirth
- Sphincter weakness in old age
- Prostate cancer
- Benign prostatic hypertrophy
- Spinal cord disease, paraplegia

Oliguria or anuria
- Hypovolaemia (dehydration or shock)
- Acute renal failure caused by acute glomerulonephritis
- Bilateral ureteric obstruction (retroperitoneal fibrosis)
- Detrusor muscle failure (bladder outlet obstruction or neurological disease)

Hesitancy

Hesitancy is a delay between attempting to initiate urination and the actual flow of urine. It is a characteristic sign of bladder outlet obstruction (e.g. as a result of prostatic hypertrophy).

Oliguria and anuria

Patients may complain of passing only small volumes of urine. The term oliguria is used if less than 500 ml of urine is passed over 24 h. The subjective assessment of urine volume is often inaccurate and requires confirmation by 24 h urine collection and measurement. Apparent oliguria may occur in patients with bladder muscle (detrusor) failure. Consequently, it may be necessary to pass a catheter to confirm true oliguria.

Pain

Pain may originate in the kidneys, ureter, bladder or urethra. Infection of the kidneys (pyelonephritis) causes pain and tenderness in the renal angles, usually associated with fever, anorexia and nausea. Obstruction of the ureters by stones, sloughed papillae or blood may cause intense pain in the renal angle. This pain may radiate towards the groins and, in men, into the testes. Renal 'colic' caused by stones in the ureters is extremely painful, often causing the patient to double-up or roll around in a futile attempt to find relief. Bladder pain may occur in severe cystitis. The pain is of moderate severity, localised to the suprapubic region and associated with urgency and frequency.

Dysuria

Dysuria describes a stinging or burning sensation that occurs when passing urine. It is often accompanied by frequency and urgency. The most common cause of dysuria is cystitis.

Haematuria

Blood in urine may be obvious, associated with a cloudy colour or only apparent on chemical testing (microscopic haematuria). Whether the passage of blood is painful or painless may be of diagnostic assistance.

Differential diagnosis
Haematuria

Painful
- Kidney stones
- Urinary tract infection
- Papillary necrosis

Painless
- Infection
- Cancer of the urinary tract
- Acute glomerulonephritis
- Contamination during menstruation

Examination of the abdomen

Before beginning your examination ask the patient to lie flat, with the head resting comfortably on a pillow, arms lying loosely on either side. According to the demands of the particular procedure you are performing, try to expose the patient as little as possible. The 'classical' arrangement is shown in Figure 7.25 but until you gain experience it will help to have the visual clues provided by the landmarks of the entire abdomen and lower chest; subsequent illustrations reflect this.

The abdominal examination depends largely on the palpation and percussion of organs that normally lie out of reach of the examining hands. As with all other examinations, it is important to become completely familiar with the clinical anatomy of the abdomen.

The costal margin demarcates the superficial boundary between the chest and abdomen, although the domes of the diaphragm rise behind the ribs to accommodate the liver and spleen, so a full abdominal examination also includes examination of the lower half of the chest (Fig. 7.26). Familiarise yourself with the bony landmarks of the abdomen (Fig. 7.27). Feel the xiphisternum at the lower end of the sternum, then trace the outline of the costal margin formed by the seventh costal cartilage at the xiphisternum to the tip of the 12th rib. Note a distinct step in the costal margin which provides a useful landmark because it coincides with the tip of the 10th rib. Turn your attention to the bony margins of the lower abdomen. The iliac crest has a distinct anterior prominence, the anterior superior iliac spine, from which the inguinal ligament runs downward and medially to attach to a lateral prominence on the pubic bone (the pubic tubercle).

For descriptive purposes the anterior abdominal wall may be divided into four quadrants (Fig. 7.28). Trace the imaginary lines demarcating the left and right upper and lower quadrants. A vertical line extends from the xiphisternum to the pubic symphysis in the midline and a horizontal line is drawn through the umbilicus. The abdomen may also be divided into nine segments

resembling a 'noughts and crosses' matrix (Fig. 7.29). These segments are useful landmarks for ensuring a complete and systematic examination of the abdomen. A vertical line is dropped from the midclavicular points on either side and these are crossed by a horizontal line drawn in the subcostal plane and by a line joining the anterior superior iliac spines.

When locating or describing the position of the abdominal organs it is useful to recognise the anterior anatomical planes and their correlation with vertebral levels (Fig. 7.30). The xiphisternum corresponds to the

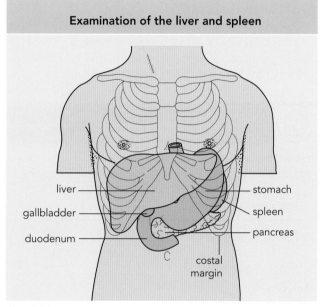

Examination of the liver and spleen

liver — stomach
gallbladder — spleen
duodenum — pancreas
costal margin

Fig. 7.26 The liver and spleen lie protected under the ribs and so the lower one-half of the chest must be exposed in order to examine them.

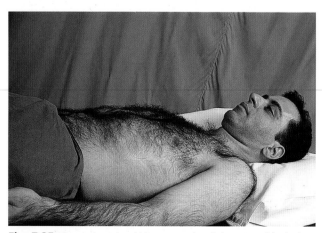

Fig. 7.25 The patient should be exposed as little as possible during your examination.

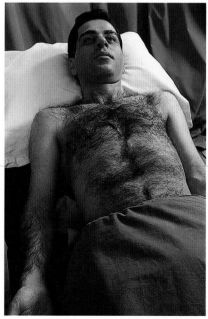

Fig. 7.27 The bony landmarks of the anterior abdominal wall.

level of T9. The transpyloric plane lies midway between the suprasternal notch and the pubis, approximately a hand's breadth below the xiphoid cartilage. This plane corresponds to the vertebral level of L1 and passes through the pylorus, the long axis of the pancreas, the duodenojejunal flexure and the hila of the kidneys. The subcostal plane coincides with the level of L3 and is defined by a line joining the lowest point of the thoracic cage on either side. A line joining the highest points of the iliac crest corresponds to the level of L4.

INSPECTION OF THE ABDOMEN

Contours

Expose the patient to the groins and observe the symmetry of the abdomen from the foot of the bed. The normal abdomen is concave and symmetrical and moves gently with respiration. Next, move to the patient's right and view the abdomen tangentially. From this position it is easier to pick out the subtle changes of contour and shadow. In thin individuals you may notice the pulsation of the abdominal aorta in the midline above the umbilicus. Ask the patient to raise the head a few inches off the pillow. This tenses the rectus abdominis, which becomes firm and prominent on either side of the midline.

Abnormal contours and distension of the abdomen may be caused by a number of mechanisms (Fig. 7.31). Establish whether the swelling is generalised or localised. Fluid and gaseous distension is generalised and symmetrical (Fig. 7.32). Fluid gravitates towards the flanks causing the loins to bulge, and the umbilicus, which is normally inverted, may become everted when massive ascites distends the abdomen beyond its normal compliance. In thin individuals, the contour of an enlarged liver may be visible below the right costal margin. A midline fullness in the upper abdomen may indicate disease of the stomach (e.g. carcinoma), pancreas (e.g. pancreatic cysts) or an abdominal aortic aneurysm.

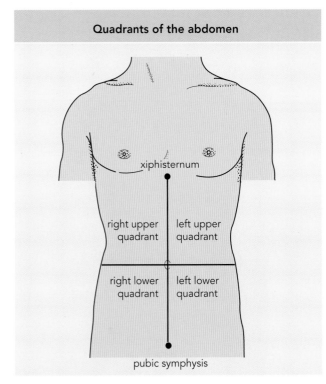

Fig. 7.28 The quadrants of the anterior abdominal wall.

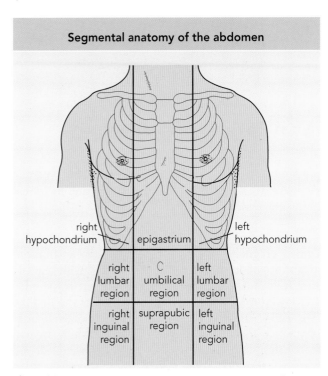

Fig. 7.29 The nine segments of the anterior abdominal wall.

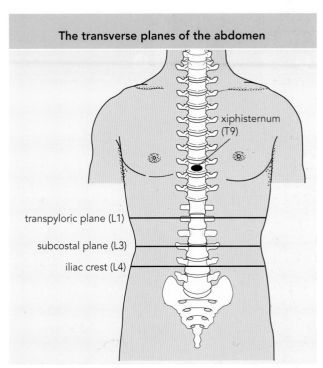

Fig. 7.30 The transverse planes and their equivalent vertebral levels.

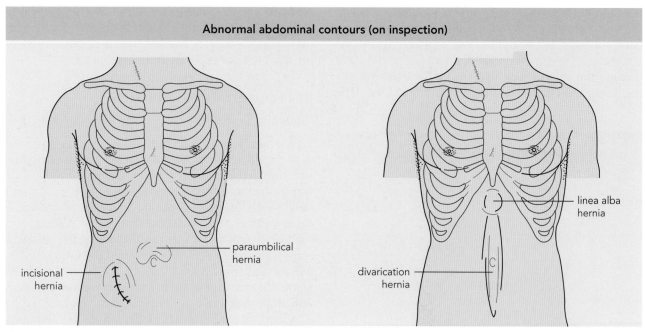

Abnormal abdominal contours (on inspection)

incisional hernia

paraumbilical hernia

linea alba hernia

divarication hernia

Fig. 7.31 Some abnormal abdominal contours.

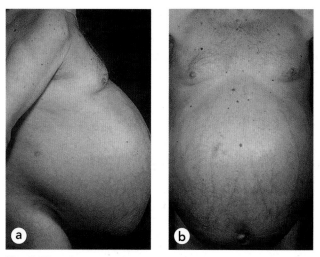

Fig. 7.32 The characteristic appearance of gross ascites: (a) lateral, (b) anterior view.

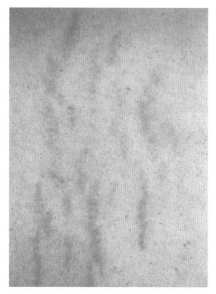

Fig. 7.33 Striae gravidarum appear after childbirth.

Suprapubic fullness may reflect an enlarged uterus (pregnancy or fibroids), ovaries (cysts or carcinoma) or a full bladder. The periodic rippling movement of bowel peristalsis may be observed in intestinal obstruction, especially in thin individuals. This is referred to as a visible peristalsis.

Abnormal bulges may appear when intra-abdominal pressure is raised and may be revealed by tensing the abdominal muscles. If the muscles of the recti are abnormally separated on either side of the midline (divarication of the recti), tensing the abdominal muscles causes a longitudinal bulge to appear in the midline (Fig. 7.31). The appearance of a more localised bulge just above or below the umbilicus occurs with a paraumbilical hernia (Fig. 7.31). Direct and indirect inguinal herniae may also become prominent when intra-abdominal

pressure is raised by coughing. Surgical scars are potential points of weakness in the abdominal wall and incisional herniae may develop under the scar.

Skin

During pregnancy the abdominal wall skin is stretched and after childbirth many women are left with tell-tale stretch lines (striae gravidarum) that arc across the mid- and lower abdominal wall on either side of the midline (Fig. 7.33). Stretch marks similar to those occurring after pregnancy may occur in patients successfully treated for ascites. In Cushing's syndrome, excessive adrenal corticoid secretion thins the skin and purplish striae appear on the abdominal wall even in the absence of a

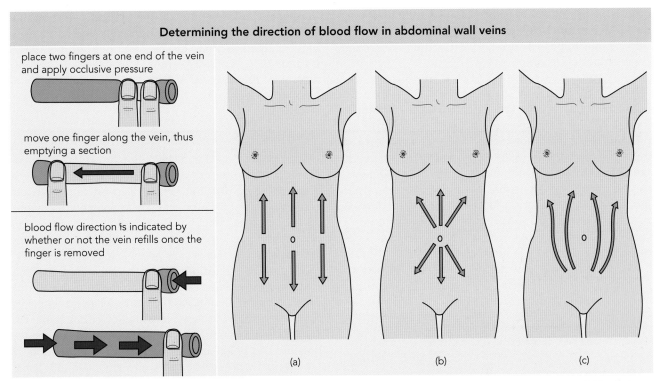

Determining the direction of blood flow in abdominal wall veins

place two fingers at one end of the vein and apply occlusive pressure

move one finger along the vein, thus emptying a section

blood flow direction is indicated by whether or not the vein refills once the finger is removed

(a)

(b)

(c)

Fig. 7.34 Determining the direction of blood flow in abdominal veins. (a) Normal blood flow pattern and those characteristic of (b) portal hypertension and (c) obstruction of the inferior vena cava.

pregnancy. In acute haemorrhagic pancreatitis, there may be a bluish discoloration of either the flanks (Grey Turner's sign) or the periumbilical area (Cullen's sign), which results from seepage of bloodstained ascitic fluid along the fascial planes and into the subcutaneous tissue. A similar appearance may occur after rupture of an ectopic pregnancy.

Look for veins coursing over the abdominal wall: they are rarely prominent in health. If veins are visible, map the direction of flow by emptying the vein with the index finger of one hand while attempting to prevent refilling by applying occlusive pressure more proximally over the vein. The direction of flow helps distinguish normal from abnormal flow patterns (Fig. 7.34). In portal hypertension and inferior vena caval obstruction, the venous return to the liver or vena cava is redirected through abdominal wall collaterals that provide an alternative route to the right atrium. These veins dilate and may be seen coursing across the abdominal wall. It is possible to distinguish collaterals caused by portal hypertension from those caused by inferior vena caval obstruction by mapping the direction of flow in these vessels.

Look for surgical scars, which should have a fleshy red or pink colouring in the first year after an operation, becoming white as the scar tissue matures. Common locations of surgical scars are shown in Figure 7.35.

PALPATION OF THE ABDOMEN

Although the intra-abdominal organs are normally impalpable, in diseased states palpation and percussion

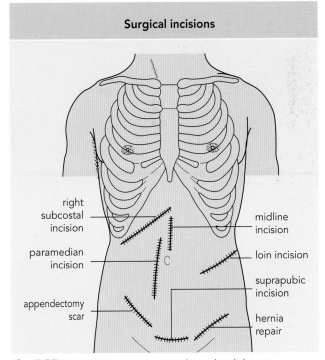

Surgical incisions

right subcostal incision

paramedian incision

appendectomy scar

midline incision

loin incision

suprapubic incision

hernia repair

Fig. 7.35 Surgical scars seen commonly on the abdomen.

provide substantial clinical information. These procedures are difficult to perform if the patient is not relaxed. If the abdominal wall muscles are tense, ask the patient to bend the knees and flex the hips (Fig. 7.36). This helps to relax the abdomen. Always warm your hands before palpating the abdomen and use the fingertip and palmar aspects of the fingers; a single-handed technique may be used but you may prefer to use both hands, the upper hand applying pressure, while the lower hand concentrates on feeling (Fig. 7.37).

Light palpation

Before laying a hand on the abdomen ask the patient to localise any areas of pain or tenderness. If these are present, begin the examination in the segment furthest from the discomfort. Start light palpation by gently pressing your fingers into each of the nine segments, sustaining the light pressure for a few seconds while gently exploring each area with the fingertips. Tenderness may be reflected by grimacing, so with every move of your hand briefly look to see the patient's facial response.

Gentle palpation will detect tenderness caused by inflammation of the parietal peritoneum. In peritonitis, the patient flinches on even the lightest palpation and there is reflex rigidity, guarding and rebound tenderness. Light palpation may localise an area of peritoneal inflammation, thereby helping to establish a differential diagnosis. It is unusual to feel the abdominal organs or large masses on light palpation unless they are grossly enlarged.

Deep palpation

Once you have used light palpation to explore for areas of tenderness and muscle tension, the sequence is repeated using firm but gentle deep pressure with the palmar surface of the fingers. Deep palpation is helpful for palpating abdominal masses, and healthy individuals often report pain on deep pressure of the abdomen. If the patient is relaxed it is usually possible to press deeply into the abdomen. While doing so try to imagine the anatomy underlying your hand (Fig. 7.38). In thin individuals, the descending and sigmoid colon may be felt as an elongated tubular structure in the left loin and lower quadrant. The sigmoid is mobile and can readily be rolled under the fingers. The colon can usually be distinguished from other structures because of its firm stool content. It has a putty-like consistency and can be indented with the fingertips. The 'mass' also becomes less obvious after the passage of stool. In thin individuals, the abdominal aorta may be felt as a discrete pulsatile structure in the midline, above the umbilicus. The rectus muscles may be mistaken for an abnormal fullness or the edge of a mass. Tensing the abdominal muscles causes the rectus to become more prominent, whereas intra-abdominal masses are less easy to feel.

Abdominal masses and enlargement of the liver, spleen and kidneys may also be felt by deep palpation. Any abnormal fullness, firmness or discrete mass should be localised by careful palpation of shape, mobility, consistency and movement with respiration. Localisation helps determine which organ may be involved. Determine whether there is any deep tenderness, suggesting stretching of the capsule of either the liver or kidney, or early peritoneal inflammation or infiltration. A large

Palpation of the abdomen

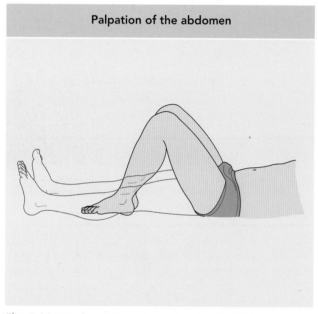

Fig. 7.36 Palpation of the abdomen may be aided if the patient is asked to flex the hips. This helps to relax the anterior abdominal wall.

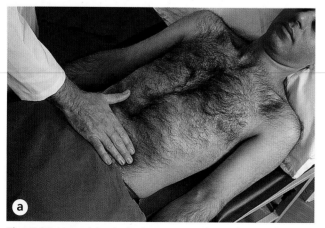

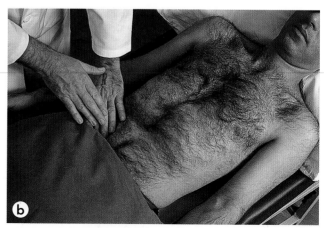

Fig. 7.37 Light abdominal palpation is performed using one (a) or both hands (b).

Structures that may be felt on deep palpation

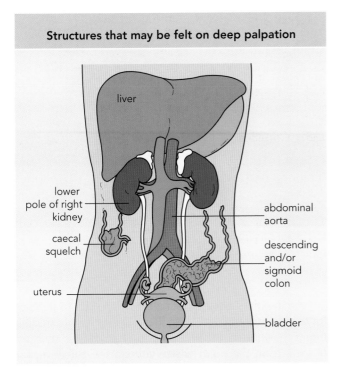

Fig. 7.38 On deep palpation of the abdomen, these structures may be felt.

pulsatile structure in the midline above the umbilicus indicates an aortic aneurysm or a transmitted impulse to a mass overlying the aorta. These can usually be distinguished using the index finger of either hand to sense whether the movement is pulsatile or transmitted (Fig. 7.39).

PALPATION OF THE ORGANS

The solid organs (liver, pancreas, kidneys and spleen) are normally out of reach of the examining hand. The stomach, small intestine and colon are soft, pliable and impalpable. In chronic fibrosing diseases of the liver (e.g. micronodular cirrhosis) or kidneys (e.g. chronic glomerulonephritis), these organs shrink even further from reach. However, they may become palpable when enlarged.

EXAMINING THE LIVER

Palpating the liver

Examine the liver with the surface anatomy in mind. Visualise its upper margin as a line passing just below each nipple on either side and imagine the lower margin spanning a line from the tip of the 10th rib on the right to a point just below the left nipple (Fig. 7.40). The upper surface of the organ is tightly apposed to the undersurface of the diaphragm and examination takes advantage of the movement of the liver with respiration. The initial aim of the examination is to define the outline of the lower edge of the right lobe, which is normally tucked along the inner surface of the right costal margin. The edge of the

Distinction between aortic pulsation and movement of an overlying structure

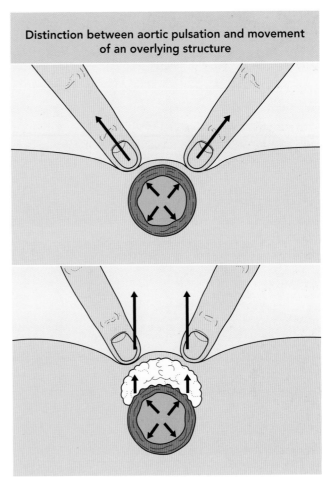

Fig. 7.39 Palpating the aorta. The direction of the pulsation indicates whether it arises directly from the aorta (above) or is transmitted by a mass overlying the tissues (below).

The surface anatomy of the liver

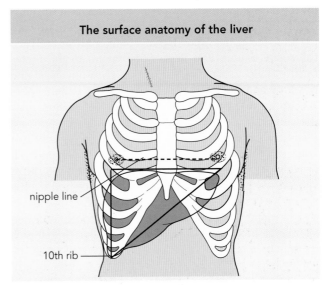

Fig. 7.40 The surface anatomy of the liver.

smaller left lobe nestles under the lower left rib cage and is often impalpable even when the organ is generally enlarged.

Examine from the patient's right and use either the fingertips or the radial side of the index finger to explore

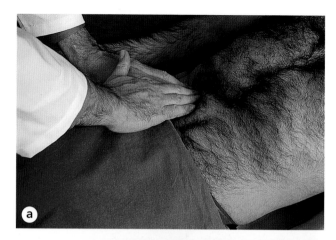

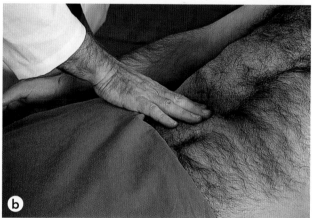

Fig. 7.41 Liver palpation. A two-handed (a) and single-handed (b) technique using the radial surface of the index finger(s) to feel for the lower liver edge as it descends during inspiration.

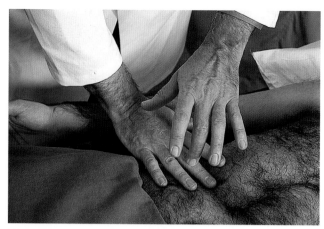

Fig. 7.42 Positioning of the hand when percussing for the lower border of the liver.

for the liver edge under the costal margin. Point the ends of the index, middle and ring fingers in an upward position, facing the liver edge, at a point midway between the costal margin and iliac crests, lateral to the rectus muscle (Fig. 7.41). Press the fingertips inwards and upwards and hold this position while the patient takes a deep inspiration. Near the height of inspiration relax the inward pressure slightly but maintain upward pressure. As the fingers drift upwards feel for the liver edge slipping under them as the organ descends. If no edge is felt, repeat the manoeuvre in a stepwise fashion, each time moving the starting position a little closer to the costal margin. If the liver is impalpable at this point, you should repeat the procedure more laterally in line with the anterior axillary line. In patients of thin or medium build a normal liver edge may be palpable just below the right costal margin at the height of inspiration. Repeat the palpation in the midline and below the left costal margin where the lower edge of the middle and left lobes should not be palpable. A single-handed technique may also be used (Fig. 7.41). The radial surface of the index finger is positioned below and parallel to the costal margin and this surface is used to explore for the lower liver edge as it descends during inspiration.

At this point in the examination it is useful to percuss for the lower liver edge. With the long axis of your middle finger positioned parallel to the right costal margin, percuss from the point where you started palpating for the liver (Fig. 7.42). This point normally overlies bowel and should sound resonant. Repeat the percussion in a stepwise manner, each time moving the finger closer to the costal margin until the note becomes duller. This should coincide with the costal margin. Ask the patient to inspire deeply; the dullness should move down as the liver descends.

Next, find the position of the upper margin of the liver so that you can assess the liver span. The upper margin cannot be palpated because it lies high in the dome of the diaphragm, but it can be located by noting the change in percussion note from the resonance of the lungs to the dullness of the liver. The upper margin of the liver usually lies deep to the sixth intercostal space. Percuss the third space and then percuss each succeeding interspace until you detect the transition from resonance to dullness (Fig. 7.43). On deep inspiration the percussion interface should descend by either one or two interspaces as the lungs expand and the liver descends. Liver size is proportional to body size. Measure the liver span in the midclavicular line; in women this should measure 8–10 cm and in men, 10–12 cm.

Downward displacement of the liver In patients who have hyperinflated lungs (e.g. emphysema), the diaphragm is flattened and the liver is pushed down so that the edge may be easily palpable below the costal margin (Fig. 7.44). Percussion reveals that the upper border of the liver is depressed and that the liver span is within normal limits.

Abnormal liver shape The right lobe of the liver may be abnormally shaped, with an elongated tongue-like projection pointing towards the right iliac crest (Fig. 7.45). This anatomical variant, known as a Riedel's lobe, is more common in women and feels like a mobile mass on the right side of the abdomen arising from under the

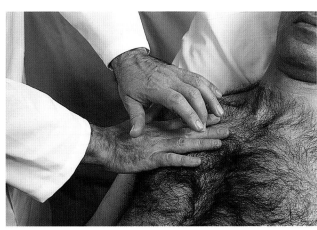

Fig. 7.43 Percussion of the upper border of the liver.

Liver pushed down by hyperinflation

hyperinflated
lungs

costal
margin

Fig. 7.44 When the lung fields are markedly hyperinflated, the liver is pushed down and the lower border may be readily palpable, although the span is normal.

Riedel's lobe

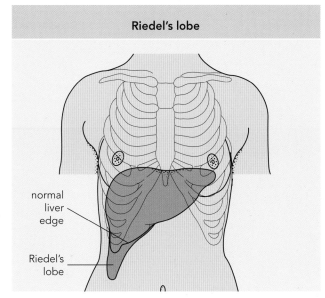

normal
liver
edge

Riedel's
lobe

Fig. 7.45 A Riedel's lobe is a normal variant of shape. The elongated 'tongue' is palpable and must be distinguished from a pathological cancer.

Dx Differential diagnosis

Hepatomegaly

- Macronodular cirrhosis
- Neoplastic disease (primary and secondary cancer, myeloproliferative disorders)
- Infections (viral hepatitis, tuberculosis, hydatid disease)
- Infiltrations (iron, fat, amyloid, Gaucher's disease)

---

costal margin and moving with respiration. A Riedel's lobe is commonly mistaken for an enlarged right kidney and if in doubt this can be resolved by ultrasound scanning.

Enlargement of the liver Liver enlargement is usually described as mild, moderate or massive (Fig. 7.46). If the liver is enlarged, trace the shape of the liver edge and decide whether it is smooth or irregular, whether the consistency is soft, firm or hard and whether or not the organ is tender. The presence of a palpable spleen suggests cirrhosis with portal hypertension or infiltrating diseases of the reticuloendothelial and haemopoietic systems.

Small livers The lower margin of the liver may not be palpable because of fibrosis or atrophy of the organ. This may be difficult to detect clinically but should be suspected

if the liver edge is not palpable and if, on percussion, the dullness of the lower liver margin is detected well above the costal margin (Fig. 7.47). Atrophy of the liver may be the result either of severe acute liver damage, perhaps caused by fulminant viral hepatitis or hepatotoxic poisons, or of chronic disease causing fibrosis and micronodular cirrhosis (e.g. alcoholic cirrhosis).

General signs of liver disease

The liver has considerable functional reserve but as this is exhausted the patient develops characteristic signs of liver failure. Look for jaundice in the sclerae, which are normally a brilliant white colour. Mild jaundice may be difficult to discern in artificial light and in dark-skinned patients the sclerae may be slightly pigmented. With deepening jaundice the skin becomes yellow, and in chronic, severe obstructive jaundice the skin may appear almost green in colour.

In patients with chronic liver disease, localised vascular dilatation results in the appearance of vascular spiders (spider naevi) (see Fig. 3.11). These consist of a central

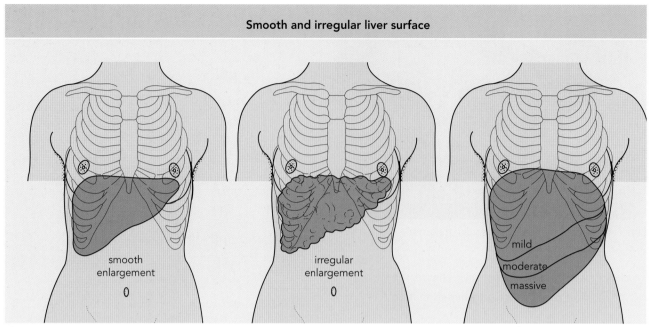

Smooth and irregular liver surface

smooth
enlargement

irregular
enlargement

mild
moderate
massive

Fig. 7.46 Liver enlargement. Enlargement of the liver can be smooth (e.g. fatty liver) or irregular (e.g. macronodular cirrhosis, tumour infiltration).

Symptoms and signs

Signs of liver disease

General examination
- Nutrition status
- Pallor (blood loss)
- Jaundice
- Breath fetor of liver failure
- Xanthelasmata (chronic cholestasis)
- Parotid swelling (alcohol abuse)
- Bruising (clotting diathesis)
- Spider naevi
- Female distribution of body hair

Mental state
- Wernicke's or Korsakoff's psychosis
- Flapping tremor of hepatic encephalopathy
- Inability to copy a five-pointed star

Hands
- Leuconychia (hypoproteinaemia)
- Liver flap
- Palmar erythema
- Dupuytren's contractures
- Mild finger clubbing

Chest
- Gynaecomastia
- Right-sided pleural effusion

Abdomen
- Dilated veins
- Liver or spleen enlargement
- Ascites
- Testicular atrophy

Percussion of shrunken liver

resonance well
above costal
margin

Fig. 7.47 Atrophy of the liver may be detected by percussing the lower border. The area of resonance will extend above the costal margin.

arteriole from which branch a series of smaller vessels, in a pattern resembling spider legs. Spider naevi are found in the territory drained by the superior vena cava; common sites include the neck, face and dorsa of the hands. The central arteriole can be occluded with a pencil tip and on release of the pressure the vessels rapidly refill from the centre.

Severe hepatocellular disease associated with portosystemic shunting can result in hepatic encephalopathy.

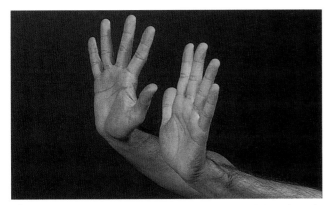

Fig. 7.48 To elicit a flapping tremor in hepatic encephalopathy, ask the patient to outstretch the arms with the hands extended at the wrist and metacarpophalangeal joints. This position is held for 20 seconds.

Often there are accompanying signs of portal hypertension, such as splenomegaly and ascites, but the physical sign characteristic of hepatic encephalopathy is a 'flapping tremor'. Ask the patient to stretch out both arms and hyperextend the wrists with the fingers held separated (Fig. 7.48). A coarse, involuntary flap occurs at the wrist and metacarpophalangeal joints. A further sign is sleepiness and this may progress to coma. Encephalopathic patients often have difficulty copying a picture of a five-pointed star and they may struggle to complete a simple 'dot-to-dot' diagram.

The severity of liver disease is categorised by the Child–Pugh classification (see 'symptoms and signs' box), which assigns points to the clinical and biochemical findings to reach a score. The score is a guide to prognosis.

Risk factors

Cirrhosis

- Alcoholism
- Chronic hepatitis B
- Chronic hepatitis C
- Chronic biliary disease (sclerosing cholangitis, primary biliary cirrhosis)
- Iron overload
- Autoimmune disease
- Copper overload

Differential diagnosis

Hepatic encephalopathy

- Protein load (acute bleed, dietary binge)
- Diuretics and electrolyte abnormalities
- Development of hepatocellular cancer
- Toxins or drugs (alcohol binge, sedatives, opiates)
- Infection

Differential diagnosis

Portal hypertension

Presinusoidal
- Portal vein block
- Schistosomiasis
- Cystic fibrosis

Sinusoidal and postsinusoidal
- Cirrhosis
- Veno-occlusive disease
- Hepatic vein block (Budd–Chiari syndrome)

PALPATING THE GALLBLADDER

Conclude the liver palpation by feeling for the gallbladder. Imagine the position of the fundus, which lies under the point where the rectus abdominis muscle intersects the costal margin. This surface marking coincides with the tip of the right 9th rib.

Using gentle but firm pressure palpate the gallbladder area by pointing the tips of the fingers towards the organ while the patient inspires deeply (Fig. 7.49). When the gallbladder is inflamed (cholecystitis), the most striking physical sign is tenderness and guarding over the gallbladder region. The patient experiences intense pain, winces and interrupts the breath as your fingers make contact with the descending organ (Murphy's sign).

The normal gallbladder is impalpable and only becomes palpable when obstructed and distended with bile. The

Symptoms and signs

Child–Pugh classification of severity of liver disease

Parameter	Points assigned		
	1	2	3
Ascites	Absent	Slight	Moderate
Albumin (g/l)	>35	28–35	<2.8
INR (clotting)	<1.7	1.8–2.3	>2.3
Encephalopathy	None	Grade 1–2	Grade 3–4

Score
- 5–6 = Grade A (well-compensated disease)
- 7–9 = Grade B (significant functional disturbance)
- 10–15 = Grade C (decompensated liver disease)

Prognosis (%)

	1 year	2 year
Grade A	100	85
Grade B	80	60
Grade C	45	35

Palpating the gallbladder

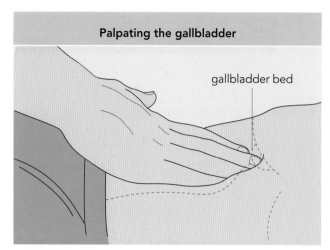

Fig. 7.49 Palpating the gallbladder bed.

Courvoisier's law

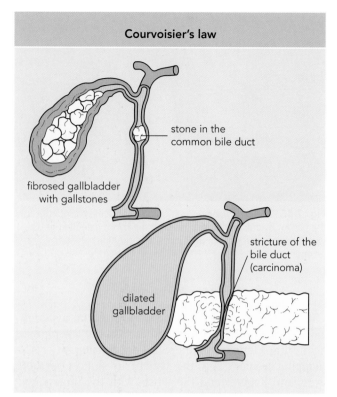

Fig. 7.50 If jaundice is caused by impaction of a gallstone in the bile duct, the fibrosed, stone-filled gallbladder does not dilate. However, if jaundice is caused by a bile duct stricture the healthy gallbladder dilates and can be palpated as a soft mass arising from behind the 9th right rib anteriorly.

distended organ is contiguous with the lower border of the liver and moves with respiration. In the absence of jaundice, a palpable gallbladder suggests obstruction of the cystic duct with the formation of a mucocele. Obstruction of the bile duct by a stone causes jaundice but the gallbladder is rarely palpable because stone formation is associated with chronic cholecystitis and the thickened, fibrosed gallbladder wall does not distend. Jaundice associated with a palpable gallbladder usually implies biliary obstruction caused by a carcinoma of either the head of the pancreas or the common bile duct. In this case the organ is not diseased and is able to dilate (Courvoisier's law) (Fig. 7.50). Remember, however, that exceptions to this rule do occur.

PALPATING THE SPLEEN

The normal spleen cannot be felt and only becomes palpable once it has doubled in size. The spleen enlarges from under the left costal margin towards the right iliac fossa in a downward and medial direction. Often only the tip of the spleen can be felt as it enlarges, although in moderate and massive splenomegaly the organ can be felt well below the costal margin.

Before palpating for the spleen, wrap the palmar surface of your left hand around the back and side of the lower rib cage to provide support and lift the spleen anteriorly. Start the examination from the region of the umbilicus. Position the fingers of the right hand obliquely across the abdomen, with the fingertips pointing at the left costal margin and towards the axilla (Fig. 7.51). The general technique is similar to that described for the liver. Using a moderate amount of pressure, press the index and middle fingers inwards and upwards and hold this steady while asking the patient to breathe in deeply. At the midpoint of the inspiratory effort, lessen the inward pressure but maintain the upward pressure, allowing the fingers to drift in the direction of the descending spleen. The notched leading edge of an enlarged spleen can be

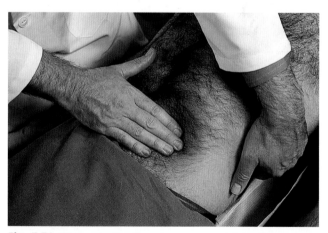

Fig. 7.51 When palpating the spleen use your left hand to support the ribcage posteriorly, while the fingertips of your right hand explore the leading edge of the organ.

felt passing under the fingers and glancing off at the height of inspiration.

If the spleen is impalpable at the starting point of the examination, move the fingertips progressively closer to the left lower rib cage. Make a final pass at the lower costal margin with the fingers probing just under the rib cage. Some clinicians prefer to palpate the spleen with the patient rolled into the right lateral position, with their knees drawn up to relax the abdominal muscles.

Percussion of spleen

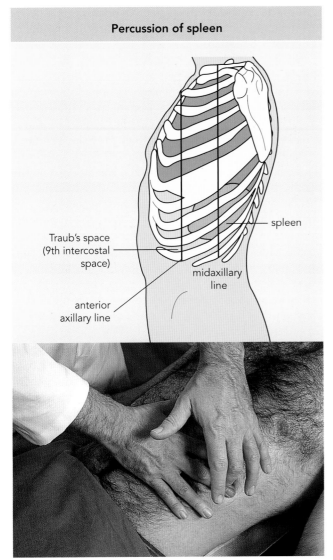

Fig. 7.52 After palpating for the spleen, percuss for the enlarged organ in the 9th intercostal space anterior to the anterior axillary line.

Description of splenomegaly

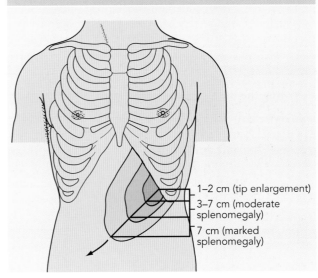

1–2 cm (tip enlargement)
3–7 cm (moderate splenomegaly)
7 cm (marked splenomegaly)

Fig. 7.53 The different degrees of splenomegaly.

Symptoms and signs

Differentiation between splenomegaly and palpation of the left kidney

Kidney	Enlarged spleen
• Moves late in inspiration	• Moves early in inspiration
• Possible to get above upper pole	• Impossible to get above a spleen
• Smooth shape	• Notched leading edge
• Resonant to percussion	• Dull to percussion in Traub's space
	• Enlarges towards umbilicus

Differential diagnosis

Splenomegaly

- Portal hypertension
- Infections (malaria, subacute bacterial endocarditis, tuberculosis, typhoid)
- Chronic lymphatic leukaemia
- Chronic myeloid leukaemia
- Myelofibrosis
- Gaucher's disease
- Haemolytic anaemia

At this point in the examination it is useful to percuss for splenic dullness. The tip of a normal spleen lies posterior to the anterior axillary line and is bounded anteriorly by the gas-filled stomach and colon. Percuss the 9th intercostal space anterior to the anterior axillary line (Traub's space) (Fig. 7.52). This space overlies bowel and is normally tympanitic but as the solid spleen enlarges this area becomes less resonant, eventually sounding dull with more marked splenomegaly.

An enlarged spleen is readily distinguished from other organs in the region, such as the left kidney. Note whether there is tenderness and assess the degree of enlargement, using a ruler to measure the distance from the left costal margin to the tip of the spleen (Fig. 7.53). Splenomegaly may be caused by stimulation and hypertrophy of the reticuloendothelial elements, congestion with blood or by infiltration by abnormal cells.

EXAMINING THE RENAL SYSTEM

Like the examination of the liver, the kidney examination is aided by systemic signs that reflect impaired function of the organ. In acute renal failure, there is oliguria (<500 ml/24 h) and signs of fluid overload. The clinical syndrome is dominated by a rapidly progressive deterioration of biochemical tests of function (raised blood urea, creatinine and potassium) occurring over hours or days (see 'differential diagnosis' box – acute renal failure). When renal failure develops over weeks, months or years, systemic signs appear (see 'differential diagnosis' and 'symptoms and signs' boxes – chronic renal failure).

Palpating the kidneys

Pole to pole the kidneys extend from the vertebral level of T12 to L3 and the larger right lobe of the liver displaces the right kidney 2 cm lower than the left. Viewed from the rear, the kidneys lie in the renal angle formed by the 12th rib and the lateral margin of the vertebral column (Fig. 7.54). The adrenal glands perch on the upper pole of each kidney.

The kidneys are not usually palpable through the thickness of the abdominal wall and abdominal contents, although in thin individuals a normal-sized kidney may be felt. The right kidney is easier to palpate because it lies lower than the left. A normal kidney has a firm consistency and a smooth surface.

When examining the kidneys, position the patient close to the edge of the bed and examine each kidney from the patient's right, bearing in mind the surface anatomy. The kidneys are retroperitoneal organs and deep bimanual palpation is required to explore for them. When examining the left kidney, tuck the palmar surfaces of the left hand posteriorly into the left flank and nestle the fingertips in the renal angle (Fig. 7.55a). Position the middle three fingers of the right hand below the left costal margin, lateral to the rectus muscle and at a point opposite the posterior hand (Fig. 7.55b). To examine the right kidney, tuck your left hand behind the right loin and position the fingers of your right hand below the right costal margin, lateral to rectus abdominis. Palpate for the lower pole of each kidney in turn. The aim of the manoeuvre is briefly to trap the lower pole of the kidney between the fingers of both hands as the organ moves up and down with deep respiration. The spleen is closely associated with the diaphragm and thus moves early in respiration but the kidneys lie lower down and they only descend towards the end of inspiration. Ask the patient to inspire deeply; press the fingers of both hands firmly together, attempting to capture the lower pole as it slips through the fingertips. This technique is known as balloting the kidney (Fig. 7.55b). If the kidney is palpable the rounded lower pole can be felt slipping between the opposing fingers as the patient breathes in and out.

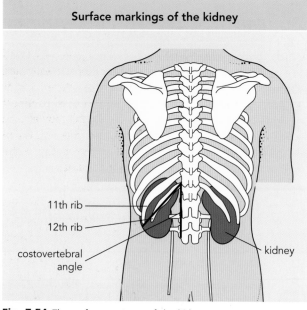

Surface markings of the kidney

11th rib
12th rib
costovertebral angle
kidney

Fig. 7.54 The surface anatomy of the kidneys.

 Differential diagnosis

Acute renal failure

- Shock (hypovolaemic, septic or cardiogenic)
- Acute glomerulonephritis
- Toxins or drugs (ethylene glycol, carbon tetrachloride)
- Acute haemoglobinuria or myoglobinuria
- Acute renal vein thrombosis

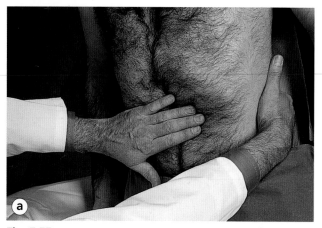

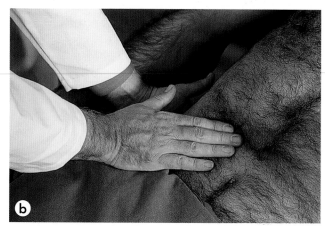

Fig. 7.55 Positioning the hands when palpating (a) the left and (b) the right kidney.

Symptoms and signs
Signs of chronic renal failure

- Sallow complexion
- Anaemia (normocytic, normochromic)
- Uraemic fetor
- Deep acidotic breathing (Kussmaul respiration)
- Hypertension
- Mental clouding
- Uraemic encephalopathy (flapping tremor)
- Pleural and pericardial effusion
- Pericardial rub (pericarditis)
- Evidence of fluid overload or depletion
- Renal masses (polycystic kidneys)
- Large bladder (chronic bladder outlet obstruction)

Differential diagnosis
Chronic renal failure

- Chronic glomerulonephritis
- Systemic hypertension
- Diabetes mellitus with nephropathy
- Chronic obstructive uropathy
- Polycystic disease of the kidneys
- Analgesic nephropathy

The kidney may be tender, especially when acutely infected (pyelonephritis) or obstructed (hydronephrosis). This may be apparent on bimanual palpation, although a more specific sign is 'punch' tenderness over the renal angles. To test this response sit the patient forward and place the palm of the left hand over the renal angle. Then, using moderate force, punch the dorsal surface of the hand with the ulnar surface of the clenched right fist (Fig. 7.56). Perform this test for each kidney in turn and assess the patient's reaction.

It is important to distinguish kidney enlargement from splenomegaly on the left and hepatomegaly on the right. The principal cause of bilateral enlargement is polycystic disease of the kidney, whereas unilateral enlargement suggests a malignant tumour (e.g. hypernephroma).

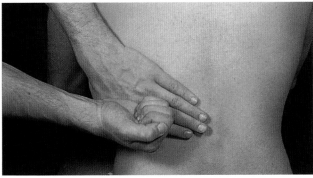

Fig. 7.56 Assessing the punch tenderness over the renal angles.

PALPATING THE AORTA

The descending aorta emerges through the aortic hiatus in the diaphragm and hugs the vertebral bodies until it bifurcates into the common iliac arteries at the level of L4, which approximates to a point just below the umbilicus. It lies adjacent to the inferior vena cava and gives off a number of major tributaries that feed the major abdominal organs (Fig. 7.57). The aorta can be palpated between the thumb and finger of one hand or by positioning the fingers of both hands on either side of the midline at a point midway between the xiphisternum and the umbilicus (Fig. 7.58). Press the fingers posteriorly and slightly medially and feel for the pulsation of the abdominal aorta against your fingertips. This pulsation can be felt in thin individuals but it is usually impalpable in muscular or obese patients.

An abdominal aortic aneurysm may be felt as a large pulsatile mass above the level of the umbilicus. The abdominal aorta may also become abnormally prominent in elderly people when marked curvature of the spine displaces it anteriorly and laterally.

PERCUSSION OF THE ABDOMEN

At this stage of the examination you will have percussed the liver and spleen. General percussion of the abdomen is used to establish whether abdominal distension is caused by gas or fluid. Percussion is also used to detect an overfilled bladder. The stomach, small bowel and colon fill the entire anterior abdomen and the percussion note of the anterior abdomen wall between the costal margins and iliac crests is normally tympanic.

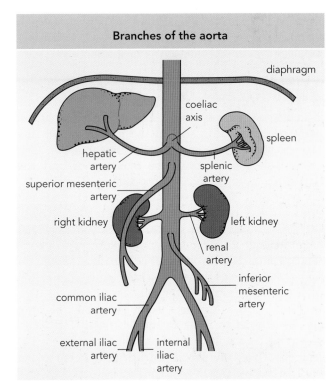

Fig. 7.57 The abdominal aorta and its branches.

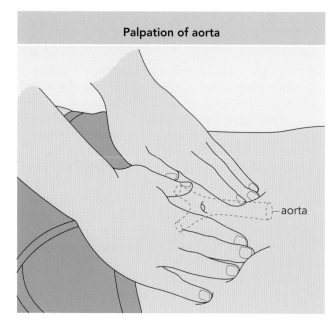

Palpation of aorta

Fig. 7.58 Palpation of the aorta at a point midway between the umbilicus and the xiphisternum.

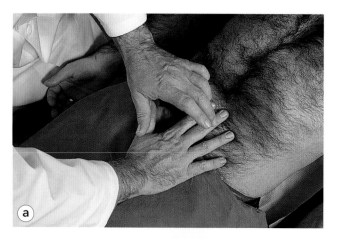

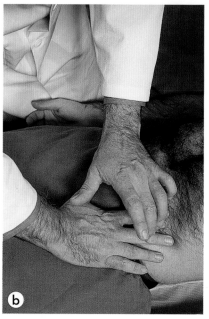

Fig. 7.59 When percussing for ascites, (a) begin in the midline with your finger parallel to the lateral wall of the abdomen and (b) continue towards the left flank. A change in the percussion note indicates a gas–fluid interface.

Percussion to detect ascites

Abdominal distension is usually caused either by gaseous dilatation of the bowel or abnormal accumulation of fluid. In the supine position, gas accumulates more centrally, whereas fluid gravitates into the flanks. The gas-filled normal bowel tends to float above ascites, so the gas–fluid interface characteristic of ascites is detected by a change in the percussion note from the resonance overlying bowel to the dullness of fluid. The presence of ascites can be confirmed by altering the patient's posture and demonstrating a change in the position of the gas–fluid interface.

A change in percussion note (shifting dullness) is easiest to assess by percussing from an area of resonance to an area of dullness. With the patient supine, percuss in the midline at the level of the umbilicus with the fingers parallel to the lateral wall of the abdomen (Fig. 7.59a). This point overlies gas-filled bowel and the percussion note should be tympanic. Progressively reposition your hand approximately 2 cm to the left and repeat the percussion towards the left flank (Fig. 7.59b). The note should remain tympanic until you reach the lateral abdominal wall. A distinct transition zone between tympany and dullness, a gas–fluid interface, should be marked lightly with a water-soluble marking pen. Now ask the patient to roll into the right lateral position. This allows the fluid to gravitate to the right flank and the gas-filled bowel to rise into the left flank (Fig. 7.60). Repeat the percussion from the midline towards the left flank. The tympany should extend well lateral to the interface marked in supine examination.

Percussion to detect a distended bladder

If the bladder outlet is obstructed and the detrusor muscle fails, the organ distends and emerges above the pubic bone from its usual position deep within the pelvis. The suprapubic area is usually tympanic and a dull sound on percussion here is a useful clinical sign of bladder distension.

Use the general principle of percussing from resonance to dullness to check for bladder enlargement. Percuss from the level of the umbilicus, parallel to the pubis (Fig. 7.61) and progress down the midline towards the pubic bone. The note should remain tympanic to the pubic bone. A level of dullness above this landmark indicates the upper margin of a distended bladder or possibly enlargement of the uterus. An enlarged bladder is felt as a rounded fullness, whereas an enlarged uterus is felt as a more distinct solid structure.

Shifting dullness of ascites

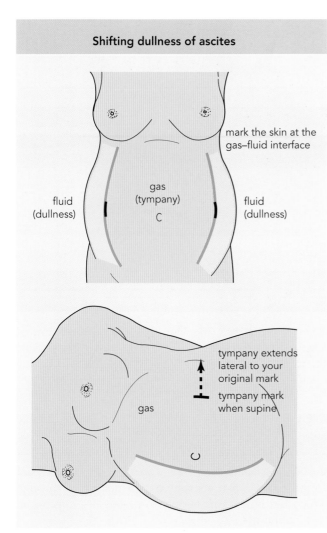

mark the skin at the gas–fluid interface

gas (tympany)
C

fluid (dullness)

fluid (dullness)

tympany extends lateral to your original mark

tympany mark when supine

gas

Fig. 7.60 To confirm the presence of ascites, roll the patient into the right lateral position because this causes fluid to settle in the dependent right flank, whereas gas-filled bowel floats above to fill the left flank. A shift in the positions of dullness and tympany indicates free fluid.

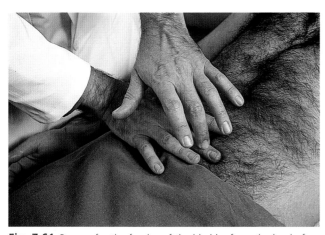

Fig. 7.61 Percuss for the fundus of the bladder from the level of the umbilicus.

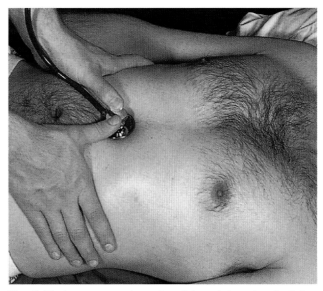

Fig. 7.62 If you suspect obstruction of the pyloric outlet, check for a 'succussion splash' by simultaneously listening in the epigastrium and shaking the upper abdomen from side to side.

AUSCULTATION OF THE ABDOMEN

The sounds generated by the abdomen are gurgling noises caused by the intestinal peristalsis moving gas and fluid through the bowel lumen. These are best assessed by auscultation.

Listening for bowel sounds

Place the diaphragm of the stethoscope on the mid-abdomen and listen for intermittent gurgling sounds (borborygma). These peristaltic sounds occur episodically at 5–10s intervals, although longer silent periods may occur. Keep listening for approximately 30s before concluding that bowel sounds are reduced or absent.

The absence of any bowel sounds can indicate intestinal paralysis (paralytic ileus); this is always associated with abdominal distension. Rapidly repetitive bowel sounds (often termed 'active' bowel sounds) may be normal but they may also be an early sign of mechanical obstruction if they are associated with a colicky abdominal pain. In progressive bowel obstruction, large amounts of gas and fluid accumulate and the bowel sounds change in quality to a higher pitched 'tinkling'. This is an ominous sign of impending bowel paralysis.

Auscultation may also be helpful when diagnosing obstruction of gastric outflow. In pyloric obstruction, the stomach distends with gas and fluid; this can be detected by listening for a 'succussion splash'. Steady the diaphragm of the stethoscope on the epigastrium and shake the upper abdomen for the splashing sound characteristic of gastric outflow obstruction (Fig. 7.62).

Listening for arterial bruits

Position the diaphragm of the stethoscope over the abdominal aorta and apply moderate pressure (Fig.

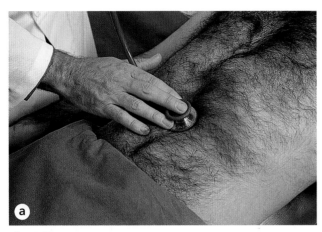

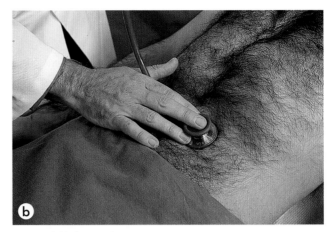

Fig. 7.63 Position of the stethoscope when listening for bruits in (a) the aorta and (b) the renal artery.

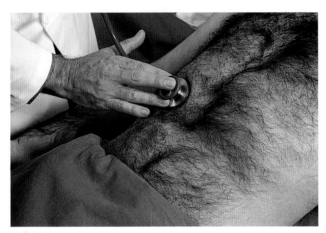

Fig. 7.64 Position of the stethoscope when listening for a liver bruit.

7.63a). The heart sounds may be transmitted to this area but aortic flow should be silent. A distinct systolic murmur (a bruit) indicates turbulent flow and suggests arteriosclerosis or an aneurysm.

Listen for renal arterial bruits at a point 2.5 cm above and lateral to the umbilicus (Fig. 7.63b). The presence of a renal bruit suggests congenital or arteriosclerotic renal artery stenosis or narrowing caused by fibromuscular hyperplasia.

AUSCULTATION OVER THE LIVER AND SPLEEN

Conclude the auscultation by listening over the liver (Fig. 7.64) and spleen. A soft and distant bruit heard over an enlarged liver is always abnormal, suggesting either primary liver cell carcinoma or acute alcoholic hepatitis. Secondary liver tumours do not transmit bruits. Occasionally, a creaking 'rub' may be heard over the liver or spleen. This indicates inflammation of the outer capsule of the organ and adjacent peritoneum, perhaps caused by perihepatitis or perisplenitis. More rarely, carcinomatous infiltration of the capsule and surrounding structures may be the cause.

Examining the groin

The spermatic cord, inguinal lymph nodes and femoral artery occupy the groin. A swelling in the groin is usually the result of either an inguinal or femoral hernia or due to enlarged lymph nodes.

INGUINAL CANAL AND FEMORAL SHEATH

During male fetal development the testis and spermatic cord migrate from the abdomen into the scrotum through the inguinal canal. This passage occludes after the descent of the testes but it remains a potential route through which the bowel can herniate in later life, causing an inguinal hernia.

The inguinal canal passes downward and medially from the internal to the external ring, running above and parallel to the inguinal ligament, which forms its lower border (Fig. 7.65). The internal ring lies immediately above the point at which the inguinal ligament and femoral artery intersect. The femoral artery lies at the midfemoral point, which is located midway between the anterior superior iliac spine and the symphysis pubis. The external ring lies immediately above and medial to the pubic tubercle. The femoral artery enters the femoral triangle from behind the inguinal ligament and is enclosed in a fascial sheath. This sheath also accommodates the femoral vein, which lies medial to the artery, and the femoral canal, which is a small gap immediately adjacent and medial to the vein. The femoral canal is plugged with fat and a lymph node (Cloquet's gland) and it is a potential pathway for the formation of a direct femoral hernia.

Examining herniae

An indirect inguinal hernia forms when bowel or omentum protrudes through a lax internal ring and finds its way into the inguinal canal. Bowel may force its way through the external ring and may even slip into the scrotum (Fig. 7.66).

An inguinal hernia usually presents as a lump in the groin or the scrotum that is most prominent when the

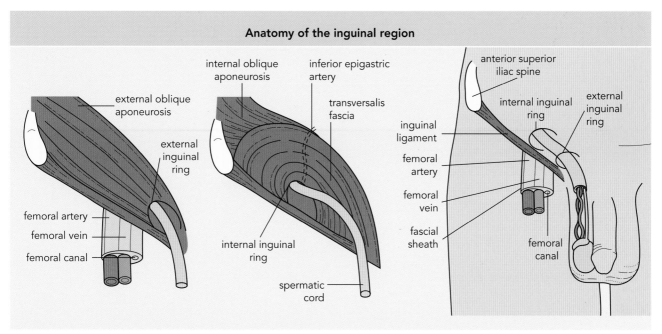

Anatomy of the inguinal region

external oblique
aponeurosis

internal oblique
aponeurosis

inferior epigastric
artery

anterior superior
iliac spine

external
inguinal
ring

transversalis
fascia

internal inguinal
ring

external
inguinal
ring

inguinal
ligament

femoral
artery

femoral artery

femoral vein

femoral
vein

femoral canal

internal inguinal
ring

fascial
sheath

femoral
canal

spermatic
cord

Fig. 7.65 The anatomy of the inguinal canal and femoral sheath.

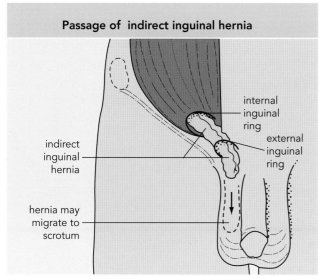

Passage of indirect inguinal hernia

internal
inguinal
ring

external
inguinal
ring

indirect
inguinal
hernia

hernia may
migrate to
scrotum

Fig. 7.66 An indirect hernia enters through the internal ring and exits through the external ring.

intra-abdominal pressure is raised (e.g. when standing or coughing). The hernia may reduce spontaneously when the patient lies down, so it is best to examine the hernia with the patient standing. Place two fingers on the mass and ascertain whether or not an impulse is transmitted to your fingertips when the patient coughs. Most herniae can be reduced manually, so attempt this by gently massaging the mass towards the internal ring. Once the hernia is fully reduced, occlude the internal ring with a finger pressing over the femoral point. Ask the patient to cough. An indirect inguinal hernia should not reappear until you release the occlusion of the internal ring.

A direct inguinal hernia develops through a weakness in the posterior wall of the inguinal canal. These herniae

seldom force their way into the scrotum and, once reduced, their reappearance is not controlled by pressure over the internal ring.

When an inguinal hernia extends as far as the external ring it may be confused with a femoral hernia. The distinction is made by establishing the relationship of the hernia to the pubic tubercle: an inguinal hernia lies above and medial to the tubercle, whereas a femoral hernia lies below and lateral.

Examining the anus, rectum and prostate

RECTUM AND ANUS

The rectum is a curved segment of the bowel, approximately 12 cm long, lying in the concavity of the mid- and lower sacrum (Fig. 7.67). The upper two-thirds of the anterior rectum but not the posterior surface is covered by peritoneum. The anterior rectal peritoneum reflects onto the bladder base in men, it forms the rectouterine pouch (known as the pouch of Douglas) in women and is filled with loops of bowel. Anterior to the lower one-third of the rectum lie the prostate, bladder base and seminal vesicles in men and the vagina in women. The anus is 3–4 cm long and joins the rectum to the perineum. The anal wall is supported by powerful sphincter muscles, the voluntary external and involuntary internal sphincters, which constrict to provide tone and continence (Fig. 7.68). The rectal mucosa can be directly visualised through a proctoscope or sigmoidoscope but a great deal may be learned by palpation of the anus, rectum and prostate.

Anatomical relationships of the rectum in males and females

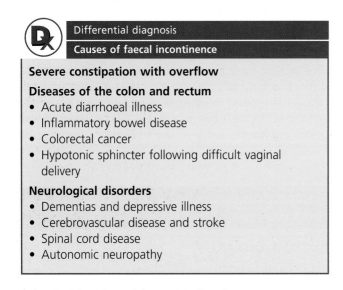

Fig. 7.67 The relationship of the anterior rectum to the prostate gland and bladder base in men (left) and the posterior vaginal wall and uterine cervix in women (right).

Dx Differential diagnosis

Causes of faecal incontinence

Severe constipation with overflow

Diseases of the colon and rectum
- Acute diarrhoeal illness
- Inflammatory bowel disease
- Colorectal cancer
- Hypotonic sphincter following difficult vaginal delivery

Neurological disorders
- Dementias and depressive illness
- Cerebrovascular disease and stroke
- Spinal cord disease
- Autonomic neuropathy

The anal sphincters

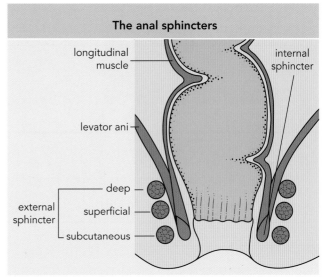

Fig. 7.68 The internal and external anal sphincters.

Rectal examination should not be unduly painful and it is important to explain this to the patient, along with your reasons for performing it. The examination will promote a feeling of rectal fullness and it may stimulate a desire to evacuate. Tell the patient to expect this. Always work with an assistant and always glove both hands.

Position the patient in the left lateral position with the hips and knees well flexed and the buttock positioned at the edge of the bed (Fig. 7.69). The positions around the anal opening are described by the positions around the clock face (Fig. 7.70). Gently separate the buttocks to expose the natal cleft and anal verge (Fig. 7.71). Inspection of the natal cleft and anal verge may reveal skin tags, pilonidal sinuses, warts, fissures, fistulas,

external haemorrhoids or prolapsed rectal mucosa (Fig. 7.72). A bluish discoloration of the perineal skin suggests Crohn's disease. The anal skin is innervated with pain fibres and anal pain and tenderness are suggestive of infection (e.g. perianal abscess), fissure and fistula-in-ano or thrombosis of an external haemorrhoid.

Lubricate your index finger with a clear, water-soluble gel (e.g. K-Y jelly) and press the fingertip against the anal verge with the pulp facing the 6 o'clock position (Fig. 7.71). Slip your finger into the anal canal and then insert it into the rectum, directing the tip posteriorly to follow the sacral curve (Fig. 7.73). With your finger fully

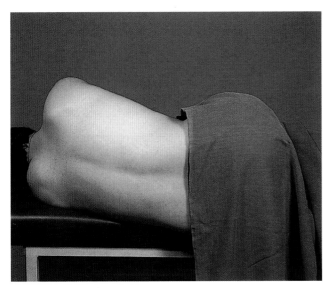

Fig. 7.69 The correct position of the patient before a rectal examination.

The clock face positions around the anus

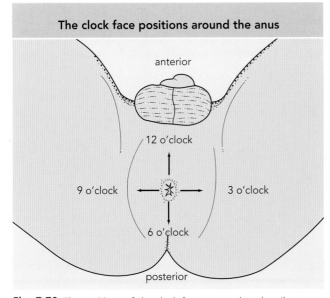

anterior

12 o'clock

9 o'clock   3 o'clock

6 o'clock

posterior

Fig. 7.70 The positions of the clock face are used to describe positions around the anus.

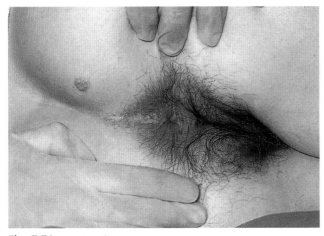

Fig. 7.71 Exposing the anus.

introduced, check on anal tone by asking the patient to squeeze your finger with the anal muscles. Then gently sweep the finger through 180° using the palmar surface of the finger to explore the posterior and posterolateral walls of the rectum. Rotate the finger round to the 12 o'clock position. This is accomplished more easily by adopting a half-crouched position and simultaneously pronating your wrist. This position allows you to sweep the finger across the anterior and anterolateral walls of the rectum. The normal rectum feels uniformly smooth and pliable. In men, the prostate can be felt anteriorly and in women it may be possible to feel the cervix as well as a retroverted uterus.

On rectal palpation you may feel an intrinsic tumour caused by a carcinoma or polyp. Perirectal sepsis causes marked rectal wall tenderness and an abscess may be felt pointing into the lumen. The anterior rectal peritoneal reflection straddles both the anterior rectum itself and the structures lying in front of it. Consequently, malignant or inflammatory lesions of the peritoneum may be felt through the anterior wall of the rectum.

Withdraw your finger from the rectum and anus and check the glove tip for stool. There may be melaena, blood or pus and you may notice the pale, greasy stools characteristic of malabsorption.

PROSTATE

The prostate gland is examined during the rectal examination. The normal prostate measures approximately 3.5 cm from side to side and protrudes 1 cm into the rectum (Fig. 7.74a). The gland has a rubbery, smooth consistency and a shallow longitudinal groove separates the right and left lobes. It should not be tender to palpation but the patient may experience the urge to urinate.

Red flag – urgent referral
Prostate enlargement

- Asymmetric enlargement
- Stony hard consistency
- Discreet nodularity

Palpation of the prostate aims to assess size, consistency, nodularity and tenderness. The assessment of prostatic size is learnt through experience. Benign hypertrophy of the prostate is common in men over 60 years old. The enlargement is smooth and symmetrical and the gland feels rubbery or slightly boggy (Fig. 7.74b). A cancerous prostate may feel asymmetric, with a stony hard consistency, and discrete nodules may be palpable (Fig. 7.74c). Marked prostatic tenderness suggests acute prostatitis, a prostatic abscess or inflammation of the seminal vesicles. If prostatic infection is suspected, attempt to massage the organ from within the rectum in order to squeeze prostatic fluid towards the urethral meatus, where it can be collected for microscopy and culture.

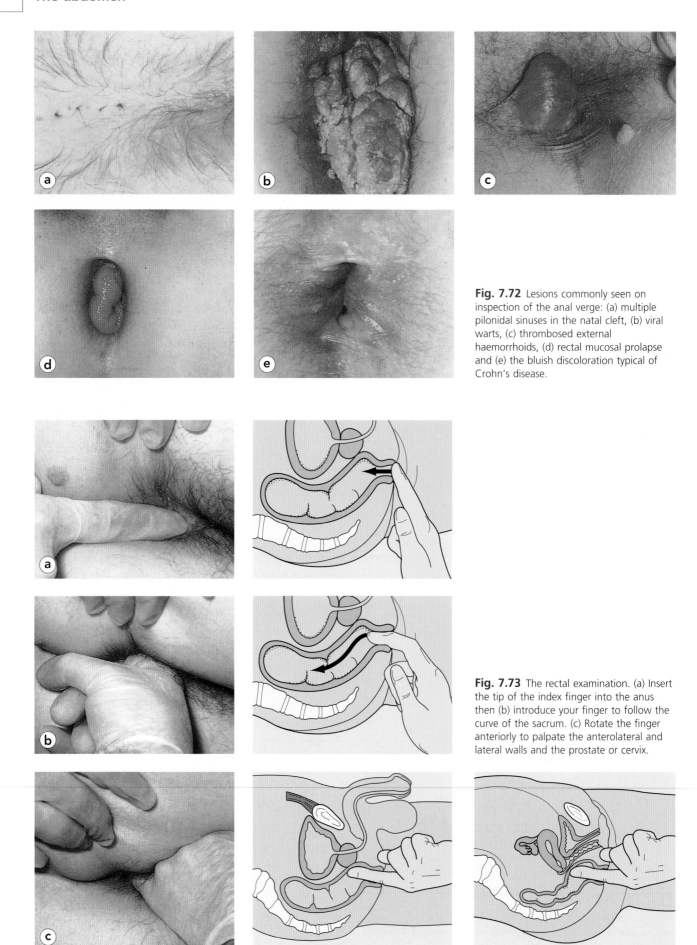

Fig. 7.72 Lesions commonly seen on inspection of the anal verge: (a) multiple pilonidal sinuses in the natal cleft, (b) viral warts, (c) thrombosed external haemorrhoids, (d) rectal mucosal prolapse and (e) the bluish discoloration typical of Crohn's disease.

Fig. 7.73 The rectal examination. (a) Insert the tip of the index finger into the anus then (b) introduce your finger to follow the curve of the sacrum. (c) Rotate the finger anteriorly to palpate the anterolateral and lateral walls and the prostate or cervix.

Palpating the normal and abnormal prostate

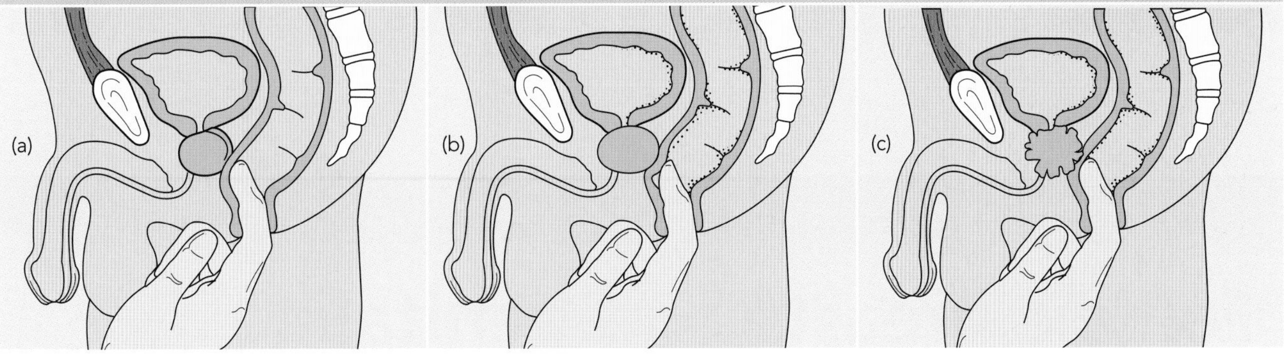

Fig. 7.74 (a) The normal prostate felt through the anterior rectal wall has a median sulcus separating the two lateral lobes. (b) The median sulcus may become indistinct in a benign hypertrophied prostate and the gland feels firm and smooth and bulges more than 1 cm into the lumen. (c) A carcinomatous prostate feels hard and irregular and the median sulcus is obliterated.

Examination of elderly people
Abdominal examination in elderly people

- On inspection of the abdomen there may be asymmetry caused by kyphoscoliosis of the spine
- Osteoporosis and deformity of the rib cage causes the costal margin to migrate towards the pelvis, making abdominal examination more difficult
- If the patient is hard of hearing or dyspraxic there may be difficulty obtaining the cooperation needed to palpate the liver and spleen
- Constipation in the elderly often manifests with the impression of a mass in the left lower quadrant (this can be re-assessed after an enema to induce evacuation)
- An ectatic aorta is often palpable and scoliosis often displaces the aorta, giving a false impression of an aortic aneurysm
- Consider an aneurysm if the aorta is assessed to be >5 cm in diameter at its widest (readily confirmed on ultrasound)

- Aortic bruits are more common in the elderly, reflecting atherosclerosis or aneurysm
- Leaking aneurysm presents as backache; rupture presents as an acute abdominal emergency with shock, abdominal distension, poor distal perfusion and asymmetrical pulses
- Benign or malignant prostatic hypertrophy in older men predisposes to bladder outlet obstruction, detrusor instability and failure, urinary retention and infection
- Acute urinary retention is a common cause of acute 'unexplained' confusion in the elderly – always examine for an enlarged bladder in elderly patients presenting with confusion, delirium, incontinence or fever
- Faecal incontinence may be associated with dementia, chronic constipation with overflow, laxative abuse and disordered sphincteric function
- A rectal examination and plain abdominal x-ray usually clarifies faecal impaction in the elderly

Review
Framework for the routine examination of the abdomen

General examination
- Nutrition and hydration
- Peripheral oedema (hypoproteinaemia)
- Leuconychia or koilonychia
- Signs of liver disease

Inspection
- Shape and symmetry
- Scars and striae
- Abdominal wall veins and flow pattern
- Visible peristalsis
- Hernias (paraumbilical, inguinal)

Palpation (nine segments)
- Light palpation to assess tenderness
- Deeper palpation for masses

- Liver, spleen, kidneys
- Bladder, uterus, aorta

Percussion
- Upper and lower liver margins
- Spleen (Traub's space)
- Shifting dullness (ascites)
- Suprapubic dullness (bladder)

Auscultation
- Bowel sounds
- Aortic and renal bruits
- Hepatic and splenic rubs

Rectal examination
- Rectal mucosa
- Prostate, uterus

8

Female breasts and genitalia

The clinical assessment of the reproductive system is often neglected in routine examinations because of patients' discomfort and embarrassment and because of doctors' reluctance to conduct the genital examination as a routine procedure. The case history and examination intrude into patients' most intimate boundaries, so careful scripting is necessary to reassure the patient. The sensitivity associated with the examination is further heightened when dealing with patients of the opposite sex. A chaperone should always be close at hand when a member of the opposite sex is examined.

It is reassuring to remember that the majority of patients feel reasonably comfortable discussing sexual problems with their doctor; this stems from a cultural acceptance that doctors deal with all aspects of bodily function and an understanding that the doctor–patient relationship is confidential and professional. It is important to establish trust and competence when assessing the genital tract. Undergraduate courses in gynaecology, obstetrics and genitourinary medicine provide the opportunity to learn the examination techniques required for a thorough examination.

Structure and function

PUBERTY

The transition from childhood to adolescence is regulated by hormones secreted by the hypothalamic–pituitary axis. During puberty there is a rapid spurt in growth, accounting for approximately 25% of the final adult height. Secondary sexual characteristics develop and sexual awareness is aroused.

The age of puberty varies and parents and teenagers often worry about what they perceive as a delayed growth spurt. A number of factors determine the onset of puberty. Over the past 150 years there has been a progressive fall in the age of the first menstrual period (menarche). This is thought to reflect the effects of improving nutrition and general health on the onset of puberty. There is evidence that body weight is an important trigger for puberty:

moderately overweight girls tend to enter puberty earlier than their lean contemporaries. Abnormal weight loss (such as occurs with anorexia nervosa or a debilitating illness) causes delay of the menarche or cessation of established periods altogether (amenorrhoea).

Adolescent development can be assessed using pubertal milestones defined by Tanner (Fig. 8.1). For girls this is based on breast development and the growth of pubic hair. Puberty in girls begins between 8 and 13 years of age. The average age of the menarche is 12.5 years and most girls will have menstruated by the age of 14.5 years.

Hormonal changes in puberty

Puberty is established by the activation of the neuroendocrine axis. The cerebral cortex plays a central role in the initial activation of the hypothalamus, which stores gonadotrophin-releasing hormone (GnRH). This hormone is released into the hypothalamo-hypophyseal portal system and is carried to the anterior lobe of the pituitary gland where it stimulates the release of sex hormones. During childhood, GnRH secretion is inhibited and loss of this inhibition signals the onset of puberty (Fig. 8.2). Pulsatile release of GnRH provides the signal for the pulsatile release of follicle-stimulating hormone (FSH) and luteinising hormone (LH) from the pituitary gland which, in turn, stimulates the gonads. The hormonal products of the female gonads then exert their specific influences on the reproductive organs and induce the development of secondary sexual characteristics. Breast growth (telarche) in women is followed by the menarche and the establishment of the menstrual cycle.

Breast development

Oestrogen secretion from the developing ovaries is the prime stimulus for breast development. Initially, there is widening of the areola with a small mound of breast tissue developing beneath it. This is followed by progressive enlargement of the breasts until the full adult size is attained (Fig. 8.1).

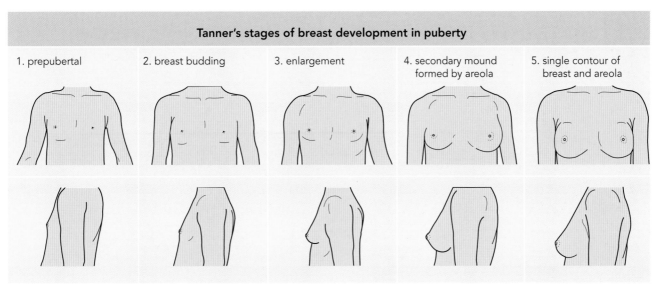

Tanner's stages of breast development in puberty

1. prepubertal
2. breast budding
3. enlargement
4. secondary mound formed by areola
5. single contour of breast and areola

Fig. 8.1 Stages of breast development. Development from the preadolescent stage (1) begins initially with a widening of the areola and the development of subareolar tissue (2). Progressive expansion occurs (3–4) until adult size is attained (5).

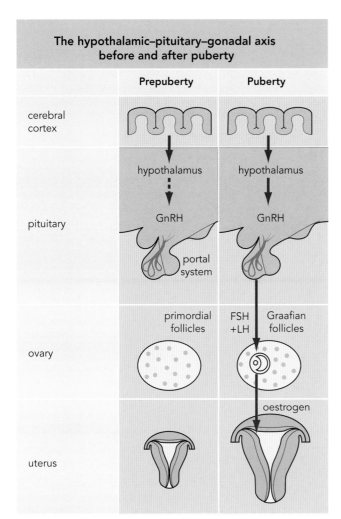

The hypothalamic–pituitary–gonadal axis before and after puberty

	Prepuberty	Puberty
cerebral cortex		
pituitary	hypothalamus ↓ GnRH	hypothalamus ↓ GnRH portal system
ovary	primordial follicles	FSH +LH Graafian follicles
uterus		oestrogen

Fig. 8.2 The hypothalmic–pituitary–gonadal axis. In childhood, gonadotrophin-releasing hormone (GnRH) secretion is inhibited (left). Loss of GnRH inhibition induces puberty and provides the signal for the release of follicle-stimulating hormone (FSH) and luteinising hormone (LH). FSH and LH stimulate the gonads and exert cyclical changes in the uterine endometrium (right).

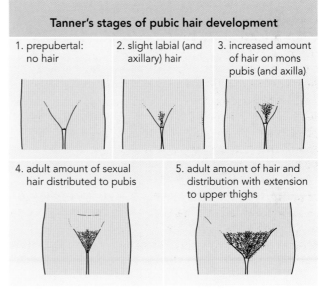

Tanner's stages of pubic hair development

1. prepubertal: no hair
2. slight labial (and axillary) hair
3. increased amount of hair on mons pubis (and axilla)
4. adult amount of sexual hair distributed to pubis
5. adult amount of hair and distribution with extension to upper thighs

Fig. 8.3 Pubic hair development. Development from the preadolescent (1) begins with the growth of sparse straight hair along the medial borders of the labia (2). Further growth of darker coarser curlier hair continues (3–4) until the typical inverted triangular distribution of the adult female is seen (5).

Pubic hair growth

In both males and females, growth of the pubic hair is regulated by adrenal androgens, with an additional contribution of testicular androgen in the male. In females, the pattern of pubic hair growth has a characteristic inverted triangular appearance (Fig. 8.3).

Ovarian and menstrual cycle

The cyclical release of FSH and LH from the pituitary is reflected in serum concentration changes. Ovulation occurs in response to these changes and this in turn

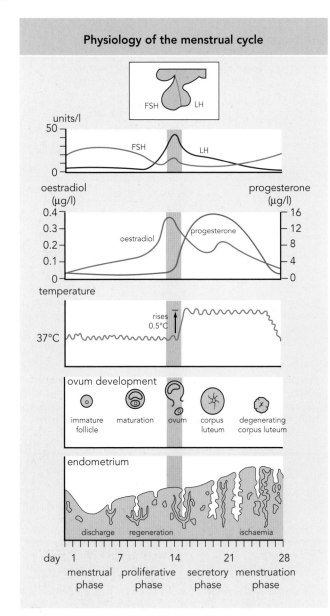

Fig. 8.4 Physiological changes associated with the menstrual cycle.

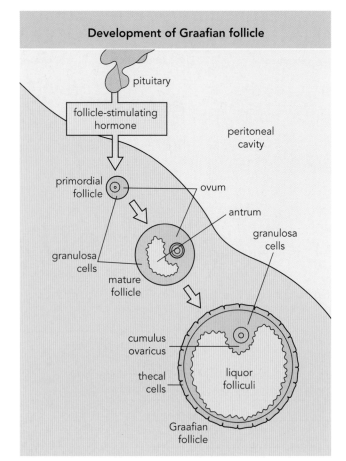

Fig. 8.5 Development of a mature ovarian follicle.

hormone in the second phase of the ovulatory cycle. The granulosa cells of the corpus luteum express LH receptors which are also capable of binding human chorionic gonadotrophin (HCG), a hormone secreted by the fetal syncytiotrophoblast. In the absence of fertilisation, HCG does not appear in the circulation, and by about the 23rd day of the cycle, the corpus luteum starts to atrophy. Progesterone levels fall, allowing the re-expression of FSH secretion and the initiation of another cycle. If conception has not occurred, menstruation commences. This is caused by an intense vasospasm in the arterioles feeding the superficial layers of the endometrium, which causes hypoxic necrosis of this tissue. The tissue is then expelled through the vagina.

Climateric and menopause

By about the age of 40 years, the number of functional oocytes has fallen to the point where sex hormone synthesis is reduced. This signals the onset of the climacteric, which over a period of years culminates in the cessation of menstruation (the menopause). Initially, FSH levels increase in an attempt to stimulate follicular ripening; later, anovulatory cycles develop with irregular menstrual bleeding; finally, at about the age of 50 years, menstruation ceases. Loss of hormonal feedback results in high serum levels of FSH and LH (Fig. 8.6). Serum levels of these hormones are used as a test for the

regulates cyclical changes in the uterine endometrium (Fig. 8.4). In each cycle, a few 'selected' dormant ovarian follicles become responsive to FSH, with usually only a single dominant follicle maturing to the point of ovulation (Fig. 8.5). The primordial follicle consists of a large oocyte surrounded by a flattened follicular epithelium. In the few responsive follicles, FSH stimulates the proliferation of granulosa cells which secrete an oestradiol-rich fluid that accumulates in the follicle (the antrum). As the follicle grows, it is surrounded by a specialised layer of thecal cells which are derived from the ovarian stroma. The responsive follicle grows to attain a preovulatory size of 2–3 cm. In midcycle there is a surge of both FSH and LH (Fig.8.4); the LH surge is thought to trigger the events leading to the extrusion of the ovum from the ovary.

Extrusion of the ovum leaves behind the corpus luteum (Fig. 8.4), which secretes progesterone, the dominant sex

Chapter

Physiological changes in the menopause

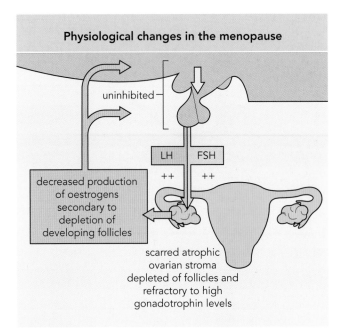

Fig. 8.6 Loss of hormonal feedback in the menopause. The hypothalamus tries to compensate for the falling oestrogen level by increasing production of follicle-stimulating hormone (FSH) and luteinising hormone (LH).

Muscles underlying the breast

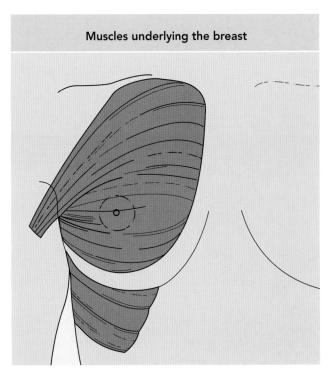

Fig. 8.7 The breast overlies pectoralis major and serratus anterior muscles.

climacteric and menopause. The decline in oestrogen production results in atrophy of the breasts, genital organs and bone. Vasomotor instability may result in hot flushes.

Breast structure and function

The breasts overlie the pectoralis major and serratus anterior muscles and extend from the second to sixth ribs (Fig. 8.7). It is convenient to divide the breast into four quadrants by horizontal and vertical lines intersecting at the nipple (Fig. 8.8). A lateral extension of breast tissue (the axillary tail of Spence) extends from the upper outer quadrant towards the axilla.

Each breast is formed from 15–20 glandular lobules embedded in a supporting bed of fatty and fibrous tissue that gives shape to the organ (Fig. 8.9). Fibrous septa known as Cooper's (suspensory) ligaments separate the lobules and provide support by attaching between the subcutaneous tissue and the fascia of the muscles. Each glandular lobule drains into the nipple through a lactiferous duct. This duct is surrounded by myoepithelial cells that can contract to eject milk into the nipple. The nipple is infiltrated with smooth muscle that contracts in response to sensory and tactile stimuli, causing the nipple to become erect. Surrounding the nipple is the pigmented areola. Sebaceous glands (the glands of Montgomery) provide local secretion. Extra nipples with breast tissue may occur along a primordial 'milk line' which extends from the axilla to the groin (Fig. 8.10).

Segmental anatomy of the breast

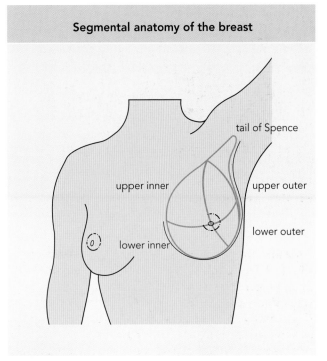

Fig. 8.8 For descriptive purposes, the breast is divided into four quadrants and a tail (of Spence).

LYMPHATIC DRAINAGE OF THE BREAST

As breast cancer spreads to regional lymph nodes, it is important to appreciate lymphatic drainage because the discovery of affected nodes implies a more serious prognosis and influences the mode of treatment. In general, the lymphatics follow the blood supply, yet there

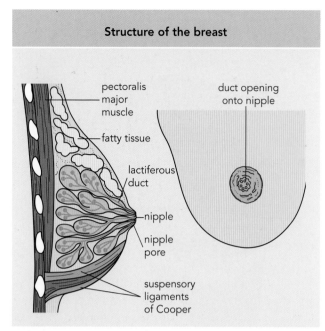

Fig. 8.9 The breast is formed by glands with their ducts opening individually through the nipple. Fatty tissue shapes the breast and the fibrous (Cooper's) ligaments provide support.

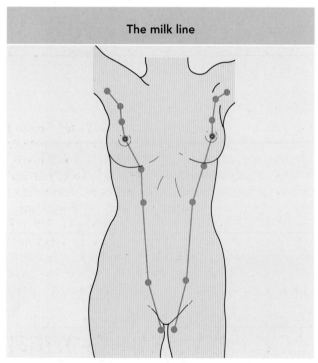

Fig. 8.10 Supernumerary nipples and breast tissue may appear along the milk line.

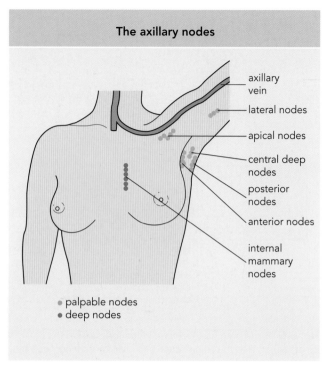

Fig. 8.11 Diagrammatic representation illustrating the position of the axillary lymph nodes.

is a free connection between the lymphatics of the one breast, and sometimes with the other. Nonetheless, the lateral part of the breast usually drains towards the axillary group of nodes and the medial half towards the internal mammary chain. The axillary nodes are arranged into five groups, each of which must be examined (Fig. 8.11). The vast interconnection of lymphatics predisposes to widespread metastatic spread, with nodes in the opposite axilla becoming affected. Even the abdominal nodes may be involved.

FUNCTION OF THE BREAST

During puberty, glandular growth is primarily under the trophic influence of oestradiol and progesterone. Throughout pregnancy, the breasts enlarge further under the influences of rising concentrations of oestrogens, progesterone, placental lactogen and prolactin secreted by the anterior pituitary. A darkish ring (secondary areola) appears around the areola during pregnancy. Suckling by the newborn child stimulates a neuroendocrine reflex that causes further release of prolactin as well as oxytocin (from the posterior pituitary). Oxytocin (which also has a uterine-contracting action) stimulates contraction of the myoepithelial cells surrounding the lobules and lactiferous ducts, causing the expression of milk (Fig. 8.12). The effect of sucking on the nipple sustains lactation. Feeding mothers produce approximately 1 litre of milk daily. When the child is weaned, the sucking reflex is lost and lactation dries up.

Symptoms of breast disease

PAIN

Throughout the menstrual cycle there are cyclical, trophic and involutional changes in the glandular tissue. This dynamic response of the tissue to changes in hormones may cause breast pain and tenderness which fluctuates predictably with the menstrual cycle, usually more

The suckling reflex in lactation

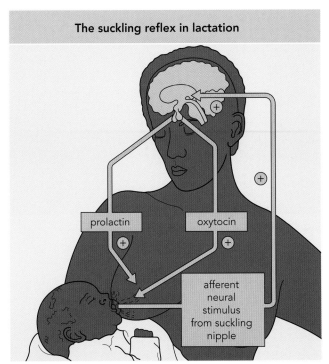

prolactin   oxytocin

afferent
neural
stimulus
from suckling
nipple

Fig. 8.12 Sucking sends an afferent stimulus to the anterior and posterior pituitary, resulting in the release of prolactin and oxytocin.

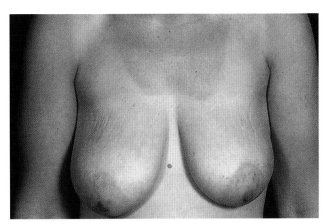

Fig. 8.13 Initially, inspect the breast from the front with the patient sitting with her arms comfortably resting at her sides.

towards the end of a cycle. A painful breast in the first few months of lactation is almost always due to a bacterial infection of the gland and is characterised by fever as well as redness and tenderness over the infected segment. Ask about local trauma, as fat necrosis may cause pain, and also consider thrombophlebitis of the veins (Mondor's disease).

DISCHARGE

Patients may present with an abnormal nipple discharge. Determine whether the fluid is clear, opalescent or bloodstained. In men, and women who have never conceived, a discharge is always abnormal. However, after childbearing, some women continue to discharge a small secretion well after lactation has stopped. The inappropriate secretion of milk (galactorrhoea) is caused by a deranged prolactin physiology. A blood discharge should always alert you to the likelihood of an underlying breast cancer.

BREAST LUMPS

A patient may present after discovering a breast lump by self-examination. This discovery causes great alarm because the patient will usually associate the lump with breast cancer.

Examination of the breast

You will usually examine the breast in the course of the chest examination. In asymptomatic women, you will need to decide whether to include a full breast examination as part of your routine examination. Male doctors must always examine in the presence of a female nurse or chaperone. The aim of examination is to check for breast lumps and it is reasonable to recommend a formal breast examination in asymptomatic women over the age of 40 years. Before examining the patient, suggest to her that the general examination of the chest offers a good opportunity to check the breasts for lumps. Remember to inform her of your findings (reassurance is the best of all medicines). Many techniques have been described, yet the principles remain similar.

INSPECTION

The patient should undress to the waist. Position yourself in front of the patient, who should be sitting comfortably with her arms at her side (Fig. 8.13). Note the size, symmetry and contour of the breasts, the colour and venous pattern of the skin. Observe the nipples and note whether they are symmetrically everted, flat or inverted. If there is unilateral flattening or nipple inversion, ask whether this is a recent or long-standing appearance. In fair-skinned women, the areola has a pink colour but darkens and becomes permanently pigmented during the first pregnancy. Ask the patient to raise her arms above

| Differential diagnosis |
| Breast lumps |

Benign
- Fibroadenoma (mobile)
- Simple cyst
- Fat necrosis
- Fibroadenosis (tender 'lumpy' breasts)
- Abscess (painful and tender)

Malignant
- Glandular
- Areolar

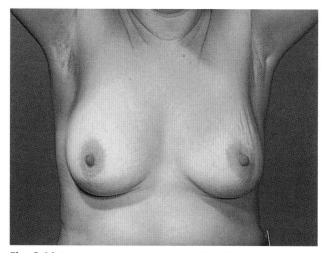

Fig. 8.14 To accentuate any asymmetry of the breast ask the patient to raise her arms above her head.

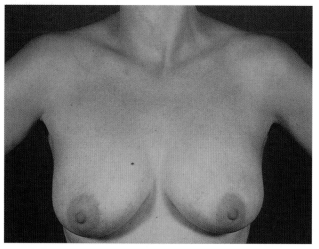

Fig. 8.15 Another technique for accentuating the breast contours is by pressing the hands against the hips.

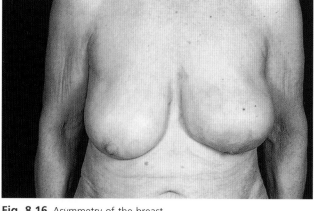

Fig. 8.16 Asymmetry of the breast.

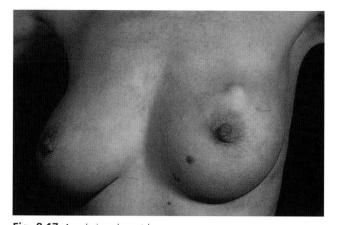

Fig. 8.17 An obvious breast lump.

Red flag – urgent referral
Signs suggestive of breast cancer (see also Fig. 8.18)

- Skin dimpling
- Everted, flat or retracted nipple

her head and then press her hands against her hips (Figs 8.14, 8.15). These movements tighten the suspensory ligaments, exaggerating the contours and highlighting any abnormality. In men, the nipple should lie flat on the pectoralis muscle.

ABNORMALITIES ON INSPECTION

In normal women there may be some asymmetry of the breast and nipples, ranging from unilateral hypoplasia to a mild but obvious asymmetry (Fig. 8.16). You may be struck by an obvious lump (Fig. 8.17), retraction or gross deviation of a nipple (Fig. 8.18), prominent veins or oedema of the skin with dimpling like an orange skin (peau d'orange). Abnormal reddening, thickening or ulceration of the areola should alert you to the possibility of Paget's disease of the breast, a specialised form of breast cancer (Fig. 8.19). Male gynaecomastia is an important physical sign and may be spotted on inspection as a swelling of the areola or, in more florid cases, the development of obvious breasts (see Ch. 9).

BREAST PALPATION

During the chest examination the patient will be lying on the examination couch with her arms resting comfortably at her side or held above her head. Palpate the breast tissue with the palmar surface of the middle three fingers, using an even rotary movement to compress the breast tissue gently towards the chest wall (Fig. 8.20). Examine each breast by following a concentric or parallel trail that creates a systematic path that always begins and ends at a constant spot (Fig. 8.21). An obsessive and systematic exploration of all the breast tissue ensures that small lumps which could be easily missed are not. If the breasts are abnormally large or pendulous, use one hand to steady the breast on its lower border while palpating

Signs suggestive of breast cancer

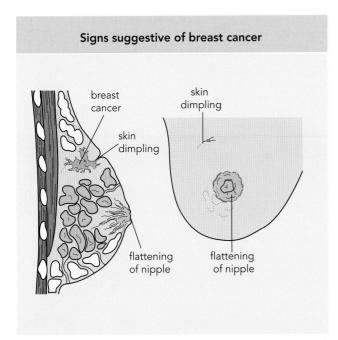

Fig. 8.18 Signs suggestive of breast cancer. Nipples may be everted, flat or retracted.

with the other. The texture of normal breast tissue varies from smooth to granular, even knotty; only experience will teach you the spectrum of normality. Texture may also vary with the menstrual cycle; nodularity and tenderness often increases towards the end of a cycle and during menstruation. Remember that breast texture is normally symmetrical and a comparison of the two breasts may help you to judge whether an area is abnormal or not.

To examine the axillary tail of Spence, ask the patient to rest her arms above her head. Feel the tail between your thumb and fingers as it extends from the upper outer quadrant towards the axilla (Fig. 8.22). If you feel a breast lump, examine the mass between your fingers and assess its size, consistency, mobility and whether or not there is any tenderness.

In men, palpation helps distinguish true from 'pseudo' gynaecomastia (obesity with fatty breast). In true gynaecomastia a disc of breast tissue can be felt under the areola. Unlike fat, breast tissue has a distinctly lobular texture and may be tender to palpation.

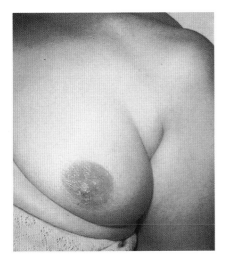

Fig. 8.19 Typical appearance of Paget's disease of the breast with reddening and scaling of the areolar skin.

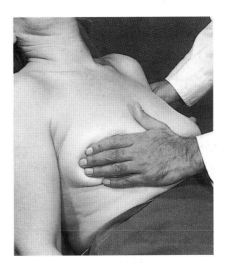

Fig. 8.20 Palpate the breast with the middle three fingers, rotating around the point of contract while pressing firmly but gently towards the chest wall.

Suggested directions of breast palpation

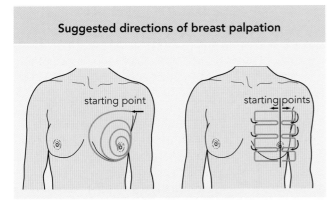

Fig. 8.21 Trace a systematic path either by following a concentric circular pattern (left) or examining each half of the breast sequentially from above down (right).

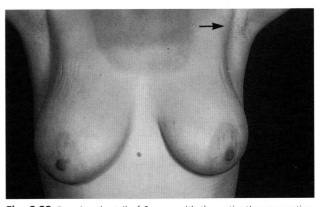

Fig. 8.22 Examine the tail of Spence with the patient's arms resting above the head. Use your thumb and first two fingers to trace the extension of breast tissue between the upper outer quadrant and the axilla.

NIPPLE PALPATION

Hold the nipple between thumb and fingers and gently compress and attempt to express any discharge (Fig. 8.23). If fluid appears, note its colour, prepare a smear for cytology and send a swab for microbiology.

LYMPH NODE PALPATION

The axillae can be palpated with the patient lying or sitting. When examining the left axilla in the sitting position, the patient may rest her (or his) left hand on your right shoulder while you explore the axilla with your right hand. Alternatively, there are different techniques for exposing the axilla. You may choose to abduct the arm gently by supporting the patient's wrist with your right hand and examining with the other hand (Fig. 8.24). The opposite hands are used to examine the other axilla. Slightly cup your examining hand and palpate into the apex of the axilla for the apical group of nodes. Small nodes may be felt only by rotating the exploring fingertips firmly against the chest wall. Next, feel for the anterior group of nodes along the posterior border of the anterior axillary fold, the central group against the lateral chest wall and the posterior group along the posterior axillary fold. Finally, palpate along the medial border of the humerus to check for the lateral group of nodes and inspect the infraclavicular and supraclavicular spaces for lymphadenopathy. If you feel nodes, assess the size, shape, consistency, mobility and tenderness.

ABNORMAL PALPATION

Breast lumps

Although there are clinical features that may favour a benign lesion rather than malignancy, all breast lumps should be investigated for possible malignancy. Common benign lumps include fibroadenomas, fibroadenosis, benign breast cysts and fat necrosis. A fibroadenoma is usually felt as a discreet, firm and smooth lump that is mobile in its surrounding tissue (endearingly referred to as a 'breast mouse'). Fibroadenosis is a bilateral condition characterised by 'lumpiness' of the breasts, which may be tender, especially in the premenstrual and menstrual phases of the cycle. Cancerous lesions usually feel hard and irregular and, unlike benign lesions, may be fixed to the skin or the underlying chest wall muscle. Special tests such as mammography, needle aspiration and biopsy may be necessary to differentiate benign from malignant diseases.

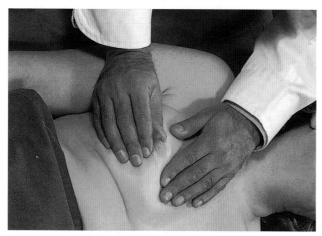

Fig. 8.23 Inspection of the nipple.

 Risk factors

Risk factors for breast cancer

- Family history – (10%)
- Genetic mutations – (5–10% BRCA1, BRCA2 positive)
- Endogenous hormones – oestrogen
- Long-term hormone replacement therapy
- Age at menarche (higher risk with earlier menarche)
- Parity – nulliparous women at higher risk

Breast abscess (mastitis)

This usually occurs during lactation and is generally caused by blockage of a duct. The temperature is raised and the skin of the infected breasts inflamed (Fig. 8.25). Palpation may reveal an area of tenderness and induration. If an abscess forms, you usually feel an extremely tender fluctuant mass.

Abnormal nipple and areola

A bloodstained nipple discharge suggests an intraductal carcinoma or benign papilloma. Unilateral retraction or distortion of a nipple should also alert you to the possibility of malignancy, especially if the abnormality is relatively recent. A unilateral red, crusty and scaling areola suggests Paget's disease of the breast (Fig. 8.19).

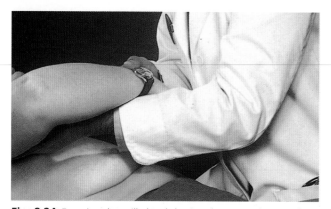

Fig. 8.24 Exposing the axilla by abducting the arm and supporting it at the wrist.

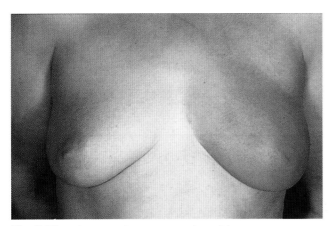

Fig. 8.25 Erythema overlying an area of mastitis.

This disorder should alert you to a likely ductal carcinoma underlying the areola. Blockage of the sebaceous glands of Montgomery may cause retention cysts.

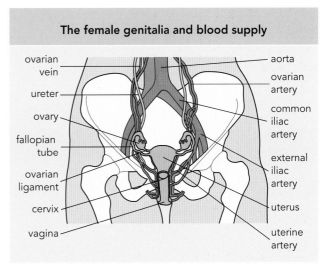

The female genitalia and blood supply

ovarian vein · aorta · ureter · ovarian artery · ovary · common iliac artery · fallopian tube · external iliac artery · ovarian ligament · cervix · uterus · vagina · uterine artery

Fig. 8.26 The female pelvis and internal genitalia.

Symptoms and signs

Breast examination

Inspection
- Symmetry and contour
- Venous pattern of skin
- Nipples (asymmetry, inversion)
- Areola (chloasma, skin ulceration, thickening)

Breast palpation
- Texture
- Symmetry
- Tenderness
- Masses (mobility, size)
- Tail of Spence

Lymph node palpation
- Axillary nodes (five groups)
- Contralateral axillary nodes
- Infraclavicular and supraclavicular nodes

Palpable lymph nodes

If you detect axillary lymphadenopathy, suspect malignancy if the nodes are hard, nontender or fixed. Infection of axillary hair follicles or breast tissue may cause tender lymphadenitis. Look carefully for a local primary site of infection such as an abrasion caused by shaving the axilla. Occasionally, patients with longstanding fibrocystic disease may have mild axillary node enlargement.

Structure of the genital tract

The female reproductive organs include the ovaries, fallopian tubes, uterus and vagina. These organs lie deep in the pelvis (Fig. 8.26), occupying the space between the

---

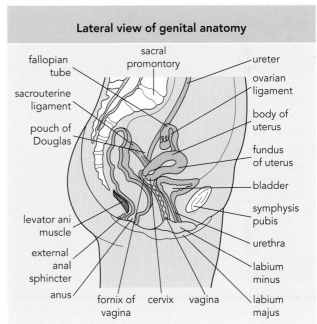

Lateral view of genital anatomy

fallopian tube · sacral promontory · ureter · sacrouterine ligament · ovarian ligament · pouch of Douglas · body of uterus · fundus of uterus · bladder · levator ani muscle · symphysis pubis · external anal sphincter · urethra · anus · labium minus · fornix of vagina · cervix · vagina · labium majus

Fig. 8.27 Lateral view of the female internal genitalia showing the relationship to the rectum and bladder.

rectum posteriorly and the bladder and ureter anteriorly (Fig. 8.27). The female internal genitalia can be inspected through the vagina, the cervix can be palpated directly or through the anterior rectal wall, and the uterus, fallopian tubes and ovaries can be examined using the technique of bimanual palpation.

VULVA

The external genitalia in the female is termed the vulva (Fig. 8.28). This comprises a fat pad that overlies the symphysis pubis (the mons pubis), a pair of prominent hair-lined skin folds extending on either side from the mons to meet posteriorly in the midline in front of the

The anatomy of the external genitalia

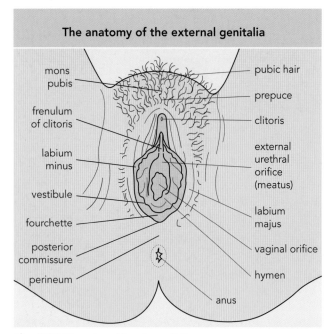

Fig. 8.28 The external female genitalia.

The pelvic floor

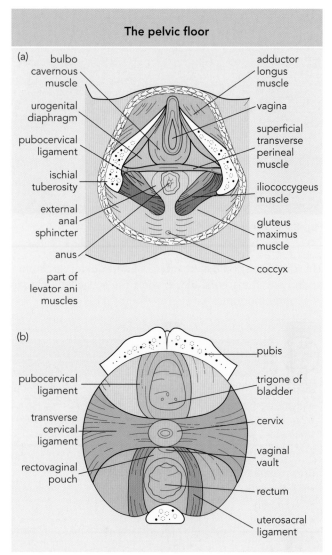

Fig. 8.29 The pelvic floor supports the pelvic organs. (a) Superficial perineal muscles. (b) Fascia and ligaments.

anal verge (the labia majora), and a pair of hairless, flat folds lying adjacent and medial to the labia majora (the labia minora). The labia minora converge anteriorly in front of the vaginal orifice, with each splitting into two small folds that meet in the midline. The anterior folds from either side merge to form the prepuce; the posterior folds form the frenulum. A nub of erectile tissue (the clitoris) lies tucked between the frenulum and prepuce. Posteriorly, the labia minora fuse to form a distinct ridge known as the fourchette. The labia minora demarcate the vestibule, which contains the urethral meatus and vaginal orifice. Bartholin's glands are a pair of pea-sized mucous glands that lie deep to the posterior margin of the labia minora and empty through a duct into the vestibule, providing lubrication of the introitus. Bartholin's glands may become infected if the ducts are obstructed, resulting in painful swelling and abscess formation.

The vulva rests on the pelvic floor, which is formed by a complex arrangement of muscles that support the rectum, vagina and urethra (Fig. 8.29).

VAGINA

The vagina is a tube-shaped passage connecting the vulva to the cervix of the uterus. Its opening in the vulva (the introitus) lies between the urethra and anus. The vagina is inclined in an upward and posterior direction. A connective tissue septum separates the vagina anteriorly from the bladder base and urethra and posteriorly from the rectum. The uterine cervix pouts through the upper vault of the vagina and divides the blind end of the vagina into the anterior, posterior and lateral fornices (Fig. 8.30). These thin-walled fornices provide a convenient access point for examining the pelvic organs.

UTERUS

The uterus is a muscular, pear-shaped organ consisting of the cervix, body and fundus (Fig. 8.31). The adult uterus is usually angled forward from the plane of the vagina (anteverted) and bends forward on itself at the junction of the internal os and the body (anteflexion) (Fig. 8.32a). In some women the uterus assumes different positions: an anteverted uterus may lie retroflexed (Fig. 8.32b) and a retroverted uterus may be anteflexed (Fig. 8.32c) or retroflexed (Fig. 8.32d).

The vaginal surface of the cervix is covered by stratified squamous epithelium. The uterus is covered with peritoneum which reflects anteriorly onto the bladder, posteriorly onto the rectum and laterally to form the broad ligaments. The peritoneum covering the posterior uterus and upper vagina reflects onto the anterior rectal wall forming a blind pocket: the Pouch of Douglas. The cuboidal cells lining the uterine cavity (the endometrium) respond to the hormonal changes of the menstrual cycle.

The fornices of the vagina

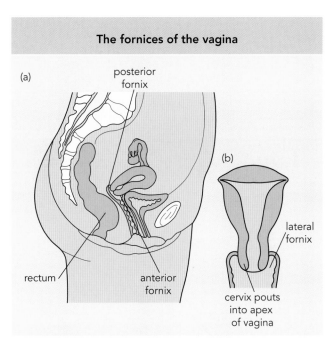

Fig. 8.30 The cervix projects into the vagina, creating the anterior, posterior (a) and lateral fornices (b).

The uterus

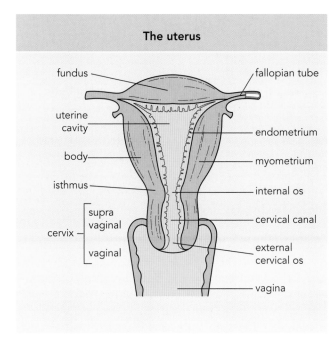

Fig. 8.31 Section through the pear-shaped, muscular uterus showing the cervix, isthmus, body (corpus) and fundus. The mucosa is called the endometrium. The cervical canal has an internal and external os.

Different positions of the uterus

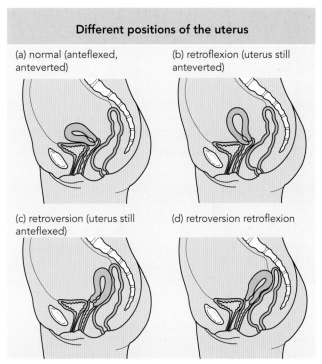

Fig. 8.32 The different anatomical positions of the uterine body within the pelvis. (a) The normal uterus is angled forward from the plane of the vagina (anteverted) and bends forward on itself (anteflexed). In some women the uterus assumes different positions: (b) retroflexed, anteverted; (c) retroverted, anteflexed; (d) retroverted, retroflexed.

Ovarian ligaments and adnexal structures

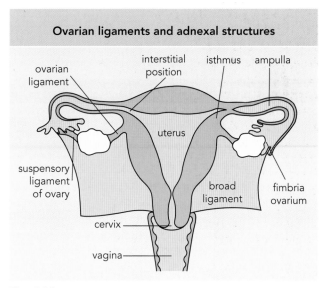

Fig. 8.33 Coronal section of the uterus and fallopian tubes showing the ligamentous attachments of the ovary.

ADNEXAE

The adnexae refers to the fallopian tubes, ovaries and their connective tissue attachments.

Fallopian tubes

The fallopian tubes insert into the upper outer uterus (the cornu) and project laterally along the free edge of the broad ligaments curving around the ovaries (Fig. 8.33).

The tubes vary in length from 8 cm to 14 cm and open into the peritoneum through the trumpet-shaped infundibulum. The entrance to the fallopian tube (the ostium) is bounded by fringe-like fimbria that overlie the ovary and help to capture the ovum when it is expelled in midcycle. The ovum moves along the fallopian tube by a combination of peristalsis and the wafting action of the cilia on the mucosal lining cells.

Ovaries

There are two ovaries. Each is oval in shape and usually rests in a slight depression in the side wall of the pelvis. The ovary is not lined by peritoneum; it measures 3 cm long, 2 cm wide and 1 cm thick. The ovarian ligament connects the ovary to the cornu of the uterus. The connective tissue stroma of the ovary contains graafian follicles at various stages of development, the corpus luteum, which develops after ovulation, and the corpus albicans, a relic of a degenerating corpus luteum.

Pelvic fascia and ligaments

The connective tissue overlying the muscular floor of the pelvis condenses into ligaments that stabilise and support the pelvic organs by attachments to the pelvis. The cardinal ligaments (Mackenrodt's ligaments) span laterally, connecting the cervix and upper vagina to the bony pelvis. The uterosacral ligaments pass posteriorly and backwards from the posterolateral cervix, attaching to the periosteum overlying the sacroiliac joints and the midsacrum. The pubocervical fascia extends forward from the cardinal ligament, joining to the pubic bone on either side of the bladder. These pelvic ligaments and the muscular floor of the pelvis may become lax and weaken, allowing the pelvic organs to drop and prolapse (Fig 8.34; and see Fig. 8.49).

The broad ligament is formed from the peritoneum that suspends from the lateral wall of the uterus to the lateral wall of the pelvis. The fallopian tubes, ovarian ligament, uterine and ovarian vessels and lymphatics run in the broad ligament.

Symptoms of genital tract disease

There may be initial reluctance to discuss genital and sexual disorders but with gentle coaxing you should be able to lead the patient towards a frank account of her sexual history. The degree to which you pursue the history depends on the relevance to the patient's problems. Organic and psychological disorders may affect sexual function and this may be important, although not central, to the presenting disease. Cardiac and respiratory disease may interfere with normal sexual activity; after a myocardial infarct there is often concern about recommencing a normal sex life. Reduction or loss of libido is common in acute and chronic illness. Patients with psychological disorders such as anorexia nervosa or depression may present with a primary complaint of loss of libido or a menstrual disorder. In contrast, patients suffering from primary sexual problems may present with physical symptoms, such as abdominal pain, that may camouflage the underlying sexual problem.

The genital-sexual history commonly follows the urinary history. You may find that asking about previous pregnancies or the pattern of the menstrual cycle provides a suitable platform for more detailed questioning.

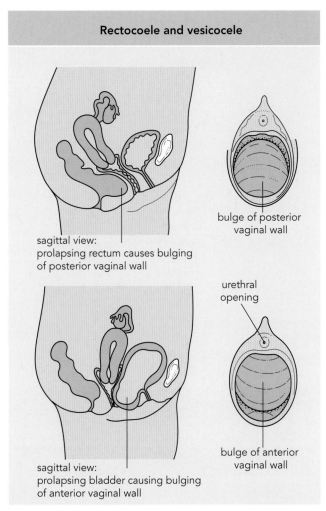

Rectocoele and vesicocele

sagittal view: prolapsing rectum causes bulging of posterior vaginal wall

bulge of posterior vaginal wall

urethral opening

sagittal view: prolapsing bladder causing bulging of anterior vaginal wall

bulge of anterior vaginal wall

Fig. 8.34 Pelvic floor examination. (a) Prolapsing rectum causes bulging of posterior vaginal wall. (b) Prolapsing bladder causing bulging of the anterior wall.

MENSTRUAL HISTORY

Establish the age of the menarche

As a result of the wide variation in the age of the menarche, parents and children may be unduly concerned about delay. Most European and North American girls start menstruating by the age of 14.5 years (range 9–16 years). Body weight appears to play a role and the menarche occurs at an average weight of 48 kg. If there is anxiety about delayed menarche or primary amenorrhoea, ask whether or not pubic and axillary hair growth and breast development have commenced. By the age of 14 years, secondary sexual characteristics should have appeared. If the menarche has not occurred and there are no other signs of sexual development, it is reasonable to consider organic causes of primary amenorrhoea, such as gonadal dysgenesis (Turner's syndrome), congenital anatomical abnormalities of the genital tract (e.g. absence, uterine hypoplasia, vaginal hypoplasia), polycystic ovaries or pituitary or hypothalamic tumours in childhood. If secondary sexual characteristics have appeared, reassure the patient that investigation is usually only necessary if the menarche has not occurred by the age of 16 years.

Determine the pattern of the menstrual cycle

Throughout the childbearing years, women should be encouraged to specify the starting date of each menstrual period (i.e. the date when bleeding commences). Record the starting date of the most recent period. The duration of the menstrual cycle is calculated from the first day of bleeding to the first day of bleeding in the next menstrual cycle. This cycle may vary from 21 to 35 days in normal women but the average duration is 28 days. Most healthy, fertile women have regular, predictable cycles that vary in duration by 1 or 2 days. Once regular periods are established, concern is soon aroused if there is deviation from the norm.

Questions to ask

The menstrual cycle

- Age of menarche?
- Age of telarche?
- Do you use the contraceptive pill or hormone replacement therapy?
- Length of cycle?
- Days of blood loss?
- Number of tampons or pads used per day?
- Are there clots?
- Has there been a change in the periodicity of the cycle?

Blood loss from menstruation averages approximately 70 ml (range 50–200 ml). Attempts to assess menstrual loss are rather inaccurate, yet there are indicators: women with heavy periods saturate rather than stain tampons or pads, whereas the passage of large and frequent clots suggests excessive bleeding. The only accurate method for assessing menstrual loss is to weigh absorbent pads before and after each change.

Attempt to classify any change or abnormality in the menstrual cycle. First establish whether the cycles are regular and, if so, calculate the cycle length and attempt to assess whether the periods are scanty or heavy. Bear in mind contraceptive practices because the patient's intrinsic rhythms will be masked if she is taking a cyclical contraceptive pill or undergoing hormone replacement therapy (HRT) (Fig. 8.35). The most common irregularities include failure to menstruate at the expected time (secondary amenorrhoea). Cycles may be infrequent and scanty (oligomenorrhoea), unusually frequent (polymenorrhoea), excessively heavy (menorrhagia) or frequent and heavy (polymenorrhagia). Bleeding after intercourse is termed postcoital bleeding. If regular cycles are interrupted by days of spotting or blood-tinged discharge, this is known as intermenstrual bleeding.

Effect of LH and FSH on ovarian hormone synthesis

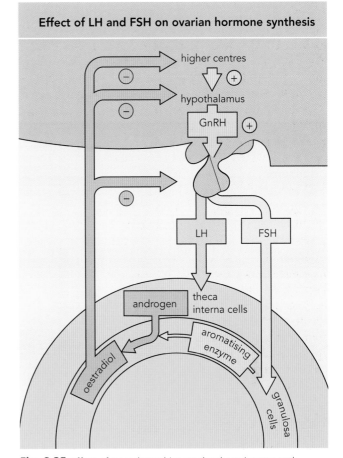

Fig. 8.35 Effect of gonadotrophins on the theca interna and granulosa cells which produce the ovarian hormones.

Secondary amenorrhoea

Develop the case history by considering possible causes of secondary amenorrhoea. Pregnancy and lactation are the most common causes. The patient may suspect a pregnancy: there may be clues such as early morning nausea and vomiting, urinary frequency and tender enlarged breasts. Stress, anxiety, depression, bereavement and a change of environment may interrupt the cyclical release of sex hormones by the hypothalamic–pituitary axis. Consider fear of pregnancy, which is a common cause of delayed menstruation. Not only do patients with excessive weight loss due to anorexia nervosa present with amenorrhoea but highly trained long-distance athletes may also stop menstruating. Enquire about contraceptive practices as 'post pill' amenorrhoea is well recognised. Consider the menopause in women entering the climacteric years. This is often heralded by a change in the cyclical pattern, reduced menstrual flow and the onset of menopausal symptoms such as hot flushes and dryness of the introitus and vagina. In the absence of an obvious cause for amenorrhoea, consider diseases of the hypothalamus, pituitary and ovary.

Differential diagnosis
Secondary amenorrhoea

Physiological
- Pregnancy
- Lactation

Psychological
- Anorexia nervosa
- Depression
- Fear of pregnancy

Hormonal
- Post contraceptive pill
- Pituitary tumours
- Hyperthyroidism
- Adrenal tumours

Ovarian
- Polycystic ovaries
- Ovarian tumour
- Ovarian tuberculosis
- Constitutional disease
- Severe acute illness
- Chronic infections or illnesses
- Autoimmune diseases

Abnormal patterns of uterine bleeding

Oligomenorrhoea Oligomenorrhoea is the term used to describe infrequent or scanty menstrual periods. This pattern may be normal between the menarche and the establishment of a regular menstrual pattern and is also a feature of the climacteric as the menopause approaches. In some women, the oligomenorrhoea of puberty persists into adult life. Ascertain whether the infrequent, scanty periods are a change from the normal pattern or a pattern present from puberty. If oligomenorrhoea presents as a distinct change in the menstrual pattern, consider the same factors implicated in the differential diagnosis of secondary amenorrhoea.

Dysfunctional uterine bleeding This term is used to describe frequent bleeding or excessive menstrual loss that cannot be ascribed to local pelvic pathology (e.g. fibroids, pelvic inflammatory disease, carcinoma, polyps). Establish whether the abnormal cyclical pattern is regular or irregular. Regular dysfunctional bleeding may present as menorrhagia, epimenorrhoea or polymenorrhoea. The predictability of these abnormal cycles usually implies that ovulation is occurring, although this needs to be confirmed. Irregular dysfunctional bleeding usually implies that ovulation has ceased; the menstrual rhythm is lost and the cyclical pattern is replaced by unpredictable bleeding of varying severity.

Intermenstrual and postmenopausal bleeding Patients may complain of vaginal bleeding unexpectedly between normal periods or after the menopause. Enquire about sex hormone therapy, as 'breakthrough bleeding' may occur with hormone treatment. Diseases of the uterus and cervix may present with abnormal bleeding, so consider disorders of the mucosa (e.g. endometritis, carcinoma, endometrial polyps) or submucosa (e.g. submucosal leiomyomas, fibroids). Postcoital bleeding usually indicates local cervical or uterine disease (carcinoma or a cervical polyp).

Vaginal discharge

Vaginal discharge is a common complaint during the child-bearing years. Many women notice slight soiling of the underwear at the end of the day; this is a normal physiological response to the cyclical changes occurring in the glandular epithelium of the genital tract and it is likely to become more profuse in pregnancy. A physiological discharge is scanty, mucoid and odourless. Pathological discharge is usually trichomonal or candidal vaginitis. The discharge may irritate the vulval skin causing itching (pruritus vulvae) or burning. Attempt to assess the severity of the discharge by ascertaining whether the discharge merely stains the underwear or is heavier and requires protective pads.

Differential diagnosis
Vaginal discharge

Physiological
- Pregnancy
- Sexual arousal
- Menstrual cycle variation

Pathological
- Vaginal
  - candidosis (thrush)
  - trichomoniasis
  - Gardnerella associated
  - other bacteria (e.g. caused by a retained tampon)
  - postmenopausal vaginitis
- Cervical
  - gonorrhoea
  - nonspecific genital infection
  - herpes
  - cervical ectopy
  - cervical neoplasm (e.g. polyp)
  - intrauterine contraceptive device

Questions to ask
Vaginal discharge

- How long has the discharge been present?
- Is the discharge scanty or profuse?
- Is extra protection necessary or does the discharge simply spot or stain?
- What is the colour and consistency?
- Is there an odour?
- Is the discharge bloodstained?
- Is there associated lower abdominal pain and fever?
- Is there itching or burning of the vulval area?

The nature of the discharge may be helpful. With vaginitis caused by *Candida albicans* the discharge is white, has a curd-like appearance and consistency (Fig. 8.36) and causes intense itching. Vaginitis caused by *Trichomonas vaginalis* usually presents with a profuse opaque or cream-coloured, frothy discharge that has a characteristic 'fishy' smell (Fig. 8.37). The trichomonal discharge may cause vulval irritation and is occasionally accompanied by burning on micturition: this is caused by inflammation of the urethral meatus. If the patient complains of a profuse, foul-smelling discharge, consider a retained foreign body (e.g. a tampon). Cervical infection due to gonorrhoea, *Chlamydia trachomatis* or nonspecific cervicitis may present with a discharge but, unlike vaginitis, these rarely cause itching or burning of the vulva.

Pain

Gynaecological disorders should always be considered in women presenting with lower abdominal pain. If the pain predictably occurs immediately before and during a period, the likely cause is dysmenorrhoea. This is a suprapubic, boring or cramp-like pain caused by intense pelvic congestion; it occurs a day or two before menstruation or with uterine contraction during the shedding and expulsion of the endometrium. Severe dysmenorrhoea should alert you to the possibility of endometriosis, a disorder resulting from cyclical changes (including withdrawal bleeding) occurring in endometrial tissue implanted in ectopic sites (e.g. in the fallopian tubes or peritoneum).

Ovulation may cause a unilateral iliac fossa or suprapubic pain in midcycle that lasts a few hours (mittelschmertz). Severe iliac fossa pain should warn you of the possibility of a haemorrhage into an ovarian cyst or torsion of a cyst. If the pain is preceded by a missed period, and especially if there is shock, you should also consider the possibility of a ruptured ectopic pregnancy. If the lower abdominal pain is accompanied by a vaginal discharge, fever, anorexia and nausea, consider acute infection of the fallopian tubes (acute salpingitis).

Dyspareunia

Pain on intercourse (dyspareunia) may be caused by either psychological or organic disorders. Try to distinguish vaginal spasm that makes penetration difficult (vaginismus) from pain occurring once penetration has occurred. Assess whether the pain is superficial (suggesting a local vulval cause or a psychological spasm) or deep (suggesting inflammatory or malignant disease of the cervix, uterus or adnexae). After the menopause, the vulva and vagina become dry and atrophic and this may cause discomfort on intercourse.

PSYCHOSEXUAL HISTORY

A satisfactory sex life is an important component of a healthy emotional relationship. In an unmarried woman, ask whether she has had intercourse. Patients may complain of loss of sex drive (libido), failure to achieve orgasm, pain or difficulty with intercourse and ambivalence about sexual preference. These symptoms and personal problems are often camouflaged behind other symptoms such as nonspecific abdominal pain, depression, fatigue or headache. It requires shrewd clinical judgement to recognise the underlying psychosexual problem. Tactfully enquire about the sexual history.

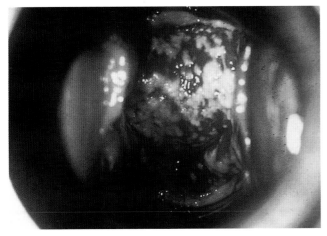

Fig. 8.36 Vaginal candidiasis has a curd-like appearance.

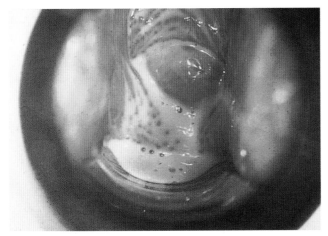

Fig. 8.37 Trichomoniasis.

Questions to ask

Psychosexual history

- Are you able to develop satisfying emotional relationships?
- Do you have satisfying physical relationships?
- Are you heterosexual, homosexual or ambivalent?
- Do you use contraception and, if so, what form?
- Do you have problems achieving arousal?
- Do you experience orgasm?

OBSTETRIC HISTORY

Enquire whether the patient has ever been pregnant and whether there were fertility problems. Record the number of completed and unsuccessful pregnancies. If the patient has miscarried, record the maturity of the pregnancy at the time of miscarriage. Ask about complications during pregnancy (e.g. hypertension, diabetes) and problems associated with labour and the period after delivery (the puerperium).

? Questions to ask

Obstetric history

- Have you ever been pregnant and, if so, how often?
- Did you have any problems falling pregnant?
- How many children do you have?
- Have you miscarried and, if so, at what stage of pregnancy?
- Were there any complications in pregnancy (e.g. high blood pressure or diabetes)?
- Was the labour normal or did you require forceps assistance or a caesarean section?

Examination of the female genital tract

Examination of the genitalia is intrusive; nonetheless, most women are psychologically prepared if they are seeking attention for a gynaecological disorder. In the course of taking the history you should already have established a rapport with your patient and if there are gynaecological symptoms the examination should follow naturally.

Before the examination, take the time to explain the need for the examination and the procedure. If you have no reason to suspect a painful examination, reassure the patient that there should be little discomfort. If there is a suggestion of vaginitis or pelvic inflammatory disease, explain that there may be a little discomfort and that the patient should inform you if there is pain. While ensuring the patient's comfort and privacy you should always be accompanied by a nurse who can provide reassurance for the patient and assist you with the procedure (e.g. speculum examination, cervical smears).

Before the examination, ask the patient to empty her bladder. This adds to the comfort of the examination and excludes a full bladder in the differential diagnosis of suprapubic and pelvic swellings. Ensure that a clean gown is available and that there are satisfactory facilities for the patient to undress.

GENERAL EXAMINATION

Before examining the genital tract you should perform a general examination. Excessive facial hair (hirsutism) may be normal but if overly excessive may provide a clue

to an endocrine imbalance. Anaemia may occur with menstrual disorders and you may recognise syndromes that are commonly associated with menstrual disorders (e.g. thyrotoxicosis, myxoedema, Cushing's syndrome, anorexia nervosa, other serious chronic diseases). You will have examined the breasts during the chest examination and assessed the development of secondary sexual characteristics.

Examination of the abdomen

A full abdominal examination precedes the vulval and vaginal examination. Although the uterus and adnexae lie deep within the protective confines of the pelvis, abnormalities may be apparent above the pubis. Lower abdominal tenderness occurs in pelvic inflammatory disease and enlargement of the uterus or ovaries may present with a palpable lower abdominal mass. Large ovarian cysts may fill the abdomen; this presentation is readily mistaken for ascites. Careful abdominal percussion helps distinguish ascites from a cystic ovarian tumour. A large ovarian cyst displaces the bowel laterally, and on percussion there is central dullness with resonance in the flanks (Fig. 8.38). This contrasts with ascites, which is characterised by central resonance and dullness in the flanks.

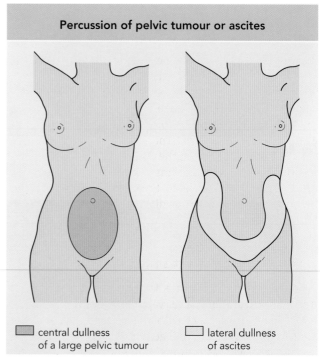

Percussion of pelvic tumour or ascites

central dullness of a large pelvic tumour

lateral dullness of ascites

Fig. 8.38 Careful examination of the abdomen allows differentiation between large ovarian cysts and ascites. An ovarian cyst displaces the bowel towards the flanks: the central abdomen is dull, whereas the flanks are more resonant. This contrasts with ascites, in which the flanks are dull and the central abdomen tympanitic.

Assessing the height of the fundus in pregnancy

week	height of uterus
12	palpable above pubic bone
16	midway between symphysis and umbilicus
20	lower border of umbilicus
28	midway between umbilicus and xiphisternum
34	just below xiphisternum
38–40	height drops as fetal head engages pelvis

Fig. 8.39 The maturity of a pregnancy can be assessed by examining the height of the fundus.

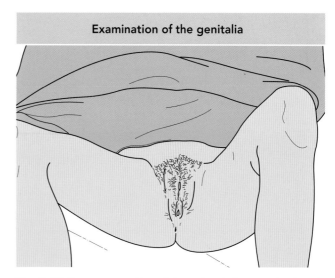

Examination of the genitalia

Fig. 8.40 The correct position of the patient before examination of the genitalia.

Abdomen in pregnancy

After the 12th week of the pregnancy, the uterus becomes palpable above the symphysis pubis, making it possible to assess the maturity of the fetus from the height of the fundus (Fig. 8.39).

Examining the external genitalia

This examination is usually performed on a conventional examination couch. The nurse should prepare and position the patient for the examination. The patient lies supine with the hips and knees flexed and the heels close together. Help the patient to abduct the thighs to allow adequate access to the external genitalia (Fig. 8.40). Use a blanket or sheet to cover the abdomen and mons pubis. Ensure good general lighting; you will also require a direct light source to focus on the vulva. When examining the vulva and vagina, wear disposable plastic gloves on both hands.

INSPECTION AND PALPATION OF THE VULVA

Explain that you are going to examine the labia and the area surrounding the vaginal opening. Maintain intermittent eye contact with the patient. Uncover the mons to expose the external genitalia. The pattern of hair distribution over the mons pubis provides a useful measure of sexual development. Once puberty is complete the mons and outer aspects of the labia majora should be well covered with hair. Systematically examine the labia majora, labia minora, the introitus, urethra and clitoris.

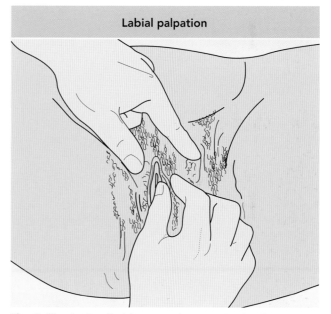

Labial palpation

Fig. 8.41 Palpating the labia majora between the thumb and index finger.

The labia majora on either side lie in close contact in the midline. Gently separate the labia with the fingers of your left hand and inspect the medial aspect, which should be pink and slightly moist. Palpate the length of the labia majora between index finger and thumb (Fig. 8.41); the tissue should feel pliant and fleshy. Next, examine Bartholin's glands between the index finger and thumb (Fig. 8.42). The right index finger palpates from the entrance of the vagina while the thumb palpates the outer surface of the labia majora posteriorly. A normal Bartholin's gland is not palpable.

To expose the vestibule, separate the labia minora. The vestibular tissue should be supple and slightly moist.

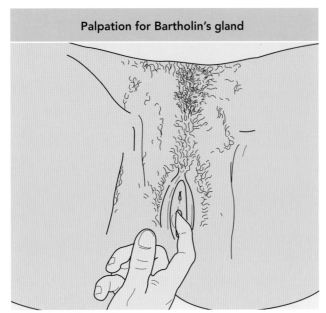

Palpation for Bartholin's gland

Fig. 8.42 Palpating Bartholin's gland with the index finger just inside the introitus and the thumb on the outer aspect of the labium majus.

Separation of the labia minora exposes the vaginal orifice and urethra.

After the menopause the skin and subcutaneous tissue of the external genitalia become atrophic and the mucosa loses its moist texture. These involutional, atrophic changes are normal and result from the loss of ovarian hormones.

Abnormalities of the vulva

A confluent, itchy, red rash on the inner aspects of the thighs and extending to the labia suggests candidiasis (Fig. 8.43). This is often associated with a vaginal discharge and should alert you to the possibility of diabetes or recent treatment with broad-spectrum antibiotics. A vaginal discharge due to candidiasis or a trichomonal infection may irritate the vulval skin, causing redness and tenderness (vulvitis).

The vulva is a common site for boils (furuncles) to appear. These are tender to palpation and should be distinguished from sebaceous cysts, which are firm, rounded, yellowish and nontender, with an apical punctum indicating the opening of the blocked duct.

Many papular vulval lesions are caused by sexually transmitted infections. Crops of small, painful, vulval and perianal papules and vesicles that ulcerate suggest a herpes simplex infection (Fig. 8.44). You may notice multiple genital warts (condylomata acuminata), which can coalesce to form large irregular tissue masses (Figs 8.45, 8.46). Most genital warts are caused by a human papillomavirus. The lesions usually occur on the fourchette and may extend onto the labia, into the vagina, and posteriorly onto the perineum. Flat, round or oval papules covered by a grey exudate suggests lesions of secondary syphilis (condylomata lata) (Fig. 8.47).

Vulval ulceration has a wide differential diagnosis. The most common ulcerating lesions include carcinoma of the vulva or macerated, ulcerating herpetic warts. Acute vulval ulceration occurring with mouth and tongue ulcers and inflamed red eyes suggests Behçet's syndrome. A firm painless labial ulcer suggests the chancre of primary syphilis, whereas broad, moist ulcerating papules covered by grey slough suggest secondary syphilis. Suspect granuloma inguinale (caused by *C. trachomatis*) in women from tropical and subtropical regions presenting with vulval nodules and inguinal lymphadenopathy. The nodules coalesce and ulcerate, forming a large ulcer with rolled edges which must be distinguished from carcinoma. Chancroid, caused by *Haemophilus ducreyi*, is another sexually-transmitted ulcerating disease affecting the vulva.

Leucoplakia is a potentially malignant, hypertrophic skin lesion affecting the labia, clitoris and perineum. The skin thickens, feels hard and indurated and is distinguished from surrounding tissue by its white colour.

Bartholin's glands are palpable if the ducts obstruct. This results in a painless cystic mass or an acute (Bartholin's) abscess: a hot, red, tender swelling in the posterolateral labia majora deep to the posterior end of the labia minora (Fig. 8.48).

Examination of the vagina

If the patient has an intact hymen, you may choose to examine the genitalia indirectly through the rectum. If the woman has an intact hymen but uses vaginal tampons, it is usually possible to perform a single digit vaginal examination.

Before proceeding with the internal examination, separate the labia to expose the vestibule and ask the patient to 'bear down' and exert a downward force on the vulva. If the pelvic floor is stable and the muscles intact, bulges and swellings should not appear through the vaginal walls below the introitus. If there is muscle weakness, the posterior bladder wall may prolapse, causing a bulge (a cystocele) along the anterior vaginal wall (see Fig. 8.34). If the rectum prolapses, this may

Differential diagnosis
Vulval ulceration

Squamous cell carcinoma

Infections
- Syphilitic chancre
- Secondary syphilis
- Granuloma inguinale (Chlamydia)
- Chancroid (*Haemophilus ducreyi*)
- Ulcerating herpetic warts

Behçet's syndrome

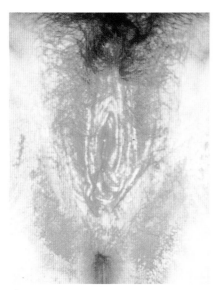

Fig. 8.43 Primary cutaneous candidosis of the vulva.

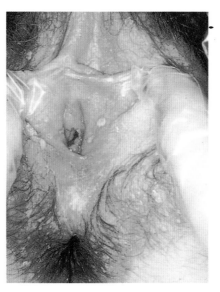

Fig. 8.44 Herpes simplex vesicles in the perianal region, fourchette and inner surface of the labia minora.

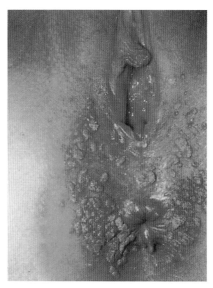

Fig. 8.45 Multiple perianal warts (condylomata acuminata) encroaching onto the labia.

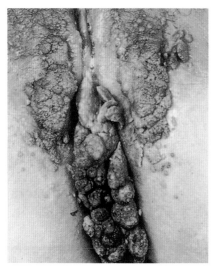

Fig. 8.46 Perianal warts.

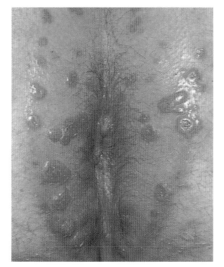

Fig. 8.47 Condylomata lata caused by secondary syphilis tend to occur in moist areas of the body and are prevalent in the vulva and perineum.

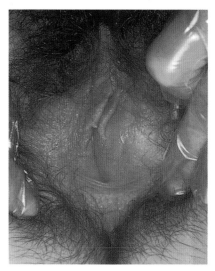

Fig. 8.48 Swelling of posterolateral perineum caused by Bartholin's abscess.

cause a bulge (a rectocele) in the posterior vaginal wall. Uterine prolapse may also occur (Fig. 8.49).

A full vaginal examination includes inspection with a speculum, followed by a bimanual examination of the uterus and adnexae. Before continuing the examination, explain that you are about to inspect the vagina and cervix with a speculum.

SPECULUM EXAMINATION

The speculum is designed for inspection of the cervix and vaginal walls. In addition, the speculum provides access to the cervix and fornices for bacteriological swabs and

cervical smears. If you anticipate taking samples, use water as a lubricant for your gloved fingers and the speculum because lubricant gels may interfere with the processing and analysis of samples.

A bivalve speculum (e.g. Cusco's) is the instrument most commonly used to inspect the vagina (Fig. 8.50). Thoroughly familiarise yourself with its operation before examining a patient. The instrument is made of either stainless steel or plastic, and is available in different sizes. There are two blunt, rounded, elongated blades hinged at the base. In the closed position, the tips of the blades appose, allowing the closed blades to slide safely into the slit-shaped introitus and into the tubular vagina.

Uterine prolapse

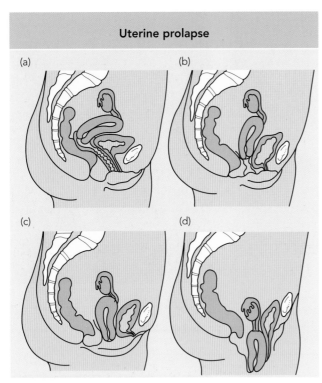

(a)   (b)

(c)   (d)

Fig. 8.49 Uterine prolapse. (a) Normal uterus. (b) First- and (c) second-degree prolapse of the uterus. (d) Complete prolapse of the uterus.

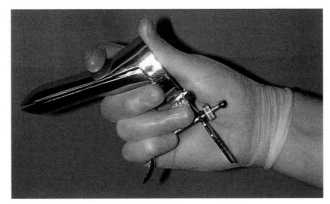

Fig. 8.50 A bivalve Cusco's speculum used for examining the vaginal walls and cervix.

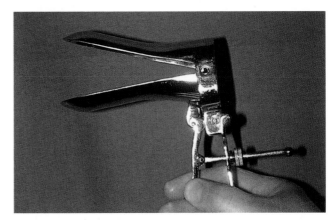

Fig. 8.51 Speculum held in the open position with a lock-nut.

The blades open when the thumbpiece is squeezed (Fig. 8.51) and, once positioned in the vagina, a hinged screw and nut arrangement fixes the blades in the open position.

Warm the blades under a stream of tepid water. The most convenient hand position for holding the speculum is illustrated in Figure 8.50. Explain to the patient that you are about to insert the instrument and reassure her that the procedure should be painless. Use the index and middle fingers of the free hand to separate the labia and expose the introitus (Fig. 8.52a). Position these two fingers just inside the introitus, pressing gently towards the perineal body. Slide the closed blades obliquely over the fingers into the introitus and introduce the instrument into the vagina, directing it to follow the line of the long axis of the vagina, maintaining a posterior angulation of approximately 45° (Fig. 8.52b). While inserting the instrument, rotate it in a clockwise direction until the anterior and posterior blades run along the length of the anterior and posterior vaginal walls with the handles pointing towards the anus (Figs 8.52c,d). Maintain a downward pressure on the speculum and press on the thumbpiece to hinge the blades open (Fig. 8.52e) to expose the vaginal vault and cervix (Fig. 8.52f).

Adjust the light source to illuminate the vagina. If the cervix is not immediately visible, arc the blades anteriorly to bring the cervix into view. If you have difficulty finding the cervix, withdraw the blades a little and reposition the speculum in a more horizontal plane. Make any minor adjustments necessary to establish the optimal position for visualising the cervix, then tighten the thumbscrew to secure the position.

Examination of the cervix

The position of the cervix relates to the position of the uterus (see Fig. 8.32). The cervix usually points posteriorly and the uterus lies in an anterior plane (anteversion). Conversely, the cervix may point anteriorly with the uterus in a posterior retroverted position. There are also intermediate positions between these two. The cervix should lie centrally along the long axis of the vagina projecting 1–3 cm into the vagina. The shape of the external os changes after childbirth. In nulliparous women, the os is round, whereas after childbirth, the os may be slit-like or stellate (Fig. 8.53).

Inspect the colour of the cervix. The colour varies according to the position of the meeting point, usually in the region of the external os, of the squamous epithelium covering the vaginal surface of the cervix and the mucosal lining of the cervical canal. The surface of the cervix is pink, smooth and regular, and resembles the epithelium

Speculum examination of the vagina

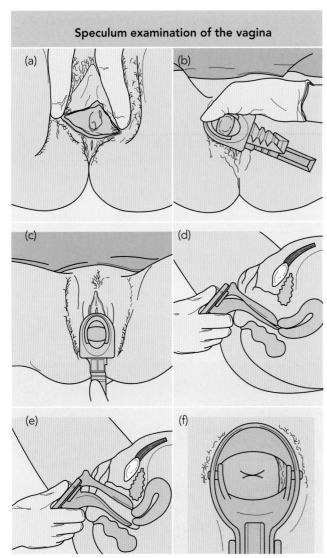

Fig. 8.52 (a) Expose the vaginal opening, (b) direct the closed speculum into the vagina, (c) rotate the speculum as it penetrates the long axis. (d) Final position of the fully inserted speculum. (e) Open the blades. (f) Search for the cervix and os.

External os

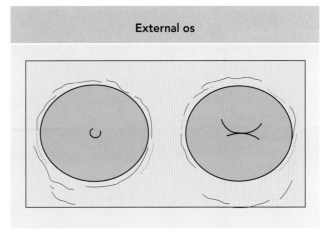

Fig. 8.53 In nulliparous women, the external os is round (left); it becomes slit-shaped (right) after birth of a child.

distinguished from early cervical cancer, so cytology should always be performed.

ABNORMALITIES OF THE CERVIX

An eccentric cervix suggests disease of the uterus or the adnexae. Nabothian cysts may develop if there is obstruction of the endocervical glands. These are seen as small, round, raised white or yellow lesions which only assume importance if they become infected. There may be a cervical discharge. If there is a pungent odour, suspect an infective cause and swab the area. An inflamed cervix covered by a mucopurulent discharge or slough is characteristic of acute and chronic cervicitis; the mucosa looks red rather than pink and, if the cervicitis follows pregnancy, you may notice laceration and pouting of the endocervical mucosa (ectropion). Cherry-red friable polyps may grow from the cervix (a source of vaginal bleeding after intercourse). Ulceration and fungating growths suggest cervical carcinoma.

Cervical smear

Cytologists can detect premalignant cells or established cervical cancer by examining a preparation of cells scraped from the surface of the cervix. The technique is routine in the course of the speculum examination. The demonstration of premalignant cells provides the opportunity for cancer prevention: the early detection of cancer allows for a higher, successful cure rate.

Before proceeding with the smear, prepare three clean glass microscope slides. Accurate labelling of the specimens is critical: slides with frosted glass at one end are preferable, for this allows you to write the patient's name and number clearly on the slide. Prepare the slide, mark with the patient's details, and label 'cervical smear'. Explain to the patient that you are about to take a smear. The cervical smear is performed after inspecting the cervix. A specially-designed disposable wooden spatula

of the vagina. In early pregnancy the cervix has a bluish colour caused by increased vascularity (Chadwick's sign). During pregnancy, the squamocolumnar junction may migrate beyond the external os and onto the cervix, retreating back, a few months after childbirth, into the cervical canal. Periodically, after pregnancy, the squamocolumnar junctions fail to regress into the os, giving the appearance of an erosion (ectopy). Failure to regress during fetal development may give rise to a congenital erosion. Cervical 'erosions' are not ulcerated surfaces but a term used to describe the appearance of the cervix when the endocervical epithelium extends onto the outer surface of the cervix. The columnar epithelium appears as a strawberry-red area spreading circumferentially around the os or onto the anterior or posterior lips. Cervical ectopy cannot be confidently

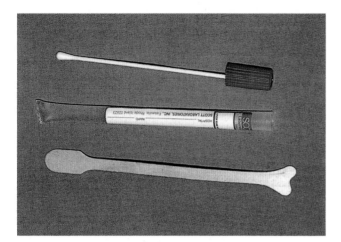

Fig. 8.54 Spatula with bifid end used for cervical cytology. Transport medium for microbiology, and swab.

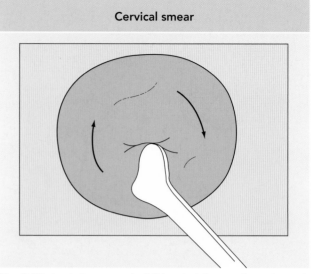

Cervical smear

Fig. 8.55 Cervical meatus. The bifid end of the spatula is advanced to the external os and cervical cells are harvested by rotating the spatula around the circumference of the os.

with a bifid end at one side and a rounded end at the other is used (Fig. 8.54). The bifid end is used to harvest the cervical cells. Introduce the spatula through the speculum and position the bifid end at the os (Fig. 8.55). The desquamating cells are collected by rotating the spatula around the circumference of the os and the lips of the cervix. Withdraw the spatula and spread the cervical material onto the labelled glass slide by stroking each side of the bifid end of the spatula along the glass. The cervical cells and some mucus should cling to the glass. Immediately spray the slides with fixative or fix them by immersion in 95% alcohol.

Taking vaginal swabs

If the patient has a vaginal discharge, use the speculum examination to take a swab for culture. You can use a conventional throat swab; insert the cotton wool end into the secretion (e.g. the region of the cervical os and vaginal pool) and allow the tip sufficient time to soak up secretion. Remove the swab, place it in a suitable transport medium and send the specimen immediately to the laboratory for processing.

Removing the speculum

After inspecting the cervix, undo the thumbscrew and simultaneously withdraw the speculum and rotate the open blades in an anticlockwise direction to ensure that the anterior and posterior walls of the vagina can be inspected. Near the introitus, allow the blades to close, taking care not to pinch the labia or any hairs while withdrawing the speculum.

Internal examination of the uterus

The speculum examination is followed by the vaginal examination. Explain that you are about to perform an internal examination of the uterus, tubes and ovaries.

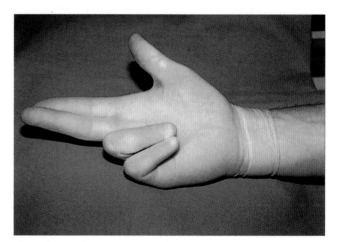

Fig. 8.56 The finger position used for performing a vaginal examination.

Again, expose the introitus by separating the labia with the thumb and forefinger of the gloved left hand and gently introduce the gloved and lubricated right index and middle fingers into the vagina, remembering that the organ is directed backwards in the direction of the sacrum. The thumb is abducted to allow maximum use of the length of the index and middle fingers; the ring and little finger are flexed into the palm (Fig. 8.56). Palpate the vaginal wall as you introduce your fingers. The walls are slightly rugose, supple and moist.

CERVIX

Locate the cervix with the pulps of your fingertips. The cervix should feel firm, rounded and smooth. Assess the mobility of the cervix by moving it gently and palpate the fornices. This procedure should be painless.

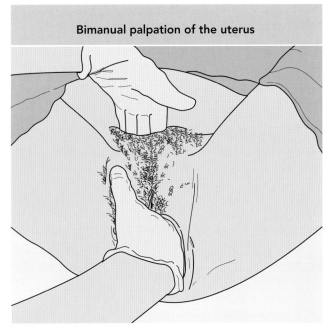

Fig. 8.57 The bimanual technique used to palpate the uterus. The vaginal fingers lift the cervix, while the other hand dips downwards and inwards to meet the fundus.

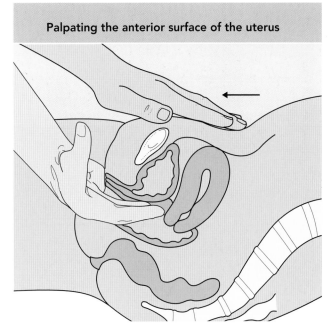

Fig. 8.58 By placing the vaginal fingers in the anterior fornix it is possible to examine the anterior surface of the uterus.

Abnormalities of the cervix

In pregnancy, the cervix softens (Hegar's sign). If there is tenderness on movement (known as 'excitation tenderness'), suspect infection or inflammation of the uterus or adnexae; or if the patient is shocked, suspect an ectopic pregnancy. You may palpate an ulcer or tumour already noted on the speculum examination.

UTERUS

Next, palpate the uterus. A bimanual technique is used to assess the size and position of the organ (Fig. 8.57). Position the palmar surface of your free hand on the anterior abdominal wall about 4 cm above the symphysis pubis. Attempt to 'capture' the uterus gently between your apposing fingers. Use your internal fingers to elevate the cervix and uterus in the direction of the external hand while simultaneously pressing the fingertips of the external hand in the direction of the internal fingers. Using this displacement technique an anteverted fundus should be palpable just above the symphysis. Assess its size, consistency and mobility, and note any masses and tenderness.

Further exploration may be helped by re-examining the uterus with your fingers positioned in the anterior fornix (Fig. 8.58); this permits the vaginal fingers to examine the anterior surface of the uterus while the abdominal fingers explore the posterior wall. If the uterus is retroverted, the fundus is more difficult to feel through the abdominal wall; nevertheless, it might become more readily palpable if the vaginal fingers are positioned in the posterior fornix.

Abnormalities of the uterus

If the uterus appears to be uniformly enlarged, consider a pregnancy, fibroid or endometrial tumour. Fibromyomas (fibroids) are common benign uterine tumours which may be single or multiple and may vary in size. Single, large uterine fibroids are felt on abdominal examination as a firm, nontender, well-defined rounded mass arising from the pelvis. On bimanual palpation, the mass appears contiguous with the cervix: the two structures move together. Multiple fibroids give the uterus a lobulated feel. Occasionally, the fibroid is pedunculated and is felt as a mobile pelvic mass which is readily confused with a mass arising from the adnexae.

ADNEXAE

Palpate the left and right adnexae in turn. Note, the adnexae are difficult to palpate in obese women. Place the fingers of your abdominal hand over the iliac fossa while readjusting the vaginal fingers into the lateral fornix and positioning the finger pulps to face the abdominal fingers (Fig. 8.59). Remembering the anatomy of the ovaries and fallopian tubes, gently but firmly appose the fingers of either hand by pressing the abdominal hand inward and downward, and the vaginal fingers upwards and laterally. Feel for the adnexal structures as the interposed tissues slip between your fingers. The manoeuvre should be relatively painless, although palpation of the ovaries might elicit some tenderness. Yet again, reassure you patient that any discomfort she feels is normal. If you feel an adnexal structure, assess its size, shape, mobility and tenderness. Ovaries are firm,

Palpating the adnexae

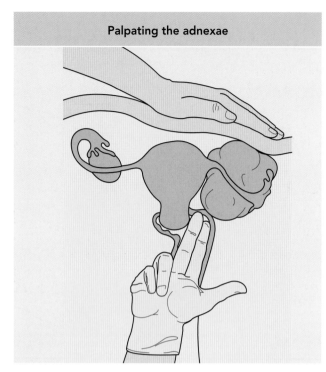

Fig. 8.59 Positioning the vaginal and abdominal fingers to palpate the adnexal structures.

ovoid, and often palpable. Normal fallopian tubes are impalpable.

Abnormalities of the adnexal structures

The most common causes of enlarged ovaries include benign cysts (e.g. follicular or corpus luteal cysts) and malignant ovarian tumours. Ovarian tumours are either unilateral or bilateral. Cysts feel smooth and the wall may be compressible. Occasionally, ovarian tumours are large enough to be palpable on abdominal examination and may fill the lower and mid-abdomen, creating the impression of ascites.

In acute infections of the fallopian tubes (salpingitis), there is lower abdominal tenderness and guarding, and, on vaginal examination, marked tenderness of the lateral fornices and cervix. The acute pain makes palpation of the adnexae difficult. In chronic salpingitis, the lower abdomen and lateral fornices are tender, yet the uterus and adnexae may be amenable to examination. If the uterus is retroverted and fixed by adhesions, it may be possible to feel thickening and swelling of the tubes extending to the ovaries. If the tubes are blocked, there may be cystic swelling of the tubes (hydrosalpinx) or they may become infected and purulent (pyosalpinx).

After completing the bimanual examination, withdraw your fingers from the vagina and inspect the glove tips for blood or discharge. Re-drape the genital area and reassure the patient that the examination is complete and that you will discuss the findings in the consulting room once she is dressed.

Examination of elderly people
Breasts and genital tract

- There is rapid fall in sex hormone synthesis after the menopause, resulting in changes in the structure and function of the genitalia
- There is progressive involution of the breast tissue and, as the acinar tissue atrophies, the breasts become more pendulous
- The risk of breast cancer remains at any age, including the very old
- After the menopause there is loss of vulval adipose tissue, and reduction in vaginal secretion results in drying of the mucosal surface
- The atrophy of tissue of the introitus results in vestibular narrowing, increased susceptibility to urinary tract infection and dyspareunia

- Loss of sex hormones results in altered hair distribution and androgen dominance may be apparent with male pattern facial hair growth, mild to moderate male pattern baldness and loss of the female pattern labial hairline
- Despite involutional changes, many older women maintain libido and remain sexually active into the later years of life
- Atrophy of the vagina and introitus can be prevented by hormone replacement therapy and topical oestrogen application
- Vaginal lubrication can be enhanced by using water-soluble lubricant jellies

Framework for the routine examination of female breasts and genitalia

General examination
- Endocrine syndrome
- Hirsutism, acne
- Breast examination
- Routine abdominal examination
- Inguinal lymph nodes

Vulva
- Inspection and palpation of the vulva
- Bartholin's gland palpation

Vagina
- Digital examination
  - cervix
  - cervical tenderness

- fornices
- pouch of Douglas

Uterus
- Bimanual palpation
  - body and fundus
  - adnexal region
  - ovaries

Speculum
- Inspect cervix and os
- Take cervical smear
- Bacterial swab for culture
- Inspect vaginal mucosa as speculum withdrawn

9

The male genitalia

Unlike the female genitalia, the male organs are readily accessible for examination. As for women, taking a sexual case history and examining a male is embarrassing and intrusive, so care must be taken to ensure confidentiality, privacy and comfort. An overview of structure and function will help you gain confidence when taking a history and examining the genitalia and will aid the interpretation of symptoms and signs.

Structure and function

The male genitalia include the penis, scrotum, testes, epididymides, seminal vesicles and prostate gland (Fig. 9.1). The penis provides a common pathway to the exterior for both urine and semen. In fetal development, the testes develop close to the kidneys and slowly migrate caudally, emerging at the external inguinal ring in the eighth month of development and descending into the scrotum in the ninth month. The neural, vascular and lymphatic supply to the testes also arise from near the kidney and the migrating testes drag these structures through the inguinal canal into the scrotum. This has important clinical implications, as renal pain is often referred to the scrotum and the natural route for lymphatic spread of testicular cancer is to para-aortic (rather than inguinal) nodes.

PUBERTY

In boys, puberty starts 1–2 years later than in girls. The onset of male puberty is signalled by an increase in testicular volume and this is followed approximately one year later by a spurt in linear growth and an increase in muscle bulk.

Hormonal changes in puberty

Testosterone feedback to the hypothalamus can inhibit the hypothalamic–pituitary axis release of luteinising hormone (LH) and follicle-stimulating hormone (FSH). In the child, this feedback is especially sensitive and even low levels of circulating gonadal steroids are sufficient to inhibit the secretion of FSH and LH. Male puberty is initiated by a fall in the sensitivity of the hypothalamus to inhibition at low levels of circulating sex hormones. By resetting the sensitivity of the feedback to the hypothalamus, FSH and LH are released, thereby exerting their trophic effects on their target cells in the testes.

Throughout male puberty, LH levels increase slowly and steadily (Fig. 9.2), whereas FSH levels increase more sharply in early puberty, with a more gentle increase afterwards. FSH stimulates the Sertoli cells and regulates the growth of seminiferous tubules and spermatogenesis. As most of the testis is formed of tubules, the increased testicular volume in puberty is largely under the control of FSH. LH stimulates the Leydig (interstitial) cells which synthesise testosterone from cholesterol (Fig. 9.3). Testosterone circulates bound to sex hormone-binding

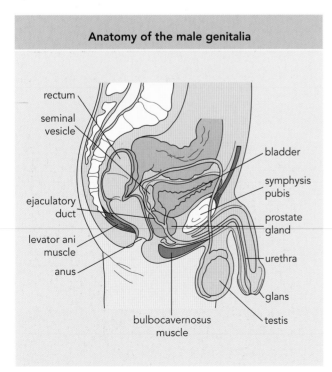

Anatomy of the male genitalia

rectum
seminal vesicle
ejaculatory duct
levator ani muscle
anus
bulbocavernosus muscle
bladder
symphysis pubis
prostate gland
urethra
glans
testis

Fig. 9.1 The male genitalia include the external organs, seminal vesicles and the prostate gland.

globulin (SHBG). The linear growth spurt follows closely behind the surge of testosterone. Some testosterone is converted to oestradiol in the Leydig cells and other extragonadal tissue sites. The effects of testosterone are shown in Table 9.1. The importance of oestrogen in males remains unclear, although it does regulate the synthesis of SHBG.

Development of secondary sexual characteristics

Tanner described the pubertal development of the male genitalia and pubic hair growth (Fig. 9.4). Initially, the testes enlarge and the scrotal skin becomes thin and red (stage 2). The enlargement of the phallus occurs later in the growth spurt and is associated with thickening, crinkling and pigmentation of the scrotal skin (stage 3). Increasing levels of gonadal and adrenal androgens stimulate the growth of pubic, axillary and facial hair. Pubic hair begins to develop as sparse, long, slightly curly hair at the base of the phallus (stage 4). Later, coarser, curlier hair extends to cover the symphysis pubis and finally extends to the inner thigh and along the linea alba (this constitutes the male escutcheon) (stage 5).

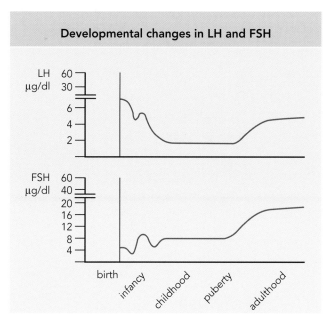

Fig. 9.2 Changes in LH and FSH secretion before, during and after puberty.

Table 9.1 Effects of testosterone

- Stimulates the development of secondary sexual characteristics
- Controls libido
- Anabolic effect causes muscle growth and fat deposition
- With growth hormone, stimulates linear growth in adolescence
- With erythropoietin, stimulates red cell production

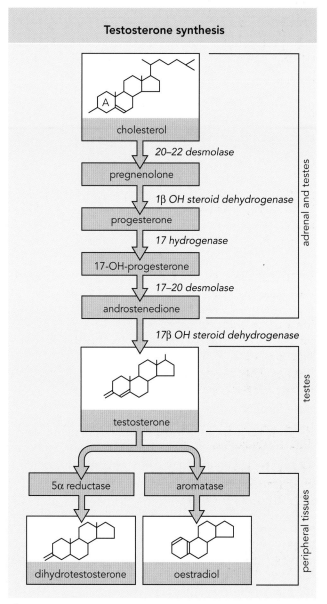

Fig. 9.3 Biochemical pathway in the synthesis of testosterone from cholesterol.

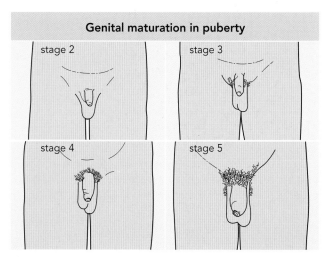

Fig. 9.4 Tanner's five stages of male genital maturation (Stage 1 preadolescence is not shown).

Histology of the testis

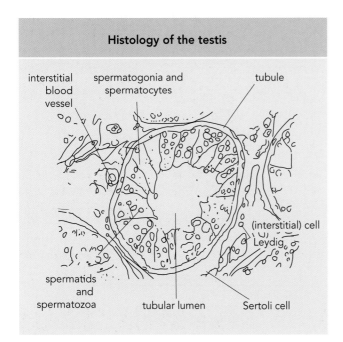

Fig. 9.5 Histological section through a testis shows seminiferous tubules, developing sperm, Leydig and Sertoli cells.

The hypothalamic–pituitary–testicular axis

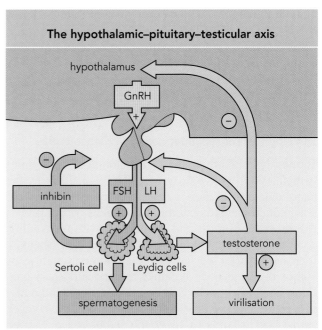

Fig. 9.6 The hypothalamic–pituitary–gonadal axis. Pulsatile release of GnRH stimulates the anterior pituitary to secrete LH and FSH, which stimulate the Leydig and Sertoli cells, respectively.

Male fertility

The male testis is composed of a network of tightly coiled and convoluted seminiferous tubules that drain through the rete testis into the epididymis. Spermatozoa develop from the germinal epithelium of the seminiferous tubules which lie in close contact with the Leydig and Sertoli cells (Fig. 9.5). LH binds to the Leydig cells, stimulating the production of testosterone from cholesterol. FSH binds to the Sertoli cells, stimulating the synthesis of inhibin, a peptide hormone that inhibits FSH production by the pituitary (Fig. 9.6). The development from immature spermatogonia to mature spermatozoa takes 72 days. The passage of the sperm through the epididymis to the ejaculatory ducts takes a further 14 days, during which time the spermatozoa become motile.

Spermatogenesis occurs most efficiently when the ambient testicular temperature is 36°C. The smooth muscle of the scrotum and spermatic cord alters the position of the testicles in relation to the external inguinal ring to maintain (under various conditions of heat and cold) an optimal temperature for spermatogenesis.

PENIS

The penis consists of the two sponge-like cylinders, the corpora cavernosa, forming the dorsal and lateral surfaces, and the corpus spongiosum, which ends in a bulbous expansion, the glans penis (Fig. 9.7). The urethra passes through the corpus spongiosum. The skin covering the corpora extends over the glans to form the prepuce.

Tactile and psychogenic stimuli cause sexual arousal. An autonomic (parasympathetic) reflex causes increased arterial flow through branches of the pudendal artery to

Anatomy of the penis

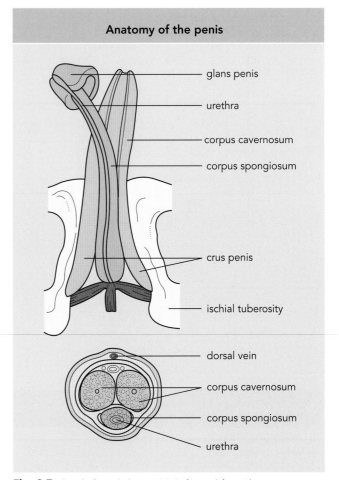

Fig. 9.7 The shaft and glans penis is formed from the corpus spongiosum and the corpus cavernosum.

the penis and fills the corpus spongiosum. The organ assumes the erectile position necessary for vaginal penetration. The reflex is completed by a sympathetic neural outflow that results in contraction of the ejaculatory ducts and the bladder neck, causing ejaculation of semen and orgasm. This is followed by increased tone in the arterioles and sinusoids of the corpora, diversion of blood away from the penis and, finally, detumescence.

SCROTUM AND ITS CONTENTS

Before attempting to examine the testis and epididymis, it is important to understand the structure of these organs. The scrotum is a muscular pouch that holds the testes. A septum separates the left and right testicles. The scrotal skin is thin, pigmented and crinkled and lined by the dartos muscle. This permits considerable contraction and relaxation of the scrotum, which helps keep the optimal temperature for spermatogenesis.

The left testis almost always lies lower than the right. Each testis is ovoid in shape, measuring approximately 4 × 3 × 2 cm. A fibrous capsule, the tunica albuginea, invests the testis. The seminiferous tubules converge and anastomose posteriorly to form the efferent tubules which converge to form the head of the epididymis (Fig. 9.8). This, in turn, gives rise to the body and tail which drain into the vas deferens. The vas deferens passes through the inguinal canal (Fig. 9.9), joining the seminal vesicles, which, in turn, converge to form the ejaculatory duct. The epididymis attaches along the posterior border and upper pole of the testis. Both the testis and the epididymis have vestigial remnants of fetal development known as the appendix testis and hydatid of Morgagni, respectively. These occasionally twist and can cause severe testicular pain.

Lymphatics from the penile and scrotal skin drain to the inguinal nodes. Examination of the groin nodes is an integral part of the genital examination, especially if there is an ulcer or discharge.

PROSTATE

The structure of the prostate is described in Chapter 7. The organ envelops the first part of the urethra and the ejaculatory ducts from the seminal vesicles, which open into the prostatic urethra. The prostate secretes a specialised fluid that provides lubrication before intercourse and serves also to increase the volume of the ejaculate.

Symptoms of genital tract disease

Like women, men may choose either to express their symptoms openly or to expose the problem in a less obvious manner. Moreover, the doctor may feel embarrassed to broach the sensitive issues of sexual orientation, sexual function, sexually transmitted disease and possible exposure to HIV. Learn to ask direct questions with sensitivity while maintaining the firm impression that you are both confident and decisive when talking about what is, after all, another normal bodily function.

At the outset of your history-taking, you will already have ascertained whether the patient is single or married

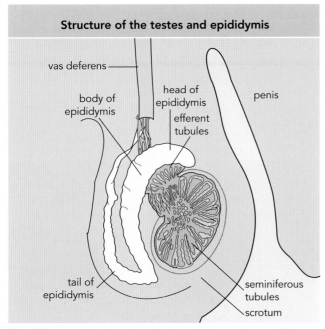

Structure of the testes and epididymis

vas deferens
body of epididymis
head of epididymis
efferent tubules
penis
tail of epididymis
seminiferous tubules
scrotum

Fig. 9.8 Coronal section through the testis shows the seminiferous tubules of the testis converging to form the efferent tubules, which then give rise to the head, body and tail of the epididymis and the vas deferens.

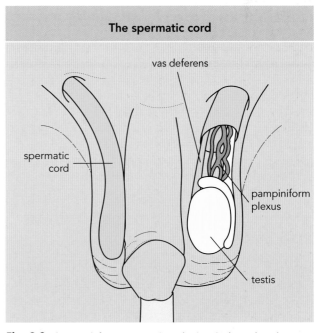

The spermatic cord

vas deferens
spermatic cord
pampiniform plexus
testis

Fig. 9.9 The vas deferens passes into the inguinal canal as the spermatic cord, which then converges on the seminal vesicles. The pampiniform vascular plexus surrounds the spermatic cord.

and if he has fathered any children. The genital and sexual history follows on naturally from the urinary tract history (see Ch. 7). Ask about penile discharge, pain or swelling of the testes and ability to enjoy normal sexual relations. These questions should provide the cue for a shy or inhibited patient to talk about sexual or genital problems. Depending on the nature of the presenting symptoms, you may wish to ask about homosexual contact. You may feel uneasy about phrasing the question but in societies in which AIDS is acknowledged as a problem, the majority of patients understand the importance of the question and most often will not take offence to a question like 'Have you ever had a homosexual partner?' or 'Do you practise safe sex?' If a genital or sexual symptom becomes apparent, assure the patient of the confidentiality of the interview and attempt to analyse the problem in greater depth.

URETHRAL DISCHARGE

A urethral discharge is a common presenting symptom. Remember that a discharge of smegma from a normal prepuce is very different from a discharge caused by urethritis. In urethritis, the patient may notice staining of his underwear and complain of urinary symptoms such as burning or stinging when passing urine. Sexually transmitted disease is a common cause of urethral discharge and patients concerned about sexually transmitted disease will usually mention fear of it. If this information is not forthcoming, ask the patient directly

about the possibility of contact with sexually transmitted disease. Ask about a recent episode of gastroenteritis, for urethritis may follow a few weeks later. Reiter's syndrome (Fig. 9.10) is the most florid manifestation of this association and is characterised by a urethral discharge, balanitis, painful joints (arthritis and tendinitis) and bilateral conjunctivitis.

Differential diagnosis
Urethral discharge

Physiological
• Sexual arousal

Pathological
• Gonococcal urethritis (incubation 2–6 days)
• Nongonococcal urethritis
• Idiopathic nonspecific urethritis
• *Chlamydia trachomatis*
• *Trichomonas vaginalis*
• *Candida albicans*
• Posturinary catheter
• Reiter's syndrome (may follow gastroenteritis) includes arthritis and conjunctivitis

GENITAL ULCERS

The appearance of an ulcer or 'sore' always raises the spectre of sexually transmitted disease. Consequently, this possibility is likely to alarm your patient even though ulcers are not always caused by sexual transmission. Enquire discreetly about possible contact with sexually transmitted disease or casual sexual encounters. Ask whether the ulcer is painful and try to assess a possible incubation period. Herpetic ulcers tend to recur and may be preceded by a prodrome of a prickly sensation or pain in the loins. There may be a clear history of contact with a partner infected with herpes and sexual transmission may affect the mouth or anus as well as the penis. Exotic ulcerating venereal infections occur in the tropics and it is important to obtain a careful history of foreign travel and possible sexual contact.

Questions to ask
Urethral discharge

• Is there a possibility of recent exposure to a sexually transmitted disease?
• How long ago might you have had such a contact (incubation period)?
• Does your partner complain of a vaginal discharge?
• Have you experienced joint pains or gritty, red eyes?
• Have you recently suffered from gastroenteritis?

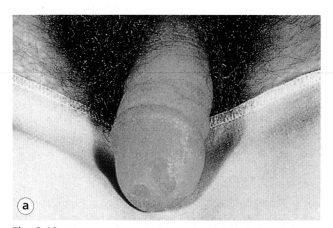

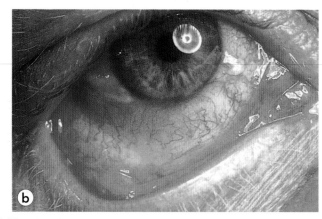

Fig. 9.10 Reiter's syndrome is characterised by (a) circinate balanitis and (b) conjunctivitis.

TESTICULAR PAIN

Inflammation or trauma to the testes causes an intense visceral pain that may radiate towards the groin and abdomen. Testicular pain has a deep boring quality often accompanied by nausea. The pain may be accompanied by swelling and be aggravated by movement or even light palpation. Painless swelling of a testis should alert you to the possibility of a cystic lesion or malignancy.

Questions to ask
Testicular pain

- Was the pain preceded by trauma?
- How rapidly did the pain develop?
- Was the pain preceded by a fever or swelling of the salivary glands (mumps)?
- Was the pain preceded by burning on micturition or a urethral discharge?

Differential diagnosis
Testicular pain

- Trauma
- Infection (mumps orchitis)
- Epididymitis
- Testicular torsion
- Torsion of epididymal cyst

IMPOTENCE

The term impotence refers to a spectrum of sexual dysfunction ranging from loss of libido, failure to obtain or to maintain an erection, to inability to achieve orgasm. Impotence is often a manifestation of emotional disturbance; therefore, you should try to assess whether the patient is depressed, anxious about sexual encounters or troubled by emotional aspects of the relationship. Fear of causing pregnancy and concern about a contagious disease such as AIDS may serve to cause impotence. Take a careful drug and alcohol history; alcoholism is an important cause of impotence and many widely

Differential diagnosis
Drug-related causes of impotence

- Major tranquillisers (phenothiazines)
- Lithium
- Sedatives (barbiturates, benzodiazepines)
- Antihypertensives (methyldopa, clonidine)
- Alcohol
- Oestrogens
- Drug abuse (heroin, methadone)

prescribed drugs are associated with impotence. An obvious association with organic disease may be apparent in patients presenting with concomitant cardiovascular, respiratory or neurological symptoms.

INFERTILITY

Primary infertility refers to a failure to achieve conception, whereas secondary infertility refers to a difficulty or a failure to conceive, although there has been at least one successful conception in the past. Male infertility accounts for approximately one-third of childless relationships. Consequently, both partners are evaluated when couples present with infertilty. Ask about the duration of infertility and whether the patient has ever managed to conceive. As many couples have little understanding of the timing of ovulation and conception, you should enquire in some depth about the frequency and timing of intercourse and about attempts to time intercourse to coincide with the female partner's fertile period. Ask about drugs, as antimetabolites used in cancer treatment or sulfasalazine used in colitis may cause subfertility.

Questions to ask
Infertility

- Have you or your partner ever conceived?
- Do you have difficulty obtaining or maintaining an erection?
- Do you ejaculate?
- Do you understand the timing of ovulation in your partner?
- Are you on any medication that may cause impotence or sperm malfunction (e.g. sulfasalazine)?
- Have you noticed any change in facial hair growth?
- Have you ever had cancer treatment?

Examination of the male genitalia

This examination usually follows the abdominal examination and you will already have approached the area when examining the groin and hernial offices. Although a detailed genital examination is usually only undertaken when the patient complains of appropriate symptoms, it is advisable to check the testes in the course of a routine examination as 'opportunistic screening' may occasionally reveal a testicular tumour. Explain that you would like to examine the penis and testes and offer reassurance that the examination will be quick and gentle. Like any other examination, your confidence, or lack of it, soon becomes apparent to the patient. If you have a good knowledge of the anatomy and physiology already outlined, you will soon master a quick but thorough examination. It is advisable for women doctors to examine the genitalia with a chaperone close at hand.

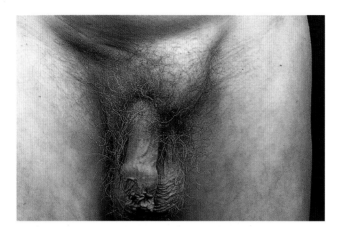

Fig. 9.11 Hernias may only become apparent when the patient stands.

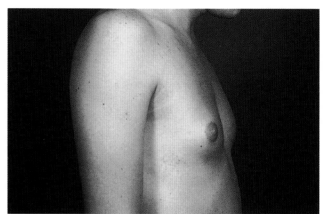

Fig. 9.12 Typical appearance of male gynaecomastasia.

It is usual practice to wear disposable plastic gloves for hygienic reasons and to emphasise the strictly clinical nature of the examination. The genitalia are usually examined with the patient lying but remember that varicoceles and scrotal hernias may only be apparent when the patient stands; it is advisable to check for scrotal swellings in the standing position if the diagnosis is unclear with the patient lying down (Fig. 9.11). Avoid creating a feeling of total nakedness by covering part of the thighs.

GENERAL EXAMINATION

You will already have performed a general examination and noted the distribution of facial, axillary and abdominal hair. In testicular malfunction (hypogonadism), there may be loss of axillary hair, the pubic hair distribution may start to resemble the distinctive female pattern and there is a typical facial appearance with wrinkling around the mouth. You will have also checked the breast and noted whether or not gynaecomastia was evident (Fig. 9.12).

EXAMINATION OF THE PENIS

Normal penis

The length and thickness of the flaccid penis vary widely and bear no relationship either to potency or to fertility. The dorsal vein of the penis is usually prominent along the dorsal midline. Gently retract the foreskin (prepuce) to expose the glans penis. The foreskin should be supple, allowing smooth and painless retraction. There is often a trace of odourless, curd-like smegma underlying the foreskin. Examine the external urethral meatus, which is a slit-like orifice extending from the ventral pole of the tip of the glans. Use your index finger and thumb to squeeze the meatus gently open. This should expose healthy, glistening pink mucosa. If the patient has complained of a urethral discharge, try to elicit this sign. The patient may be able to 'milk' the shaft of the penis

Differential diagnosis
Male gynaecomastia

Physiological
- Puberty
- Old age

Pathological
- Hypogonadism
- Liver cirrhosis
- Drugs (spironolactone, digoxin, oestrogens)
- Tumours (bronchogenic carcinoma, adrenal carcinoma, testicular tumours)
- Thyrotoxicosis

to express the secretion; if not, you may try to express a discharge by 'milking' the shaft of the penis from the base towards the glans. If a discharge appears, swab the area with a sterile bud and immerse the specimen in a transport medium for quick dispatch to the microbiology laboratory.

Abnormalities of the penis

Prepuce The prepuce may be too tight to retract over the glans (phimosis). If the prepuce is tight but retracts and catches behind the glans, oedema and swelling may occur, preventing the return of the foreskin (paraphimosis). If left untreated, the swelling and congestion may result in gangrene.

Glans Hypospadias (Fig. 9.13) is a developmental abnormality causing the urethral meatus to appear on the inferior (ventral) surface of the glans (primary hypospadias), penis (secondary hypospadias) or even the perineum (tertiary hypospadias). Inflammation of the glans is termed balanitis (Fig. 9.10); if there is inflammation of the glans and prepuce, the term balanoposthitis is used. Genital (herpetic) warts may be seen on the glans.

Urethral discharge This is one of the most common genital disorders in men and is caused by urethral

Hypospadias

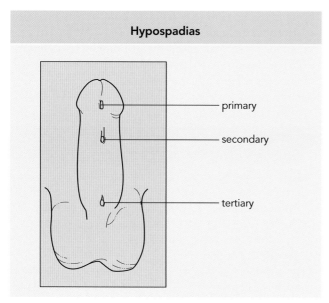

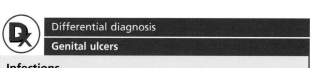

Fig. 9.13 Hypospadias: a developmental abnormality. The urethral meatus opens on the ventral surface of the penis.

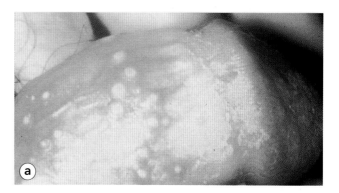

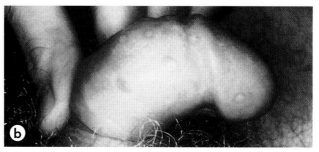

Fig. 9.14 After 4–5 days incubation, a crop of relatively painless herpetic vesicles appear on the penis (a). Vesicles rupture, with the development of painful superficial erosions with a characteristic erythematous halo (b).

inflammation (urethritis). The cause of a urethral discharge cannot be confidently predicted from appearance, although gonorrhoea is likely to cause a profuse purulent discharge. Nongonococcal urethritis may also be caused by urethral infection or be associated with Reiter's syndrome.

Dx **Differential diagnosis**

Genital ulcers

Infections
- Genital herpes
- Syphilis (chancre, mucous patches, gumma)
- Tropical ulcers

Balanitis
- Severe candidiasis
- Circinate balanitis (Reiter's syndrome)

Drug eruption
- Localised fixed drug eruption
- Generalised (Stevens–Johnson syndrome)

Carcinoma

Behçet's syndrome

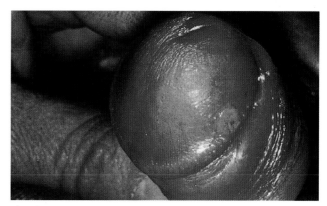

Fig. 9.15 The primary chancre of syphilis may occur on the glans, prepuce or shaft.

Penile ulcers Ulceration of the glans or, more rarely, the shaft of the penis may occur in a number of disorders. Examine the ulcer and always palpate the groins for inguinal lymph node involvement because the skin of the penis drains to this group of nodes. The most common cause is herpetic ulceration. Characteristic painless vesicles occur 4–5 days after sexual contact (Fig. 9.14). The vesicles often rupture, causing painful superficial erosions with a characteristic erythematous halo. The confluence of these erosions may cause discrete ulcers

that can become secondarily infected. The urethral meatus may be affected causing dysuria. If there is a possible history of sexually transmitted disease, consider syphilis (primary chancre) (Fig. 9.15) and in the tropics consider chancroid, lymphogranuloma venereum and granuloma inguinale. Infrequently, fixed drug reactions may cause penile ulceration. Squamous cell carcinoma may present as an ulcer of the penis or the scrotum.

Priapism Occasionally, a patient may present with a painful and prolonged erection. This pathological erection is termed priapism. Most often there is no obvious cause but predisposing factors such as leukaemia, haemoglobinopathies (e.g. sickle cell anaemia) and drugs (aphrodisiacs) should be considered.

EXAMINATION OF THE SCROTUM

Inspect the scrotal skin, which is pigmented when compared with body skin. The left testis lies lower than the right but the impression of both testes is readily identified (Fig. 9.16). The tone of the dartos muscle is influenced by ambient temperature. Consequently, the normal scrotal appearance varies with temperature.

Ensure that your hands are warm before palpating the testis. Use gentle pressure, sufficient to explore the bulk of the tissue without causing pain. Throughout the examination, watch the patient's facial expression, for this should reassure you that the examination is not causing undue discomfort. Compare the left and right testes because many testicular disorders are unilateral. Feel the testicle between your thumb and first two fingers (Fig. 9.17). Note the size and consistency of the testis. The organ has a pliant, soft rubbery consistency and there should not be much tenderness. Next, palpate the epididymis, which is felt as an elongated structure along the posterolateral surface of the testicle (Fig. 9.18).

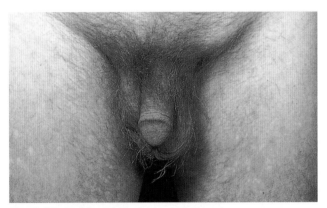

Fig. 9.16 The left testis lies lower than the right.

The epididymis normally feels smooth and is broadest superiorly at its head.

Finally, roll with the finger and thumb the vas deferens, which passes from the tail of the epididymis to the inguinal canal through the external inguinal canal. This structure is smooth and nontender and is felt leading from the epididymis to the external inguinal ring.

Abnormalities of the scrotum

If one-half of the scrotum appears smooth and poorly developed, consider an undescended testis (cryptorchidism). This appearance of the scrotum helps to distinguish a maldescent from a retractile testis, in which the testis has descended but retracts vigorously towards the external inguinal ring. The retracted testis will be difficult to palpate.

The scrotal skin may be red and inflamed; a common cause is candidiasis (Fig. 9.19). Small yellowish scrotal lumps or nodules are common and usually represent sebaceous cysts.

Swellings in the scrotum

Decide whether the swelling arises from an indirect inguinal hernia or from the scrotal contents. It is possible to 'get above' a testicular swelling but not a scrotal hernia (Fig. 9.20). An intrinsic swelling may arise from enlargement of the testis, testicular appendages and epididymis or by an accumulation of fluid in the tunica vaginalis, the double membrane that invests the testes.

Palpate the swelling between the thumb and first two fingers and decide whether the swelling is solid or cystic.

Cystic swelling Cystic accumulations are caused by entrapment of fluid in the tunica vaginalis (a hydrocele) or accumulation of fluid in an epididymal cyst and are

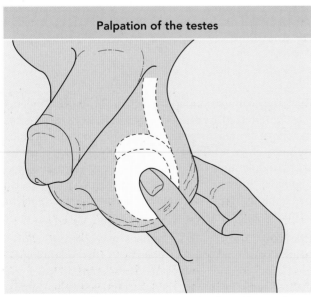

Fig. 9.17 Palpate the testis between your thumb and first two fingers.

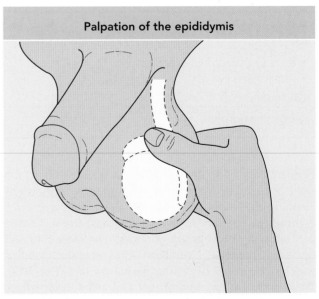

Fig. 9.18 The epididymis is felt along the posterior pole of the testis.

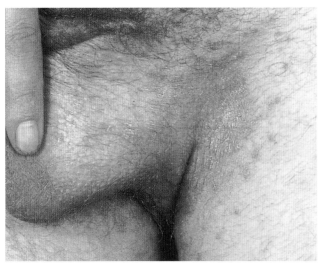

Fig. 9.19 Candida infection of the scrotum often extends to the groin and thigh.

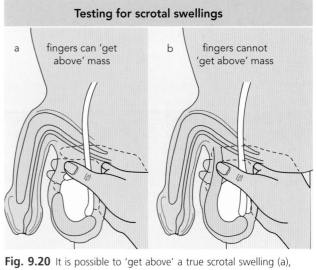

Fig. 9.20 It is possible to 'get above' a true scrotal swelling (a), whereas this is not possible if the swelling is caused by an inguinal hernia that has descended into the scrotum (b).

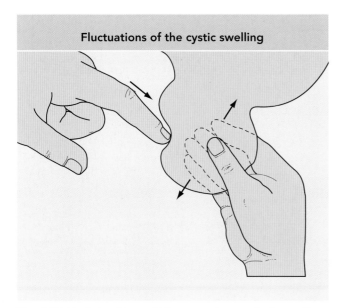

Fig. 9.21 To distinguish a solid from a cystic mass, fix the swelling between finger and thumb of one hand and use the index finger of the other hand to invaginate at right angles.

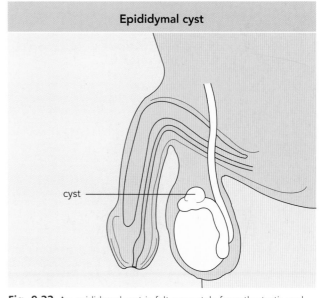

Fig. 9.22 An epididymal cyst is felt separately from the testis and lies posteriorly.

typically fluctuant. Steady the mass between the thumb and first two fingers of one hand and use the index finger of the other hand to invaginate the mass in a second plane (Fig. 9.21). The tense fluid-filled cyst will fluctuate between finger and thumb in response to the pressure change. Cystic lesions usually transilluminate. Darken the room and place a pen-torch light up against the swelling. A fluid-filled cyst spreads a bright red glow into the scrotum, whereas this does not occur with solid tumours. Remember that if the cyst wall is abnormally thickened or the effusion is bloodstained, transillumination may not occur. Next, try to distinguish between a hydrocoele and an epididymal cyst. As the epididymis lies behind the body of the testis, an epididymal cyst is felt as a distinct swelling behind the adjoining testis (Fig.

9.22). In contrast, a hydrocele surrounds and envelops the testis, which becomes impalpable as a discrete organ (Fig. 9.23). The distinction between an epididymal cyst and hydrocele is not always clear and the two may occur together.

Varicocele Varicoceles occur in 5–8% of normal adult males and are almost always left sided (Fig. 9.24). A varicocele results from a varicosity of the veins of the pampiniform plexus, a leash of vessels surrounding the spermatic cord, and is caused by abnormality of the valve mechanism of the left testicular vein, which drains into the left renal vein (the right drains directly into the inferior vena cava). Most varicoceles do not cause symptoms and are discovered as an incidental finding.

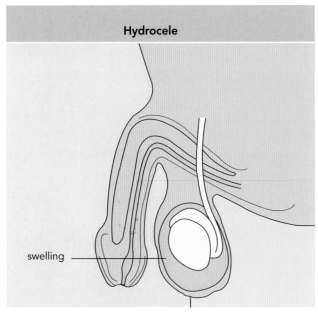

Fig. 9.23 A hydrocele surrounds the entire testis, which cannot, therefore, be felt as a discrete organ.

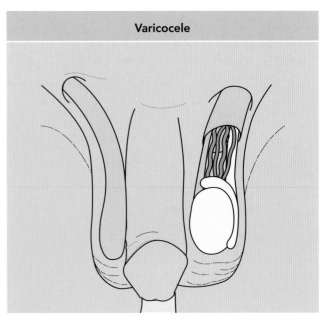

Fig. 9.24 A left-sided varicocele has the texture of a 'bag of worms' when palpated. The mass is separate from the testis and epididymis.

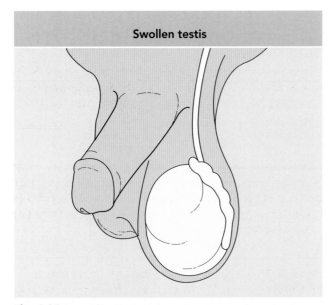

Fig. 9.25 In orchitis, the testis is swollen, tense and very tender. Usually only one testis is involved.

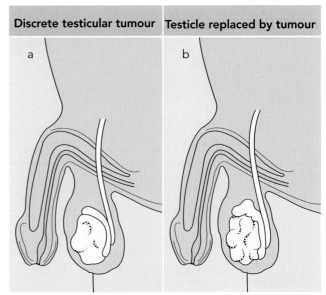

Fig. 9.26 Carcinoma may present as a discrete mass within a testis (a) or may expand to replace the entire organ (b).

However, patients may rarely present with scrotal swelling, discomfort or infertility. Examine the patient in the standing position – the varicocele feels like a 'bag of worms'. Ask the patient to cough while you palpate the varicocele – a characteristic feature is transmission of the raised intra-abdominal pressure to the varicocele, which is felt as a discrete cough impulse. The varicocele is separate from the testis. The ipsilateral testis is usually smaller than expected. A varicocele usually empties when the patient lies supine.

Solid swellings As with cystic swellings, use your knowledge of the anatomy to distinguish between a testicular and an epididymal mass. Diffuse, acutely painful swelling usually occurs in acute inflammatory condition such as orchitis (Fig. 9.25) or torsion of the testis. These acute emergencies are usually readily distinguishable from a solid or discrete swelling of the body of the testis. Solid masses may be smooth or craggy, tender or painless but, whatever the character, carcinoma must be the first differential diagnosis (Fig. 9.26). Other solid masses include tuberculomas and syphilitic gummas. Solid tumours of the epididymis are due to chronic inflammation (usually tuberculous epididymitis) and are usually benign. The epididymis feels hard and craggy (Fig. 9.27) and is not unduly tender.

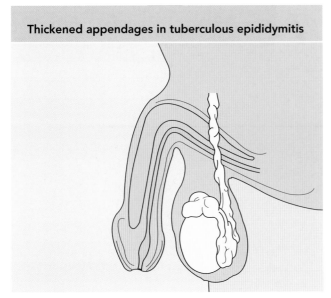

Thickened appendages in tuberculous epididymitis

Fig. 9.27 In tuberculous epididymitis, the epididymis is firm and thickened and the cord may feel beaded.

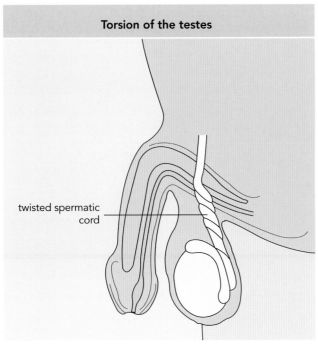

Torsion of the testes

twisted spermatic cord

Fig. 9.28 Torsion of the testicle on the spermatic cord impairs the blood supply. The affected testis is swollen, tender and lies higher than expected. The overlying scrotal skin is often reddened and oedematous.

Torsion of the testis

This usually occurs in young boys and presents with severe scrotal pain that usually radiates to the inguinal region and lower abdomen. On examination, the scrotal skin overlying the affected testis may be reddened, with the affected testis lying higher than the unaffected testis (Fig. 9.28). The testis may be very tender and the spermatic cord may feel thickened and sensitive to palpation. The

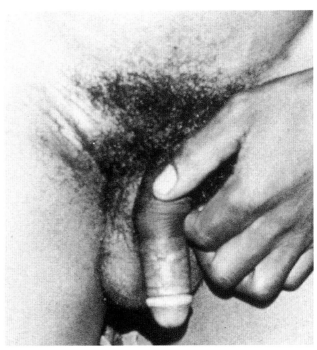

Fig. 9.29 In lymphogranuloma venereum, the inguinal lymph nodes enlarge.

opposite testis may have an abnormal lie because it is not uncommon for both testes to be abnormally positioned. The presentation and findings may be confused with orchitis and testicular torsion.

Scrotal oedema

Scrotal oedema usually occurs when there is diffuse oedema (anasarca) caused by severe congestive heart failure or hypoproteinaemia such as in nephrotic syndrome. The scrotal tissue becomes stretched and taut with pitting of the skin.

EXAMINATION OF THE LYMPHATICS

The skin lymphatics of the penis and scrotum drain towards the inguinal nodes; you should complete your genital examination by feeling for nodes in the groin, which are felt deep to the inguinal crease. The testicular lymphatics drain to intra-abdominal nodes. Special tests such as computerised tomography or lymphangiography are necessary to evaluate the testicular lymphatics.

Enlarged inguinal nodes

Enlarged nodes occur in infective and malignant disorders affecting the skin of the penis and scrotum. The primary chancre of syphilis is usually associated with lymphadenopathy. The nodes are typically mobile, rubbery and not tender. The most florid forms of inguinal lymphadenopathy occur in patients with lymphogranuloma venereum (Fig. 9.29).

Examination of elderly people

Genitalia in elderly males

- Men remain sexually active well into the later years of life
- Impotence and loss of libido commonly accompany chronic disease such as heart failure and respiratory and renal/prostatic disease
- Always consider drugs when elderly patients complain of impotence or loss of libido (e.g. antihypertensive medication)
- While women stop ovulating by the sixth decade, most men continue to produce sperm well into the eighth and ninth decades
- Benign prostatic hypertrophy of its own accord does not affect genital function; prostatectomy may result in retrograde ejaculation or nerve damage and impotence.
- Hydrocele and varicocele are common causes of testicular swelling in elderly men but testicular cancer is rare

Review

Framework for the routine examination of the male genitalia

- Note pattern of hair distribution
- Stage sexual development
- Examine abdomen generally
- Examine inguinal lymph nodes
- Inguinal hernias?
- Retract foreskin
- Examine glans penis and meatus
- Check for urethral discharge
- Examine the scrotum
  - inspect scrotal skin
  - check lie of testes (left lower than right)
  - palpate the testes and epididymis
  - check scrotal swellings for fluctuation and transillumination
  - palpate the spermatic cord within the scrotum

10

Bone, joints and muscle

The skeleton provides protection for the internal organs along with a strengthening and support system for the limbs. The presence of joints in the limbs and spine permits movement of what would otherwise be rigid structures. The cartilage interposed between the bone surfaces of a joint cushions the forces that are generated during movement. Joint strength is enhanced by ligaments that are either incorporated into the joint capsule or independent of it. Movement at the joint is achieved by contraction of the muscles passing across it.

The tubular arrangement of the long bones achieves maximal resistance to a bending force while economising on the amount of material used in its construction. The lines of the trabeculae in cancellous bone match the lines of stress encountered at those particular points. The surface markings and contours of bone are determined by external forces and the origins of tendons and ligaments.

Cartilage consists of a collection of rounded cells (chondroblasts) embedded in a matrix. There are three

Structure and function

BONE

Long bones are hollow with an outer layer of compact bone arranged, on the surface, into flat layers of lamellae and, more deeply, as concentric rings traversed by longitudinal passages (the Haversian canals) (Fig. 10.1). The central cavity of a long bone is occupied by bone marrow. At the ends of the long bones, a meshwork (cancellous bone) forms with marrow in its interstices. The arrangement of the meshwork is determined by the stresses to which the bones are exposed. Between adjacent Haversian canals and their surrounding concentric rings, the bony lamellae are arranged more haphazardly. In the spaces between these bony lamellae lie osteocytes.

Formation of bone is controlled by osteoblasts, and its destruction by osteoclasts. The osteocytes, derived from osteoblasts, are concerned with the exchange of calcium between bone and the extracellular fluid. Collagen, synthesised by osteoblasts and fibroblasts, forms the major part of the bone matrix. The calcium content of bone is mainly composed of crystals of hydroxyapatite. Approximately 1% of the calcium and phosphate of bone is in equilibrium with the extracellular fluid. Only osteoclastic resorption can release the remainder. The exchange of calcium between bone and extracellular fluid is controlled by parathormone and calcitriol, a metabolite of vitamin D.

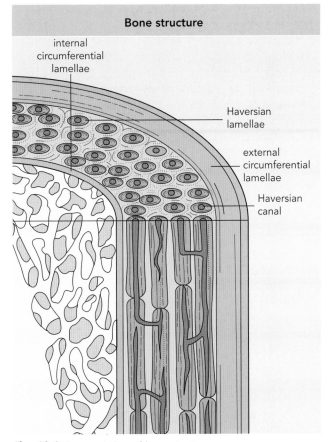

Fig. 10.1 Representation of bone structure.

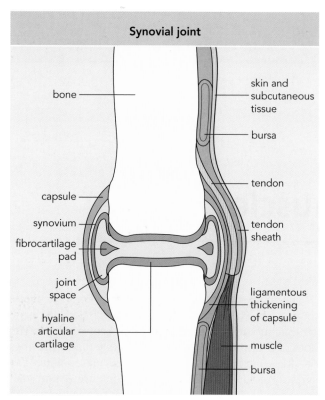

Fig. 10.2 Cross-section of a synovial joint.

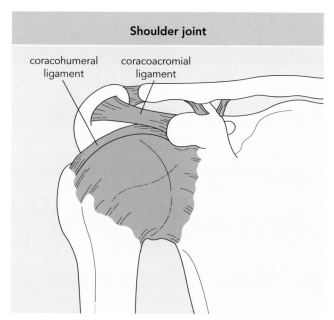

Fig. 10.3 The shoulder joint and the attachments of the coracohumeral ligament.

main types: hyaline, elastic and fibrocartilage. Hyaline cartilage is found on the articular surface of joints, in the costal cartilages and in the larynx, trachea and bronchi. Hyaline cartilage combines elasticity with a capacity to resist external forces. With increasing age, cartilage water content falls, with a consequent deterioration in tensile stiffness, fracture strength and fatigue resistance. Fibrocartilage is predominantly composed of fibrous tissue and is a part of the tendon at the point of its insertion into bone (Sharpey's fibres). It is also found in certain joints. Elastic cartilage has a concentrated network of elastic fibres that give its structure considerable flexibility. It is found in the pinna and in some of the laryngeal cartilages.

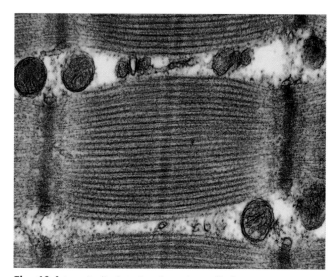

Fig. 10.4 Longitudinal section through myofibrils.

JOINTS

Joints can be classified into those allowing free movement (diarthroses), those that are fixed (synarthroses) and those that permit limited movement (amphiarthroses). In diarthroses (synovial joints), a space exists between the bone surfaces, allowing movement of one bone against the other (Fig. 10.2). Further classification of these joints can be made according to the type of movement that occurs (e.g. ball and socket, hinge). A synovial joint is enclosed by a collagenous capsule attached to the bone at some distance from the joint. The inner surface of the capsule is lined by a fluid-producing membrane. Localised thickenings of the capsule, the ligaments, connect the adjacent bones. Other ligaments blend into the capsule

at one end but are attached to bone at the other (Fig. 10.3) or remain totally independent of the joint capsule.

The synovial membrane is one cell thick. One type of cell ingests foreign or autologous material that has entered the joint; another synthesises and secretes the synovial fluid. Synovial fluid is a dialysate of plasma with the addition of hyaluronate proteoglycan. The ratio of the concentration of a synovial fluid protein to its serum concentration is determined by molecular size. The synovial fluid provides both nutrition for the articular cartilage and lubricates the joint surfaces.

Temporary synarthroses (synchondroses) are found at the growing points of long bones in the form of epiphyseal cartilage. The sutures of the skull are synarthroses, the bony margins being joined by fibrous tissue.

Amphiarthroses are permanent joints. A good example is the intervertebral disc of the spine. An outer layer of dense concentric bundles of collagen, the annulus fibrosus, encloses a core of hydrated compact tissue, the nucleus pulposus.

MUSCLE

A motor neuron innervates 100–1000 skeletal muscle fibres. Within the muscle fibre is a recurring anatomical structure, the sarcomere, consisting of thin filaments that are composed of actin and thick filaments composed of myosin (Fig. 10.4). During the contraction and relaxation of muscle, the thin and thick filaments move in relationship to one another. All the fibres of a particular motor unit have similar properties. Muscle fibres are divided into fast and slow twitch (type I and type II) according to their speed of contraction, although in humans a continuum of twitch speed exists.

Slowly contracting motor units are innervated by slowly conducting nerve fibres with a low threshold and firing frequency. Rapidly contracting motor units are innervated by axons that conduct rapidly but have a high threshold. The strength of muscle contraction can be altered either by varying the number of motor units recruited or by altering their firing frequency. The recruitment process begins with small units and progresses to larger. Firing frequency ranges from 10 to 20 Hz for slow units and up to 100 Hz for fast units. Slow twitch muscles have a high myoglobin content, producing a reddish appearance. Slow twitch fibres use oxidative mechanisms for energy formation; fast twitch fibres employ glycolysis. The former are fatigue-resistant, the latter rapidly fatiguable. In general, slow units provide sustained muscle tension over long periods, of the sort required to maintain a particular posture, whereas fast units allow short-lived, sudden muscle contraction.

Symptoms of bone, joint and muscle disorders

BONE

Pain

Bone pain has a deep, boring quality. The pain is focal in the presence of a bone tumour or infection but diffuse in generalised disorders (e.g. osteoporosis). The pain of a fracture is sharp and piercing and exacerbated by movement but relieved by rest.

JOINTS

Joint symptoms include pain, swelling, crepitus and locking.

Differential diagnosis
Bone pain

Focal pain
- Fracture or trauma
- Infection
- Malignancy
- Paget's disease
- Osteoid osteoma

Diffuse pain
- Malignancy
- Paget's disease
- Osteomalacia
- Osteoporosis
- Metabolic bone disease

Risk factors
Age-related osteoporosis

- Female
- Premature loss of gonadal function
- Family history of osteoporosis
- Thin body habitus
- Decreased physical activity
- Low calcium intake
- Smoking
- High alcohol intake
- Nulliparity

Pain

In an arthritic disorder, pain is usually the most prominent complaint. Important aspects to determine are the site and severity of the pain, whether it is acute or chronic, how it is influenced by rest and activity and whether it appears during a particular range of movement.

Ask the patient to point to the maximal site of pain. Although irritation of structures close to the skin produces well-localised pain, disturbance of deeper structures produces pain that is poorly localised and eventually segmental in distribution.

The segments to which the pain is referred (the sclerotomes) differ somewhat from dermatomal distributions. Consequently, deep pain can be felt at a point some distance from the affected structure, that is, referred pain. Where joint disease exists, misinterpretation of the site of the disease process can follow (Fig. 10.5). Spinal pain can also be referred. Abnormal function in the upper cervical spine can lead to pain over the occipital region, whereas disorders of the lower lumbar spine may lead to upper lumbar back pain stemming from the fact that the posterior longitudinal ligament is innervated by the upper lumbar nerves.

Severity of joint pain is difficult to judge, depending, as it does, on the patient's personality. Osteoarthritis and

Joint pain

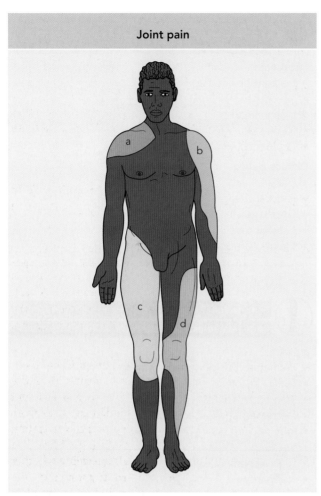

Fig. 10.5 Distribution of pain arising from (a) the acromioclavicular or sternoclavicular joints, (b) the scapulohumeral joint, (c) the hip joint and (d) the knee joint.

rheumatoid arthritis typically result in chronic pain with periodic exacerbation; septic arthritis or gout produce an acutely painful joint.

Inflammatory joint disease tends to cause pain on waking, improving with activity but returning at rest. Mechanical joint disease (e.g. caused by osteoarthritis) leads to pain that worsens during the course of the day, particularly with activity.

For certain joint disorders (e.g. at the shoulder), pain is apparent only during a specific range of movement. If confirmed by examination, this selectivity can be valuable in differential diagnosis.

Swelling and crepitus

If the patient has noticed joint swelling, elicit for how long it has been present, whether there is associated pain and whether the swelling fluctuates. A noisy joint is not necessarily pathological. Introspective individuals are likely to interpret periodic clicking in a joint, in the absence of pain, as having pathological significance. It does not. Crepitus is a grating noise or sensation; it can have both auditory and palpable qualities. Fine crepitus is more readily felt than heard, but crepitus stemming from advanced degeneration of a large joint (e.g. the hip) is readily audible.

Locking

A joint locks if ectopic material becomes interposed between the articular surfaces. It is particularly associated with damage to the knee cartilages. Ascertain if the locking occurs at a particular point during movement of the joint.

MUSCLE

Muscle symptoms include pain and stiffness, weakness, wasting, abnormal spontaneous movements and cramps.

Pain and stiffness

Muscle pain tends to be deep, constant and poorly localised. If caused by local muscle disease, it is likely to

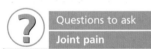

Questions to ask

Joint pain

- Where is the maximal site of pain?
- Does the pain change during the course of the day?
- Has the pain been there for a short or long time?
- Does the pain get better or worse with movement?

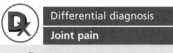

Differential diagnosis

Joint pain

- Inflammatory
  - rheumatoid arthritis
  - ankylosing spondylitis
- Mechanical
  - osteoarthritis
- Infective
  - pyogenic
  - tuberculosis
  - brucellosis
- Traumatic

Differential diagnosis

Muscle pain

- Inflammatory
  - polymyositis
  - dermatomyositis
- Infective
  - pyogenic
  - cysticercosis
- Traumatic
- Polymyalgia rheumatica
- Neuropathic
  - e.g. Guillain–Barré syndrome

be exacerbated by contraction of the muscle and relieved by rest. If the patient complains more of muscle stiffness (particularly of the lower limbs) than pain, suspect the possibility of spasticity caused by an upper motor neuron lesion.

Weakness

A complaint of global weakness is more likely in neurotic individuals than in patients with neurological disorders.

Important questions to ask include the distribution of the weakness, whether it appears related to any pain in the limb, whether it fluctuates and whether it is static or progressive. A complaint of predominant proximal weakness suggests the possibility of primary muscle disease (e.g. polymyositis or myopathy). A predominantly distal weakness is more likely to be neuropathic. If the weakness is fluctuant, and particularly if it worsens during the course of activity, you will need to consider myasthenia gravis when you come to examine the patient (see also Ch. 11). Weakness caused by sudden entrapment of a peripheral nerve (e.g. a traumatic radial nerve palsy) will be stable or even improving by the time the patient seeks medical attention. In other conditions the weakness is progressive (e.g. motor neuron disease).

Questions to ask
Muscle weakness

- Is the weakness global or focal?
- Is the weakness secondary to a painful limb?
- Does the weakness fluctuate?
- Is the weakness increasing in severity?

Wasting and fasciculation

Both these features form an important part of the examination, but both may have been noticed by the patient and volunteered during history-taking. If the patient describes muscle twitching, ascertain whether the movement has occurred in several different muscles or whether it has been confined to one area, most likely the calf.

Cramps

Cramps are seldom of pathological significance. They are usually confined to the calves and can be triggered by forced contraction of the muscle.

General principles of examination

BONE

Whichever structure is being examined, ensure that it is completely exposed and that the patient is comfortably positioned. Determine whether there is any abnormal

angularity. Is there limb shortening? Look for tenderness by gently palpating those parts of the bone close to the skin surface.

JOINTS

You need to follow a strict routine with joint examination, incorporating inspection, palpation and assessment of the movement of the joint.

Inspection

Things you are looking for include swelling, joint deformity, overlying skin changes and the appearance of the surrounding structures.

Swelling Causes of joint swelling include effusions, thickening of the synovial tissues and of the bony margins of the joint. Differentiation of these causes is achieved by palpation. If you suspect joint swelling, compare it with the joint of the opposite limb. Particularly note if the swelling appears to be of the joint itself or of the adjacent structures.

Deformity Deformity results either from misalignment of the bones forming the joint or from alteration of the relationship between the articular surfaces. If misalignment exists, a deviation of the part distal to the joint away from the midline is called a valgus deformity and a deviation towards the midline a varus deformity (Fig. 10.6). If a deformity exists you will need later to determine whether it is fixed or mobile. Partial loss of contact of the articulating surfaces is called subluxation, and complete loss dislocation. Although these are usually traumatic, they can also be seen in inflammatory joint disease, particularly rheumatoid arthritis. Swan neck, Boutonnière and mallet are descriptive terms used for deformities of

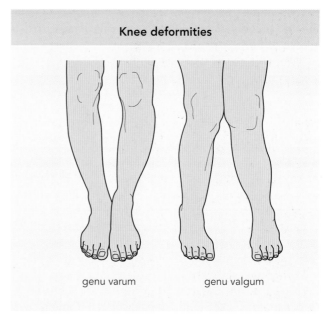

Knee deformities

genu varum   genu valgum

Fig. 10.6 Genu varum (left) and genu valgum (right).

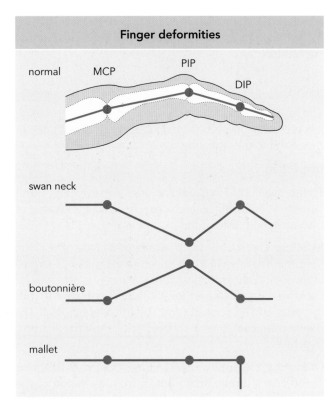

Finger deformities

normal

MCP   PIP

DIP

swan neck

boutonnière

mallet

Fig. 10.7 Deformities of the finger in rheumatoid arthritis.

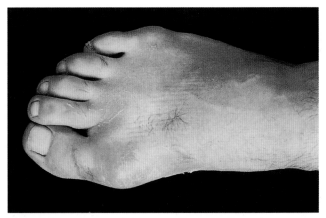

Fig. 10.8 Acute gout of the first metatarsophalangeal joint.

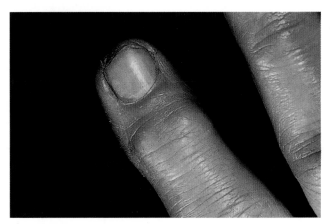

Fig. 10.9 Osteoarthritis of the DIP joint.

the metacarpophalangeal and interphalangeal joints of the hand (Fig. 10.7).

Skin changes You should palpate the skin over a joint to assess its temperature rather than relying simply on its colour. Redness of the skin over a joint implies an underlying acute inflammatory reaction (e.g. gout) (Fig. 10.8).

Changes of adjacent structures The most striking change adjacent to a diseased joint is wasting of muscle. Assess muscle bulk above and below the affected joint, making a comparison with the opposite limb if that is spared. Wasting of quadriceps is particularly conspicuous in severe disease of the knee joint.

Palpation

During palpation of a joint, assess the nature of any swelling, whether there is tenderness and whether the joint is hot.

Swelling The method of examining for an effusion will be described for the individual joints. Your first step is to determine the consistency of any swelling. Is the swelling hard, suggesting bone deformities secondary to osteoarthritis? Certain sites are particularly susceptible to osteoarthritic change (e.g. the distal interphalangeal joints of the hand) (Fig. 10.9). A slightly spongy or boggy swelling suggests synovial thickening and is particularly associated with rheumatoid arthritis. An effusion is fluctuant, that is, the fluid can be displaced from one part of the joint to another. Swellings may also arise adjacent

to a joint. Again determine their consistency. Soft fluctuant swellings suggest enlarged bursae. Harder swellings occur in rheumatoid arthritis and gout.

Tenderness Carefully palpate the joint margin and adjacent bony surfaces together with the surrounding ligaments and tendons. Your task is to discover whether any tenderness is within the joint or outside it, and whether the tenderness is focal or generalised. In an acutely inflamed joint, the whole of its palpable contours will be tender. If there is derangement of a single knee cartilage, tenderness will be confined to the margin of that cartilage. In degenerative joint disease, you may find tenderness in structures adjacent to the joint. Tenderness close to the joint may reflect primary pathology in bone (e.g. osteomyelitis) or in the tendon sheath (e.g. De Quervain's tenosynovitis) (Figs 10.10, 10.11).

Temperature For a small joint, for example, in the finger, assess temperature with the finger tips, using an unaffected joint in the same or the other hand for comparison. For a larger joint, for example, the knee, rub the back of your hand across the joint then compare with the other limb. If the contralateral joint is also affected, carry your hand above and below the joint margins to make the comparison.

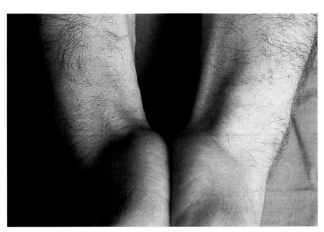

Fig. 10.10 De Quervain's tenosynovitis of the wrist.

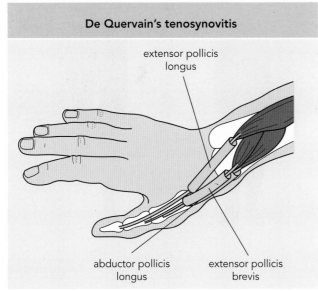

Fig. 10.11 De Quervain's tenosynovitis. The tendons of abductor pollicis longus and extensor pollicis brevis are inflamed.

Neutral position

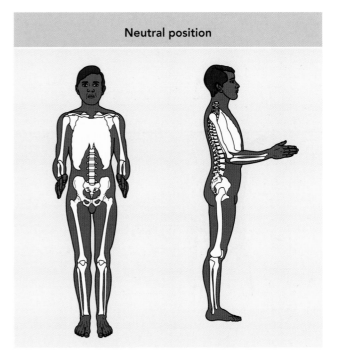

Fig. 10.12 The neutral position from which joint measurement is performed.

Range of joint movement

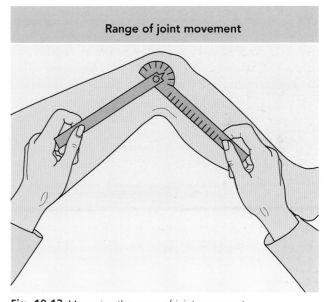

Fig. 10.13 Measuring the range of joint movement.

Joint movement

Next proceed to examine the range of movement of the joint, whether movement is limited by pain and whether there is instability.

To define the range of joint movement, start with the joints in the neutral position, defined as the lower limbs extended with the feet dorsiflexed to 90°, and the upper limbs midway between pronation and supination with the arms flexed to 90° at the elbows (Fig. 10.12). For accurate measurement of joint movement you will need a goniometer (Fig. 10.13) but for routine purposes your eye should allow a reasonably true estimate. Movement of a joint is either active (i.e. induced by the patient) or passive (i.e. induced by the examiner). Sometimes you need to assess both but you will generally assess active movements in the spine but passive movements in the limb joints. Restriction of active compared with passive movement is usually due to muscle weakness.

From the neutral position, record the degrees of flexion and extension. If extension does not normally occur at a joint (e.g. the knee) but is present, describe the movement as hyperextension and give its range in degrees. Sometimes there is restriction of the range of movement. For example, if the knee fails by 30° to reach the extended position, describe this as either a 30° flexion deformity or as a 30° lack of extension (Fig. 10.14). For the ankle and wrist, extension is described as dorsiflexion and flexion as plantar and palmar flexion, respectively. For a ball and socket joint, you will need to record the range of flexion, extension, abduction, adduction and internal and external

Flexion deformity

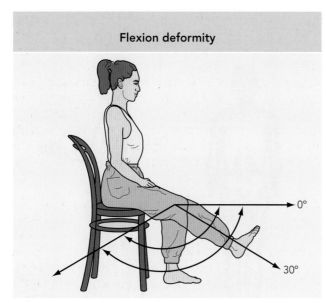

Fig. 10.14 30° flexion deformity of the knee.

Types of joint movement

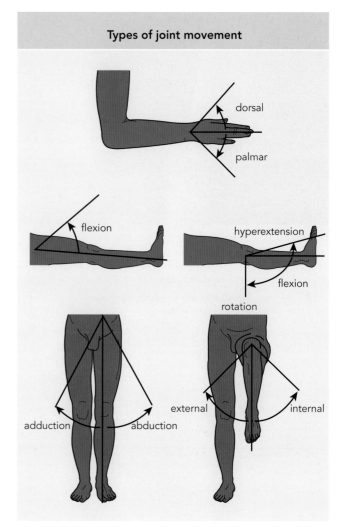

Fig. 10.15 Description of joint movement according to the type of joint.

rotation (Fig. 10.15). The range of joint movement varies between individuals: an excessive range of movement can be constitutional as well as pathological. Carefully note if pain occurs during joint movement. In joint disease, pain is likely to occur throughout the range of movement. In certain disease processes around the joint (e.g. in the ligaments or bursae), pain can be restricted to a particular range or type of movement. Damage of either the articular surfaces or of the ligaments related to a joint can lead to instability. You will discover this partly by finding that the joint can be moved into abnormal positions and partly, particularly for the knee joint, by observing the joint as the patient walks.

GALS

A screening history and examination process for the musculoskeletal system has been devised for undergraduate use (GALS – gait, arms, legs and spine).

SCREENING HISTORY

- Have you any pain or stiffness in your muscles, joints or back?
- Can you dress yourself completely without difficulty?
- Can you walk up and down stairs without difficulty?

If the answers to all three questions are negative, significant musculoskeletal abnormality is unlikely.

SCREENING EXAMINATION

- Gait – Inspect the patient walking, turning and walking back.
- Spine – Inspect the patient from three positions from behind, from the side, then ask the patient to bend forwards and touch the toes, and finally from in front

ask the patient to try to place the relevant ear on each shoulder in turn (lateral neck flexion).
- Arms – From in front ask the patient to place both hands behind the head, elbows back.
  - Place both hands by the side, elbows straight.
  - Place both hands out in front, palms down, fingers straight.
  - Turn both hands over. Make a tight fist with each hand.
  - Place the tip of each finger onto the tip of the thumb in turn.
  - The examiner then squeezes across the second to the fifth metacarpals to elicit tenderness.
- Legs – Inspect from in front (with the patient standing).
  - Inspect with the patient lying flat.
  - Flex each hip and knee while holding the knee (confirming full knee flexion without knee crepitus).
  - Passively internally rotate each hip in flexion (checking for pain and restricted movement).

- Press on each patella for tenderness and palpate for an effusion.
- Squeeze across the metatarsals for tenderness due to metatarsophalangeal disease.
- Inspect both soles for callosities reflecting abnormal weight-bearing.

RECORDING FINDINGS

Normal response to the screening questions can be recorded as:

Pain   0
Dress   ✓
Walk   ✓

Results of the physical examination can be recorded if gait (G) is normal, there are no abnormalities to the appearance (A) of the areas inspected (i.e. no swelling, deformity, wasting, abnormal position or skin change) and no abnormalities of movement (M) of the arms (A), legs (L) or spine (S) as follows:

G   ✓
            A   M
A   ✓   ✓
L   ✓   ✓
S   ✓   ✓

Any abnormality is recorded as an X and described in more detail.

MUSCLE

The methods for examining individual muscles will be given in the section on regional examination. Initially your assessment will include inspection, palpation, then testing of muscle power.

Inspection

Look for evidence of muscle wasting, for signs of abnormal muscle bulk and for spontaneous contractions.

Wasting Remember that striking muscle wasting can accompany joint disease (e.g. wasting of the small hand muscles in rheumatoid arthritis and wasting of the quadriceps in virtually any arthropathy affecting the knee joint). If there is no significant joint disease, wasting (other than caused by a profound loss of body weight) reflects either primary muscle disease or disease of its innervating neuron. Make allowances for the age of the patient and his or her occupation. Some thinning of the hand muscles occurs in elderly people but is not accompanied by weakness. If you suspect wasting of one limb, measure the circumference of that limb and compare it with its fellow. For example, for the thigh, mark the line of the medial cartilage of the knee joint, measure up, for example, 20 cm, on each thigh and record the circumference of the legs at that point.

Increased muscle bulk Usually abnormal muscle bulk reflects the patient's obsession with his own bodily strength (it is almost always a man). There are rare conditions that lead to muscle hypertrophy. If the enlargement is due to increase in muscle bulk, it is called true hypertrophy and is seen, for example, in congenital myotonia. If the increased bulk is due to fatty infiltration (and you will then discover the muscle is actually weak), it is called pseudohypertrophy. This finding is characteristic of certain of the muscular dystrophies (e.g. Duchenne's).

Spontaneous contractions Completely expose the muscle when looking for evidence of spontaneous contraction. Make sure the patient is warm and relaxed. Shivering brought on by cold can be difficult to distinguish from fasciculation. Spontaneous movements can occur with both upper and lower motor neuron lesions. In the former, particularly at the spinal level, you may see either flexor or extensor spasms of the legs, either at the hips or knees. The movements can occur spontaneously or be triggered by attempting to move the patient and are often painful. Fasciculation produces episodic muscle twitching that can be subtle in small muscles. It is a feature of lower motor neuron lesions but can also be seen in normal individuals. Fasciculation is intermittent. Wait for a few minutes before deciding it is absent. It is particularly important to determine whether the fasciculation is confined to a single muscle or whether it is more widely distributed. The former may reflect the result of cervical radiculopathy or be physiological (particularly if confined to the calves); the latter suggests a diagnosis of motor neuron disease.

Palpation

Muscle palpation is of limited value. If the muscle is infected or inflamed it is likely to be tender. Most myopathies are painless but there are exceptions (e.g. the acute myopathy occurring in alcoholics). Muscle tenderness can also occur in neurogenic disorders (e.g. the peripheral neuropathy of thiamine deficiency can lead to marked calf tenderness).

Testing muscle power

You should follow the UK Medical Research Council classification (p. 363) when testing and recording muscle power. Remember to make allowance for sex, age and the patient's stature. If the muscle itself, or the joint that it moves, is painful then power will be correspondingly limited. Patterns of muscle weakness are particularly important in neurological diagnosis. Is the weakness global, does it predominate distally or proximally in the limb, does its distribution fit with either a peripheral nerve or root distribution? Sometimes muscle power is decidedly fluctuant: there is a sudden give, alternating with more effective contraction. Although this pattern can occur in myasthenia gravis, it is usually the reflection of a nonorganic disability. If muscle fatigue is a prominent symptom assess it objectively. For example, for the deltoid, ask the patient to abduct the shoulder to 90°. Test power immediately, then after the patient has held that posture for 60 seconds.

You will need to be selective when deciding which muscles to test. Your choice will be guided partly by the patient's complaints, both in terms of their distribution and their quality.

REGIONAL STRUCTURE, FUNCTION AND EXAMINATION

Temporomandibular joints

Ask the patient to open and close the jaw. If the temporomandibular joints are lax, there may be considerable side-to-side movement. Now palpate the joint margins by placing your fingers immediately in front of and below the tragus. As the patient opens the jaw, palpate the head of the mandible as it moves forwards and downwards. In temporomandibular joint dysfunction, the joint capsule is tender and chewing is painful. The generalised arthritic disorders seldom affect this joint.

The spine

STRUCTURE AND FUNCTION

The primary curvatures of the spine, in the thoracic and sacral regions, are determined by differences in height of the anterior and posterior aspects of the vertebrae at these levels. The secondary curvatures of the cervical and lumbar regions depend more on the relative heights of the anterior and posterior aspects of the intervertebral discs. The nucleus pulposus allows an even distribution of applied force onto the annulus fibrosus and the hyaline laminae covering the opposing vertebral bodies.

Forward flexion and extension occur at all levels of the spine but are maximal at the junction of the atlas with the occiput and in the lumbar and cervical regions. Lateral flexion is greatest at the atlanto-occipital junction, occurs to some extent in the lumbar and cervical regions, but minimally in the thoracic region. Rotation other than at the atlantoaxial joints, is determined by the shape of the apophyseal joints and is maximal at the thoracic level.

Examination of the spine

With the patient undressed to the underwear, ask the patient to stand upright. Assess the posture of the whole spine before examining its component parts. An increased flexion is called kyphosis, increased extension, lordosis and a lateral curvature, scoliosis. Gibbus refers to a focal

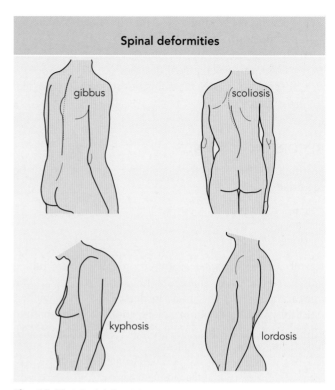

Fig. 10.16 Spinal deformities.

flexion deformity (Fig. 10.16). Using the position of the spinous processes tends to underestimate the degree of scoliosis, as the spines rotate towards the midline. The scoliosis is accentuated when the patient bends forwards.

For each spinal level, start by inspection and follow by palpation to elicit any tenderness. Finally, assess the range of movement and determine whether it is restricted by pain.

CERVICAL SPINE

The examination is best achieved with the patient sitting. Note any deformity, then palpate the spinous processes. A cervical rib is sometimes palpable in the supraclavicular fossa. Obliteration of the radial pulse by downward traction of the arm does not reliably predict the presence of a cervical rib or band.

Examine active then passive movements. For flexion, ask the patient to bring the chin onto the chest and for extension ask them to bend the head backwards as far as possible. Observe both these movements from the side. For lateral flexion, stand in front of or behind the patient and ask the patient to bring the ear towards the shoulder first on one side, then the other. For rotation, stand in front or over the patient asking the patient to look over one shoulder then the other (Fig. 10.17). Note whether any movement triggers pain either locally or in the upper limb. Repeating the movements while applying gentle pressure over the vertex of the skull may trigger pain or paraesthesiae in the arm if there is a

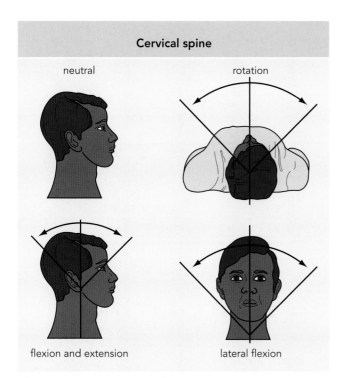

Fig. 10.17 Movements of the cervical spine.

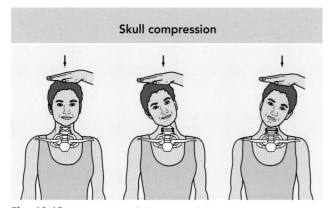

Fig. 10.18 Compression of the vertex of the skull to reproduce cervical root pain. Compression with the head in the neutral position (left) or laterally flexed to the right is painless (middle). With the head flexed to the left (right), the side of the root compression, downward pressure is painful.

critical degree of narrowing at an intervertebral foramen (Fig. 10.18).

THORACIC SPINE

Sit the patient with the arms folded across the chest, then ask the patient to twist as far as possible first to one side then to the other. The range of movement is best appreciated from above. Next measure chest expansion. A movement of at least 5 cm should occur and provides an assessment of the mobility of the costovertebral junction. Palpate the spinous processes for any tenderness and assess any deformity.

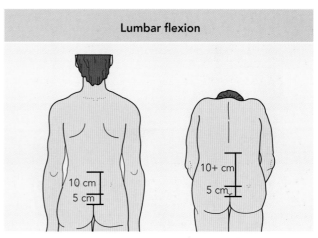

Fig. 10.19 Measuring lumbar flexion.

LUMBAR SPINE

Having inspected the lumbar spine and tested for tenderness, assess the range of movement. While standing at the patient's side, ask the patient to touch the toes, keeping the knees straight. To assess the contribution made to flexion by the lumbar spine, mark the spine at the lumbosacral junction, then 10 cm above and 5 cm below this point. On forward flexion the distance between the two upper marks should increase by approximately 4 cm, the distance between the lower two remaining unaltered (Fig. 10.19). Now assess extension, again from the side, then lateral flexion. For this, stand behind the patient and ask the patient to slide the hand down the outside of the leg, first on one side and then on the other (Fig. 10.20).

SACROILIAC JOINTS

Palpate the joints, which lie under the dimples found in the lower lumbar region. To test whether movement at the joint is painful, first press firmly down over the midline of the sacrum with the patient prone (Fig. 10.21) then, with the patient supine, forcibly flex one hip while maintaining the other in an extended position.

NERVE STRETCH TESTS

Nerve stretch tests are carried out to determine whether there is evidence of nerve root irritation, usually as a consequence of prolapse of a lumbar disc.

Straight leg raising

With the patient supine, carefully elevate the extended leg at the hip. Normally, 80–90° of flexion is possible.

Restriction of movement can occur with both spinal and hip disease. In the presence of nerve root irritation at the L4 level or below, straight leg raising evokes pain as the sciatic nerve is stretched (Fig. 10.22). If the foot is now dorsiflexed, the pain increases (Bragard's test).

Thoracolumbar spine

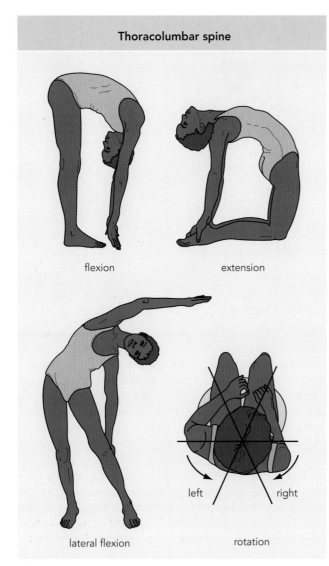

flexion   extension

left   right

lateral flexion   rotation

Fig. 10.20 Movements of the thoracolumbar spine.

Sacroiliac joint

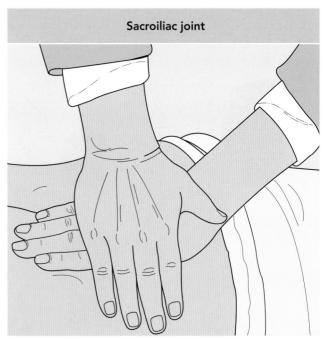

Fig. 10.21 Assessing the sacroiliac joint.

Return the foot to the neutral position, then flex the knee. The hip can now be flexed further before pain reappears but if the knee is then extended, the pain increases (Lasegue's test).

Femoral stretch test

Turn the patient into the prone position. First flex the knee. If this fails to trigger pain, extend the leg at the hip. A positive response, with pain in the back extending into the anterior thigh, suggests irritation of the second, third or fourth lumbar root on that side (Fig. 10.23).

Clinical application

Back pain can arise from disease processes in the vertebrae, from degenerative changes in the joints between the vertebrae, from degeneration or actual prolapse of the intervertebral disc and from the ligaments and muscles supporting and moving the spine.

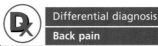

Differential diagnosis

Back pain

- Muscle or ligamentous strain
- Degenerative intervertebral disc
- Spondylolisthesis
- Arthritis
  – osteoarthritis
  – rheumatoid arthritis
  – ankylosing spondylitis
- Bone infection
  – pyogenic
  – tuberculous
- Trauma
- Tumour
- Osteochondritis
- Metabolic bone disease

Questions to ask

Back pain

- Is the pain confined to the back or does it radiate to the upper or lower limb?
- Is the pain exacerbated by coughing or sneezing?
- Did the pain begin suddenly or gradually?

PROLAPSED INTERVERTEBRAL DISC

A prolapse of disc material is most likely to occur either in the cervical (principally at C5/6) or the lumbar (principally at L5/S1) region. Once nerve root irritation occurs, likely symptoms include local and referred pain, with sensory

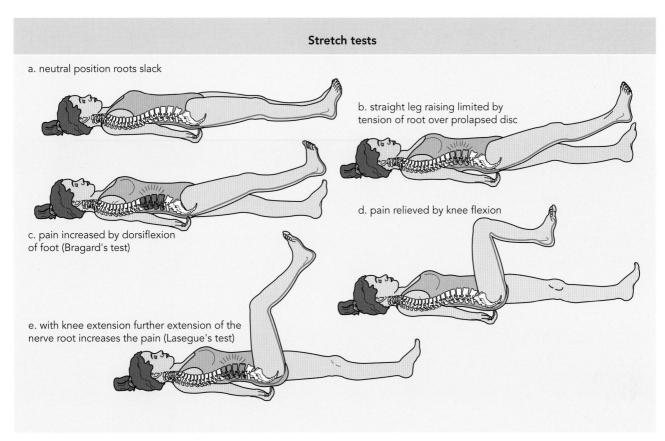

Fig. 10.22 Stretch tests: (a) neutral position, (b) straight leg raising, (c) Bragard's test, (d) knee flexion and (e) Lasegue's test.

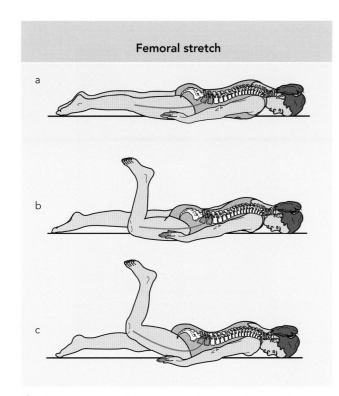

Fig. 10.23 (a) Femoral stretch. The pain may be triggered by (b) knee flexion alone or (c) in combination with hip extension.

and motor symptoms in the limb. The pattern of distribution of sensory change, weakness or reflex change allows prediction of the affected nerve root (Fig. 10.24).

OTHER CONDITIONS

Ankylosing spondylitis

In ankylosing spondylitis the patient, usually male, complains of spinal pain and stiffness, the latter improving with exercise. The sacroiliac joints are affected initially. Increasing loss of spinal mobility can lead to a thoracic kyphosis combined with loss of the lumbar lordosis (Fig. 10.25).

Rheumatoid arthritis

This complaint commonly involves the upper cervical spine. Synovitis affecting the cruciate ligament allows posterior subluxation of the odontoid peg. Compression of the upper cervical cord is a potential hazard, producing a tetraparesis (Fig. 10.26).

Spinal tumours

Spinal tumours are usually metastatic from prostate, breast, bronchus or kidney. Initially, there is local severe rest pain, sometimes with a referred component caused by spinal root compression. Later, focal neurological signs appear.

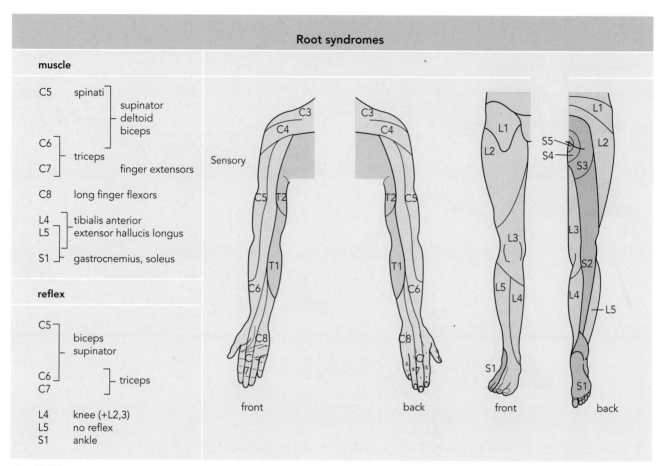

Fig. 10.24 Sensory, motor and reflex changes in cervical and lumbar root syndromes.

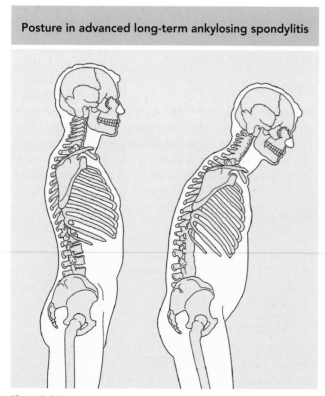

Fig. 10.25 Posture in advanced long-term ankylosing spondylitis on the right with control subject on the left.

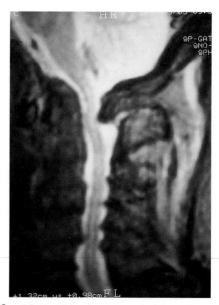

Fig. 10.26 Axial T$_2$-weighted MRI scan showing atlantoaxial dislocation.

Tuberculosis

This disease most commonly involves the thoracic or lumbar spine. The infective process begins in the anterior margin of the vertebral body with early involvement of the disc space. Vertebral collapse with gibbus formation and paraspinal abscess follow. Symptoms include back pain and deformity with evidence of spinal cord compression.

TRAUMATIC LESIONS

Cervical spine injuries include atlantoaxial dislocation, fractures of the arch of the atlas and compression fractures of the vertebral bodies. Complications include spinal instability and neurological damage.

Fractures around the cervicothoracic junction are easily missed unless the shoulders are well depressed at the time of the radiograph.

Thoracic and lumbar spine injuries include compression fractures and fractures of the transverse processes. Pathological fractures commonly occur at this level. Complications include paraplegia (with thoracic fractures) and haemorrhage into the retroperitoneal space.

The shoulder

STRUCTURE AND FUNCTION

Movement of the shoulder takes place both at the glenohumeral and the scapulothoracic joints. For abduction, the first 90° of movement takes place at the glenohumeral joint. This is achieved by contraction first of supraspinatus (0–30°) then of deltoid (30–90°). Abduction of the shoulder beyond 90° requires rotation of the scapula, which is achieved by contraction of trapezius. Adduction is principally due to pectoralis major and latissimus dorsi. Forward flexion depends mainly on pectoralis major and the anterior fibres of the deltoid, extension on latissimus dorsi, teres major and the posterior fibres of the deltoid. Lateral rotation is accomplished by contraction of infraspinatus and medial rotation by pectoralis major, latissimus dorsi and the anterior fibres of the deltoid. Immediately above the glenohumeral joint lies the subacromial bursa and the rotator cuff, which is formed by the tendons of the supraspinatus, infraspinatus and subscapularis.

INSPECTION AND PALPATION

Inspect the contour of the shoulder and its surrounding structures. Small effusions in the shoulder are difficult to detect. Anterior dislocation results in a forward and downward displacement with alteration of the shoulder contour (Fig. 10.27). Posterior dislocation is obvious. Fracture of the clavicle and anterior dislocation of the sternoclavicular joint are usually readily visible. Look at the deltoid to see if it is wasted. Then inspect the periscapular muscles. The bulk of the supraspinatus and infraspinatus is easily assessed.

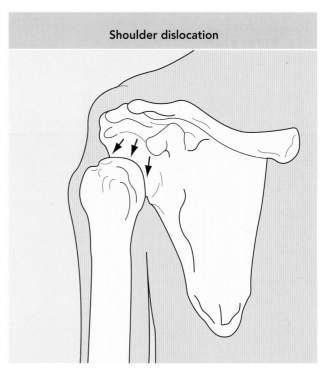

Shoulder dislocation

Fig. 10.27 Dislocation of the shoulder.

Palpate the shoulder and sternoclavicular joints for tenderness.

JOINT MOVEMENT

Remember that most movement at the shoulder involves both the glenohumeral joint and rotation of the scapula across the thorax. You will test flexion and extension, internal and external rotation, abduction and adduction (Fig. 10.28). When testing abduction, anchor the scapula with your free hand, to ensure that over the first 90° only glenohumeral movement is allowed (Fig. 10.29). Test first passive then active movement. During abduction, note particularly if pain occurs. Is the pain present throughout the movement or only over a particular range? With a frozen shoulder (attributed to capsulitis of the glenohumeral joint), pain is accompanied by restriction of all glenohumeral movements.

Painful arc syndrome

The painful arc syndrome causes pain on shoulder elevation. As the arm is elevated, elements of the rotator cuff, comprising the tendons of the supraspinatus, infraspinatus and subscapularis, come into contact with the undersurface of the acromion. Inflammation of one of the muscles, particularly the supraspinatus or of the subacromial bursa, causes pain in the region of the shoulder, with a painful arc of movement during abduction (Fig. 10.30). Pain is absent initially, develops during abduction as elements of the cuff come into

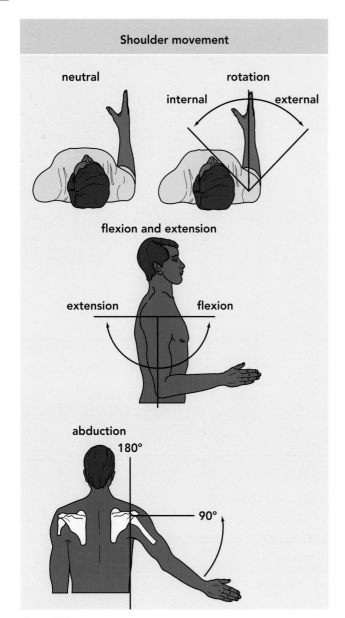

Shoulder movement

neutral

rotation
internal   external

flexion and extension

extension   flexion

abduction
180°

90°

Fig. 10.28 Testing shoulder movement.

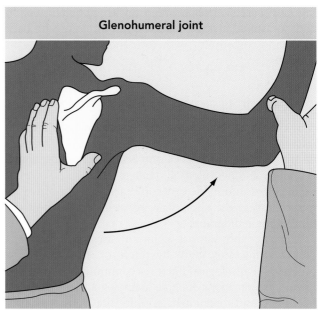

Fig. 10.29 Testing shoulder abduction at the glenohumeral joint.

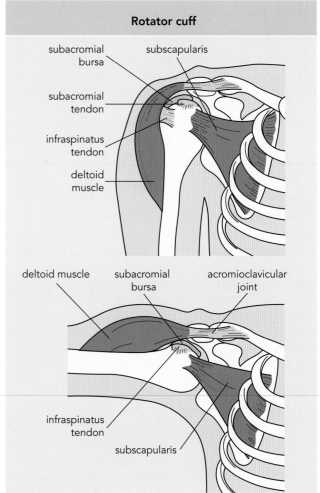

Rotator cuff

subacromial bursa

subscapularis

subacromial tendon

infraspinatus tendon

deltoid muscle

deltoid muscle   subacromial bursa   acromioclavicular joint

infraspinatus tendon

subscapularis

Fig. 10.30 The rotator cuff apparatus.

contact with the undersurface of the acromion, then disappears in the final part of abduction as the tendons fall away from the acromion.

Bicipital tendonitis

In bicipital tendonitis, tenosynovitis involves the long head of the biceps. The patient complains of pain in the anterior aspect of the shoulder and arm. The pain is reproduced by palpating the tendon or by contracting the muscle.

Traumatic lesions

These include dislocation, fracture dislocation and fractures of the neck of the humerus. Dislocations are usually anterior, less commonly posterior. With the

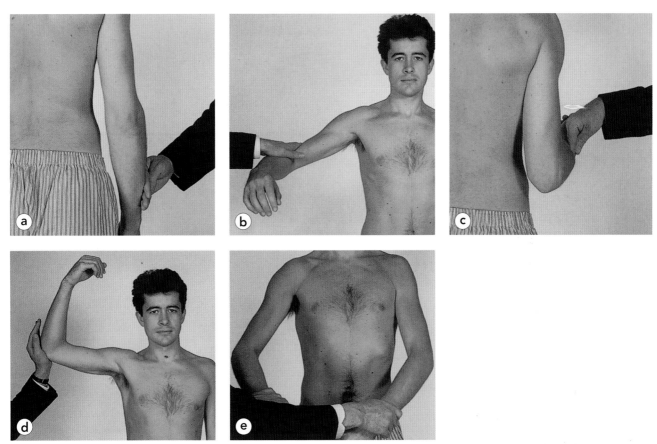

Fig. 10.31 Testing the major muscles concerned with shoulder movement. (a) Supraspinatus, (b) deltoid, (c) infraspinatus, (d) latissimus dorsi and (e) pectoralis major.

former, the contour of the shoulder is flattened and the arm abducted. Axillary nerve damage can occur and, less often, trauma to the brachial plexus or the axillary artery.

MUSCLE FUNCTION

In the presence of any of the above conditions, muscle power is limited by concomitant pain. If shoulder movements are free and painless, the individual muscles concerned with movement around the joint can now be tested (Fig. 10.31).

Cervical radiculopathy

Cervical radiculopathy often affects the fifth nerve root. Weakness is found in the spinati, deltoid and biceps. Wasting may follow (Fig. 10.32). The biceps and supinator reflexes are depressed.

Neuralgic amyotrophy

In neuralgic amyotrophy, severe pain around the shoulder is followed by patchy weakness and wasting in the shoulder girdle muscles. One form affects the long thoracic nerve, with consequent winging of the scapula as the arm is pushed forwards (Fig. 10.33).

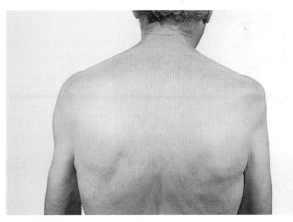

Fig. 10.32 Wasting of deltoid, infraspinatus and supraspinatus in a right C5 root lesion.

Nerve palsies

Nerve palsies affecting the shoulder are rare. A fracture of the upper end of the humerus can damage the circumflex nerve, resulting in weakness of deltoid and a small patch of numbness over the lateral aspect of the shoulder.

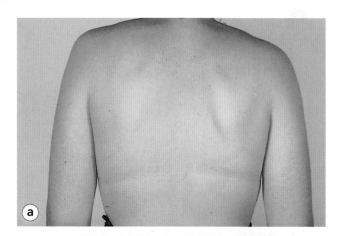

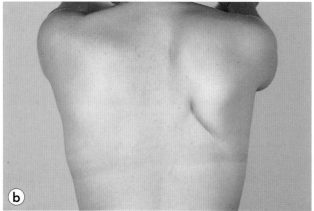

Fig. 10.33 Winging of the scapula on forward pressure.

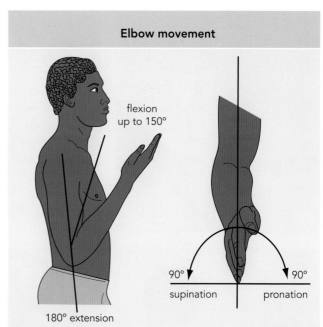

Fig. 10.34 Range of movement at the elbow.

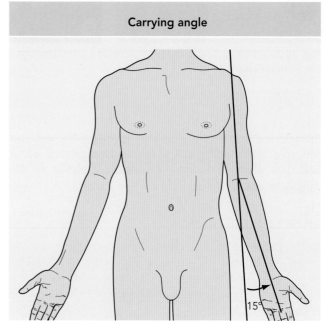

Fig. 10.35 Carrying angle of the forearm.

The elbow

STRUCTURE AND FUNCTION

There are two joints at the elbow, one involving the humerus, radius and ulna, the other joining the upper ends of the radius and ulna. Flexion or extension movement occurs at the former through a range of approximately 150°. The latter joint allows the forearm to rotate (pronation-supination) through a range of 180° (Fig. 10.34). In males, the forearm is only slightly abducted from the axis of the humerus. In females, the abduction is greater, forming a carrying angle of about 15° (Fig. 10.35).

The biceps flexes the elbow when the arm is supinated. The brachioradialis and brachialis flex the elbow in either the pronated or supinated position. Extension of the elbow is achieved by triceps, with a minor contribution from anconeus (Fig. 10.36). Supination is produced by contraction of the supinator and pronation by the combined action of pronator teres and pronator quadratus.

INSPECTION AND PALPATION

Inspect the joint from behind, comparing its alignment with the other arm. An effusion produces a swelling on either side of the olecranon. Swelling of the olecranon bursa can follow trauma or occurs in association with rheumatoid arthritis. Now palpate the subcutaneous border of the ulna, a common site for rheumatoid nodules (Fig. 10.37). Move on to palpate the lateral and medial epicondyles (Fig. 10.38). Inflammation of the extensor and flexor origins at these respective sites (tennis elbow and golfer's elbow) leads to pain in the region of the elbow exacerbated by forced wrist extension

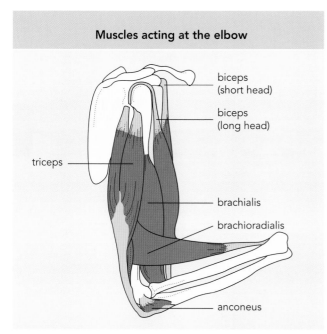

Fig. 10.36 Flexors and extensors of the elbow.

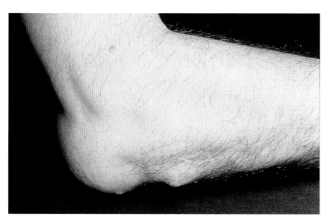

Fig. 10.37 Olecranon bursitis, rheumatoid nodule.

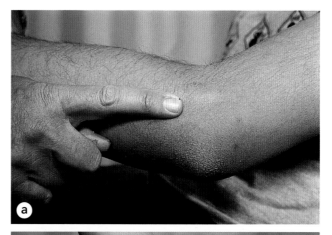

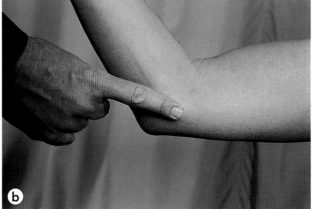

Fig. 10.38 Eliciting tenderness in a case of lateral (a) and (b) medial epicondylitis.

for the former and forced wrist flexion for the latter. Immediately inside the medial epicondyle is the ulnar groove, within which you can palpate the ulnar nerve. The nerve tends to thicken at this site even in normal individuals.

JOINT MOVEMENT

Flexion and extension at the elbow allow a total range of movement of approximately 150°. Supination and pronation both occur through a range of approximately 90°.

TRAUMATIC LESIONS

These include dislocations, fractures of the radial head and of the distal humerus. Dislocation is usually in a posterolateral direction. Both ulnar and median nerve damage can occur. Fractures of the head of the radius typically follow a fall onto an outstretched hand.

MUSCLE FUNCTION

Test the principal muscles concerned with elbow flexion and extension, together with pronation and supination (Fig. 10.39).

A lesion of the C6 nerve root is common (Fig. 10.40). Muscles that can be affected include the biceps, brachioradialis, supinator and triceps. In practice, triceps weakness predominates, with depression or loss of the triceps reflex. Any loss of sensation occupies the thumb and index finger.

The forearm and wrist

STRUCTURE AND FUNCTION

Movements of the wrist comprise flexion, extension and ulnar and radial deviation (Fig. 10.41). Flexion–extension movements of the fingers occur at both

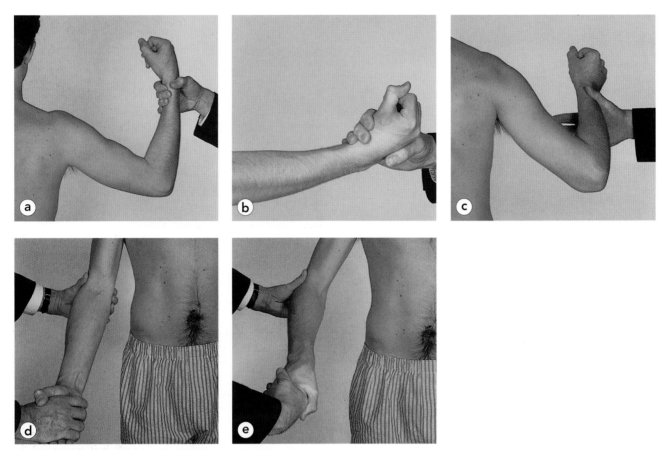

Fig. 10.39 Examining the muscles acting at or around the elbow joint. (a) Biceps, (b) brachioradialis, (c) triceps, (d) supinator and (e) pronator.

C6 root		
Muscles affected	**Dermatomal changes**	**Reflex changes**
biceps brachioradialis supinator triceps		(biceps) triceps

Fig. 10.40 C6 root syndrome.

INSPECTION AND PALPATION

Compare the size of the forearms, but remember that the dominant forearm tends to be rather larger. Compare the two wrists for size and for any evidence of swelling or deviation. Malunion of a distal fracture (Colles') leads to extension deformity. If the patient describes a wrist strain, carefully palpate in the region of the anatomical snuff box. Localised tenderness suggests a diagnosis of a fractured scaphoid. In De Quervain's tenosynovitis, inflammation of the tendons of the abductor pollicis longus and extensor pollicis brevis causes wrist pain, with localised tenderness and crepitus as the tendon moves through its sheath (see Fig. 10.11).

JOINT MOVEMENT

From the neutral position test flexion of the wrist (approximately 90°) then extension (approximately 70°). A comparison of the degree of dorsiflexion between the two wrists is best achieved by asking the patient to press the palms together while elevating the elbows so that the forearms are in a straight line. The range of palmar flexion can be similarly compared with the back of the hands pressed together. Now assess radial and ulnar deviation of the wrist. Wrist involvement is common in rheumatoid arthritis. Besides pain and limitation of movement,

the metacarpophalangeal and the interphalangeal joints.

The major flexors of the wrist are flexor carpi radialis and ulnaris. The major extensors are extensor carpi ulnaris and extensor carpi radialis longus and brevis. The long flexors and extensors of the fingers and thumb, by virtue of passing over the wrist joint, also exert a minor effect there.

Wrist movements

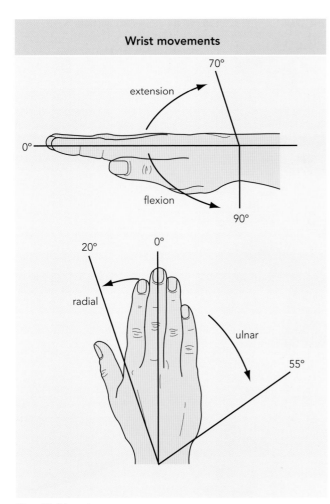

Fig. 10.41 Wrist movements.

stretching of the ulnar collateral ligament allows the head of the ulna to subluxate upwards (Fig. 10.42).

TRAUMATIC LESIONS

Fractures usually occur through the distal radius or ulna, typically after a fall on an outstretched hand. Colles' fracture is sited about 1–2 cm above the distal end of the radius. The fracture is displaced dorsally. Smith's fracture is one at this site which is displaced in the opposite direction.

Deformity is common after a Colles' fracture leading to shortening of the radius. Carpal tunnel syndrome can occur as a late complication.

Wrist sprains are commonplace. The wrist may be painful and swollen but radiographs reveal no bony

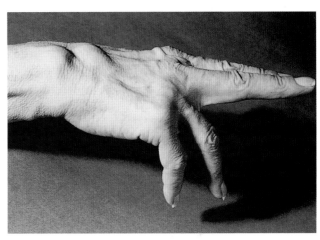

Fig. 10.42 Elevation of the ulnar head in rheumatoid arthritis. The flexion deformity of the fourth and fifth digits is the result of rupture of their extensor tendons.

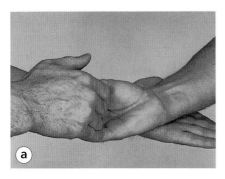

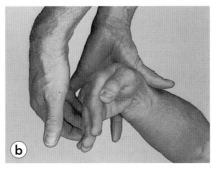

Fig. 10.43 Examining some of the muscles of the forearm. (a) Flexor carpi radialis, (b) flexor carpi ulnaris, (c) extensor carpi ulnaris and (d) extensor carpi radialis longus.

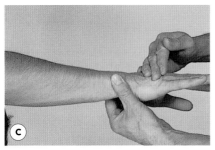

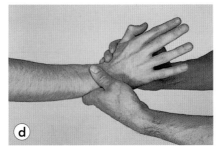

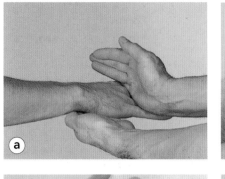

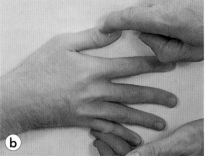

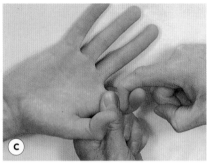

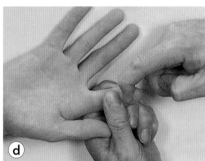

Fig. 10.44 Examining the long finger flexors and extensors. (a) Extensor digitorum, (b) extensor pollicis longus, (c) flexor digitorum sublimis and (d) flexor digitorum profundus.

injury. Treatment consists of immobilisation in a plaster.

MUSCLE FUNCTION

Now test the muscles acting at the wrist (Fig. 10.43) and the long flexors and extensors of the fingers (Fig. 10.44).

A C7 root lesion affects the triceps together with wrist and finger extension. The triceps jerk may be depressed and sensory loss, if present, occurs over the middle finger.

A radial palsy most commonly results from damage to the nerve in the spiral groove. There is weakness of the supinator, brachioradialis and wrist and finger extension (Fig. 10.45). The brachioradialis component of the supinator reflex is depressed.

Sensory loss is often slight, mainly involving an area of skin in the region of the anatomical snuff box.

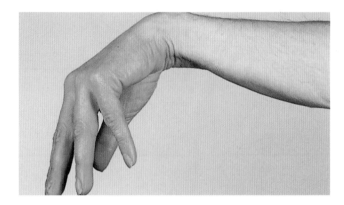

Fig. 10.45 Wrist and finger drop in a left radial palsy.

The small muscles of the hand control fine movements of the thumb and fingers. The thenar eminence muscles consist of abductor pollicis brevis, flexor pollicis brevis and opponens pollicis. Contained in the hypothenar eminence are abductor digiti minimi, flexor digiti minimi and opponens digiti minimi. Finally, there are the lumbrical muscles, the dorsal and palmar interossei and adductor pollicis. The lumbricals extend the fingers at the interphalangeal joints (with additional more complex actions), the interossei principally abduct and adduct the fingers, whereas the adductor pollicis adducts the thumb.

The hand joints

INSPECTION AND PALPATION

A good way to examine the hands both for joint and muscle function is to ask the patient to sit opposite you

The hand

STRUCTURE AND FUNCTION

The metacarpophalangeal joints allow abduction and adduction movements when the fingers are extended (Fig. 10.46). Abduction of the thumb carries it away from the plane of the palm of the hand and adduction towards it. Extension moves the thumb radially in the plane of the hand, flexion in the ulnar direction. Opposition rotates the thumb, bringing its palmar surface into contact with the fifth finger (Fig. 10.47).

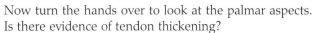
with the hands spread on a flat surface. You are looking for signs of joint deformity and whether any deformity is generalised or focal. If the latter, are particular joints affected? While inspecting the joints, remember to look at the state of the skin and whether the nails are deformed.

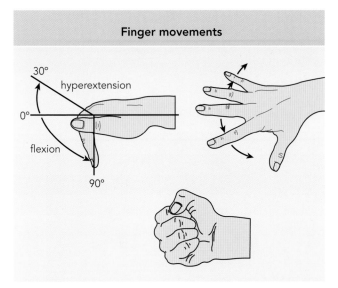

Fig. 10.46 Finger movements at the metacarpophalangeal (left and right) and at the interphalangeal joints (below).

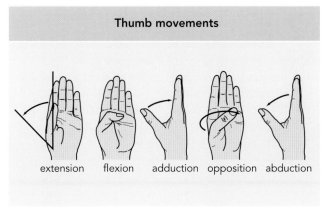

Fig. 10.47 Movements of the thumb.

Now turn the hands over to look at the palmar aspects. Is there evidence of tendon thickening?

Now carefully palpate the joints. Is there joint tenderness? Assess the quality of any swelling (Fig. 10.48). Can you feel any nodules along the tendon sheaths?

In early rheumatoid arthritis, slight swelling of the proximal interphalangeal joints is accompanied by tenderness (Fig. 10.49). At a later stage of the condition, substantial deformities occur (see Fig. 10.7) accompanied by wasting of the small hand muscles. If the changes predominate in the distal interphalangeal joints, carefully inspect the nails for signs suggesting a diagnosis of psoriasis (Fig. 10.50). In osteoarthritis, nodules (Heberden's nodes) typically appear over the distal interphalangeal joints but are also seen at the proximal interphalangeal joints (Bouchard's nodes) (Fig. 10.51).

Osteoarthritis commonly affects the carpometacarpal joint of the thumb in combination with changes in the

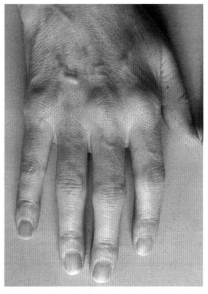

Fig. 10.49 The hand in early rheumatoid arthritis.

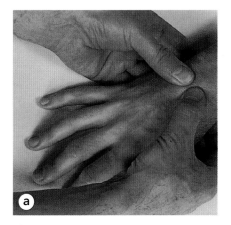

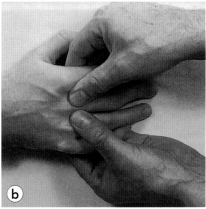

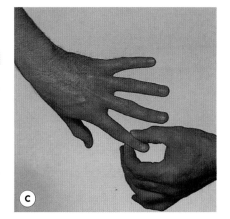

Fig. 10.48 Palpating the wrist (a), metacarpophalangeal (b) and interphalangeal (c) joints.

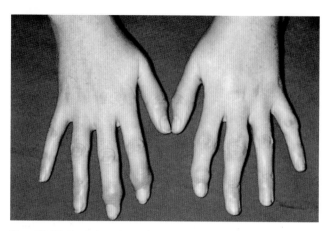

Fig. 10.50 Psoriatic arthropathy.

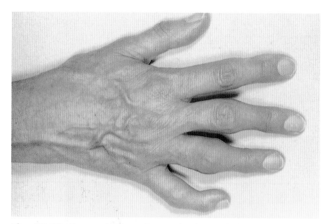

Fig. 10.51 Osteoarthritis at the proximal interphalangeal joints.

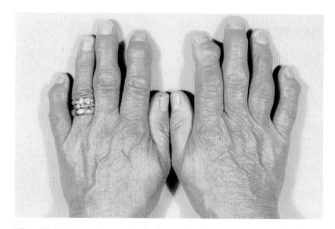

Fig. 10.52 The square hand of osteoarthritis.

distal interphalangeal joints resulting in the appearance of a 'square hand' (Fig. 10.52).

Nodule formation on a flexor tendon can lead to the tendon being caught in a localised narrowing of the sheath. The result, trigger finger, is a flexion deformity from which the finger can be extended only by force (Fig. 10.53).

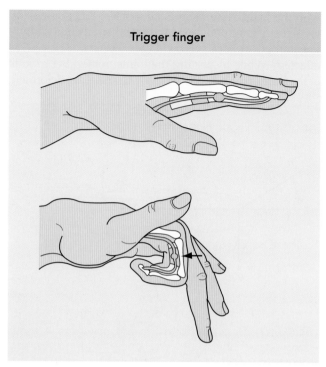

Trigger finger

Fig. 10.53 Trigger finger. The thickened area becomes trapped in an area of narrowing of the tendon sheath (arrow).

? Questions to ask

Weakness of the hand

- Is the weakness associated with joint pain?
- Is the weakness confined to the muscles supplied by the median or ulnar nerve?
- If the weakness is global, are both hands or just one hand affected?
- Is there accompanying sensory loss?

TRAUMATIC LESIONS

Hand injuries include tendon damage and fractures. Severed extensor or flexor tendons require suturing to facilitate healing.

Fractures include those of the phalanges, with or without dislocation, and of the carpal and metacarpal bones. Scaphoid fractures are easily missed on radiography, requiring oblique views for their detection. Typically they produce pain, swelling and tenderness in the region of the anatomical snuff box, usually after a fall on an outstretched hand. Avascular necrosis is a recognised complication.

MOVEMENT

Test the range of movement in the thumb and fingers. For abduction and adduction of the fingers, outlining the fingers on blank paper gives a quantitative assessment of the degree of their abduction from the neutral position.

The hand muscles

Muscle and joint function cannot always be conveniently separated. A generalised joint disorder (e.g. rheumatoid arthritis) may well lead to wasting of the small hand muscles caused by disuse, or may lead to focal wasting caused by entrapment of a particular nerve (e.g. the median).

INSPECTION

First inspect the dorsum of the hands. In this position, all the muscles that are visible are supplied by the ulnar nerve. In elderly people, muscle bulk in the hand reduces but without accompanying weakness. Wasting produces guttering between the extensor tendons, hollowing between the index finger and thumb and loss of the convexity of the hypothenar eminence. Look for fasciculation. Now turn the hands over and inspect the palmar surfaces. For the first time, you have the opportunity to assess the bulk of muscles supplied by the median nerve by examining the thenar eminence. By now you have determined whether there is any small muscle wasting, whether it is bilateral or unilateral and, if unilateral, whether it is global or confined to the distribution of the median or ulnar nerve.

TESTING POWER

Start with a muscle supplied by the ulnar nerve. A good choice is the first dorsal interosseous (Fig. 10.54). If the muscle is weak, test two other readily accessible muscles supplied by the nerve, the adductor pollicis and abductor digiti minimi. Now move on to muscles supplied by the median nerve. Start with abductor pollicis brevis then proceed to test opponens pollicis (Fig. 10.55).

Clinical application

If the weakness is confined to the muscles of the thenar eminence, you are dealing with a distal median nerve lesion, most probably within the carpal tunnel. Weakness with or without wasting of the muscles of the thenar eminence is accompanied by a characteristic failure of the

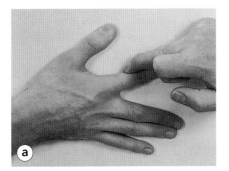
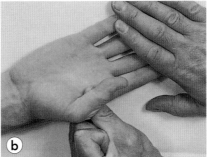
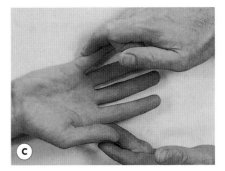

Fig. 10.54 Testing some of the small muscles supplied by the ulnar nerve. (a) First dorsal interosseous. With the fingers flat, the patient is trying to abduct the index finger against resistance. (b) Adductor pollicis. The patient is forcibly adducting the thumb towards the palmar surface of the index finger. (c) Abductor digiti minimi. The patient is abducting the little finger against resistance.

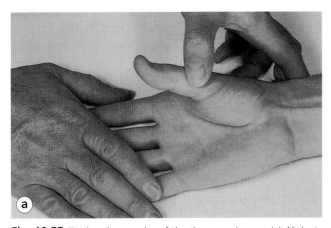
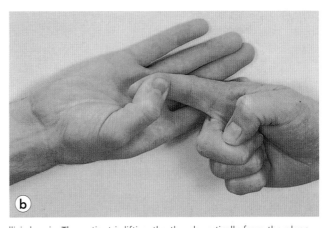

Fig. 10.55 Testing the muscles of the thenar eminence. (a) Abductor pollicis brevis. The patient is lifting the thumb vertically from the plane of the palm of the hand. (b) Opponens pollicis. Against resistance, the patient is trying to touch the base of the little finger with the tip of the thumb.

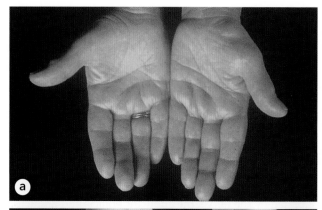

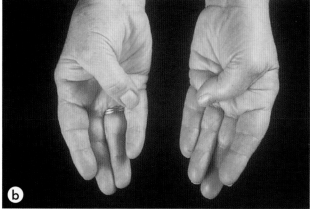

Fig. 10.56 Carpal tunnel syndrome. Wasting of the left thenar eminence (a). Failure of opposition of the left thumb (b).

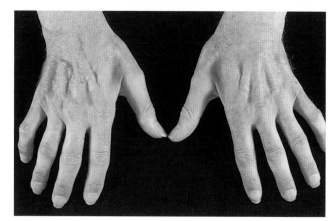

Fig. 10.57 Bilateral ulnar nerve lesions.

thumb to rotate during attempted opposition (Fig. 10.56). The carpal tunnel syndrome predominates in women, often triggered by pregnancy. Although usually idiopathic it can be triggered by other conditions, including rheumatoid arthritis, acromegaly, myxoedema and previous wrist fracture. Typically, the patient complains of nocturnal pain and paraesthesiae. The symptoms are often felt diffusely in the hand and forearm rather than being confined to the digits supplied by the nerve. Sensory loss is often not conspicuous. Ask the patient to compare touch sensation on the two sides of the ring finger. If percussion of the median nerve at the wrist produces tingling in the digits (Tinel's sign), compression at the site of percussion is likely. The test, however, is frequently negative even in proven cases. An alternative test is to maintain forced flexion of the wrist for several minutes to see if it triggers paraesthesiae in the fingers (Phalen's sign).

If the weakness is confined to the muscles supplied by the ulnar nerve, you next need to determine the site of the lesion. The most common site is in the region of the ulnar groove at the elbow, usually the consequence of recurrent trauma and angulation, or in the cubital tunnel from pressure by the aponeurosis of flexor carpi ulnaris. The hand muscles affected include the interossei, the hypothenar muscles and the third and fourth lumbricals. A characteristic deformity affects the fourth and fifth

digits (Fig. 10.57). In addition, there should theoretically be weakness of flexor carpi ulnaris and of flexor digitorum profundus to the fourth and fifth digits. In practice, these long muscles may be spared, even though the lesion is proximal. Distal ulnar lesions occur. According to the site, there may be sparing of the muscles of the hypothenar eminence and absence of sensory change.

If there is weakness of all the small hand muscles, you are probably dealing with a proximal lesion; combined median and ulnar lesions are uncommon. If the other hand is normal, suspect a problem at the level of the brachial plexus or of the T1 root. The brachial plexus can be damaged by trauma or invaded by tumour. Damage to the upper trunk affects the fifth and sixth cervical segments, damage to the middle trunk predominantly affects fibres supplying the radial nerve, and damage to the lower trunk produces a global weakness of the hand. If the sympathetic fibres in the T1 root are involved, there will be an accompanying Horner's syndrome (Fig. 10.58).

The cervical rib (thoracic outlet) syndrome results from compression of the C8 and T1 roots or the lower trunk of the plexus by a fibrous band passing from the transverse process of the seventh cervical vertebra to the first rib. Curiously, the hand weakness affects the muscles of the thenar eminence much more than those supplied by the ulnar nerve. A typical radiological feature is beaking of the C_7 transverse process (Fig. 10.59). If you find bilateral weakness, with or without wasting, of the small hand muscles, you are dealing with a more diffuse process. (Bilateral brachial plexus lesions are rare.) You have to consider a peripheral neuropathy or a lesion of the anterior horn cell (e.g. syringomyelia or motor neuron disease) (Fig. 10.60).

The hip

STRUCTURE AND FUNCTION

The hip is a ball and socket joint allowing flexion, extension, abduction, adduction, and both internal and

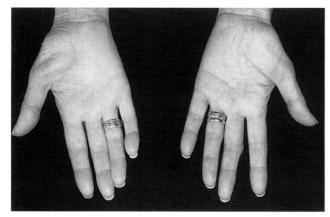

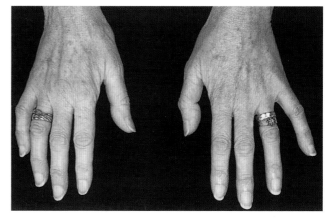

Fig. 10.58 Global wasting of the right hand (left and right), together with a Horner's syndrome (below left). Malignant invasion of the lower trunk of the brachial plexus and the T1 root.

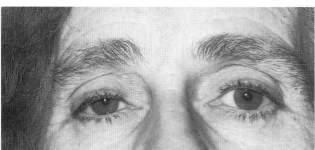

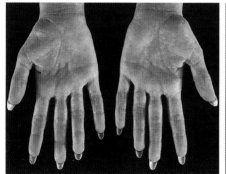

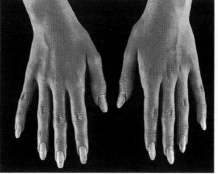

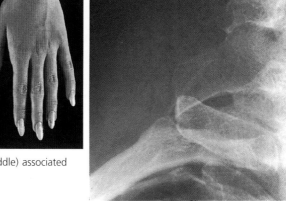

Fig. 10.59 Wasting of the small hand muscles of the right hand (left and middle) associated with beaking of the right C7 transverse process (right).

external rotation. The neck of the femur forms an angle of approximately 130° with the shaft.

Muscles acting at the hip joint may have additional actions on the spine or knee. The psoas major passes from the lumbar spine to the lesser trochanter of the femur. In addition to flexing the hip, it flexes the lumbar spine. The iliacus passes from the iliac fossa, part of the hip bone, and inserts principally into the lesser trochanter (Fig. 10.61). It acts as a hip flexor. The glutei arise mainly from the ileum. The gluteus maximus is a pure hip extensor; the other glutei principally act as abductors. The thigh is externally rotated by the obturator and adducted by the adductor majoris. Several muscles connect the pelvis with the tibia and fibula. The hamstrings comprise the biceps femoris, semitendinosus and semimembranosus (Fig. 10.62). They act (apart from the short head of the

biceps) as extensors of the hip joint and flexors of the knee joint.

INSPECTION AND PALPATION

The patient should be wearing only underpants if you are to examine the hip joints satisfactorily. Begin with the patient standing. Look for evidence of shortening of one of the legs. Compensation for this is achieved by a scoliotic posture or by flexion of the longer leg. An abduction deformity is compensated by flexion of the ipsilateral knee and adduction deformity by flexing the contralateral knee (Fig. 10.63). A flexion deformity is compensated by an exaggerated lordosis.

With the patient still standing, assess the integrity of each hip joint and its surrounding muscles by asking the

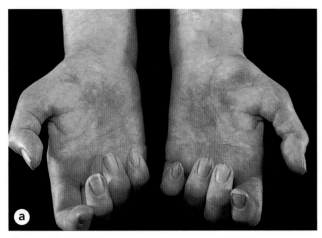

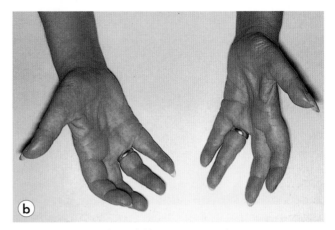

Fig. 10.60 Bilateral wasting of the small hand muscles in (a) hereditary sensorimotor neuropathy and (b) motor neuron disease.

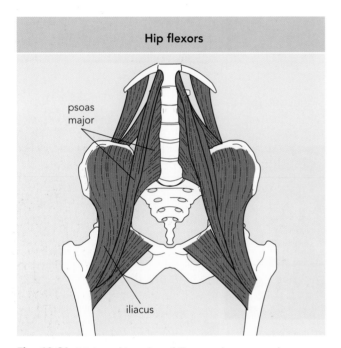

Hip flexors

psoas major

iliacus

Fig. 10.61 Origin and insertion of iliacus and psoas muscles.

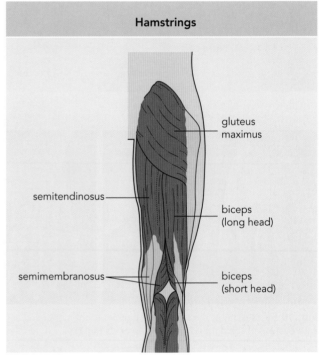

Hamstrings

gluteus maximus

semitendinosus

biceps (long head)

semimembranosus

biceps (short head)

Fig. 10.62 The hamstring muscles.

patient to stand first on one leg and then the other (Trendelenburg's test). Normally, as the foot is lifted the pelvis tilts upwards on the same side. If there is an abnormality in the hip joint or weakness of the muscle activity across it, the pelvis sinks downwards (Fig. 10.64).

Now lie the patient flat. First determine whether the iliac crests can be positioned in the same horizontal plane at right angles to the spine (Fig. 10.65). If this is not possible, there is an abduction or adduction deformity of one or other hip. Beware of the fact that flexion deformity of the hip can be concealed as the patient lies flat by a compensatory lumbar lordosis. To check for this, flex the opposite hip to its maximum, thereby eliminating the lordosis. If a flexion deformity exists, the affected leg will flex at the hip (Thomas' test) (Fig. 10.66). The joint is so deep that effusions are unlikely to be detected. To see if

there is any joint tenderness, palpate over the middle of the inguinal ligament.

MEASUREMENT OF LIMB LENGTH

When measuring limb length, you need to distinguish between true and apparent shortening. Make sure that the position of the two hip joints is comparable when measuring. The true length is measured from the anterior superior iliac spine to the medial malleolus (Fig. 10.67). If one leg is shorter, suspect pathology in or around the hip joint of that side. Apparent length is measured from the umbilicus to the medial malleolus. A difference here, without a difference in true lengths, indicates a lateral tilt of the pelvis, most often due to adduction deformity of the hip.

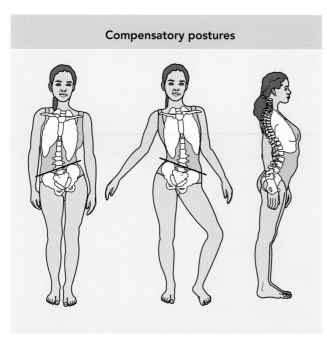

Compensatory postures

Fig. 10.63 Compensatory postures associated with (a) shortening of one leg, (b) adduction deformity of the right leg and (c) flexed deformity of the hips.

JOINT MOVEMENT

When measuring the range of hip movement, you need to ensure that the pelvis remains stationary. To do this, keep your free hand on the anterior superior iliac spine to detect any movement.

To test flexion, bend the leg, with the knee flexed, into the abdomen. Extension is best assessed by standing behind the patient and drawing the leg backwards until the point at which the pelvis starts to rotate. Abduction is measured by taking the leg outwards, again to the point where, by using the opposite hand, the pelvis is felt to move. Internal and external rotation are tested with the hip and knee flexed to 90° (Fig. 10.68).

Causes of hip pain vary, in terms of frequency, according to the age of the patient. Osteoarthritis frequently involves the hip joint. Pain is either local or referred. Movements of the joint are both restricted and painful. In advanced cases, shortening of the limb occurs with external rotation (Fig. 10.69).

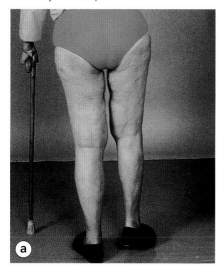

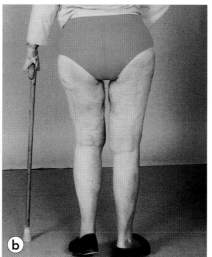

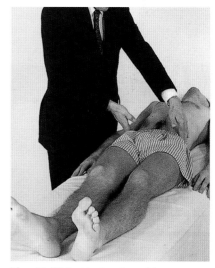

Fig. 10.64 Trendelenburg's sign. When the patient stands on the normal left leg the pelvis tilts to the left (a). When she stands on the right leg (where there was osteoarthritis at the hip) the pelvis fails to tilt to the right (b).

Fig. 10.65 Positioning the pelvis.

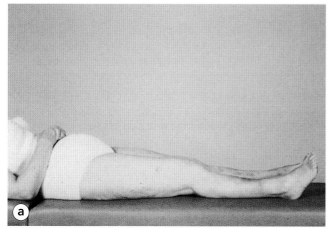

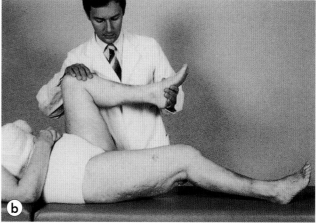

Fig. 10.66 Thomas' test. The fixed flexion deformity of the right hip can be obscured by a compensatory lumbar lordosis (a). When the lordosis is overcome by flexing the left hip, the right leg then lifts (b).

Bone, joints and muscle

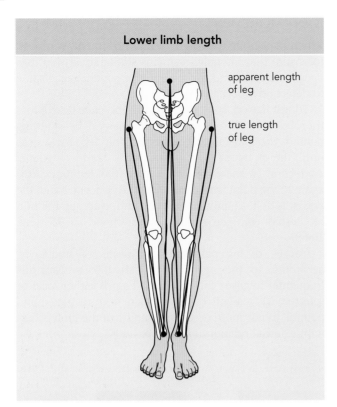

Lower limb length

apparent length
of leg

true length
of leg

Fig. 10.67 True and apparent lengths of the lower limbs.

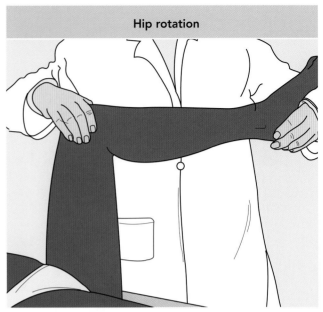

Hip rotation

Fig. 10.68 Measuring the extent of hip rotation.

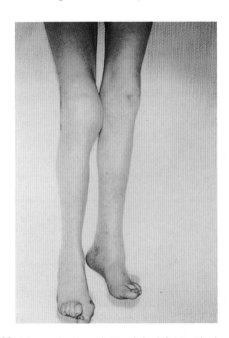

Fig. 10.69 Advanced osteoarthritis of the left hip. The leg is shortened and externally rotated.

Risk factors
Osteoarthritis

- Age
- Obesity
- Hereditary
- Trauma
- Congenital joint anomalies
- Previous inflammatory joint disease

Differential diagnosis
Knee pain

- Trauma
  - dislocation
- Arthritis
  - osteoarthritis
  - rheumatoid arthritis
- Slipped femoral epiphysis
- Osteochondritis (Perthes' disease)
- Infection
  - e.g. osteomyelitis

TRAUMATIC LESIONS

Dislocations are usually posterior and may then be accompanied by acetabular fractures. The leg is internally rotated, adducted and flexed. Sciatic nerve palsy is a potential complication. Fractures of the neck of the femur are commonplace in elderly people. The leg may be shortened and externally rotated. The condition carries a high morbidity for elderly people and has a capacity to progress to avascular necrosis of the femoral head. Fractures of the femoral shaft are either traumatic or pathological. Traction is the preferred treatment option in children but internal fixation is used for adults.

Slip of the upper femoral epiphysis occurs in adolescents, leading to pain and inability to weight bear.

Groin strains are common in people involved in sporting activities. The pain is dull, exacerbated by hip movement and is likely to be the result of tears in the fibres of the hip flexors.

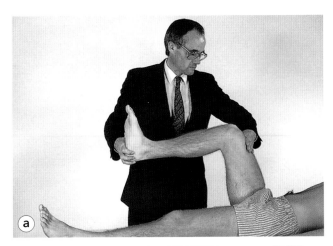

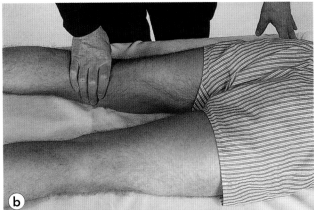

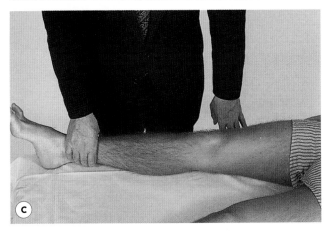

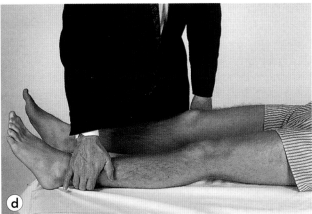

Fig. 10.70 Testing the muscles acting at the hip joint: (a) flexion, (b) extension, (c) adduction, (d) abduction.

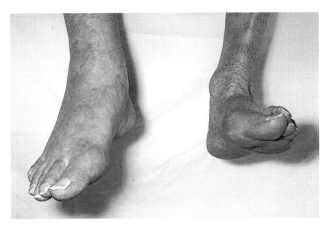

Fig. 10.71 Right sciatic palsy.

Muscle function

Test the power of hip flexion, extension, abduction and adduction (Fig. 10.70). Sciatic palsies are associated with pelvic trauma, injuries to the buttock or thigh or infiltration by tumour. The muscles supplied by the lateral popliteal component of the nerve tend to be more affected than those supplied by the medial popliteal branch (Fig. 10.71).

The knee

STRUCTURE AND FUNCTION

Although principally a hinge joint, a limited range of rotation is possible at the knee. Anteriorly, the capsule is formed by the tendon of the quadriceps femoris and the patella. At the sides, the capsule is strengthened by the medial and lateral collateral ligaments. Within the joint are the anterior and posterior cruciate ligaments passing from the tibia to the lateral and medial condyles of the femur, respectively (Fig. 10.72). Interposed between the femoral condyles and the tibia are the fibrocartilaginous semilunar cartilages. The joint capsule is lined by synovium that partly surrounds the cruciate ligaments. Communicating with the synovial cavity are bursae that are related to the insertions or origins of some of the tendons around the joint (Fig. 10.73).

Flexion-extension occurs between approximately 0° and 150° (Fig. 10.74). A minor degree of hyperextension can occur in some normal individuals. As full extension is reached, the femur rotates medially because of the longer articular surface of the medial condyle, tightening the capsular ligaments in the process. Flexion is produced by the hamstrings and extension by the quadriceps femoris.

INSPECTION AND PALPATION

With the patient standing, look for a knee deformity, either genu valgum (knock-knee) or genu varum (bow leg). Now continue your inspection with the patient lying supine. The bulk of the quadriceps muscle is a sensitive

Knee ligaments

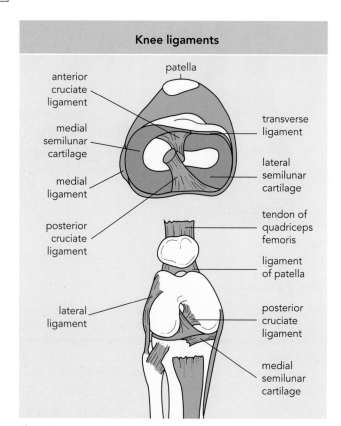

Fig. 10.72 The ligaments of the knee joint.

Knee bursa

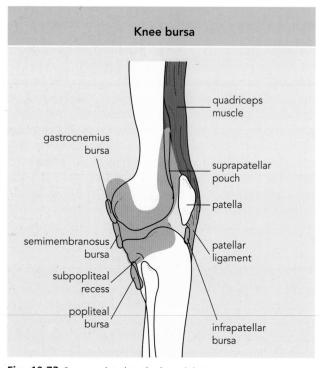

Fig. 10.73 Bursae related to the knee joint.

Knee flexion–extension

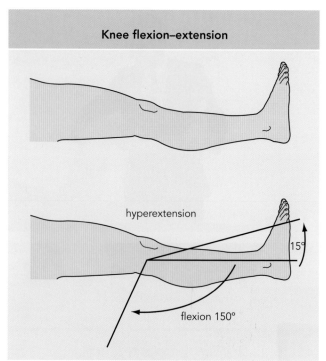

Fig. 10.74 Flexion–extension at the knee joint.

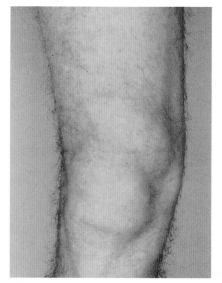

Fig. 10.75 Effusion in the suprapatellar pouch in a patient with rheumatoid arthritis.

guide to the presence of knee joint pathology. If necessary measure the thigh of each leg at a comparable distance from the joint margin. Next look for an effusion. If this is large, the swelling will extend from the suprapatellar region down either side of the patella (Fig. 10.75). Smaller effusions are detectable only by palpation. First, try ballottement: the patellar tap test. Use your left hand to force any fluid out of the suprapatellar pouch and then gently press the patella into the femur with the second and third fingers of your right hand. If there is a substantial effusion the patella will spring back against your fingers (Fig. 10.76a). For smaller effusions, look for the bulge sign. Again, force any fluid out of the suprapatellar pouch but at the same time anchor the patella with the index finger of the same hand. Next, gently stroke down between the patella and the femoral condyles, first on one side then the other. If an effusion is present, a bulge

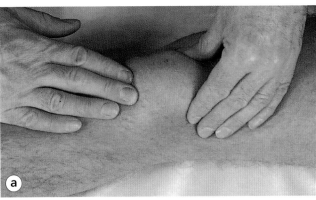

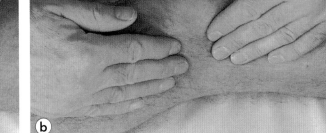

Fig. 10.76 Detection of an effusion. (a) Patellar tap. (b) Bulge sign.

appears on the other side of the knee during the manoeuvre (Fig. 10.76b).

Palpate the joint and surrounding structures, looking for any tenderness and also to assess the consistency of any swelling.

JOINT MOVEMENT

Test the range of movement with the patient lying supine. As you record the movement, palpate the joint for any crepitus. In addition, move the patella laterally and medially across the femoral condyles. Is the movement painful or does it elicit crepitus?

STABILITY

There are several important procedures that allow you to determine the integrity of the collateral and cruciate ligaments.

To test the collateral ligaments, attempt to abduct and adduct the lower leg. If there is lateral instability, record its degree (Fig. 10.77). For the assessment of cruciate ligaments, bend the knee to a slight angle, sit on the patient's foot (better to ask permission first!) then tense the lower leg first forwards then backwards. If either ligament is lax, excessive movement will occur (Fig. 10.78). Damage to these ligaments is almost always the consequence of trauma. If the ligaments rupture, a bloodstained effusion results. Damage to the synovial lining will allow the blood to track outside the joint margin.

ASSESSMENT OF THE SEMILUNAR CARTILAGES

Damage to the cartilages is common. In order to test their integrity, bend the hip and knee to 90° and grip the heel with your right hand while pressing on the medial then lateral cartilage with your left (Fig. 10.79). Now internally and externally rotate the tibia while extending the knee. If there is a cartilage tear, its engagement between the tibia and femur during the manoeuvre leads to severe pain, a clunking noise and, sometimes, actual locking of the joint (McMurray's test).

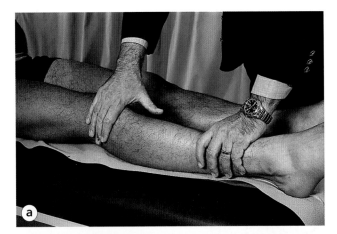

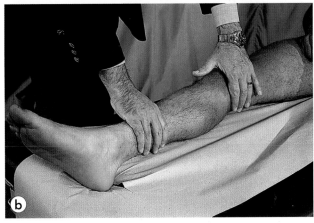

Fig. 10.77 Testing the collateral ligaments of the knee.

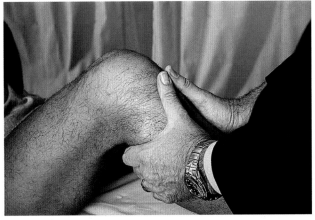

Fig. 10.78 Testing the cruciate ligaments.

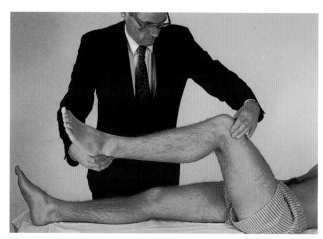

Fig. 10.79 McMurray's test.

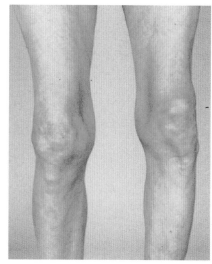

Fig. 10.80 Osteoarthritis of the knee. Bony swellings associated with quadriceps wasting.

Questions to ask
Knee pain

- Is the pain unilateral or bilateral?
- Has the patient noticed swelling of the joint?
- Does the knee lock in certain positions?

Differential diagnosis
Knee pain

- Trauma
  - fracture
  - dislocation
  - ligament damage
  - cartilage damage
- Arthritis
  - osteoarthritis
  - rheumatoid arthritis
- Osteochondritis dissecans
- Infection
  - e.g. osteomyelitis
- Bone tumours
- Referred
  - e.g. from the hip

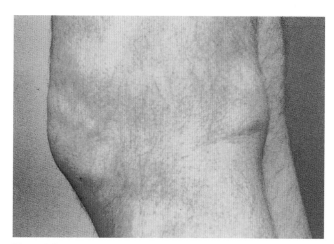

Fig. 10.81 A Baker's cyst that has partially ruptured into the calf.

In osteoarthritis, periarticular tenderness, particularly at the insertion of the capsule and collateral ligaments, is an important diagnostic clue. Later, bony swellings around the joint and secondary quadriceps wasting are common (Fig. 10.80). Remember to look at the back of the joint: the popliteal fossa. Posterior synovial protrusions (Baker's cysts) are visible here. They can complicate rheumatoid arthritis, in which additional features include effusions, synovial swelling and deformity (Fig. 10.81).

TRAUMATIC LESIONS

Ligament sprains are not associated with detectable laxity and are treated with a support bandage or plaster. With ligament rupture, the consequent joint instability necessitates surgical repair. Meniscal tears tend to occur in young people as the consequence of a twisting injury. The medial meniscus is usually affected. Effusion appears and the knee may lock, inhibiting complete extension. The torn elements are removed arthroscopically.

Patellar dislocation occurs laterally and tends to be recurrent. Total knee dislocation is unusual and generally the consequence of a road traffic accident. Fractures of the lower femur or upper tibia that involve the knee joint are complicated by joint stiffness and accelerated degenerative changes.

MUSCLE FUNCTION

Test the muscles responsible for knee extension and flexion, the quadriceps and hamstrings, respectively (Fig. 10.82). Both quadriceps weakness and wasting can accompany joint disease. If the knee joint is normal, unilateral quadriceps weakness suggests either a femoral neuropathy or an L3 root syndrome. In the latter, there is weakness of both quadriceps and the hip adductors, associated with a depressed knee jerk and sensory change over the medial aspect of the thigh and knee (Fig. 10.83).

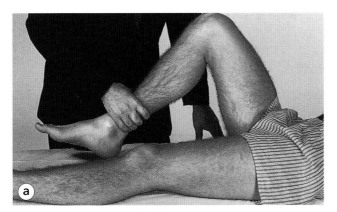

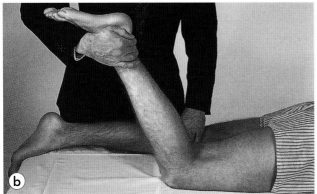

Fig. 10.82 Testing knee extension (above) and flexion (below).

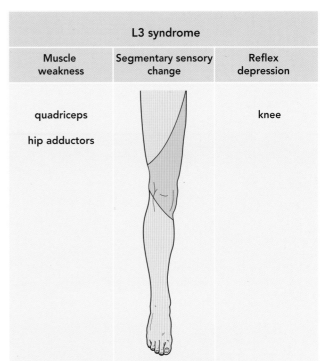

L3 syndrome		
Muscle weakness	Segmentary sensory change	Reflex depression
quadriceps hip adductors		knee

Fig. 10.83 L3 root syndrome. Motor, sensory and reflex abnormalities.

A femoral neuropathy can result from thigh trauma or haemorrhage into the psoas sheath. In diabetes mellitus, wasting of the thigh is more often the result of ischaemia of the lumbar roots rather than being caused by a femoral neuropathy. Consequently, the thigh adductors are also affected. Femoral neuropathy leads to weakness and wasting of the quadriceps, loss of the knee jerk and sensory change over the anterior thigh and the medial aspect of the lower leg (Fig. 10.84). If the nerve is damaged at the level of the psoas sheath, hip flexion is also affected. An obturator nerve palsy can follow surgery or pelvic fracture or be secondary to an obturator hernia. Weakness is confined to the thigh adductors, with altered sensation over the thigh's inner aspect.

Meralgia paraesthetica

It is worth mentioning meralgia paraesthetica. The patient complains of pain, tingling and numbness over the anterolateral aspect of the thigh. There are no motor changes. The condition is caused by compression of the lateral cutaneous nerve of the thigh at the level of the groin, and is the commonest entrapment neuropathy of the lower limb.

The ankle and foot

STRUCTURE AND FUNCTION

Movements of the ankle are essentially confined to extension (dorsiflexion) and flexion (plantar flexion). Inversion and eversion of the foot are partly achieved by movement at the subtalar joint (approximately 5°) and

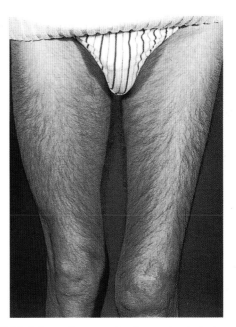

Fig. 10.84 Left femoral neuropathy after profundoplasty.

partly by movement at the midtarsal joints (20°). The predominant movements of the toes are dorsiflexion and plantar flexion (Fig. 10.85).

The main muscles of the calf are the soleus and gastrocnemius. The soleus acts purely as a flexor of the ankle, while the gastrocnemius flexes both the ankle and the knee. Of the other muscles in the posterior compartment, the tibialis posterior inverts the foot, whereas flexor digitorum longus and flexor hallucis longus flex the toes and big toe, respectively (Fig. 10.86).

The anterior compartment muscles include tibialis anterior, extensor digitorum longus, extensor hallucis

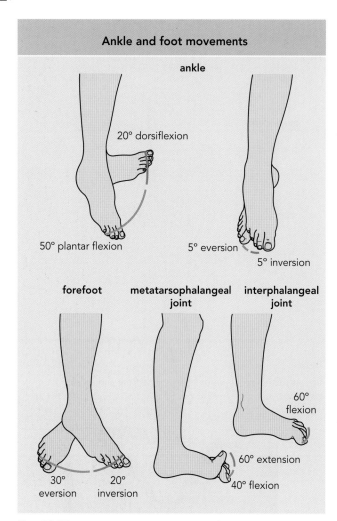

Fig. 10.85 Movements of the ankle, foot and big toe.

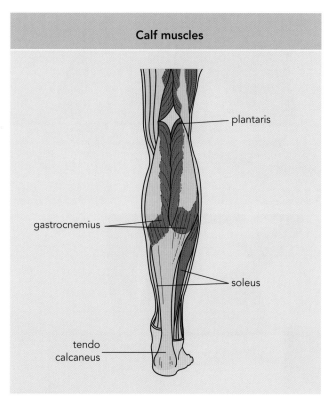

Fig. 10.86 Muscles of the calf.

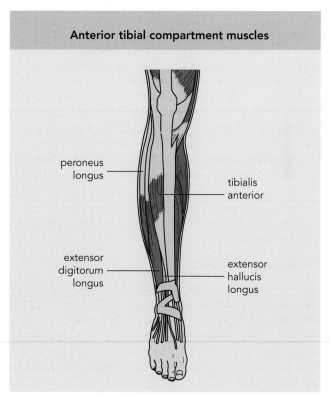

Fig. 10.87 Muscles in the anterior compartment of the leg.

longus and the peronei (Fig. 10.87). Tibialis anterior inverts the foot and dorsiflexes the ankle. The two extensors dorsiflex the toes and big toe, respectively. The peronei act as evertors of the foot.

INSPECTION AND PALPATION

To assess the alignment of the feet at the subtalar joints, look at the ankles from behind with the patient standing. In a varus deformity, the foot will be deviated towards the midline, in a valgus deformity away from it. With the patient still standing, look for any foot deformity. Is the arch of the foot exaggerated or absent? Is there deformity or swelling of the toe joints? Remember to inspect the sole of the foot as well as its dorsal aspect. Now palpate the margins of the ankle joint. In an inflammatory arthropathy, the whole joint is likely to be tender, with corresponding pain on all movement. In ankle strain, the tenderness is likely to be confined to one site with pain predominantly occurring when the joint is moved in one direction. Next palpate the heel and Achilles tendon. The latter is a fairly common site for rheumatoid nodules. To detect tenderness in the metatarsophalangeal joints, compress each one between your thumb and finger (Fig. 10.88). To test the integrity of the Achilles tendon, squeeze

the calf just below its maximal circumference. If the tendon is intact, the foot plantar flexes; if ruptured, no movement occurs.

Deformity of the foot is common. In flat foot, the longitudinal arch is lost with the consequence that most

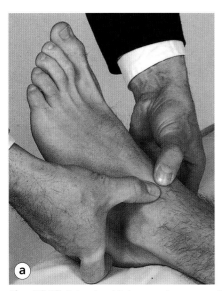 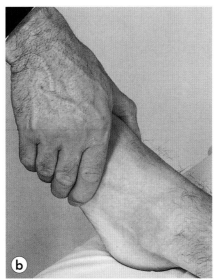 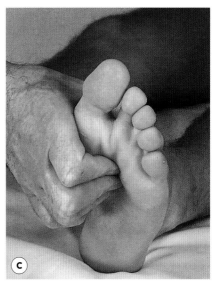

Fig. 10.88 Palpating (a) the anterior aspect of the ankle joint and (b) and (c) testing for tenderness of the metatarsophalangeal joints.

or the whole of the sole comes into contact with the ground (Fig. 10.89a). In pes cavus, the arch of the foot is exaggerated, with accompanying hyperextension of the toes (Fig. 10.89b). Hallux valgus predominates in women. It consists of abnormal adduction of the big toe at the metatarsophalangeal joint, with a bursa at the pressure point over the head of the first metatarsal (Fig. 10.89c). A hammer toe is characterised by hyperextension at the metatarsophalangeal joint with flexion at the interphalangeal joint. Painful thickenings of the skin (corns) are liable to develop at pressure points (e.g. over the proximal interphalangeal joints) (Fig. 10.89d).

Questions to ask

Foot deformities

- Has the deformity been present from birth?
- Does it affect both feet?
- Is it associated with joint pain or tenderness?

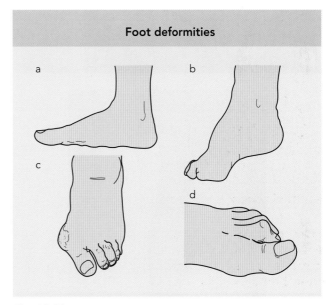
Foot deformities

Fig. 10.89 Foot deformities: (a) pes planus, (b) pes cavus, (c) hallux valgus and (d) hammer toe.

JOINT MOVEMENT

The ankle joint proper is concerned with plantar and dorsiflexion. Inversion and eversion of the foot occur both at the subtalar and midtarsal joints. To test this movement, hold the heel firmly with one hand while inverting and everting the foot with the other hand. You have already looked for tenderness in the metatarsophalangeal joints. Now test the range of flexion and extension.

TRAUMATIC LESIONS

Ankle sprains result from an inversion force typically damaging the anterior talofibular ligament. Swelling develops with pain on weight-bearing. The condition is treated by a support bandage.

Pott's fracture is a fracture-dislocation of the ankle, sometimes requiring open reduction and fixation.

Rupture of the Achilles tendon results in pain in the heel. The calf is swollen with a palpable gap in the tendon. Open operation is called for if the condition is detected early.

Osteoarthritis can affect both the ankle and the foot. In the foot, involvement of the first metatarsophalangeal joint leads either to deformity (hallux valgus) or fixation (hallux rigidus). Gout typically affects the same joint. In an acute attack, there is intense pain associated with swelling and erythema of the overlying skin (see Fig. 10.8). The reaction is secondary to deposition of urate salts within the connective tissues. If the hyperuricaemia is inadequately treated, urate deposits appear in periarticular and subcutaneous tissues. Typical sites include the first metatarsophalangeal joint, the elbow, the Achilles tendon and the ear (Fig. 10.90).

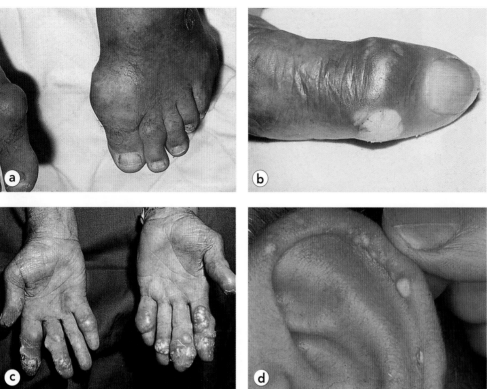

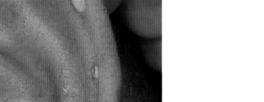

Fig. 10.90 Gouty tophi.

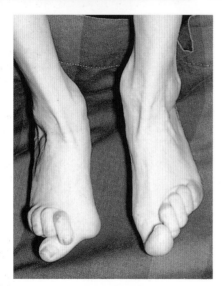

Fig. 10.91 Rheumatoid arthritis of the feet.

Rheumatoid arthritis involves both the ankle and the foot. When the disease is established, subluxation of the metatarsophalangeal joint is associated with flexion deformity at the proximal interphalangeal joints (Fig. 10.91). A variety of other inflammatory reactions can affect the ligamentous and tendon insertions around the heel. Causative agents include trauma and the seronegative arthritides.

MUSCLE FUNCTION

Test the individual muscles concerned with movement at the ankle and foot. Start with the plantar and dorsiflexors of the ankle, then of the toes (Fig. 10.92). Specifically test the extensor of the big toe, extensor hallucis longus (Fig. 10.93). Finally, test the evertors and invertors of the foot.

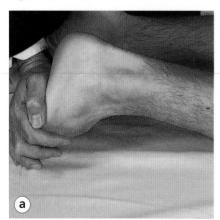
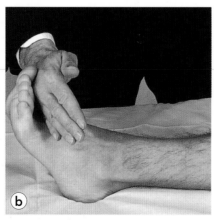
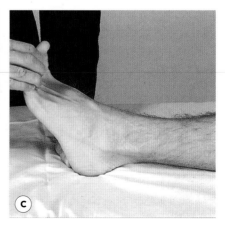

Fig. 10.92 Testing (a) and (b) plantar flexion and dorsiflexion of the ankle and (c) dorsiflexion of the toes.

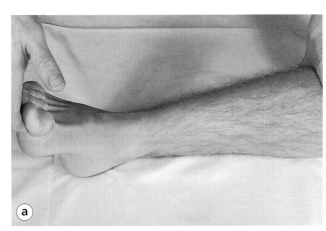

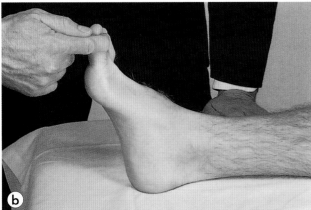

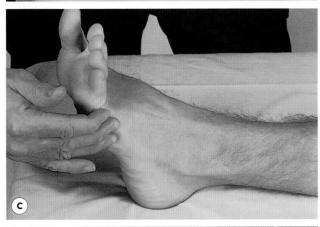

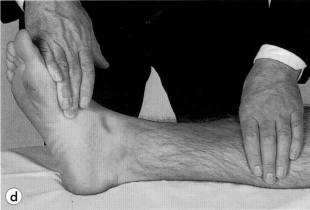

Fig. 10.93 Testing the (a) long toe flexors, (b) extensor hallucis longus, (c) peroneus longus and brevis and (d) tibialis posterior.

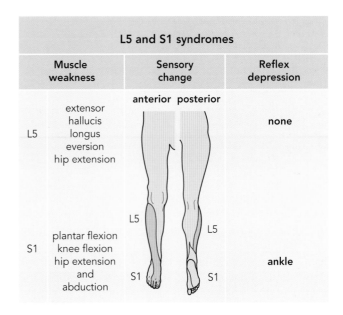

L5 and S1 syndromes		
Muscle weakness	Sensory change	Reflex depression
L5 — extensor hallucis longus eversion hip extension	anterior posterior	none
S1 — plantar flexion knee flexion hip extension and abduction		ankle

Fig. 10.94 L5 and S1 root syndromes.

Lumbar spondylosis commonly affects the L5 and S1 roots. The motor deficit with the former is often confined to extensor hallucis longus. There is no reflex change but there may be sensory change over the medial aspect of the foot. In an S1 root syndrome, there is weakness of plantar flexion of the foot (and potentially also of the calf and buttock muscles) together with a depressed or absent ankle jerk and sensory loss over the lateral border of the dorsal and plantar aspects of the foot (Fig. 10.94).

In lateral popliteal palsy, there is weakness of dorsiflexion of the foot and toes and of the foot evertors. The sensory change is often relatively inconspicuous, sometimes being confined to a small area of loss over the dorsum of the foot around the base of the first and second toes. There are no reflex changes.

Patterns of weakness in muscle disease

The pattern of weakness found in primary muscle disease differs from that seen in nerve root or peripheral nerve disorders. Conditions primarily affecting muscle include a group of genetically determined disorders (the muscular dystrophies), a group of inflammatory disorders (e.g. polymyositis), various biochemical and endocrinological dysfunctions and, finally, a further genetically determined group associated with myotonia.

Certain characteristics support a clinical diagnosis of primary muscle disease. The weakness, which is usually symmetrical, tends to predominate proximally. In the upper limbs, the periscapular muscles and deltoid are weak but the hand muscles are spared. In the lower limbs, weakness of hip flexion and extension is often conspicuous. The patient adopts a lordotic posture and has a waddling gait.

?

Questions to ask

Patterns of weakness

- Is the weakness associated with sensory symptoms or signs?
- Is there a family history of muscle disease?
- Is the weakness symmetrical?
- Is the weakness predominantly proximal or distal?

Trendelenburg's sign is likely to be positive bilaterally (see Fig. 10.64). There is particular difficulty getting upright from a lying position. Typically, the patient turns into the prone position, kneels then climbs up the legs using the upper limbs in order to extend the trunk (Gowers' manoeuvre) (Fig. 10.95). Muscle wasting and loss of tendon reflexes are late features of the myopathies. In some of the muscular dystrophies, pseudohypertrophy of muscle occurs because of infiltration by fat and connective tissue (Fig. 10.96). Distal weakness sometimes occurs in primary muscle disease, often then showing a

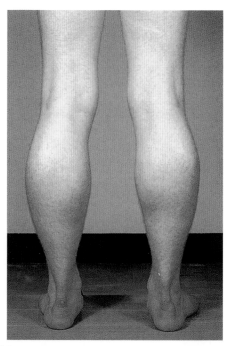

Fig. 10.96 Pseudohypertrophy of the calves.

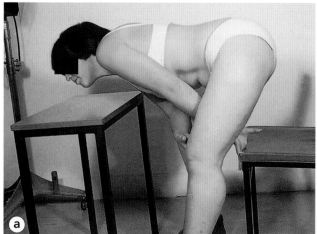

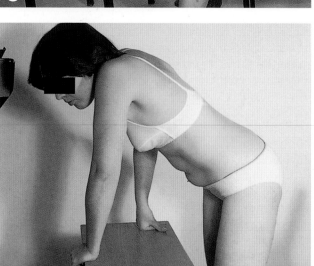

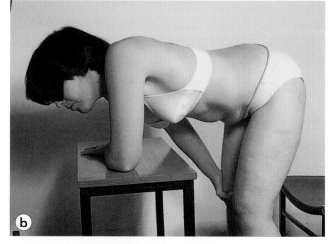

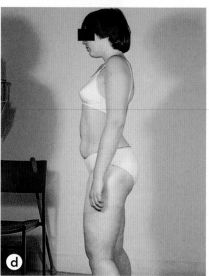

Fig. 10.95
Gowers' manoeuvre. The patient having reached a flexed position has to extend the trunk, partly by pressing on the table and partly by pressing on her thighs.

characteristic distribution. Weakness of the hands is a prominent feature of dystrophia myotonica, in which muscle weakness is accompanied by myotonia, particularly of grip.

You will have noticed how the patient walks when entering the consulting room. Having completed your limb assessment of joint and muscle you can now examine the gait formally. Remember that disease of the joints of the lower limbs can affect walking. The possibility will have been raised by the history and suggested by the joint examination. If the patient has described a substantial problem with gait, be ready to provide support when the patient starts to walk. Ask the patient to walk for a few metres, then turn and walk back towards you. You should observe both the pattern of leg movement and the posture of the arms together with control of the trunk. If gait appears normal, ask the patient to walk heel–toe, that is, 'as if on a tightrope'. If the patient appears nervous, walk alongside them.

SPASTIC GAIT

In a hemiplegia (Fig. 10.97a), the arm is held flexed and adducted while the leg is extended. In order to move the leg, the patient tilts the pelvis, which produces an outward and forward loop of the leg (circumduction). Failure to dorsiflex the foot leads to it scraping along the ground. If both legs are spastic, for example, because of spinal cord disease, the whole movement is stiff, with thrusts of the trunk being used to assist locomotion.

FOOT DROP GAIT

Foot drop (Fig. 10.97b) can be either unilateral or bilateral. The former is usually the result of a lateral popliteal palsy, the latter is the consequence of a peripheral neuropathy. Increased flexion at the hip and knee allows the plantar flexed foot to clear the ground.

ATAXIC GAIT

An ataxic gait (Figs 10.97c, d) can reflect either loss of sensory information from the feet or a disorder of cerebellar function. In the former case, the patient stamps the feet down in order to overcome the instability. Consequently, patients with this problem are much more

| Questions to ask |
| Gait |

- Does the patient trip?
- Is one shoe worn out more readily than the other?
- Does the patient stagger to one particular side?
- Does the patient, despite apparently severe ataxia, seldom sustain injury?

Gait disorders

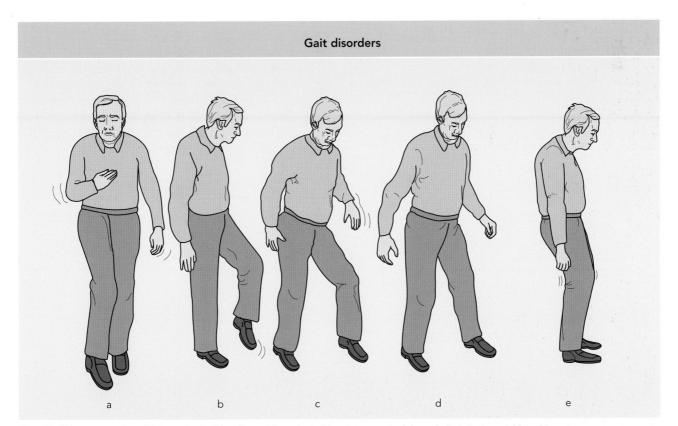

a b c d e

Fig. 10.97 Gait disorders: (a) hemiplegic, (b) unilateral foot drop, (c) sensory ataxia, (d) cerebellar ataxia and (e) parkinsonism.

unstable in the dark or with the eyes closed (positive Romberg's test).

Cerebellar disease leads to a broad-based gait that is unaffected by the presence or absence of visual information. Loss of truncal control produces erratic body movement. With unilateral cerebellar disease the patient staggers to the affected side.

WADDLING GAIT

Patients with substantial proximal lower limb weakness waddle from side to side as they walk, from a failure to tilt the pelvis when one leg is raised from the ground. There is usually an exaggerated lumbar lordosis. The findings suggest a proximal myopathy.

PARKINSONIAN GAIT

Patients with Parkinson's disease develop an increasingly flexed posture (Fig. 10.97e). Stride length diminishes and one or both arms fail to swing. There may be a problem initiating or arresting gait. Turning is difficult and requires an exaggerated number of steps.

APRAXIC GAIT

In certain conditions (e.g. normal pressure hydrocephalus) there is a particular problem with the organisation of gait even though other skilled lower limb movements are spared. The patient is liable to freeze to the ground, unable to initiate movement.

HYSTERICAL GAIT

Here, walking is erratic and unpredictable. The patient staggers wildly, often with an exaggerated movement of the arms. Falls and injuries do not exclude the possibility of a hysterical conversion reaction. There is often a violently positive Romberg's test which the patient self-corrects.

Examination of elderly people

Bones, muscles and joints

- Muscle strength declines with age; for example, grip strength falls by approximately 50% between the ages of 25 and 80 years
- Muscle bulk declines with age, for example, in the small hand muscles
- Some degree of ulnar deviation at the wrists can occur with ageing
- The range of joint movement lessens with age
- Gait becomes less certain in elderly people, with a tendency for the steps to shorten
- Elderly people tend to stand with slightly flexed hips and knees

Review

Framework for the routine examination of the musculoskeletal system

- Use GALS as a screening history and examination process
- Screening history enquires about pain or stiffness, dressing difficulty and any walking difficulty
- The screening examination assesses four areas: gait, spine, arms and legs (GALS)
- For individual joints, during a more detailed examination, a routine is followed of inspection, palpation and assessment of joint movement
- For individual muscles, the process incorporates inspection, palpation then formal testing of muscle power, using the MRC scale of 0–5
- In the lower limbs, additional stretch tests are available (straight leg raising and femoral stretch) to test for nerve root irritation in the lumbosacral region

11

The nervous system

Medical students often approach the neurological examination with trepidation, no doubt partly because of the complexities of the nervous system and partly because of the difficulties sometimes experienced in attempting anatomical localisation on the basis of abnormal physical signs. The problem for the student, however, often begins with a failure to acquire the skills necessary to elicit those signs. If they are not identified correctly, mistakes in interpretation and diagnosis inevitably follow.

This chapter summarises the examination of the central and peripheral nervous systems, although it will seldom be necessary to examine all the areas covered. Selection is influenced partly by the patient's history but also by cooperation, conscious state and level of fatigue. Certain examination techniques demand a good deal of both patient and examiner and if responses become erratic it is better to return to the examination later. Students, and sometimes doctors, are prone to examine only those areas immediately accessible with the patient supine. Remember to turn the patient over in order to assess the spine and the muscles of the shoulder and pelvic girdles. Always record your findings in full, avoiding irritating acronyms (e.g. PERLA for pupils equal, reacting to light and accommodation) and, if your examination has been limited, state exactly what you have done (rather than just 'CNS' followed by a tick). Remember that physical signs can alter, sometimes rapidly, and repeating your examination can give you useful insight into the mechanisms of certain disorders.

The cortex

STRUCTURE AND FUNCTION

On the basis of differences in histological structure, distinct areas can be identified within the cerebral cortex (Fig. 11.1). Tracts within the cortex comprise efferent pathways such as the pyramidal system, afferent pathways such as the thalamocortical projections, association fibres passing from regions within the hemisphere and commissural fibres connecting regions contralateral to one another. Surrounding the primary cortical areas for movement, sensation and vision are the cortical association areas. For example, the lateral geniculate body projects not just to the visual cortex (area 17) but also to areas 18 and 19, parts of the visual association cortex (Fig. 11.1).

The frontal lobe is separated from the parietal lobe posteriorly by the central (rolandic) sulcus, while the temporal lobe lies below the lateral (sylvian) sulcus. The

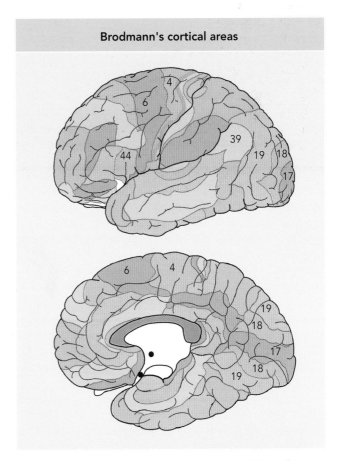

Brodmann's cortical areas

Fig. 11.1 Lateral and medial aspects of the cerebral hemisphere showing some of Brodmann's cortical areas.

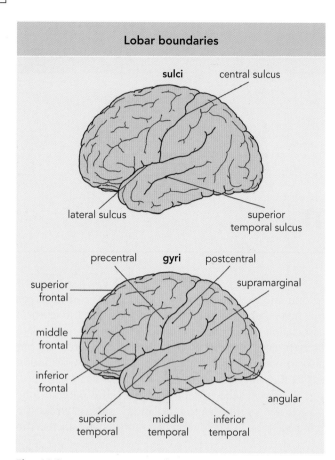

Lobar boundaries

sulci central sulcus

lateral sulcus

superior temporal sulcus

precentral **gyri** postcentral

superior frontal

supramarginal

middle frontal

inferior frontal

angular

superior temporal

middle temporal

inferior temporal

Fig. 11.2 Lateral surface of the cerebral hemisphere.

boundaries of the parietal, temporal and occipital lobes are not defined by a specific sulcus (Fig. 11.2).

The brain is supplied by paired internal carotid and vertebral arteries. The former terminate in the anterior and middle cerebral arteries, the latter in the basilar artery, which ends by forming the posterior cerebral arteries (Fig. 11.3). An anastomotic system at the base of the brain (the circle of Willis) connects these various components. The lateral surface of the cortex is supplied predominantly by the middle cerebral artery. The anterior cerebral artery supplies a strip of cortex spanning its superior margin, while the posterior cerebral artery supplies the occipital lobe and the inferior aspect of the temporal lobe (Fig. 11.4). Normal cerebral blood flow, at approximately 55 ml/100 g/min, represents approximately 15% of cardiac output. The level of blood flow is largely dependent on the $P\text{CO}_2$ of arterial blood. Vasodilatation and increased flow occur as $P\text{CO}_2$ rises. During a specific task orientated to speech, vision, hearing or motor activity, a focal increase in flow occurs in the appropriate part of the cortex.

The ventricular system contains cerebrospinal fluid (CSF) which originates predominantly in the choroid plexuses of the lateral ventricles, then circulates through the third ventricle and aqueduct before reaching the fourth ventricle. The CSF exits through the foramina of the fourth ventricle and is eventually reabsorbed through the arachnoid villae. The rate of CSF production is approximately 120 ml/24 h.

Acquisition of memory requires a number of stages. All data, whether visual or verbal, are recorded temporarily in a short-term pool. A selective and active process then passes some of the data into a long-term memory store. Finally, an active process of retrieval restores the memory to consciousness. Conventionally, memory is divided into immediate, recent and remote components, although these divisions are not absolute. Immediate or short-term memory lasts a few seconds; recent memory relates to activities or events occurring within a few hours or days and remote memory to events of the past, for example, the individual's youth. Structures particularly associated with learning storage include the hippocampi, the mamillary bodies and the dorsomedial nuclei of the thalami – the limbic system. Remote memory, however, can be retrieved even if these structures are damaged, suggesting that it is stored predominantly in the association cortex appropriate to the memory modality.

Visuospatial ability is dependent mainly on nondominant parietal lobe function. Language function is located in the left hemisphere in around 99% of right-handed individuals. For left-handed individuals, some 60% have language dominance in the left hemisphere, with 40% in the right hemisphere. Something like 80% of all left-handed individuals have mixed dominance, with language represented in both hemispheres. Within the hemisphere, a posteriorly placed area (Wernicke) is concerned with the comprehension of spoken language and an anterior area (Broca) with language output. The two are connected by the arcuate fasciculus (Fig. 11.5). The integration of the auditory and visual data required for reading and writing is achieved by the angular gyrus (area 39) (Fig. 11.1).

Questions to ask

Higher cortical function

- Has there been a change in your mood?
- Has your memory deteriorated?
- Do you have difficulty finding the right word in conversation?
- Have you ever become lost while travelling a familiar route?
- Do you have difficulty dressing?

Although certain functions can be localised to specific cortical areas, other aspects of higher cortical function are represented more diffusely.

SYMPTOMS

Many of the symptoms arising from a disorder of higher cortical function will be more evident to a close friend or relative than to the patient. Areas to cover, although

Cerebral arteries

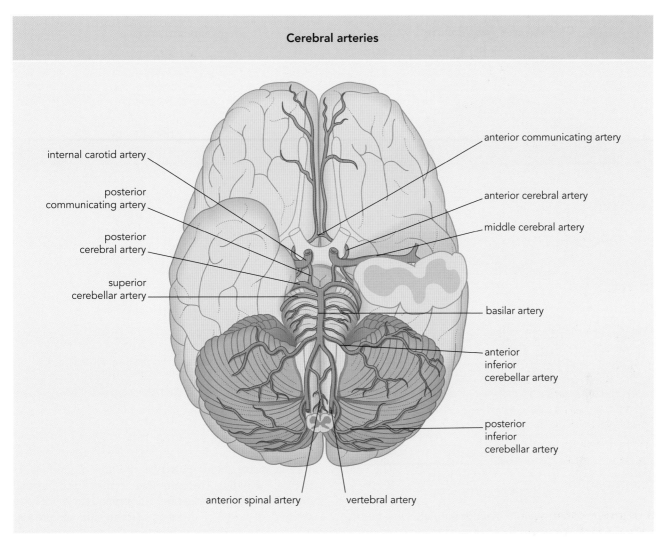

internal carotid artery

posterior communicating artery

posterior cerebral artery

superior cerebellar artery

anterior spinal artery

vertebral artery

anterior communicating artery

anterior cerebral artery

middle cerebral artery

basilar artery

anterior inferior cerebellar artery

posterior inferior cerebellar artery

Fig. 11.3 Arteries at the base of the brain.

some will be more evident during formal examination, are the following.

Mood

This can be assessed by direct questioning but also by observation of the patient's behaviour. Is the mood appropriate to the setting of the interview? Is the patient passive, apparently disinterested or even denying disability? Is there evident anxiety or a heightened state of arousal, accompanied by restlessness and pressure of talk? Does the history suggest delusions or hallucinations?

Memory

The demented patient often denies loss of memory, particularly once the condition is established. In the early stages, however, patients can retain awareness of their difficulty, and sometimes volunteer that remote memory is partly spared.

Speech

Aphasic patients usually retain insight into their word-finding difficulty. At times the defect is so substantial that history-taking from the patient becomes impossible. Listening to the history allows estimation of the degree of fluency in speech production, an assessment that will continue during the course of the examination. Patients are likely to volunteer any associated difficulty with reading (dyslexia) or writing (dysgraphia).

Geographical orientation

The first sign of geographical disorientation may be the inability to follow a familiar route. If the impairment is severe, patients can become lost in their own home but at this level of disability the problem will be volunteered by relatives rather than by the patient.

Dressing

Ask patients if they have encountered any problems while dressing. Mistakes will usually have been rectified by a relative but sometimes it is evident that the patient has lost understanding of the order and arrangement for items of dress.

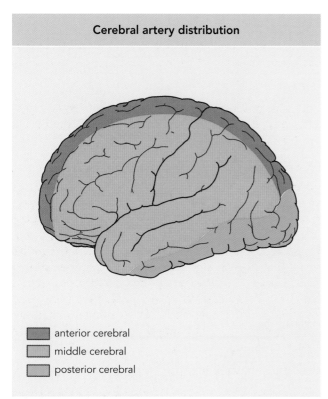

Cerebral artery distribution

anterior cerebral
middle cerebral
posterior cerebral

Fig. 11.4 The arterial supply of the lateral surface of the cerebral hemisphere.

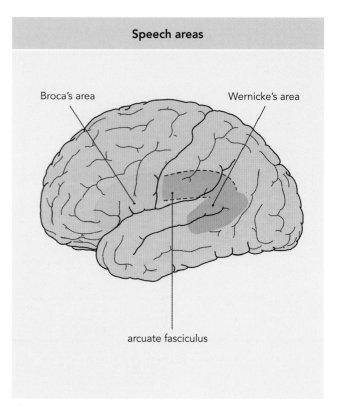

Speech areas

Broca's area

Wernicke's area

arcuate fasciculus

Fig. 11.5 Broca's and Wernicke's areas and their connecting arcuate fasciculus.

Examination

Assessment of the mental state begins as soon as the patient enters the consulting room. During the history-taking it will become apparent if there is an alteration of mood, whether there is any disturbance in the comprehension or production of speech and whether the patient has retained insight. The physical appearance can be helpful. Demented patients often have a bemused look, wondering why they are seeing a doctor. Evidence of self-neglect is usually concealed by the attentions of friends or relatives. The way in which the patient responds to questioning is of value in diagnosis. Demented patients tend to be inert and apathetic but a similar impression can be given by depressed individuals.

ORIENTATION

Begin by assessing the patient's orientation in time and space. Establish the patient's age and ask the time, date and the name of the hospital or clinic in which the interview is taking place. Ask either how long the patient has been in hospital or the duration of the interview.

MEMORY

Immediate recall

For testing recall, use digit repetition, although a normal response also requires intact attention and adequate comprehension. Start with two or three figures at 1s intervals, avoiding recognisable sequences. Normal individuals can repeat a 5–7 digit sequence. Reverse repetition of a set of digits is a more difficult process not solely dependent on memory. Normal individuals can achieve a 4–5 figure sequence. The performance of serial sevens (subtracting seven serially from 100) is dependent on many factors. An abnormal response to this test does not specifically identify the patient with dementia.

Recent memory (new learning ability)

The examination begins by asking the patient about recent events, although interpretation of the responses must take account of the patient's premorbid intelligence and level of culture. Next ask the patient to memorise three objects or, alternatively, a name, an address and a flower. Repeat the objects immediately and ask the patient to repeat them, so that they have clearly been registered. Over the next 10 min distract the patient so that there is no opportunity for mental rehearsal, then ask the patient to repeat the data. Most normal individuals can recall all the data at 10 min and 75% at 30 min. For further testing of verbal recall, give the patient a short story containing a standard number of items and, as soon as the story has been told, ask the patient to recount it.

Visual memory can be tested by displaying drawings for a 5 s period then asking the patient to reproduce the design 10 s later. Patients with visuospatial disorders will

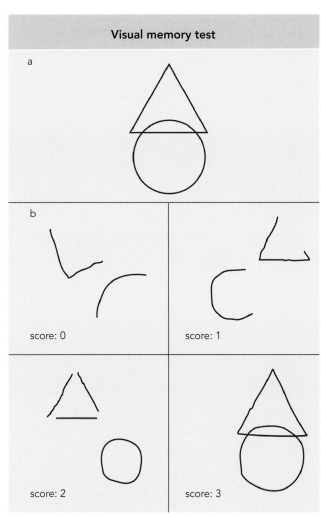

Fig. 11.6 (a) Standard design and (b) reproductions scored from 0 to 3.

Visual memory test

a

b

score: 0

score: 1

score: 2

score: 3

have problems with the task even if their visual memory is intact. The copies can be graded on a four-point scale, with a score of two, for example, indicating a recognisable design containing minor flaws and three a near-perfect or perfect reproduction. Average individuals score two or three on each test item (Fig. 11.6).

Remote memory

Ask the patient about schooling, childhood, work history, marriage and, if relevant, the ages of any children. The accuracy of the responses will need verification by a relative. Remote memory is spared in individuals with minor degrees of brain damage but will inevitably be eroded in people suffering from dementia.

INTELLIGENCE

Testing a patient's knowledge and abstract thinking must be performed in the light of their social background. Inherent in all assessments of intelligence is an estimate of the patient's premorbid ability.

Level of information

Ask the patient to give an account of recent events and their understanding of them.

Calculation

Give the patient simple addition, subtraction, multiplication, and division sums. Assessment of the results must take account of the patient's education.

Proverb interpretation

Interpretation of proverbs tests both general knowledge and capacity for abstract thinking. Proverbs of increasing complexity are read out to the patient and their interpretation recorded. A simple proverb to interpret would be 'A bird in the hand is worth two in the bush'; more difficult would be 'People in glass houses should not throw stones'. Concrete responses, typically seen in demented individuals, fail to see beyond the immediate implications of the proverb. For example, a concrete response to the second example would be that the glass would get broken.

Constructional ability

Constructional ability can be tested by asking the patient to copy designs of increasing complexity (Fig. 11.7). A scoring system can be devised, low values for which correlate well with the presence of brain damage. When assessing the patient's drawing, look for evidence of unilateral neglect, suggesting the probability of a contralateral parietal lobe syndrome.

GEOGRAPHICAL ORIENTATION

Evidence concerning this may have been forthcoming during history-taking but to test it specifically ask the patient to draw an outline of their native country, placing within it a few of the principal cities. From the figure it should be apparent whether or not the patient has an overall defect of geographical localisation or one based on neglect of one-half of the visual field (Fig. 11.8).

SPEECH AND SPEECH DEFECTS

Determine the patient's handedness. Asking which hand is used for writing is insufficient because some left-handed individuals have been taught to write with their right hand. Ask which hand is used for holding a knife, using a hair brush, using a screwdriver or for playing racket sports. Check on the family history of handedness.

Dysarthria

This is a defect of articulation without any disturbance of language function. Dysarthric patients have a normal speech content and, if they are able to write, their script will be free of dysphasic errors. Production of certain consonants depends on specific parts of the vocal

Construction test	Defect of geographical localisation

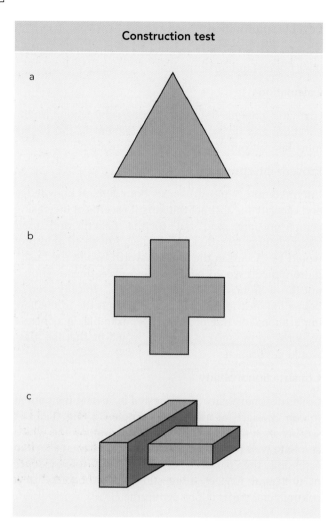

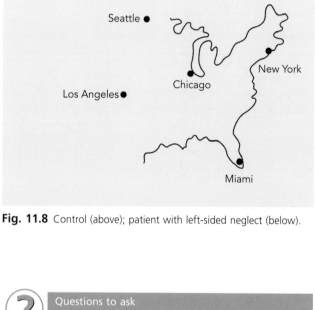

Fig. 11.7 Drawings of increasing complexity to be reproduced by the patient.

Fig. 11.8 Control (above); patient with left-sided neglect (below).

apparatus; P and B are labial sounds, D and T are lingual.

Dysphonia

Dysphonia is a defect of speech volume and is usually the result of a disorder limiting the excursion either of the muscles of respiration or of the vocal cords.

Dysphasia (aphasia)

This is a defect of language function in which there is either abnormal comprehension or production of speech or both. Much of the patient's language function will have been tested, although not deliberately, while taking the history. Seldom is there no spontaneous speech, although in certain types of dysphasia, the patient may be reduced to uttering short, meaningless phrases. Dysphasic speech lacks grammatical content, displays word-finding difficulty and contains word substitutions (paraphasias). Paraphasias are either whole word substitutions (verbal, e.g. bread for table), syllable substitutions (literal, e.g. speed for feed) or complete nonsense words (neologisms, e.g. tersh).

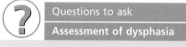

Questions to ask

Assessment of dysphasia

- What is the patient's handedness?
- Is the speech fluent or not?
- What is the level of comprehension?
- Can the patient repeat words or phrases?
- Can the patient name objects?

Fluency

Fluency may be defined as the amount of speech produced in a given period of time. Nonfluent speech, therefore, contains a limited number of words. Typically, the patient makes a greater effort in speech production, the output is often dysarthric and the phrase length limited. The overall result is a loss of rhythm and melody (dysprosody). Fluent dysphasia is near or even above normal in terms of output. Melody tends to be retained and phrase length is normal. Despite this, the patient fails to produce critical, meaningful words and output is incoherent. Verbal fluency can be formally tested by asking the patient to name as many objects as possible in a particular category (e.g. fruits and vegetables) in a set length of time.

Comprehension

In testing comprehension, increasingly complex questions can be asked but all should be answerable by a simple yes or no response. A substantial number of questions requiring randomly distributed yes or no responses are needed to avoid errors in interpretation. Avoid asking the patient to perform a skilled task; those individuals with apraxia will fail even if their comprehension is intact.

Repetition

Start by asking the patient to repeat simple words, then give sentences of increasing complexity. Patients with repetition difficulty often have a particular problem repeating 'no, ifs, ands or buts'.

Naming

A naming defect is found in virtually all dysphasic patients. Point to a succession of items, and ask the patient to name each one. Use objects commonly and less commonly encountered and mix the categories rather than restrict the test to, say, parts of the body.

READING

Reading assessment must take account of educational background. Ask the patient to read aloud, then test comprehension by asking questions requiring simple yes or no responses.

WRITING

Dysgraphia is an inevitable accompaniment of dysphasia. Begin testing writing ability by asking the patient to write single words, then sentences, initially writing them spontaneously and then in response to dictation. After checking word content, note whether the writing is crammed into one side of the page, suggesting the possibility of unilateral neglect.

PRAXIS

Apraxia is a disorder of skilled movement not attributable to weakness, incoordination, sensory loss or a failure of comprehension. The problem in movement may be confined to the limbs, to the trunk or even to the buccofacial musculature. Historically, apraxia was separated into two main categories. In ideational apraxia, destruction of the motor programming area in the supramarginal gyrus impairs the conception of an action, leading to defects in using tools or performing actions to verbal commands, though sparing the ability to mimic. Ideomotor apraxia results from separation of the motor programming area from the motor and premotor areas. Here conception of the action is spared but not the ability to perform it. The nomenclature of apraxia has become much more complex, along with the recognition that ideational apraxia is a less definable entity.

Start by asking the patient to carry out a particular task (e.g. 'pretend to use a screwdriver'). If the patient is unable to perform the task, do it yourself and then ask the patient to copy your movement. If a response is still not forthcoming, provide the object in question and ask the patient to demonstrate its use. These three tiers of command are in descending order of difficulty for the apraxic patient. Instructions that will test relevant movements include 'put out your tongue', 'pretend to whistle', 'salute' and 'show how you would use a toothbrush'. For whole body movements, ask the patient to stand to attention or stand as if about to start dancing. A more complex motor sequence is tested by asking the patient to go through a series of related movements. For example, taking the cap off a toothpaste tube, squeezing the toothpaste onto a brush, then replacing the cap.

Right–left orientation

A proportion of normal individuals have some problem with right–left orientation. Patients who are dysphasic can have problems understanding your commands. Start testing with simple tasks (e.g. 'show me your right hand') then gradually increase their complexity (e.g. 'put your left hand on your right ear').

Agnosia

Patients with visual agnosia are unable to recognise objects they see, despite intact visual pathways and speech capacity. Show objects to the patient, asking the patient to name each one and then allow the patient to manipulate the object to see if this improves recognition. Other forms of agnosia that can be tested include the ability to name and recognise individual fingers (finger agnosia) and colours (colour agnosia).

Conclusion

It is clearly not appropriate to go through such an extensive testing of higher cortical function in every patient. Screening tests have been devised that allow a rapid assessment of function. Such tests, for example, the mini mental-state test (Fig. 11.9) are useful, although their limitations need to be remembered when using them for screening purposes. A score of 20 or less suggests the possibility of a cognitive disorder, particularly dementia.

PRIMITIVE REFLEXES

At this stage it is worth testing a number of primitive reflexes (Fig. 11.10) before passing on to the cranial nerve examination.

Mini mental-state examination

Orientation

1. What is the year, season, date, month, day? (One point for each correct answer.)
2. Where are we? Country, county, town, hospital, floor? (One point for each correct answer.)

Registration

3. Name three objects taking 1 s to say each. Then ask the patient to repeat them. One point for each correct answer. Repeat the questions until the patient learns all three.

Attention and calculation

4. Serial sevens. One point for each correct answer. Stop after five answers. Alternatively, spell 'world' backwards.

Recall

5. Ask for the names of the three objects asked in Question 3. One point for each correct answer.

Language

6. Point to a pencil and a watch. Have the patient name them for you. One point for each correct answer.
7. Have the patient repeat 'No, ifs, ands or buts.' One point.
8. Have the patient follow a three-stage command: 'Take the paper in your right hand, fold the paper in half, put the paper on the floor.' Three points.
9. Have the patient read and obey the following: Close your eyes. (Write this in large letters.) One point.
10. Have the patient write a sentence of his or her own choice. (The sentence must contain a subject and an object and make some sense.) Ignore spelling errors when scoring. One point.
11. Have the patient draw two intersecting pentagons with equal sides. Give one point if all the sides and angles are preserved and if the intersecting sides form a quadrangle.

Maximum score = 30 points

Fig. 11.9 The mini mental-state test.

The glabellar tap

Tap repetitively with the tip of your index finger on the glabella. The blinking response should inhibit after three to four taps. In dementia and Parkinson's disease, the response persists.

The palmomental reflex

Apply firm and fairly sharp pressure to the palm of the hand alongside the thenar eminence. If the response is positive, contraction of the ipsilateral mentalis causes a puckering of the chin.

Pout and suckling reflexes

A positive pout response results in protrusion of the lips when they are lightly tapped by the index finger. A positive suckling reflex consists of a suckling movement of the lips when the angle of the mouth is stimulated.

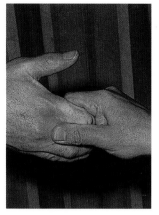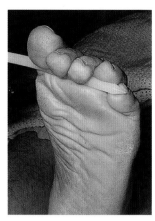

Fig. 11.10 Primitive reflexes (hand and foot grasp).

Grasp reflex

Stroke firmly across the palmar surface of the hand from the radial to the ulnar aspect. In a positive response, the examiner's hand is gripped by the patient's fingers, making release difficult. A foot grasp reflex is elicited by stroking the sole of the foot towards the toes with the handle of the patella hammer. A positive response leads to plantar flexion of the toes.

Clinical application

DEMENTIA

Dementia is defined as a disorder or progressive memory impairment coupled with at least one other cognitive deficit (aphasia, apraxia, agnosia or a defect of executive function), though in, for example, Alzheimer's disease the memory impairment may antedate the other features by some years. The majority of patients with dementia have Alzheimer's disease. Most of the remainder has either cerebrovascular disease or a mixed pathology. In the early stages of dementia, the most prominent symptoms are apathy and lack of concentration, together with defects in memory, and performance. Later, word-finding difficulty appears, with impaired comprehension and paraphasic substitutions. The patient becomes apraxic. There is a surprisingly poor correlation between the presence of dementia and the size of the cortical sulci as demonstrated on computerised tomography (CT). Ventricular size provides a better correlate (Fig. 11.11).

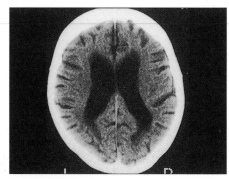

Fig. 11.11 CT scan of a patient with dementia.

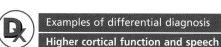

Examples of differential diagnosis

Higher cortical function and speech

- Dementia
  - Alzheimer's disease
- Amnesia
  - postherpes simplex encephalitis
- Dysarthria
  - brainstem stroke
- Dysphonia
  - myasthenia gravis
- Dysphasia
  - Broca type, Wernicke type
- Apraxia
  - corpus callosum lesions
- Grasp reflex
  - frontal lobe tumours

AMNESIA

Damage to the limbic system results in a failure to learn new memories (antegrade amnesia) associated with a defect of memory for the more recent past (retrograde amnesia). In some instances, the patient confabulates responses, particularly soon after the onset. Immediate memory remains intact. Conditions causing this picture include herpes simplex encephalitis and alcoholism. Unilateral temporal lobe lesions can have a selective effect on verbal or visual memory, according to whether the dominant or nondominant hemisphere is affected.

DYSCALCULIA

Dyscalculia can occur with bilateral or unilateral lesions. Generally, the dyscalculia is greater when the dominant hemisphere is affected.

CONSTRUCTIONAL APRAXIA AND GEOGRAPHICAL DISORIENTATION

Constructional difficulty is particularly associated with parietal lobe lesions of the nondominant hemisphere. It appears relatively early in the course of Alzheimer's disease. Geographical disorientation has a similar topographical significance.

DYSARTHRIA

Bulbar palsy

Combined weakness of the lips, tongue and palate. With palatal weakness the speech is nasal. One cause is myasthenia gravis.

Pseudobulbar palsy

Speech is hesitant and has an explosive, strangulated quality. When severe, diction is almost impossible (anarthria). Motor neuron disease can cause this picture.

Vocal cord paralysis

With unilateral paresis, speech is hoarse and of reduced volume. With bilateral paresis speech is virtually lost. If the vocal cords are adducted, there will be inspiratory stridor.

Cerebellar lesions

There is loss of speech rhythm with fluctuation in volume and inflexion. Slurring and staccato elements are found.

Dysphonia

Many patients who lose their voice do not have organic disease. In spastic dysphonia, a form of dystonia, inappropriate muscle contraction produces strained and strangulated speech.

APHASIA

Nonfluent speech is associated with anterior hemisphere lesions and fluent speech with posterior hemisphere lesions. Further differentiation is based on the results of testing comprehension, repetition and naming (Fig. 11.12).

Broca's aphasia

The output is nonfluent and usually dysarthric, comprehension is intact except for complex phrases and there are naming errors. The lesion lies in and around area 44 (Fig. 11.1) of the frontal lobe and may be vascular or neoplastic.

Transcortical motor aphasia

This is similar to Broca's aphasia except that repetition is retained. The pathological process (again, usually vascular

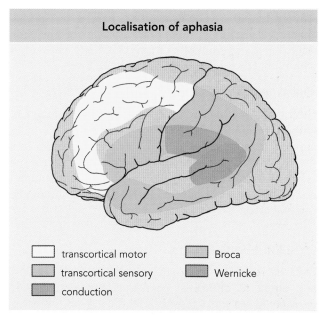

Fig. 11.12 Anatomical sites associated with the various aphasic syndromes.

or neoplastic) is located above or anterior to Broca's area.

Wernicke's aphasia

Here the patient has fluent, easily articulated speech but there are frequent paraphasias and meaning is largely absent. Comprehension and repetition are severely impaired and attempts at naming produce paraphasic errors. The patient is often described as confused.

Conduction aphasia

Conduction aphasia is fluent but not to the degree seen in Wernicke's aphasia. Interruptions to the speech rhythm are frequent but there is no dysarthria. Naming is imperfect but comprehension good. Despite this, repetition is severely abnormal. Reading, at least out loud, and writing are impaired. The condition occurs with disruption of the arcuate fasciculus connecting the posterior temporal lobe to the motor association cortex (Fig. 11.12). Cerebrovascular disease is the most common cause.

Transcortical sensory aphasia

Transcortical sensory aphasia is fluent but frequently interrupted by repetition of words or phrases initiated by the examiner (echolalia). Despite the readiness and accuracy of the patient's repetition, comprehension is severely impaired. Naming is poor and reading comprehension defective. The responsible anatomical site is less well localised than for some of the other forms of aphasia but lies in the borderlands of the temporal and parietal lobes of the dominant hemisphere.

Anomic aphasia

Anomic aphasia is fluent and interrupted more by pauses than by paraphasic substitutions. Comprehension is relatively preserved, repetition is good and naming is affected but to a varying degree. There is no specific anatomical location. Anomic aphasia can be the final stage of recovery from other forms of aphasia and is seen with both structural and metabolic brain disease.

Global aphasia

Global aphasia affects all aspects of speech function. Output is nonfluent and comprehension, repetition, naming, reading and writing are all affected, often to a severe degree. The causative pathology occupies a substantial part of the language area of the dominant hemisphere and is usually an extensive infarct in middle cerebral artery territory.

DYSLEXIA AND ALEXIA

Dyslexia refers to developmental disorders of reading, and alexia to disorders secondary to acquired brain damage. Alexia with agraphia is found with lesions of the angular gyrus of the dominant hemisphere. Alexia without agraphia in right-handed individuals is associated

with lesions affecting both the left occipital cortex and the splenium of the corpus callosum and is most commonly the result of an occlusion of the posterior cerebral artery.

AGRAPHIA

Although virtually all aphasic patients have agraphia, many patients with agraphia are not aphasic. Writing skill is also affected by motor disability, involuntary movements and visuospatial disorders.

Review

Assessment of higher cortical function

- Orientation
  - time, place and person
- Memory
  - immediate, short-term, remote
- Level of information
- Calculation
- Proverb interpretation
- Constructional ability
- Geographical orientation
- Speech
  - articulation, volume, fluency, comprehension, repetition, naming
- Reading and writing
- Praxis
- Right–left orientation
- Gnosis

APRAXIA

The pathway involved in performing a skilled task to command begins in the auditory association cortex of the dominant hemisphere then passes to the parietal association cortex, subsequently travelling forwards to the premotor cortex and finally the motor cortex itself. Interruption of this pathway at any point results in an ideomotor apraxia affecting both the dominant and nondominant hands (Fig. 11.13). The pathway from the dominant to the nondominant premotor cortex (D–D) passes through the anterior corpus callosum. A lesion there will produce an apraxia confined to the left hand. Whole body movements tend to be relatively spared even when limb ideomotor apraxia is substantial. Ideational apraxia is usually the consequence of bilateral hemisphere lesions or predominant left hemisphere dysfunction.

RIGHT–LEFT DISORIENTATION

Right–left disorientation is usually the result of a posteriorly placed dominant hemisphere lesion. Gerstmann's syndrome comprises right–left disorientation, finger agnosia, dysgraphia and dyscalculia.

The pathway for a skilled motor task

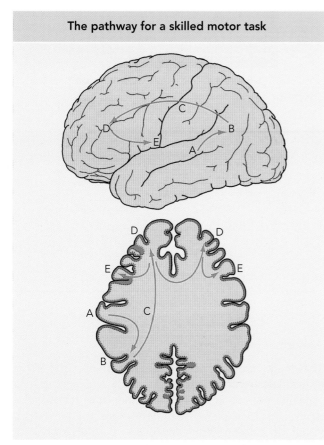

Fig. 11.13 Pathway involved in the formulation and performance of a skilled motor task.

If all four components are present, the causative pathology is likely to lie in the dominant parietal lobe, though doubt has been expressed regarding its specificity.

VISUAL AGNOSIA

One form of visual agnosia is caused by a disconnection between the visual cortex and the speech area. Patients can recognise objects and demonstrate their use but are unable to name them. Bilateral temporo-occipital lesions are the usual cause. In the other form of visual agnosia, recognition of objects fails but their use can be demonstrated if the object is placed in the hand. In other words, sensory information can bypass the defect of visual recognition, which is a consequence of damage to the visual association cortex in both hemispheres, usually vascular in nature.

PRIMITIVE REFLEXES

The palmomental reflex is found bilaterally in some normal individuals but a unilateral palmomental reflex suggests a contralateral frontal lobe lesion. Snout and suckling reflexes are elicited in patients with diffuse bilateral hemisphere disease. Bilateral grasp reflexes are of limited localising value but a unilateral response is associated with pathology in the contralateral frontal lobe. A foot grasp or tonic plantar reflex can be one of the earliest signs of a frontal lobe lesion.

The psychiatric assessment

Make sure that the patient understands who you are, and the purpose of the interview. Privacy is particularly important when sensitive issues are being explored. To begin with, avoid making notes, as this can detract from the relationship you are trying to establish with the patient. During this preliminary phase, observation of the patient's posture, gestures and facial expression may provide information regarding mood and feeling. The depressed patient appears apathetic, has little expressivity and may well be reluctant to discuss the history. The agitated patient is restless.

HISTORY OF PRESENT CONDITION

This proceeds in much the same way as history-taking from a patient with a physical complaint. Indeed, physical symptoms often predominate in those individuals with a primary psychiatric illness. Try to establish when the patient last felt well, as a means of determining the overall length of the history and as a means then of establishing the chronological order of subsequent symptoms. If necessary, interrupt the patient if there is digression into other areas, for example current social issues, through making clear that you are interested in those issues, and will wish to return to them later. Sometimes directive questions are needed to focus the patient's attention on a particular symptom, for example headache, in order to explore that symptom in greater detail. As the history proceeds, open questions will be partly replaced by closed questions, answerable by a simple yes or no response. Sometimes signs of emotional distress may appear as certain issues are raised. Rather than ignoring these, gently probe them, even if this temporarily diverts the course of the history.

Quite often, patients only indirectly refer to stressful issues by giving oblique reference to them in the course of describing their physical symptoms. Try to pick up these cues and develop the relevant issue. Failure to detect them will deter the patient from discussing them further.

Many symptoms are common to both physical and psychiatric illness but others are more specifically within the territory of psychiatry.

SPECIFIC SYMPTOMS

Mood

Enquire whether the patient, or a relative, has noticed any mood change. A particularly valuable question when screening for depression is whether the individual has lost pleasure in their normal activities (anhedonia). Supplementary to this will be enquiries regarding sleep pattern, loss of libido and suicidal ideation. Sometimes the patient denies flattening of mood, when that is all too evident from the interview. Such discrepancies should be carefully recorded.

Patients will usually complain of anxiety but sometimes its somatic manifestations, for example palpitations, sweating and tremulousness, predominate. The anxiety may be chronic and spontaneous or be triggered acutely by a specific stimulus – phobic anxiety.

Patients seldom complain of euphoria – a feeling of limitless physical and mental energy. There is likely to be a pressurised manic quality to the patient's conversation, coupled with physical restlessness.

Abnormal thoughts

These will be elicited only by sensitive questioning. The patient can be understandably reluctant to reveal certain abnormal thoughts. It may be apparent from the interview that the patient's thought pattern is difficult to follow or that abnormal thoughts have pervaded the conversation. Ask patients about paranoid ideas, in other words, whether they feel people are against them. Ask whether certain thoughts or ideas regularly intrude into their thinking, or whether they believe their thoughts are being interfered with or influenced by external agencies. Thought disorders include the following.

Delusions These are beliefs which can be demonstrated to be incorrect but to which the individual still adheres. Members of the Flat Earth Society are deluded. Often there is an element of reference, in other words that actions or words are directed specifically at that individual even if they appear on a global platform, for example television. Paranoid delusions contain a persecutory element. Delusions of worthlessness are particularly associated with depressive illness.

Obsessions These are recurrent thoughts which often result in the performance of repetitive acts (compulsions). The patient is aware that they are inappropriate but cannot resist returning to them or acting upon them. Examples of obsessional thought include convictions that a particular individual is antagonistic or that a spouse is unfaithful.

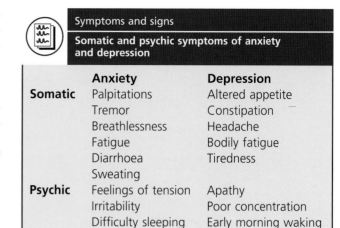

	Symptoms and signs	
	Somatic and psychic symptoms of anxiety and depression	
	Anxiety	**Depression**
Somatic	Palpitations	Altered appetite
	Tremor	Constipation
	Breathlessness	Headache
	Fatigue	Bodily fatigue
	Diarrhoea	Tiredness
	Sweating	
Psychic	Feelings of tension	Apathy
	Irritability	Poor concentration
	Difficulty sleeping	Early morning waking
	Fear	Diurnal mood swing
	Depersonalisation	Retardation
		Guilt

Abnormal perceptions

These are auditory or visual phenomena that other individuals are not aware of.

Hallucinations are experiences that have no objective equivalent to explain them. They are predominantly visual or auditory but can occur in other forms, for example of smell or taste in patients with complex partial seizures. Visual hallucinations can be unformed, for example an ill-defined pattern of lights, or formed, the individual then describing people or animals, often of a frightening aspect. Visual hallucinations are more often a feature of an organic brain syndrome, e.g. delirium tremens or adverse drug reaction, than a functional psychosis, e.g. schizophrenia. Auditory hallucinations are also either unformed or formed. They are found more often in the functional psychoses than in organic brain disease. The voices can take on a persecutory quality in schizophrenia and an accusatory element in depression. In déja and jamais vu, intense feelings of a relived experience or a sensation of strangeness in familiar surroundings occur, respectively. Both can be a feature of everyday life but when pathological are usually epileptic. Illusions are misinterpretations of an external reality: all of us have this when watching a magician at work. In depersonalisation, the individual feels a detachment from the normal sense of self; in derealisation, the individual feels a detachment from the external world. Both occur in neurotic illnesses but also, periodically, in normal individuals.

Cognition

The assessment of higher cortical function has already been discussed. It is necessary to distinguish cognitive impairment due to dementia from cognitive impairment due to delirium. In the latter there is clouding of consciousness, usually manifested as reduced awareness of, or response to, the environment.

	Questions to ask
	Psychiatric assessment

- Do you feel unduly anxious or depressed?
- Do you repeat certain tasks over and over again?
- Do you feel people are against you?
- Have you heard or seen things that are not there?
- Do you ever lose the sense of yourself or your environment?

THE FAMILY HISTORY

Begin by obtaining details of the patient's father and mother, in terms of their current age (or age at death), their own quality of health, whether they had any history of psychiatric disorder and the quality of the patient's relationship with them. Ask similar questions about the patient's siblings. Questions regarding the patient's own children are usually included in the personal history. Genetic factors are particularly strong in schizophrenia and manic-depressive psychosis.

THE PERSONAL HISTORY

Childhood

It is unlikely patients will have accurate details of their birth or early development unless there was a particular problem with them. A direct question to the patient regarding whether they were happy or unhappy in childhood is useful. Some 'happy' responses turn out to be rather less so with further delving. If there is an expression of remembered unhappiness, explore it further in terms of relationships with parents and any physical illness.

Schooling and further education

Establishing the details of this is helpful in forming an assessment of the patient's premorbid intelligence. At the same time, enquire about friendships or a tendency to isolation, and about teasing or bullying.

Sexual development

For female patients, enquire about the age of the menarche and how they attuned to adolescence in terms of menstruation and sexuality. For men, discussion should include whether their sexuality could be discussed in the home and how they acquired their sexual experience. Further issues relating to sexual development, for example homosexual experiences, are best left, at this stage, for the patient to raise.

Marital history

An overall outline includes the age of the spouse when the marriage occurred, the overall quality of the relationship, the state of the sexual relationship and details of any unease.

Occupational history

Ask how many jobs the patient has had, reasons for leaving previous posts, the quality of relationships in the workplace and the level of job satisfaction. If there has been one or more periods of unemployment, explore what effect this has had on the patient's overall welfare.

PAST MEDICAL HISTORY

This follows the usual pattern, and includes history of both physical and mental illness if these have occurred.

DRUG HISTORY

Determine alcohol consumption, but be aware of the possibility that the figure does not correspond to actual intake. Features suggesting alcohol dependency include early morning drinking, morning vomiting, taking a drink before an interview, erratic work attendance and drinking in isolation. Ask about narcotic exposure, the use of softer drugs such as cannabis and exposure to tranquillisers. If the patient is using codeine derivatives, ascertain for what purpose and the dosage.

PERSONALITY PROFILE

Evidence suggesting changing personality and mood is often better provided by colleagues, relatives or friends than by the patient. Questionnaires exist for the assessment of personality, but even without them the patient's attitude and behaviour, in terms of work and social relationships, personal drive, level of dependence, ambition and authority and response to stress will indicate the nature of the patient's personality.

Examination

The concept of the psychiatric examination needs to be interpreted broadly. A physical examination is necessary but the most telling diagnostic details will be revealed by an exploration of the patient's mental state, emerging as much from the history as from the answers to specific questions.

Clinical application

ORGANIC MENTAL STATES

In organic mental states, a specific pathological basis for the mental disorder has been established. Acute forms include the toxic confusional states, characterised by alteration of the conscious level, disordered perceptions (e.g. visual hallucinations), restlessness and thought disorder. Almost any structural or metabolic disorder can trigger the reaction. Examples include encephalitis, head injury and alcohol withdrawal. The principal chronic organic mental state is dementia.

FUNCTIONAL MENTAL STATES

In functional mental states, a specific underlying pathological or metabolic cause has not been identified. Psychotic states are those in which the individual has lost insight and neurotic states are those in which insight is preserved. The distinction is not absolute, however, and the terms are best avoided. In affective disorders, for example, anxiety, depression and mania, an alteration of mood is a major feature of the illness.

Differential diagnosis

Organic and functional mental states

- Acute anxiety state
- Chronic anxiety state
- Endogenous depression
- Reactive depression
- Manic depression
- Schizophrenia
- Obsessional states
- Conversion hysteria
- Drug- and alcohol-related disorders
- Toxic confusional state
- Dementia

Questions to ask

Mental state

- For anxiety
  - Are the symptoms provoked by particular environments?
- For depression
  - Are there suicidal thoughts?
- For schizophrenia
  - Has the patient had auditory hallucinations?
  - Does the patient believe his or her thoughts are controlled by others?

PHOBIAS

Phobias are a particular form of anxiety triggered by a specific environment or circumstance. Agoraphobia, for example, results in a fear of leaving the home, particularly if this involves entering crowded places.

DEPRESSIVE ILLNESS

Depressive illnesses include those triggered primarily by genetic or constitutional factors (endogenous) and those precipitated by adverse external events (reactive). Increasingly, the distinction is felt to be artificial.

MANIA AND HYPOMANIA

In mania and hypomania (its lesser form), there is pressure of talk and physical activity. Patients lack insight and react adversely if their grandiose schemes are questioned. In manic-depressive illness, the mood fluctuates between two extremes.

SCHIZOPHRENIA

Schizophrenia has been classified into a number of types, although the entities defined are not absolutely distinct. It is characterised by thought disorder, blunting of emotional responses, paranoid tendencies and perceptual

disorders. Thought disorder leads to irrational conversation, in which the development of ideas is either blocked or moves suddenly into unconnected channels. The emotions are blunted and the patient becomes increasingly withdrawn. Delusions are prominent and frequently contain paranoid elements. Auditory hallucinations are particularly characteristic of schizophrenia.

OBSESSIONAL STATES

In obsessional states, a preoccupation with mental or physical acts predominates. An obsessional personality displays these characteristics but not to the point where they interfere with the normal activities of life. In obsessional states, however, the relevant thought or action takes on a compulsive quality, ineffectively countered by the patient. Obsessional symptoms can feature in other psychiatric illnesses.

Symptoms and signs

The psychiatric patient

A full examination is performed to exclude any physical disorder that may contribute to the patient's condition

HYSTERIA (CONVERSION HYSTERIA)

Hysteria is a disorder in which physical symptoms or signs exist for which there is no objective counterpart and which require, in the case of signs, an elaboration on the part of the patient of which he or she is unaware. Many of the symptoms are referred to the nervous system, for example, memory loss, paralysis, unsteadiness and visual impairment. Malingerers, on the other hand, consciously elaborate their disability.

HYSTERICAL PERSONALITY

Hysterical personality is distinct from hysteria, although individuals with this personality trait may develop conversion reactions. The hysterical personality is characterised by superficiality and shallow emotional responsiveness combined with a histrionic overwrought reaction to events.

Headache and facial pain

HEADACHE

Headache is a common complaint. Often the history suffices to separate the more serious causes. The length of history is particularly important, rather then necessarily the severity of the pain. Critical issues are whether the pain is continuous or intermittent and, if the latter, what is the duration of individual attacks. There may be particular precipitants for attacks, e.g. alcohol triggering an attack of cluster headache. Accompanying symptoms should be sought, e.g. nausea or vomiting. As for any pain, it is important to determine whether there are relieving factors. Patients often find it difficult to describe the quality of their pain – it may be helpful to provide them with a list of alternatives.

Examination

With recent onset headache, careful fundoscopy is essential to exclude the presence of papilloedema. Patients will seldom be seen during a migraine attack; between attacks their physical examination will be normal. Patients with tension (muscle contraction) headaches often show focal or diffuse scalp tenderness. Patients with cranial arteritis have tenderness of the scalp vessels which are more likely to show reduced rather than absent pulsation.

Questions to ask

Headache

- How long has the headache been present?
- Is the headache continuous or episodic?
- If continuous, how long do the attacks last?
- What is the quality and severity of the pain?
- Are there any triggering or relieving factors?
- Are there any accompanying symptoms?

Differential diagnosis

Headache

- Migraine
- Tension headache
- Cluster headache
- Analgesic abuse headache
- Cranial arteritis
- Intracranial mass lesion

Red flag – urgent referral

Recent onset of headache

If accompanied by:
- scalp arterial tenderness – consider cranial arteritis
- motor, sensory or speech disorder – consider a space-occupying lesion of some sort
- papilloedema – consider space-occupying lesion or benign intracranial hypertension

FACIAL PAIN

Facial pain is commonly of psychological rather than neurological origin. The first step in analysing facial pain is to determine whether it might be related to local causes, e.g. a dental abscess or focal sinus infection. Such causes will generally be associated with revealing local symptomatology, e.g. focal facial tenderness. Some facial pain is more or less continuous, but an important cause of severe, but episodic, facial pain is trigeminal neuralgia. Again seek the quality of the pain, its duration, if it is episodic, and its severity. Ask for specific triggers, e.g. particular trigger zones on the face, palpation of which can precipitate an attack of trigeminal neuralgia. In some instances facial pain is referred from the ear.

Examination

Determine if the patient has any trigger zones. Patients experiencing trigeminal neuralgia are unlikely to allow you to examine the face.

Questions to ask

Facial pain

- Are there accompanying dental or sinus symptoms?
- What is the quality of the pain?
- If paroxysmal, does the pain have any triggers?
- Are there accompanying symptoms suggesting a psychological problem?

THE CRANIAL NERVES

The olfactory (first) nerve

STRUCTURE AND FUNCTION

The olfactory epithelium contains specialised receptor cells and free nerve endings, the latter derived from the first and second divisions of the trigeminal nerve. Unmyelinated axons from the receptor cells traverse the cribriform plate before synapsing in the olfactory bulb. From here, the olfactory tract passes backwards, dividing into lateral and medial roots in the region of the anterior perforated substance. The more important lateral root projects predominantly to the uncus of the ipsilateral temporal lobe.

Molecules derived from particular odours are absorbed into the mucus covering the olfactory epithelium. From here they diffuse via ciliary processes to the terminal processes of the receptor cells where they bind reversibly to receptor sites. This initiates an action potential in the olfactory nerve with a firing frequency related to the intensity of the stimulus.

Women have a more sensitive sense of smell than men. In both sexes, smell sensitivity declines with age. Many healthy individuals have difficulty naming or describing the quality of a particular odour even though they can distinguish it from others. The value of a particular odour for the testing of olfactory nerve function is determined principally by how selectively it stimulates the specialised receptor cells rather than the free trigeminal endings. Odours stimulating the latter include peppermint, camphor, ammonia, menthol and anisol. Highly selective stimulants of olfactory nerve endings include β-phenyl ethyl alcohol, methyl cyclopentenolone and isovaleric acid. Coffee, cinnamon and chocolate are useful everyday odours for the bedside testing of smell.

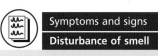

Symptoms and signs
Disturbance of smell

- Hyposmia-partial loss
- Anosmia-total loss
- Hyperosmia-exaggerated sensitivity
- Dyosmia-distorted sense

Differential diagnosis
Disturbances of olfaction

- Post-traumatic anosmia
- Postinfective anosmia
- Olfactory hallucinations in complex partial seizures

SYMPTOMS

The disturbances of smell that occur are defined in the 'symptoms and signs' box. For loss of smell, determine whether it is bilateral or unilateral.

Examination

The most convenient method for testing smell uses squeeze bottles bearing a nozzle that can be inserted into each nostril in turn. The patient is asked either to identify the smell or to describe its quality.

Clinical application

Olfaction is commonly disturbed by upper respiratory tract infection or local nasal pathology. Hyposmia can persist after an apparently banal viral illness and also after head injury. Smell sensitivity is diminished in dementia. Unilateral hyposmia is rarely the presenting symptom of a subfrontal meningioma. Olfactory hallucinations occur in complex partial seizures.

The optic (second) nerve

STRUCTURE AND FUNCTION

Two types of retinal photoreceptor, rods and cones, have been identified in humans. At the fovea only cones are found, with rods predominating in the periphery. Fibres from the nasal aspect of the fovea pass directly to the optic disc. Fibres from above and below the fovea pass

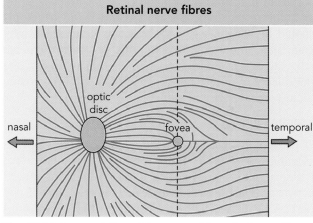

Retinal nerve fibres

nasal — optic disc — fovea — temporal

Fig. 11.14 Representation of the course of the retinal nerve fibres.

almost directly but fibres from the temporal border pass almost vertically, both superiorly and inferiorly, before arching around the other foveal fibres on their way to the optic disc (Fig. 11.14). Axons in the papillomacular bundle originate in the cones of the fovea and occupy a substantial proportion of the temporal aspect of the optic disc. Fibres from the superior and inferior parts of the periphery of the retina occupy corresponding areas in the optic nerve. As the papillomacular bundle approaches the chiasm, it moves centrally. The crossing, nasal, macular fibres occupy the central and posterior part of the chiasm.

The superior peripheral nasal fibres cross more posteriorly than the ventral fibres, which loop slightly into the terminal part of the opposite optic nerve (Fig. 11.15). Crossed and uncrossed fibres are arranged in alternate layers in the lateral geniculate body. The optic radiation extends from the lateral geniculate body to the visual (striate) cortex, area 17 (Fig. 11.1). The ventral fibres of the radiation loop forward towards the tip of the temporal lobe. The visual cortex is situated along the superior and inferior margins of the calcarine fissure, extending approximately 1.5 cm around the posterior pole. The macular representation lies posteriorly, with dorsal and ventral retina above and below the fissure, respectively. The unpaired outer 30° of the temporal field is represented in the contralateral hemisphere at the anterior limit of the striate cortex (Fig. 11.16).

Conditions of high (photopic) illumination activate cone photoreceptors, providing high spatial resolution and colour vision sense. Colour appreciation depends on three types of cone with spectral sensitivities spanning the range of colour vision. Low-illumination (scotopic) responses are mediated by rods.

SYMPTOMS

A number of questions are appropriate when assessing the patient's complaint of vision loss or alteration.

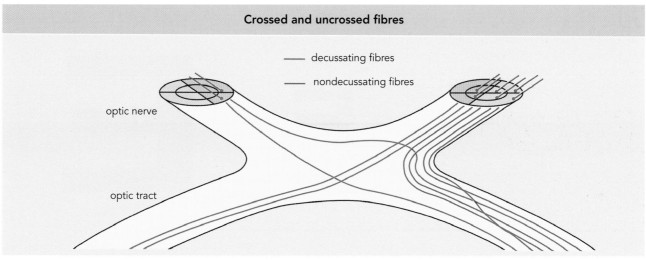

Fig. 11.15 Crossed and uncrossed fibres from the macula and the peripheral retina.

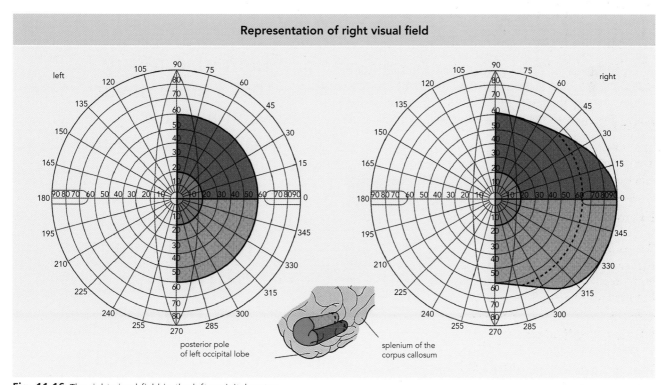

Fig. 11.16 The right visual field in the left occipital cortex.

Examination

VISUAL ACUITY

Visual acuity is tested in conditions of high illumination, producing a measure of cone function. The Snellen chart is used for testing distance vision. With the patient at the distance shown above a particular line, the visual angle subtended by a letter in that line is 5' and by individual components of the letter, 1' (Fig. 11.17).

Seat or stand the patient 6 m from the card. Ask the patient to cover each eye in turn and find which is the smallest line of print that can be read comfortably.

The visual acuity is then expressed as the ratio of the distance between the patient and the card (usually 6 m), to the figure on the chart immediately above the smallest visible line. An acuity of 6/18, therefore, indicates that, at 6 m from the chart, the patient is able to read down only to the 18 m line. Make sure the patient wears glasses if they contain a distance correction. If the patient's glasses are not available, reading through a pinhole will partly correct for any myopia. If unable to read the 60 m line at 6 m, the patient can move nearer the test type, say to 3 m. If the patient can then just read the 60 m line, the visual acuity, for that particular eye, is 3/60. A visual acuity of less than 1/60 can be recorded as counting fingers (CF),

Visual acuity

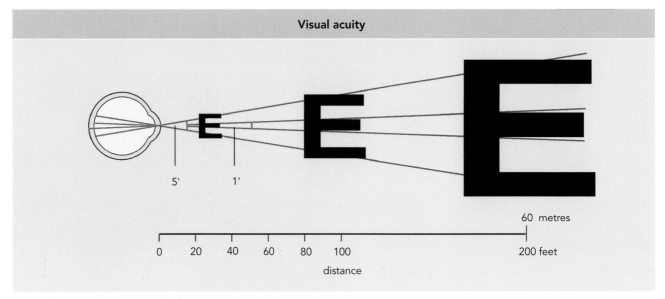

Fig. 11.17 The angles subtended by standard Snellen type.

hand movements (HM), perception of light (PL) or no perception of light (NPL). Near vision is tested using reading test types, such as that produced by the UK Faculty of Ophthalmologists (Fig. 11.18). Near visual acuity does not necessarily correlate well with distance acuity.

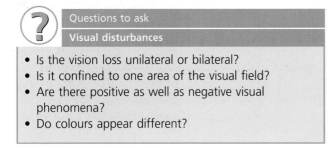

?   Questions to ask

Visual disturbances

- Is the vision loss unilateral or bilateral?
- Is it confined to one area of the visual field?
- Are there positive as well as negative visual phenomena?
- Do colours appear different?

COLOUR VISION

Tests of colour vision are designed principally to detect congenital defects. In the Farnsworth Munsell test the patient grades the shading of 84 coloured tiles. Red-green deficiency can be assessed more rapidly using the Ishihara test plates (Fig. 11.19). With the plates at about 75 cm from the eyes, which are covered in turn, ask the patient to read plates 1 to 15. If 13 or more plates are read correctly, colour vision can be regarded as normal.

VISUAL FIELDS

Retinal sensitivity diminishes with increasing distance from the fovea. Visual field mapping defines points in the visual field at which an object of a particular size or illumination is detected. The visual field is not symmetrical. It extends superiorly and medially for approximately 60°,

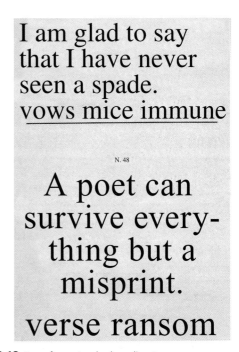

I am glad to say that I have never seen a spade.
vows mice immune

N. 48

A poet can survive everything but a misprint.

verse ransom

Fig. 11.18 Page from standard reading type.

temporally for about 100°, and inferiorly for approximately 75°. The blind spot, situated approximately 15° from fixation in the temporal field, marks the position of the optic disc. The field of vision to a coloured object, reflecting cone function, is more restricted than the field of a white object of the same size. Only the central portions of the two visual fields are binocular, the temporal margins being monocular (Fig. 11.20). Static perimetry involves the detection of a stationary target of varying brightness, while kinetic perimetry involves the detection of a moving target.

To test the visual field sit approximately 1 m from the patient. In infants or poorly cooperating adults, a

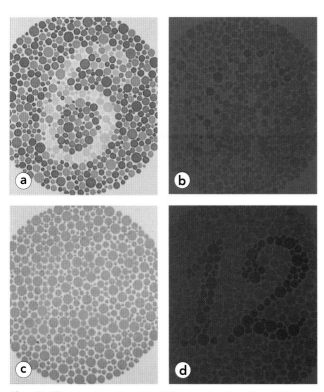

Fig. 11.19 Two plates from the Ishihara series. A patient with normal vision reads both (a) and (c) without difficulty; however, a patient with red–green deficiency is unable to read the figure 6 (b) but is able to read the figure 12 (d) correctly.

Visual fields

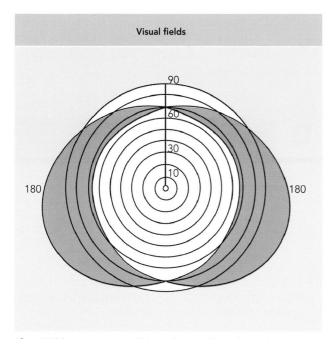

Fig. 11.20 Superimposed fields indicating binocular and monocular components.

meaningful response may be impossible to elicit or may be obtained only by using visual threat, in other words, a sudden, unexpected hand movement. For cooperative adults and older children, either finger movements or coloured objects can be used. For testing the left visual field, ask the patient to close or cover the right eye with

Visual field test

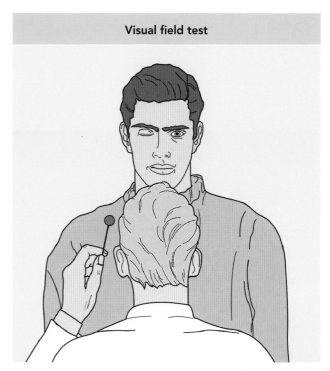

Fig. 11.21 Testing visual fields by confrontation.

the right hand, while you cover or close your left eye (Fig. 11.21). Ensure that the patient's left eye remains fixed on your right eye throughout the examination. The limits of the peripheral field can be determined by bringing the moving fingers of your right hand into the four quadrants of the patient's field. If individual half fields are full, then the target object, usually your moving fingers, should be presented in both peripheral fields simultaneously. In parietal lobe lesions, particularly of the nondominant hemisphere, a visual target presented in isolation in the contralateral field is perceived but is missed (visual

 Symptoms and signs
Types of field defect

- Absolute central scotoma
  - area around fixation in which there is no appreciation of the visual stimulus
- Relative central scotoma
  - area in which object is detected but its colour is diminished or desaturated (Fig. 11.23)
- Centrocaecal scotoma
  - extends from fixation towards the blind spot
- Bitemporal hemianopia
  - temporal halves of both fields are affected
- Homonymous hemianopia
  - a field defect in which the left or right half field is affected; in a complete right homonymous hemianopia, therefore, the temporal field of the right eye and the nasal field of the left eye are lost

Visual inattention

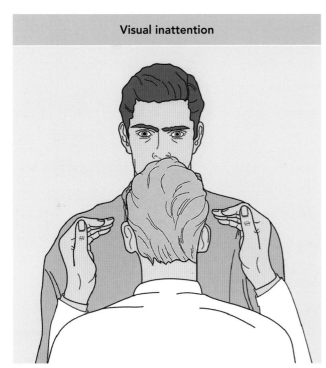

Fig. 11.22 Simultaneous presentation of finger movements in the two half fields.

Central scotoma

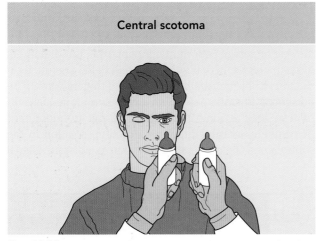

Fig. 11.23 Comparison of colour sensitivity between central and peripheral field. In this patient with a central scotoma, the red object appears brown in the central field.

suppression or inattention) when a comparable target is presented simultaneously in the ipsilateral half-field (Fig. 11.22). Peripheral field defects are often detected only if a small target object (e.g. a 10 mm red pin) is used rather than moving fingers.

Hand or finger movements are too crude a stimulus for assessing central field defects and here a small coloured object is used. It is useful to outline the blind spot first, partly because its successful identification increases confidence in one's own technique and partly because it indicates good fixation on the part of the patient. Move a red pin of some 10 mm in diameter into

the temporal field along the horizontal meridian. First explain to the patient that the object will disappear briefly then reappear and that the patient should indicate when this happens. Once you have found the position of the blind spot its shape can be mapped. Seldom will the blind spots of the patient and yourself completely coincide. Having identified the blind spot, assess the central visual field.

FUNDOSCOPY

Normally it is not necessary to dilate the pupils in order to examine the central fundus but if the patient has small pupils, or the background illumination is high, take the patient into a darkened room for the examination. If this fails to dilate the pupils sufficiently, then a mydriatic, for example, Mydrilate (1% cyclopentolate), can be instilled. This should never be done in the unconscious patient and must always be recorded in the patient's notes. Do not use mydriatics in a patient with glaucoma. Remember to reverse the effects of the mydriatic at the end of the examination by instilling 2% pilocarpine.

Ask the patient to fixate on a distant target (Fig. 11.24). If the patient wears glasses with a substantial correction, it sometimes facilitates the examination to perform it with the patient's glasses in place.

The optic disc is examined first to assess its shape, colour and clarity. The temporal margin of the disc is slightly paler than the nasal margin. The physiological cup varies in size but seldom extends to the temporal, and never to the nasal margins of the disc. The blood vessels are not obscured as they cross the disc margin, nor are they elevated (Fig. 11.25).

Differential diagnosis

Retinal and visual pathway disorders

- Anterior ischaemic optic neuropathy
- Optic neuritis
- Optic nerve compression
- Papilloedema
- Hypertensive retinopathy
- Diabetic retinopathy
- Glaucoma
- Chiasmatic compression due to pituitary tumour
- Optic tract, radiation or visual cortex lesions due to vascular disease

The vessels are examined next. The arteries are narrower than the veins and a brighter colour. They possess a longitudinal pale streak as a consequence of light reflecting from their walls. The retinal veins should be closely inspected where they enter the optic disc. In approximately 80% of normal individuals the veins pulsate. This pulsation ceases when CSF pressure exceeds

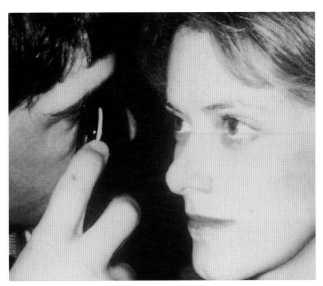

Fig. 11.24 Direct fundoscopy.

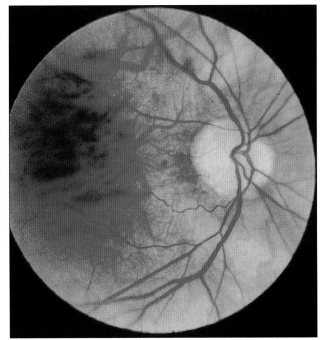

Fig. 11.26 Optic atrophy.

is examined for the presence of haemorrhages and exudates, the positions of which are best shown by a small diagram in the patient's notes, or by a description that uses the optic disc as a clock face for localisation purposes, for example, 'one large haemorrhage at 6 o'clock, one disc diameter from the disc'.

Clinical application

OPTIC ATROPHY

Optic atrophy follows any process that damages the ganglion cells or the axons between the retinal nerve fibre layer and the lateral geniculate body. It is associated with loss of bulk of the nerve and pallor of the disc (Fig. 11.26). The pallor may be diffuse or segmental. Temporal pallor is the most common form of segmental atrophy, attributable to the susceptibility of the papillomacular bundle to degenerate after optic nerve damage by compression or metabolic disturbance.

The colour of the normal optic disc is variable and the ophthalmoscopic diagnosis of optic atrophy notoriously subjective. Additional features that may help the diagnosis include the number of capillaries visible on the optic disc, and the presence of retinal nerve fibre atrophy. The former criterion has not been substantiated and detection of the latter requires considerable experience. Inspection of the retinal vessels is worthwhile. The presence of sheathing or attenuation of the retinal arterioles suggests that the optic atrophy is secondary to ischaemic optic neuropathy or central retinal artery occlusion.

PAPILLOEDEMA

Patients with papilloedema often have no visual complaints, although some describe transient obscurations

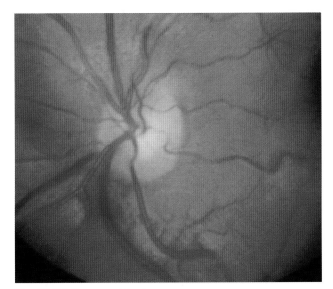

Fig. 11.25 The normal fundus.

200 mm of water. Therefore the presence of retinal venous pulsation is a very sensitive index of normal intracranial pressure. Learn to identify this physical sign. It will save countless references to 'swollen optic discs?'. The fundus

Emergency

Acute visual failure

- Unilateral – consider
  - cranial arteritis
  - optic neuritis
  - retinal detachment
  - central retinal artery occlusion
  - acute glaucoma
  - vitreous haemorrhage
- Bilateral – consider
  - cranial arteritis
  - optic neuritis

of vision either occurring spontaneously or triggered by postural change. Papilloedema is usually bilateral, although sometimes asymmetrical. Its pathogenesis remains unsettled. The term papilloedema is best reserved for patients in whom the disc swelling is secondary to raised intracranial pressure. Transmission of the raised intracranial pressure, via the subarachnoid space of the optic nerve, results in venous stasis and also interrupts both fast and slow axoplasmic flow in the optic nerve.

As papilloedema develops, swelling of the nerve fibre layer appears (best seen with a red-free light), within which haemorrhages are visible. The disc becomes hyperaemic (as a result of capillary dilatation) with a loss of definition of its margins, and retinal venous pulsation disappears (Fig. 11.27). In fully developed papilloedema there is engorgement of retinal veins, obscuration of the disc margin, flame haemorrhages and cotton wool spots (the consequence of retinal infarction). The vessels are tortuous (Fig. 11.28). Often the only visual field change at this stage is an enlargement of the blind spot (Fig. 11.29). In the later stages of papilloedema, hard exudates appear on the disc, which

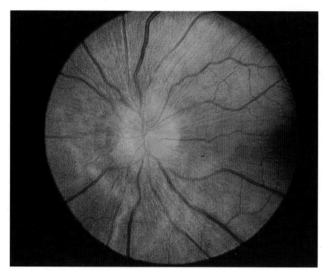

Fig. 11.27 Early papilloedema. Dilated nerve fibre bundles, superficial haemorrhages and disc hyperaemia.

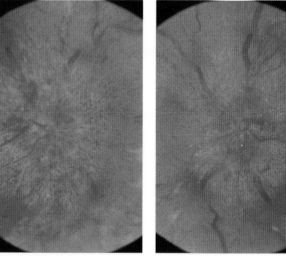

Fig. 11.28 Chronic papilloedema. Swollen optic discs, dilated capillaries, haemorrhages and cotton wool spots.

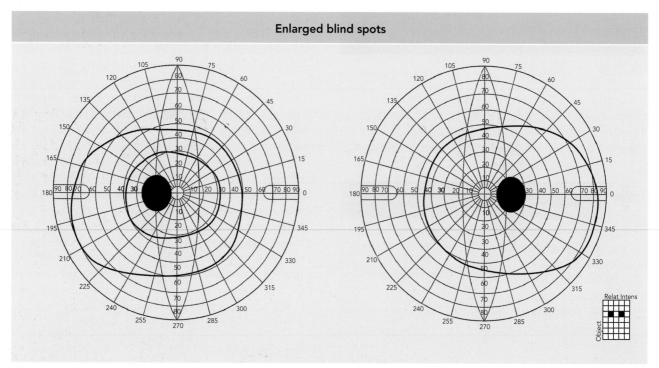

Fig. 11.29 Papilloedema. Visual fields showing bilaterally enlarged blind spots.

becomes atrophic, and other visual field abnormalities appear, including arcuate fibre defects and peripheral constriction.

Papilloedema can probably appear within 4–5 h of the development of intracranial hypertension and may not resolve for some weeks after its reduction.

OTHER FUNDUS ABNORMALITIES

Myelinated nerve fibres

A congenital anomaly in which myelinated and therefore visible nerve fibres are found at, or adjacent to, the disc margin (Fig. 11.30).

Drusen (hyaline bodies)

Drusen are thought to be derived from axonal debris and are situated in the disc anterior to the lamina cribrosa, where they appear as yellow excrescences, often distorting the disc margin. They do not usually produce visual symptoms (Fig. 11.31).

RETINAL VASCULAR DISEASE

Retinal artery and vein occlusion

After occlusion of the central retinal artery, the retina becomes pale and opaque with a cherry-red spot at the macula. The optic disc, initially swollen, becomes atrophic (Fig. 11.32). The presence of microemboli, containing either cholesterol or a fibrin–platelet mixture, establishes that the occlusion is embolic (Fig. 11.33). A branch occlusion produces a corresponding sector-shaped visual defect. In central retinal vein occlusion there is swelling of the optic disc, dilatation of the retinal veins and fundal haemorrhages (Fig. 11.34).

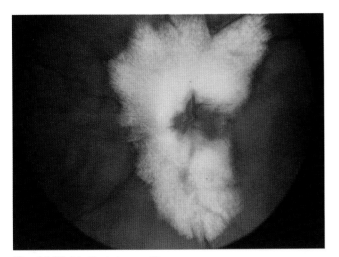

Fig. 11.30 Myelinated nerve fibres.

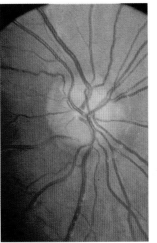

Fig. 11.31 Bilateral drusen (associated with peripapillary haemorrhage on right).

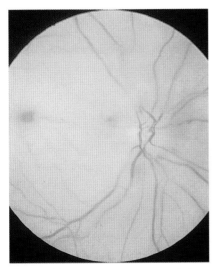

Fig. 11.32 Central retinal artery occlusion.

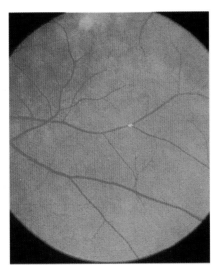

Fig. 11.33 Cholesterol embolus.

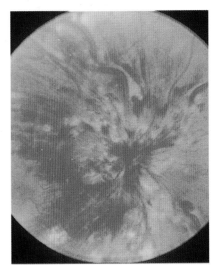

Fig. 11.34 Central retinal vein occlusion.

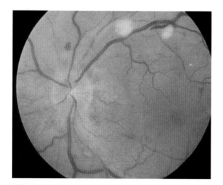

Fig. 11.35 Hypertensive retinopathy with haemorrhages, cotton wool spots and variation in arteriolar calibre.

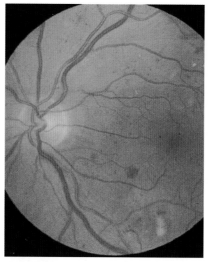

Fig. 11.36 Diabetic retinopathy. Microaneurysms, haemorrhages, exudates and cotton wool spots.

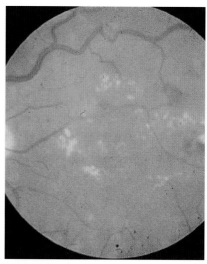

Fig. 11.37 Diabetic retinopathy. Hard exudates at the macula.

Hypertensive retinopathy

In hypertensive retinopathy, the light reflex from the arteriolar wall is abnormal and constriction of the venous wall appears at sites of arteriovenous crossing. Both the former (silver or copper-wiring) and the latter (arteriovenous nipping) are encountered in normal older individuals. A more reliable sign of hypertensive retinopathy is variation in the calibre of the retinal arterioles. As the retinopathy advances, haemorrhages and cotton wool spots appear (Fig. 11.35) and in malignant or accelerated hypertension disc swelling occurs.

Diabetic retinopathy

Diabetic retinopathy in its early stages principally affects the retinal microcirculation, producing the characteristic, although not pathognomonic, microaneurysm (Fig. 11.36). Subsequently small haemorrhages, exudates and cotton wool spots appear. Visual failure is usually due either to macular disease, in the form of oedema, infarction or lipid deposition (Fig.11.37), or to the appearance of new vessel formation (proliferative diabetic retinopathy), leading to vitreous haemorrhage and retinal detachment caused by traction of fibrous tissue (Fig. 11.38).

GLAUCOMA

Glaucoma, characterised by raised intraocular pressure, can occur either secondarily to various ocular pathologies (e.g. uveitis) or in a primary form. The latter is far more common. Resulting changes in the optic disc include enlargement of the physiological cup (particularly significant if in the vertical axis), an increase in the ratio

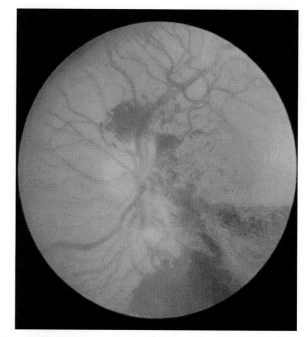

Fig. 11.38 Vitreous haemorrhage with evidence of new vessel formation at the disc margin.

of cup size to vertical disc diameter beyond 0.6 and retinal nerve fibre atrophy. Arcuate field defects accompany these changes. With advanced glaucoma there is marked undermining of the disc margins and bowing of the blood vessels (Fig. 11.39).

OPTIC NERVE DISEASE

In lesions of the optic nerve, the visual defect is monocular. Visual acuity is usually reduced and colour perception is disturbed (particularly for red–green). There is a relative afferent pupillary defect (see p. 341). The most likely visual field defect is a central scotoma (Fig. 11.40). Optic atrophy is a relatively late development in optic nerve compression. Proptosis is likely if the lesion is within the orbit.

CHIASMATIC LESIONS

Most chiasmatic syndromes are the result of compression by pituitary tumour, meningioma or craniopharyngioma. The result is a bitemporal hemianopia, although the type of defect relates to the position of the growth and its relation to the chiasm. Typically, the visual defect is asymmetrical (Fig. 11.41). In its earliest stages, the field defect can be detected only by moving a coloured target across the vertical meridian (Fig. 11.42). Patients frequently complain of blurred or double vision, a consequence of lost integration between independent nasal fields.

OPTIC TRACT AND LATERAL GENICULATE BODY LESIONS

These are uncommon. A lesion in the anterior part of the optic tract, before the homonymous fibres have joined, produces an incongruous homonymous hemianopia, that is, one in which the two half field losses are not equal (Fig. 11.43).

OPTIC RADIATION AND OCCIPITAL CORTEX LESIONS

The type of visual field loss from lesions of the optic radiation depends on their localisation. All the defects are homonymous but not necessarily congruous. In lesions affecting the temporal radiation, the superior quadrantic field is more affected than the inferior. If the defect is incongruous, the nasal loss in the ipsilateral eye is more extensive than the temporal loss in the contralateral eye (Fig. 11.44).

With parietal lobe lesions, the defect is often complete but, rarely, principally affects the inferior quadrants. Occipital lobe pathology produces congruous defects that can be total, quadrantic or scotomatous. In some instances there is macular sparing, probably because of a dual vascular supply to the macular area of the occipital cortex (Fig. 11.45). An isolated homonymous hemianopia is usually occipital in origin and almost always due to vascular disease. Temporal or parietal lobe pathology associated with visual field defects will

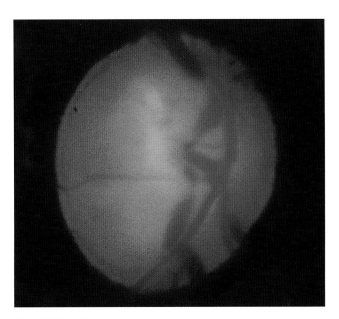

Fig. 11.39 Advanced chronic simple glaucoma.

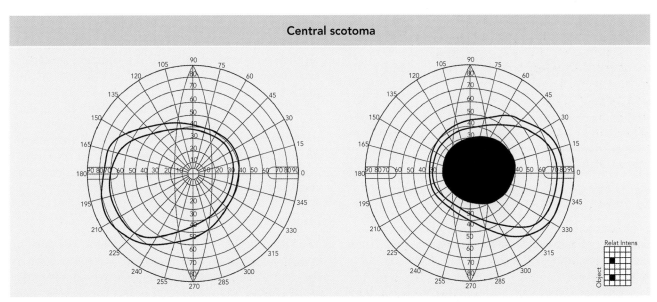

Central scotoma

Fig. 11.40 Large right central scotoma.

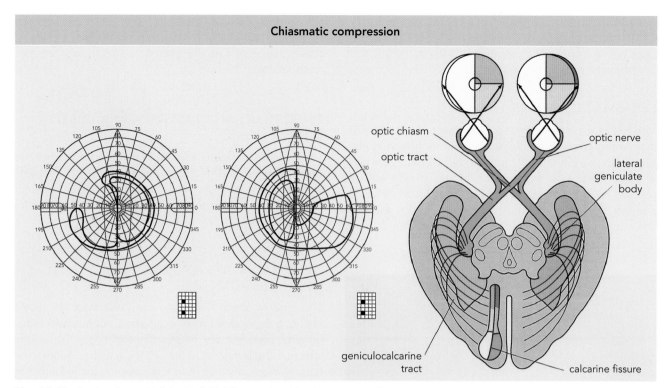

Fig. 11.41 Visual pathways (right) with field defect produced by chiasmatic compression (left).

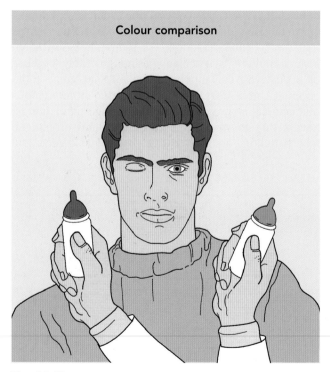

Fig. 11.42 Comparison of coloured targets in nasal and temporal fields. There is red desaturation in the temporal field of the left eye.

usually produce additional symptoms and signs. Furthermore, the pathology is often neoplastic rather than vascular.

Bilateral occipital infarction results in cortical blindness. The pupillary responses are normal. In some instances there is denial of visual disability and confabulation of visual detail (Anton's syndrome).

The oculomotor, trochlear and abducens (third, fourth and sixth) nerves

STRUCTURE AND FUNCTION

Pupillary light response pathway

The pupillary light response pathway originates in the same rods and cones that register visual stimuli. Fibres from the receptors partly decussate in the chiasm, then leave the optic tract before the lateral geniculate body on their way to the brachium of the superior colliculus and, hence, the Edinger–Westphal nucleus, via the pretectal nuclear complex (Fig. 11.46). A light stimulus to one eye triggers a bilateral, symmetrical, pupillary response. The pupillomotor fibres lie superficially in the oculomotor nerve before joining the inferior division of the nerve on their way to the ciliary ganglion. After synapsing, the fibres enter the short ciliary nerve.

Near reaction

The near reaction comprises pupillary constriction, ocular convergence and increased accommodation of the lens. The accommodation reaction is controlled by the rostral and midportion of the Edinger–Westphal nucleus. The efferent pathway passes through the

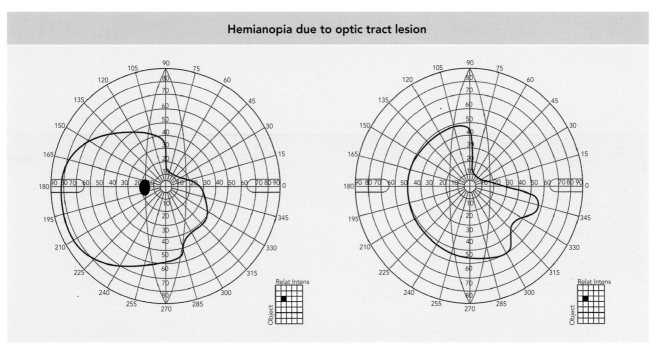

Fig. 11.43 Incongruous right homonymous hemianopia associated with a left optic tract lesion.

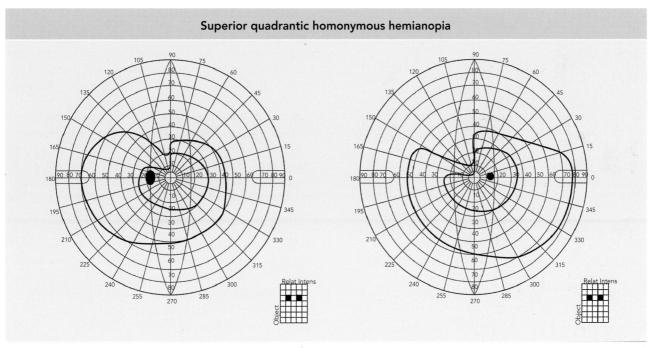

Fig. 11.44 Incongruous left superior quadrantic homonymous hemianopia associated with a lesion of the temporal part of the right optic radiation.

oculomotor nerve, ciliary ganglion and short ciliary nerve.

Ocular sympathetic fibres

The ocular sympathetic fibres originate in the hypothalamus and remain uncrossed. The first-order neurons terminate in the spinal cord in the intermediolateral cell column between the spinal segments of C8 and T2. Second-order neurons exit from the cord, principally in the first ventral thoracic root, and pass through the inferior and middle cervical ganglia before terminating in the superior cervical ganglion (Fig. 11.47). Sudomotor and vasoconstrictor fibres to the face, except for those to a small area on the forehead, run with branches of the external carotid artery. Fibres accompanying the internal carotid artery

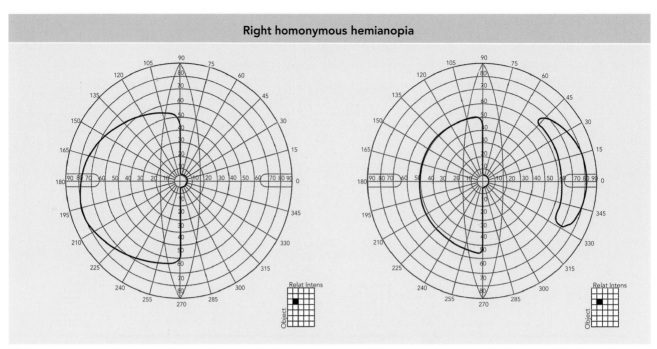

Fig. 11.45 A right homonymous hemianopia, sparing the macula and the peripheral temporal crescent of the right eye.

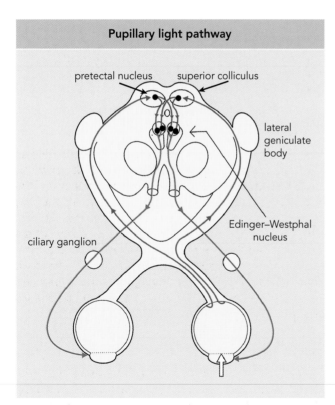

Pupillary light pathway

pretectal nucleus   superior colliculus

lateral geniculate body

ciliary ganglion

Edinger–Westphal nucleus

Fig. 11.46 Pupillary light pathway. The input from the left eye decussates at the chiasm and reaches both third nerve nuclei.

reach the pupil via branches of the ophthalmic division of the trigeminal nerve and the eyelids via branches of the ophthalmic artery. The fibres supply the dilator muscle of the iris and smooth muscle in the upper and lower lids.

Horizontal and vertical saccades

There are supranuclear, internuclear and infranuclear components in the anatomical pathways for eye movements, with different supranuclear pathways for saccadic (refixation) movements and pursuit (following) movements. Horizontal saccades originate in both the frontal and parietal lobes. Certain types of eye movement are also probably initiated in the temporal lobe. From the frontal eye fields, the principal descending pathway passes through the anterior limb of the internal capsule, continues along the ventrolateral aspect of the thalamus, decussates in the lower midbrain, then passes in the paramedian pontine reticular formation to end at the excitatory burst neurons in the pontine gaze centre (Fig. 11.48). From here, neurons project to the ipsilateral abducens nucleus and through it, via the medial longitudinal fasciculus, to the medial rectus component of the contralateral third nerve nucleus. The pathway for vertical saccades has been less clearly defined but it projects eventually to the rostral interstitial nucleus of the medial longitudinal fasciculus (Fig. 11.49), which is located at the junction of midbrain and thalamus. The nucleus receives additional ascending inputs through the medial longitudinal fasciculus and, directly, from the paramedian pontine reticular formation. From this nucleus, the pathway for downward saccades passes caudally to the third and fourth cranial nerve nuclei; that for upward saccades traverses the posterior commissure.

Pursuit movements in both the horizontal and vertical planes originate in the parieto-occipital cortex, then descend in an uncrossed pathway whose exact location remains undetermined. The path for horizontal pursuit is

The oculomotor, trochlear and abducens (third, fourth and sixth) nerves **11**

Ocular sympathetic pathway

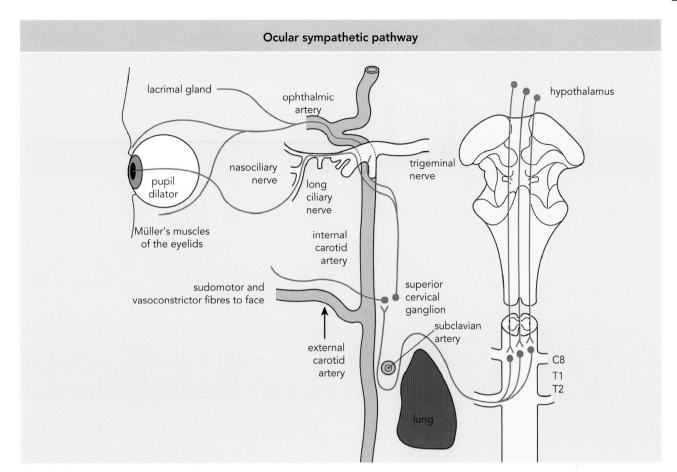

Fig. 11.47 The ocular sympathetic pathway.

known to pass through the paramedian pontine reticular formation and that for vertical pursuit is controlled, at least in part, by fibres passing rostrally through the medial longitudinal fasciculus.

The globe has an innate tendency to return to the primary position of gaze after ocular deviation, so the stimulus for a sudden horizontal or vertical movement needs to be followed by a sustained neuronal discharge to the relevant muscles if ocular deviation is to be sustained. Burst neurons trigger the initial saccade; at other times their output is suppressed by pause neurons. Simultaneously, there is inhibition of the nucleus supplying the contralateral antagonist muscle. For sustained deviation, a tonic neuronal discharge occurs that uses the same final common pathway as the burst neurons but which is influenced by other structures, including the cerebellum and the medial vestibular nucleus. A similar tonic mechanism exists for other forms of eye movement.

Saccadic movements with a velocity of up to 700°/s permit a rapid refixation of gaze from one object to another, while pursuit movements allow tracking of a slowly moving target at velocities up to 50°/s. Vestibular movements are initiated in the semicircular canals by head movement or, reflexly, by caloric stimulation. These movements maintain a stable perception of the environment during bodily movement.

Third nerve

The third nerve nucleus is located in the midbrain at the level of the superior colliculus. All its neurons project ipsilaterally, apart from those passing to the contralateral superior rectus muscle. The levators of the upper lids are supplied by a single midline nucleus. The third nerve emerges from the anterior aspect of the midbrain and lies close to the posterior communicating artery before entering the cavernous sinus, in which it runs superiorly (Fig. 11.50). It terminates in superior and inferior divisions, the latter containing pupillomotor fibres.

Fourth nerve

The fourth nerve decussates before exiting from the dorsal aspect of the midbrain, eventually innervating the contralateral superior oblique muscle. It lies immediately below the third nerve in the cavernous sinus and enters the orbit through the superior orbital fissure, along with the other nerves supplying the eye muscles.

Sixth nerve

The sixth nerve emerges from the lower border of the pons, runs beneath the petroclinoid ligament, then lies

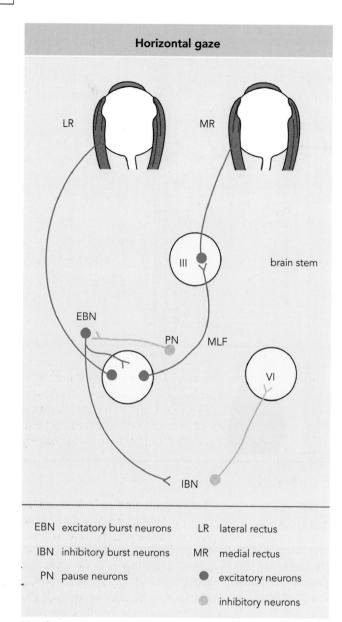

Fig. 11.48 Organisation of horizontal gaze.

Horizontal gaze

EBN excitatory burst neurons	LR lateral rectus
IBN inhibitory burst neurons	MR medial rectus
PN pause neurons	● excitatory neurons
	● inhibitory neurons

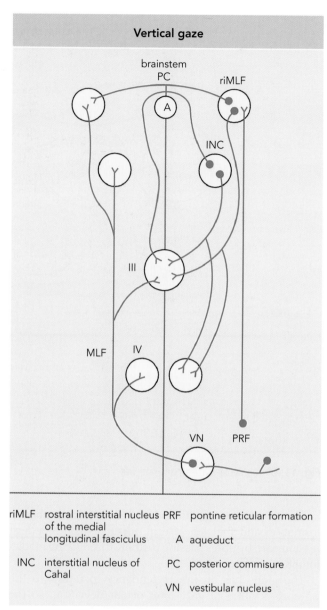

Fig. 11.49 Organisation of vertical gaze.

Vertical gaze

riMLF	rostral interstitial nucleus of the medial longitudinal fasciculus	PRF pontine reticular formation
		A aqueduct
INC	interstitial nucleus of Cahal	PC posterior commisure
		VN vestibular nucleus

close to the internal carotid artery in the medial aspect of the cavernous sinus. It supplies the lateral rectus muscle.

Nystagmus

Nystagmus is a repetitive to-and-fro movement of the eyes. In pendular nystagmus, the phases are of equal velocity, in phasic (jerk) nystagmus they differ. The slow phase of jerk nystagmus may show a linear or nonlinear time course. Vestibular dysfunction, either centrally or peripherally, is the usual cause of a jerk nystagmus in which the slow-phase is linear. In gaze-evoked nystagmus the eyes drift back from an eccentric position with a nonlinear velocity, followed by a saccadic correction. This type of nystagmus is thought to result from dysfunction of the neural integrator, the mechanism that sustains a

tonic discharge of neuronal activity during eccentric gaze.

SYMPTOMS

If the patient complains of ptosis, find out whether the problem is bilateral or unilateral and whether it fluctuates. If necessary obtain old photographs to make a comparison.

For diplopia, a number of questions may help to suggest the underlying mechanism. Weakness of the lateral or medial rectus muscles produces a horizontal diplopia. Weakness of the other eye muscles produces a vertical or oblique diplopia. The diplopia increases as the patient looks in the direction of action of the paralysed muscle.

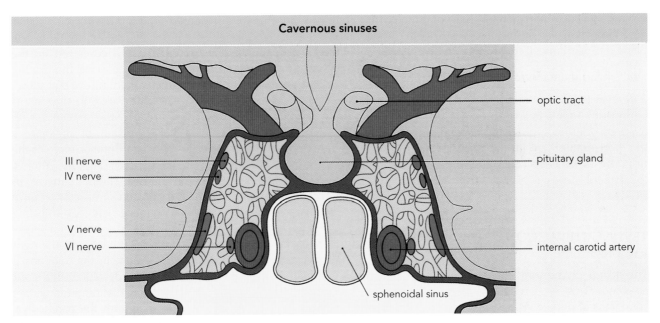

Cavernous sinuses

- optic tract
- III nerve
- IV nerve
- pituitary gland
- V nerve
- VI nerve
- internal carotid artery
- sphenoidal sinus

Fig. 11.50 Transverse section of cavernous sinuses.

Questions to ask

Diplopia

- Is the diplopia relieved by covering one or other eye?
- Is the diplopia horizontal or vertical/oblique?
- Does the diplopia increase in one particular direction of gaze?
- Does the diplopia fluctuate or is it constant?

Examination

INSPECTION OF THE EYELIDS AND PUPILS

Note the position of the eyelids. If there is a ptosis, assess its fatiguability by asking the patient to sustain upward gaze. Next examine the pupils, which normally are circular and symmetrical, although a slight difference in size (anisocoria) of up to 2 mm is seen in some 20% of the population. If there is a slight size difference, take the patient into a darkened room. A physiological anisocoria will remain unchanged. An irregular pupil is most commonly the consequence of iris disease. Ask the patient about previous ocular trauma or infection. If the pupils are markedly different in size, make sure that the patient is not using a mydriatic or meiotic in one eye alone.

Pupillary light response

Now examine the pupillary light response using a bright pencil torch. The background illumination should be low, and to prevent a near reaction the patient should fixate on a distant object. Observe the direct (ipsilateral) and consensual (contralateral) responses. A unilateral depression of the light response may be obvious but a defect of the afferent pupillary pathway is best appreciated by swinging the torch from one eye to the other. As the torch swings from, say, the right eye to the left, the pupil of the latter, which has just started to dilate because of the loss of its consensual reaction, immediately constricts.

Near reaction

If the light response is normal there is little point in testing the near reaction. If the light response is depressed, test the near reaction by asking the patient to fixate on a target (e.g. your forefinger) as it approaches the eyes. Many patients, especially elderly people, have difficulty sustaining convergence. If there is no immediate reaction, maintain convergence for a minute or so to see if a delayed reaction appears. The near reaction is additive to the pupillary light response, in other words, it can be tested in bright light.

INSPECTION OF EYE MOVEMENTS

Conjugate eye movements

Next assess conjugate eye movements. To test pursuit, ask the patient to follow a slowly moving target, first in the horizontal then in the vertical plane. If pursuit movements are slowed, brief saccades must be superimposed to allow the eyes to catch their target. The resulting movement is jerky rather than smooth. The slowing may be in one or more directions. To assess saccadic movements, ask the patient to rapidly fixate between two targets, for example, two fingers in the same plane. Saccades may be abnormal in terms of their velocity, accuracy or persistence. An overshoot or undershoot is readily detected during refixation movements. Slowing, in either initiation or performance, can occur in the horizontal or vertical plane. Inappropriate saccades will disrupt fixation. When continuous, they are described as ocular flutter if confined to the horizontal plane or opsoclonus if multidirectional.

Doll's head manoeuvre (oculocephalic reflex)

If the eyes fail to respond to a saccadic or pursuit stimulus, perform the doll's head manoeuvre. Ask the patient to fixate on your eyes, grasp the head and rotate it, first in the horizontal then in the vertical plane. An intact response (a measure of vestibular eye function) allows the patient's eyes to remain fixed on your own (Fig. 11.51).

TESTING THE ACTION OF INDIVIDUAL EYE MUSCLES

The action of the individual eye muscles can now be assessed. This is particularly relevant if the patient complains of double vision (diplopia).

In a strabismus, or squint, the axes of the eyes are no longer parallel. Esodeviation indicates that the axes are convergent and exodeviation that they are divergent. The strabismus is concomitant if the angle of deviation remains constant throughout the range of eye movement and incomitant if the angle of deviation varies. The latter is usually caused by paresis of one or more of the extraocular muscles. Now perform a cover test. In the presence of a concomitant squint, covering the fixating eye produces a movement in the squinting eye that allows it to take up fixation (unless the vision in that eye is severely depressed) (Fig. 11.52). Most patients with concomitant squint do not complain of diplopia, a symptom that suggests a disorder of one or more of the extraocular muscles or their nerve supply. After a recent oculomotor nerve paresis, altered patterns of contraction in the yoke and antagonist muscles produce characteristic deviations when alternate cover testing is performed. In the presence of a right lateral rectus weakness, the patient fixates with the left eye, the right eye tending to turn inwards because of the unopposed action of medial rectus (the primary deviation). If the left eye is now covered, increased innervation attempts are made in order to achieve fixation with the paretic eye. This abnormal stimulus spills over to the yoke muscle, the medial rectus of the left eye, which accordingly over-adducts that eye (secondary deviation). In a paralytic strabismus, secondary deviation is greater than primary (Fig. 11.53).

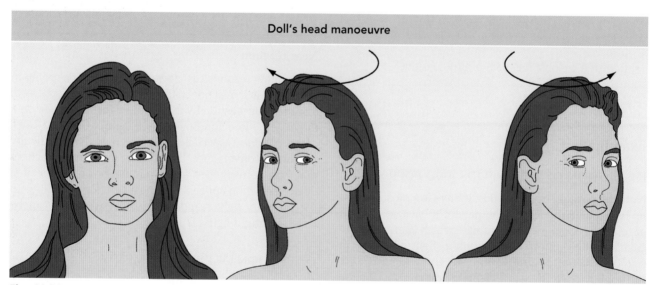

Doll's head manoeuvre

Fig. 11.51 Performing the doll's head manoeuvre in the horizontal plane.

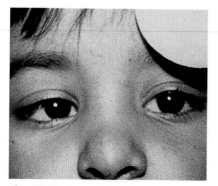
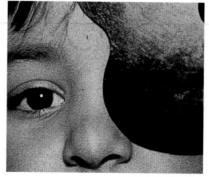
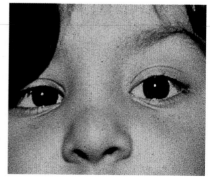

Fig. 11.52 Cover testing. There is a right esotropia that corrects temporarily when the left eye is covered.

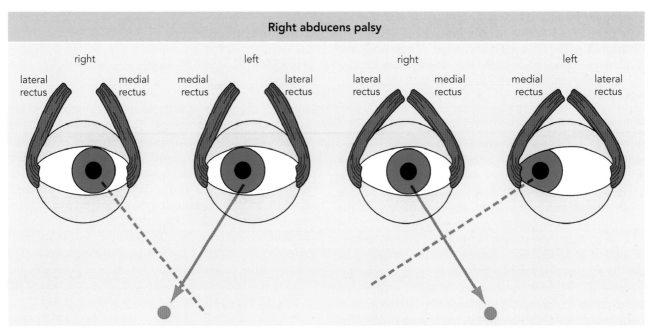

Right abducens palsy

Fig. 11.53 Right abducens palsy. The right eye tends to converge, particularly when the left eye is used for fixation. When the right eye tries to fixate, overaction of the left medial rectus occurs.

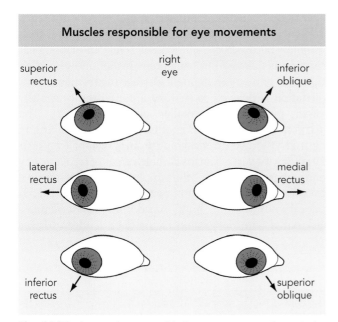

Muscles responsible for eye movements

Fig. 11.54 The muscles responsible for eye movements in particular directions.

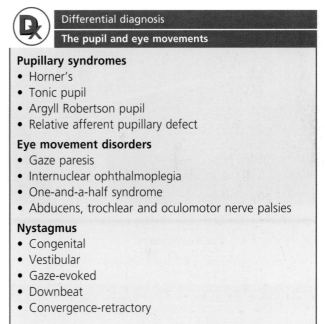

Differential diagnosis

The pupil and eye movements

Pupillary syndromes
- Horner's
- Tonic pupil
- Argyll Robertson pupil
- Relative afferent pupillary defect

Eye movement disorders
- Gaze paresis
- Internuclear ophthalmoplegia
- One-and-a-half syndrome
- Abducens, trochlear and oculomotor nerve palsies

Nystagmus
- Congenital
- Vestibular
- Gaze-evoked
- Downbeat
- Convergence-retractory

Having confirmed that the diplopia is binocular (in other words, that it disappears when one or other eye is covered) ask the patient to look in the six directions illustrated in Figure 11.54. The false image (which often appears indistinct or blurred) is peripheral to the true image and belongs to the affected eye. Having elicited the diplopia, cover first one eye, then the other, to establish to which eye the false image belongs. Observe if the patient has an abnormal head tilt as a compensation for the diplopia. To establish whether the head tilt is longstanding, examine old photographs. Finally, remember that a pattern of diplopia that is variable and difficult to interpret suggests the possibility of myasthenia gravis.

Nystagmus

Note the presence of nystagmus and whether it is pendular or jerk. Record the amplitude (fine, medium or coarse), persistence and the direction of gaze in which it occurs. Additionally, indicate whether the movement is horizontal, vertical, rotary or a mixture of several types. First-degree nystagmus to the left is a fast beating nystagmus to the left on left lateral gaze. In second- and third-degree nystagmus to the left, the same nystagmus is present on forward and right lateral gaze, respectively.

Optokinetic nystagmus

Optokinetic responses are assessed using a drum painted with vertical lines, which is rotated first in the horizontal and then in the vertical plane. As the patient looks at the drum a pursuit movement is seen in the direction of its rotation, followed by a saccade returning the eyes to the midposition. As an alternative, the patient can be asked to look at a tape measure as it is drawn across the field of gaze (Fig. 11.55). Both movements are generated by the hemisphere towards which the drum is rotating. Thus, with the drum rotating to the right, or the tape being drawn to the right, pursuit is controlled by the right parieto-occipital cortex and the correcting saccade by the right frontal cortex.

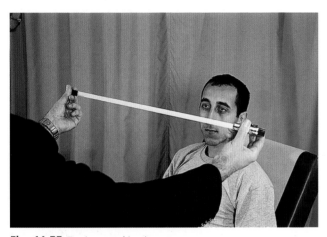

Fig. 11.55 Testing optokinetic nystagmus.

Clinical application

THE PUPIL

Horner's syndrome

Horner's syndrome results from interruption of the sympathetic fibres to the eye. The pupil is miosed and the palpebral fissure is narrowed because of mild ptosis of the upper lid and elevation of the lower lid. The pupillary asymmetry is often slight but can be accentuated by taking the patient into a darkened room. Although enophthalmos is suggested by the appearance of the eye, this is not confirmed by formal measurement. The distribution of sweating loss on the ipsilateral face depends on the site of the lesion. If there is uncertainty regarding the diagnosis, instil 4% cocaine into each eye – the normal pupil dilates, the affected pupil fails to do so (Fig. 11.56), irrespective of the site of the lesion.

Tonic pupil syndrome

The tonic pupil syndrome is usually unilateral. The affected pupil is dilated, although in longstanding cases it becomes progressively smaller. The light response is absent or markedly depressed and, consequently, in a darkened room, the affected pupil becomes smaller than its fellow because of a failure of reflex dilatation. The near reaction is delayed but sometimes is then more marked than that of the normal pupil. On relaxing the near effort, dilatation is delayed so that for a period the previously larger pupil is the smaller one (Fig. 11.57). The accommodation reaction is often sustained, resulting in blurred vision when switching from a distant to a near target or vice versa. The iris contains areas of focal atrophy and, characteristically, the pupils are hypersensitive to dilute parasympathomimetic agents (e.g. 0.125% pilocarpine). Tonic pupil syndrome is sometimes associated with depression of the deep tendon reflexes

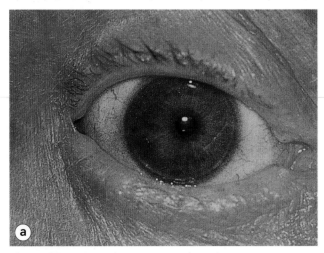

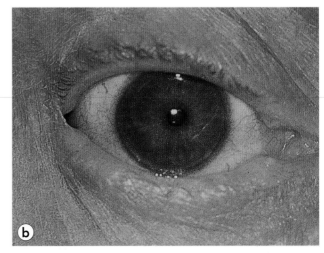

Fig. 11.56 Horner's syndrome. Before (a) and after (b) instillation of cocaine.

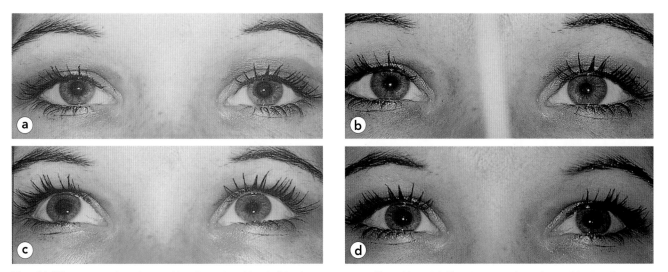

Fig. 11.57 Tonic pupil syndrome. (a) Left pupil is dilated. (b) After 1 min near effort. (c) Partial dilatation 15 s after release. (d) Virtually complete at 60 s.

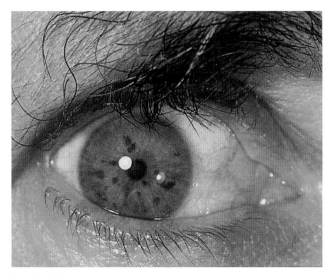

Fig. 11.58 Argyll Robertson pupil.

(Holmes–Adie syndrome) and may occur in association with various dysautonomias.

Argyll robertson pupil

The Argyll Robertson pupil is miosed, with a light response that is diminished compared with the near reaction (light-near dissociation). When the defect is fully developed, the pupil is fixed to light and fails to dilate in the dark. The pupil is often irregular with evidence of iris atrophy (Fig. 11.58). When complete, the syndrome is pathognomonic of neurosyphilis. The lesion responsible is thought to lie in the midbrain immediately above the Edinger–Westphal nucleus. A pupil of normal size with light-near dissociation can occur in other circumstances (e.g. in a blind eye).

Relative afferent pupillary defect

This results from a lesion of the afferent light reflex pathway between the retina and the optic tract. It is not found with disease of the lens or vitreous. The conducting systems of the two optic nerves are best compared by performing the swinging light test. In the presence of a unilateral optic nerve lesion, for example caused by optic neuritis, the affected pupil dilates as the torch is swung onto it from the sound eye.

DISORDERS OF EYE MOVEMENTS

Gaze paresis

In an acute frontal lobe lesion, contralateral saccadic eye movements in the horizontal plane are depressed or absent and there is limb paresis ipsilateral to the gaze palsy (Fig. 11.59). Both pursuit movements and the oculocephalic responses are spared. Saccades return later but now initiated by the contralateral frontal lobe. Subsequent damage to that frontal lobe will result in a complete horizontal saccadic palsy. A lesion at the level of the paramedian pontine reticular formation produces an ipsilateral gaze paresis for both saccadic and pursuit movement (Fig. 11.60). The limb paresis is contralateral. An ipsilateral pursuit paresis occurs with posterior hemisphere disease and is associated with a contralateral homonymous field defect.

A paresis of upward saccades, initially with relative preservation of pursuit, is a feature of the dorsal-midbrain (Parinaud's) syndrome (Fig. 11.61). Other findings include impaired convergence and dilated, light-near dissociated pupils. At a later stage upward pursuit and down gaze become affected. Causes include vascular disease and pinealoma.

OTHER SACCADIC AND PURSUIT MOVEMENT DISORDERS

Saccadic slowing, accompanied by disorganised pursuit movements, is found in both Huntington's and

Eye movements in frontal, pontine and dorsal-midbrain lesions

Fig 11.59

Fig 11.60

Fig 11.61

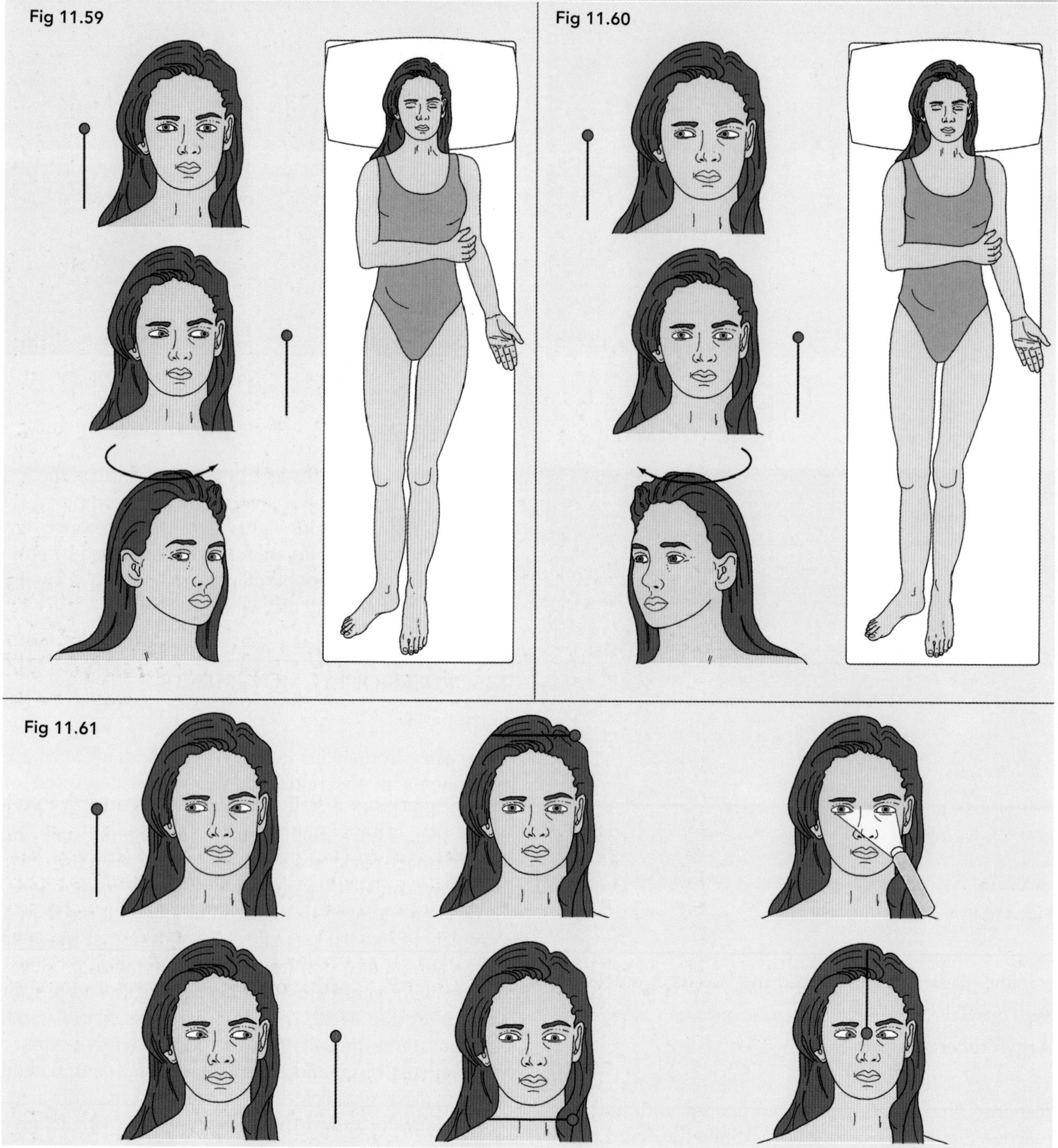

Fig. 11.59 Left frontal lobe lesion. Absent saccades to right, intact to left, preserved doll's head manoeuvre, right hemiparesis.
Fig. 11.60 Left pontine lesion. Absent saccades, pursuit and doll's head movements to the left. Right hemiparesis.
Fig. 11.61 Dorsal-midbrain syndrome. Full horizontal and downward saccades, absent upward saccades. Light-near dissociation.

Parkinson's disease. In progressive supranuclear palsy, downward saccades and pursuit fail first, followed by involvement of upward and, finally, horizontal movements. Doll's head movements are spared, at least initially (Fig. 11.62). A delay in the initiation of saccades occurs in many extrapyramidal disorders. Overshooting or undershooting saccades (hypermetria and hypometria, respectively) occur with cerebellar disease. Large or small inappropriate saccades can interrupt fixation. Causes include multiple sclerosis and cerebellar disease. Slowing of pursuit movement is most commonly caused by sedative medication.

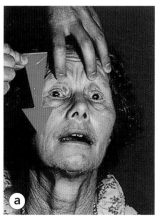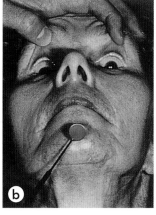

Fig. 11.62 Progressive supranuclear palsy. Failure of down gaze (a) is improved by the doll's head manoeuvre (b).

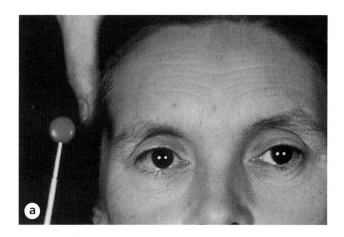

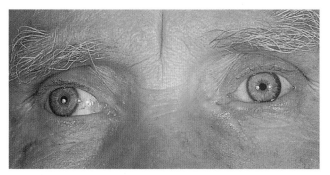

Fig. 11.63 Left internuclear ophthalmoplegia. Failure of adduction of the left eye on right lateral gaze.

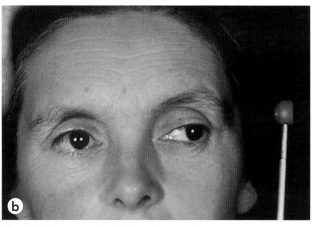

Fig. 11.64 'One-and-a-half' syndrome. Right gaze paresis with right internuclear ophthalmoplegia.

INTERNUCLEAR OPHTHALMOPLEGIA

A lesion of the medial longitudinal fasciculus leads to slowing, or total failure, of medial rectus contraction during lateral gaze (Fig. 11.63). The slowing affects all movement, whether saccadic, pursuit or reflex. To assess subtle slowing, observe the relative velocity of the two eyes while the patient rapidly fixates between two targets. There is usually an accompanying nystagmus in the abducting eye. Bilateral internuclear ophthalmoplegia is accompanied by upbeat vertical nystagmus and subtle abnormalities of vertical eye movement. Multiple sclerosis is the most common cause in younger patients, vascular disease in elderly patients.

THE 'ONE-AND-A-HALF' SYNDROME

If the lesion responsible for a unilateral internuclear ophthalmoplegia spreads into the pontine gaze centre, a more profound loss of ocular motility results. The only normal horizontal movement possible is abduction of the opposite eye (Fig. 11.64). The finding is usually the consequence of vascular disease.

ABDUCENS PALSY

A lesion of the sixth nerve nucleus produces a gaze paresis rather than an isolated lateral rectus weakness.

The latter is usually due to a lesion of the central or peripheral course of the sixth nerve but it can be caused by myasthenia or orbital disease. The eye fails to abduct. When the defect is complete, there may be a convergent strabismus because of unopposed action of the ipsilateral medial rectus (Fig. 11.65). Unilateral or bilateral sixth nerve palsies sometimes result from the effects of raised intracranial pressure (Fig. 11.66).

TROCHLEAR PALSY

Although normally a result of trochlear nerve palsy, weakness of the superior oblique muscle can occur with myasthenia or dysthyroid eye disease. An isolated trochlear nerve palsy sometimes follows a closed head injury. The head tilts to the side opposite the affected eye and the patient complains of diplopia, particularly on downward gaze. There is defective depression of the adducted eye (Fig. 11.67).

OCULOMOTOR PALSY

Nuclear oculomotor palsies tend to be either incomplete or complete but with pupillary sparing. A complete third nerve palsy cannot be nuclear unless there is

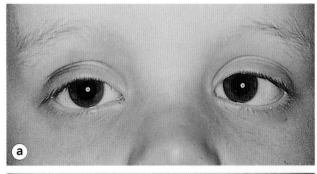

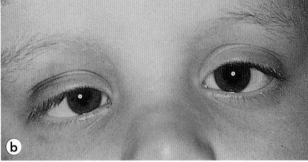

Fig. 11.65 Left sixth nerve palsy. Left esotropia on forward gaze (a). Failure of abduction of left eye (b).

involvement of the contralateral superior rectus muscle. Peripheral third nerve lesions are commonly caused by diabetes. The paresis is typically painful and pupil-sparing in about 50% of patients (Fig. 11.68). In a complete third nerve palsy there is a substantial ptosis and the eye is deviated laterally and slightly downwards. Compression of the oculomotor nerve, for example by a posterior communicating aneurysm, almost always results in pupillary dilatation (Fig. 11.69). To assess whether the fourth nerve is intact in the presence of a complete third nerve palsy, ask the patient to look down. If the superior oblique muscle is still functioning, the abducted eye shows an inwardly rotating twitch.

COMBINED PALSIES

A lesion within the cavernous sinus, for example a cavernous aneurysm, is liable to affect the oculomotor nerves in combination rather than individually. At risk are the third, fourth and sixth nerves, the first and second divisions of the trigeminal nerve and the ocular

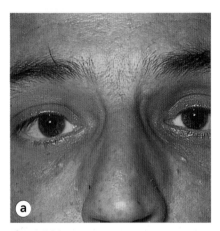

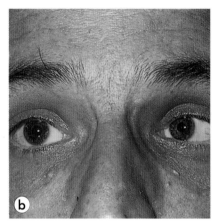

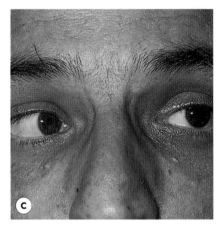

Fig. 11.66 Bilateral sixth nerve palsies. There is a tendency for the eyes to converge on forward gaze (a), with partial failure of abduction to right (b) and to left (c).

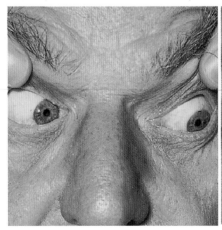

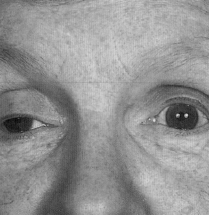

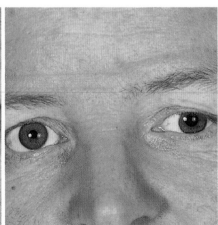

Fig. 11.67 Right superior oblique palsy.

Fig. 11.68 Pupil-sparing right oculomotor palsy caused by diabetes.

Fig. 11.69 Left third nerve paresis. The pupil is dilated.

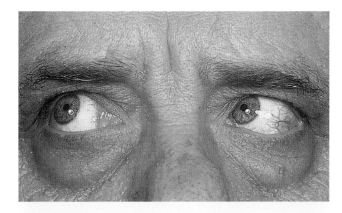

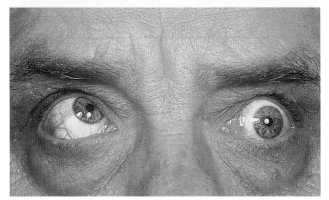

Fig. 11.70 Dysthyroid eye disease. Failure of laevoelevation of the left eye.

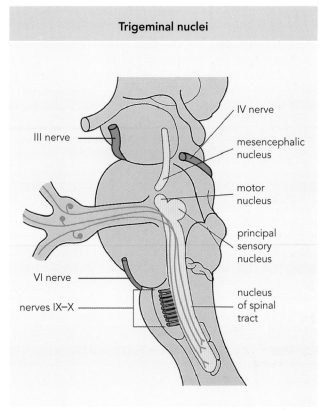

Fig. 11.71 Organisation of trigeminal nuclei within the brainstem.

sympathetic fibres. A complex, mixed ophthalmoplegia without pupillary involvement raises the possibility of myasthenia or dysthyroid eye disease (Fig. 11.70).

NYSTAGMUS

Certain types of nystagmus suggest disease at particular sites of the nervous system.

- *Pendular* – usually congenital but sometimes found in brainstem vascular disease or multiple sclerosis.
- *Vestibular* – if peripheral, usually both horizontal and rotary components and is suppressed by visual fixation. The slow phase is to the side of the lesion. If central, more variable and unaffected by fixation.
- *Gaze-evoked* – often drug-induced but also seen with disease of the cerebellum or brainstem. Vertical components indicate brainstem or cerebellar disease.
- *Down-beat* – when present on down and out gaze, very suggestive of a lesion at the foramen magnum, for example Chiari malformation.
- *Convergence-retractory* – occurs in the dorsal-midbrain syndrome. Attempts at upwards saccades produce retractory movements of the globes.
- *End-point* – physiological. Occurs at extremes of lateral gaze and can affect one eye more than the other.

The trigeminal (fifth) nerve

STRUCTURE AND FUNCTION

The motor nucleus of the nerve lies in the floor of the upper part of the fourth ventricle and receives fibres from both hemispheres, but principally the contralateral one. It also receives afferents from the sensory nuclei. Initially, the motor root remains separate, running below the gasserian ganglion before joining the mandibular division of the nerve to emerge through the foramen ovale. The principal muscles supplied by the nerve are the medial and lateral pterygoids, temporalis and masseter. Smaller muscles supplied include tensor tympani and tensor palati. Jaw closure is achieved by contraction of temporalis and masseter. Jaw opening and lateral movements are performed by the pterygoids.

There are three sensory nuclei: the main nucleus, the mesencephalic nucleus and the nucleus of the spinal tract (Fig. 11.71). Tactile stimuli are relayed through the main nucleus. From here, ascending fibres, most of which decussate, terminate in the thalamus. The spinal nucleus, continuous above with the main nucleus, extends caudally to the second cervical segment where it lies in the posterior horn continuous with the substantia gelatinosa. A rostrocaudal organisation of fibres from concentric segments over the face and head has been suggested, based on the pattern of facial sensory loss sometimes seen with lesions of the spinal tract (Fig. 11.72). Terminating in close proximity to the nucleus of the spinal tract are fibres from the seventh, ninth and tenth cranial nerves that supply cutaneous fibres to the region of the ear. The nucleus contains fibres concerned principally with pain and temperature sensation. Fibres from the nucleus decussate then ascend to the thalamus. The mesencephalic nucleus receives proprioceptive fibres from the muscles of mastication. Collaterals from the afferent fibres synapse on cells in the motor nucleus.

The sensory root accompanies the motor root through the pontine cistern before entering the gasserian ganglion, which is situated in a depression in the petrous temporal bone (Fig. 11.73). From here the ophthalmic division enters the orbit through the superior orbital fissure and the maxillary and mandibular divisions leave the skull through the foramina rotundum and ovale, respectively. The facial and scalp innervation of the three divisions is shown in Figure 11.74. In addition, the trigeminal nerve innervates the mucous membranes of the nose and mouth, certain sinuses, part of the external auditory meatus and most of the dura.

The jaw jerk

The afferent part of this reflex is formed by large afferents from muscle spindles in masseter and temporalis,

which pass to the mesencephalic nucleus in the motor rather than the sensory root. Collaterals from the axons of the unipolar mesencephalic neurons synapse with cells in the motor nucleus, producing a monosynaptic reflex arc, the efferent pathway being within the motor root.

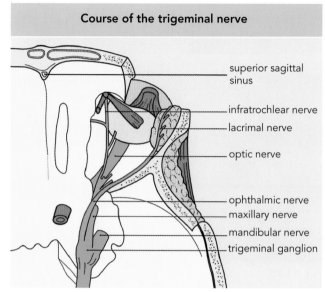

Course of the trigeminal nerve

- superior sagittal sinus
- infratrochlear nerve
- lacrimal nerve
- optic nerve
- ophthalmic nerve
- maxillary nerve
- mandibular nerve
- trigeminal ganglion

Fig. 11.73 The peripheral course of the trigeminal nerve.

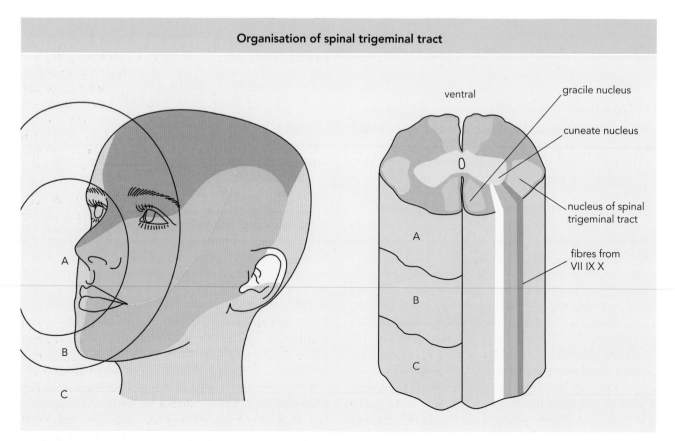

Organisation of spinal trigeminal tract

ventral

gracile nucleus

cuneate nucleus

nucleus of spinal trigeminal tract

fibres from VII IX X

Fig. 11.72 Suggested organisation of concentric segments of facial cutaneous innervation within the spinal tract.

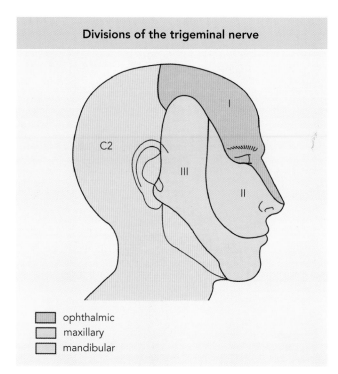

Divisions of the trigeminal nerve

☐ ophthalmic
☐ maxillary
☐ mandibular

Fig. 11.74 Cutaneous distribution of the three divisions of the trigeminal nerve.

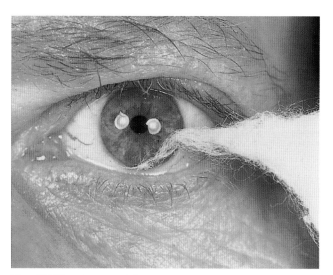

Fig. 11.75 A depressed left corneal response.

The corneal reflex

The afferent limb of the corneal reflex is contained in the ophthalmic division of the trigeminal nerve. The efferent pathway is within the seventh nerve. Stimulation of the cornea produces both an ipsilateral and a contralateral blink response, the latter being approximately 5 ms slower than the former. The central conduction time for the reflex, approximately 40 ms, indicates it is polysynaptic. Scleral, rather than corneal, stimulation results in a reflex with a considerably longer latency.

Examination

SENSORY

Details of the techniques for sensory examination are given on pp 377–380. Convenient sites for testing are the forehead, the medial aspect of the cheek and the chin. Normally, it suffices to test light touch and pinprick alone but occasionally it is necessary to assess temperature appreciation.

With the patient's eyes closed, test light touch by touching the appropriate areas of the face with a wisp of cotton wool. Avoid dragging the stimulus across the skin. A partial loss of sensation is more likely than total anaesthesia, so ask the patient to compare the stimulus with sites in other divisions of the nerve on that side, then with comparable areas on the other side of the face.

Now test pinprick sensation at the same sites. If there is sensory loss confined to the trigeminal nerve distribution, the response to this stimulus becomes normal at the level of the vertex but well above the angle of the jaw (Fig. 11.74). Again, variations in the response at different sites should be noted. As it is difficult to repeat the stimulus with equal force, minor differences of sensitivity should be ignored unless they are consistent.

THE CORNEAL RESPONSE

The corneal response is elicited by lightly touching the cornea with cotton wool. Carefully explain the procedure to the patient before proceeding. The patient's subjective reaction is assessed and the ipsilateral and contralateral blink reaction noted. Corneal sensitivity varies considerably. Patients who wear contact lenses will need to remove them first; even then dulling of the response is likely but will be symmetrical. If the response is substantially depressed, the cotton wool can be held against the cornea without provoking a reaction (Fig. 11.75). Testing the response in an unconscious patient must be done with great care. Repeated stimulation can easily traumatise the cornea.

MOTOR

Look for muscle wasting before testing the muscles of mastication. Wasting of temporalis produces hollowing above the zygoma (Fig. 11.76). Wasting of the masseter is more difficult to detect but both masseter and temporalis can be palpated while the teeth are clenched (Fig. 11.77). The power of pterygoids and of masseter and temporalis can be assessed by resisting the patient's attempts at opening and closing the jaw, respectively. Ask the patient to open the jaw first without, then with, resistance. In a

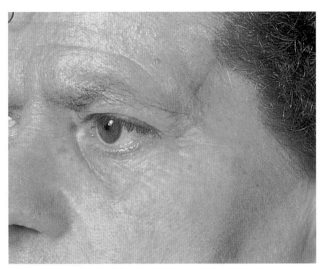

Fig. 11.76 Wasting of the temporalis producing hollowing above the zygoma.

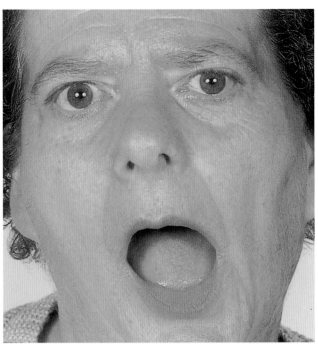

Fig. 11.78 Left trigeminal nerve lesion. Jaw deviation to the left.

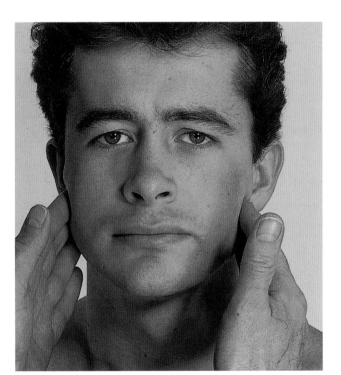

Fig. 11.77 Palpating the masseter muscles.

The jaw jerk

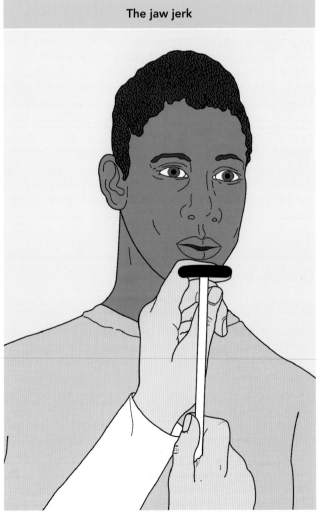

Fig. 11.79 Testing the jaw jerk.

unilateral trigeminal lesion, the jaw deviates to the paralysed side (Fig. 11.78).

THE JAW JERK

Ask the patient to open the mouth slightly. Rest your index finger on the apex of the jaw and tap it with the patella hammer (Fig. 11.79). The response, a contraction of the pterygoid muscles, varies widely in normal individuals.

Clinical application

MOTOR INVOLVEMENT

In a unilateral upper motor neuron syndrome, motor involvement of the trigeminal distribution is not usually clinically detectable. In a bilateral upper motor neuron syndrome, the jaw jerk is exaggerated.

Differential diagnosis

Facial numbness

- Malignant invasion of the trigeminal nerve
- Isolated trigeminal neuropathy
- Involvement in the lateral medullary syndrome
- Involvement with cerebellopontine angle tumours
- Sensory involvement with thalamic, capsular or cortical infarction

SENSORY INVOLVEMENT

Malignant invasion of the nerve or its ganglion results in both sensory and motor deficit, although the latter is spared initially if the ganglion is invaded. In isolated trigeminal neuropathy, motor function is spared but there is progressive loss of facial sensation. Inadvertent self-injury can result in tissue necrosis (Fig. 11.80). In spinal lesions above C2, selective loss of facial pain and temperature sense is possible, sometimes with an 'onion ring' distribution (Fig. 11.72). Loss of facial pain and temperature sense occurs ipsilaterally in the lateral medullary syndrome. Depression of light touch alone occurs with damage to the main sensory nucleus, while thalamic infarction is liable to affect all facial sensory modalities.

ALTERED CORNEAL RESPONSE

Loss of the corneal response may be the first or an early sign of trigeminal compression and should be carefully assessed in patients with unilateral facial pain or deafness. The response is depressed in a patient with a unilateral lower motor neuron facial paresis but the contralateral response is preserved.

The facial (seventh) nerve

STRUCTURE AND FUNCTION

Fibres from the seventh nerve nucleus loop around the lower end of the abducens nucleus before leaving the pons in close proximity to the acoustic nerve. Having crossed the cerebellopontine angle, the nerve enters the internal auditory meatus along with the acoustic nerve

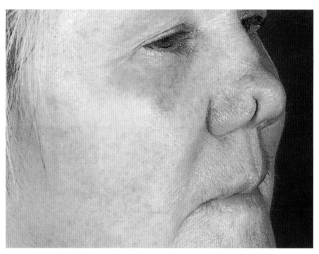

Fig. 11.80 Tissue necrosis consequent to loss of nasal sensation.

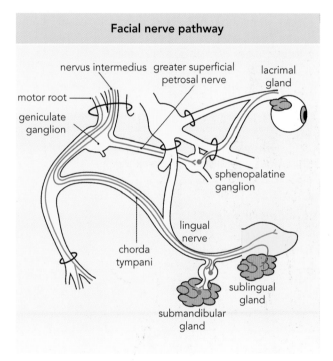

Fig. 11.81 Pathway of the facial nerve.

and the internal auditory artery and vein. Shortly afterwards, the facial nerve enters its own canal, passing forwards above the cochlea before bending sharply backwards, at which point the nerve expands to form the geniculate ganglion. Here, the greater superficial petrosal nerve leaves, eventually to reach the lacrimal gland via the sphenopalatine ganglion (Fig. 11.81). The nerve to stapedius and the chorda tympani leave the facial nerve before its exit from the stylomastoid foramen. Parasympathetic fibres in the chorda tympani supply the submandibular and sublingual glands. Special afferent fibres in the nerve supply taste sensation to the anterior two-thirds of the tongue. After leaving the stylomastoid foramen, the nerve courses through the parotid gland on its way to the muscles of facial expression. Of these, frontalis elevates the eyebrow, orbicularis oculi closes the eye and orbicularis oris the mouth, while platysma depresses the angle of the mouth. The buccinator muscle, also supplied by the facial nerve, assists in mastication.

Frontalis receives an innervation from both cortices but the muscles of the lower face are innervated solely by the contralateral hemisphere. Emotional movements receive an additional supply from other sources, including the thalamus and globus pallidus.

The sensory component of the nerve innervates the external auditory meatus, the tympanic membrane and a

small area of skin behind the ear. The taste fibres, having entered the pons, terminate in the nucleus of the tractus solitarius. From here, fibres project to the thalamus and hence the cortical gustatory area.

The intensity of a taste experience is determined by the size of the neural response. Taste buds are found in the tongue, soft palate, pharynx, larynx and oesophagus. A particular taste represents an amalgam of four primary taste functions, sweet, sour, bitter and salt, combined with any olfactory stimulating effect that the food or beverage possesses. There is some decline in taste acuity with age but to a lesser extent than occurs with olfaction.

SYMPTOMS

In a patient with a lower motor neuron facial weakness, certain questions may help to define the site of the lesion.

?	**Questions to ask**
	Facial weakness of lower motor neuron type

- Have you noticed any loss of taste on the front part of the tongue?
- Have you noticed that noises appear excessively loud in the ear on the same side?
- Does the eye on that side still water?

 | **Differential diagnosis**
---|---
 | **Facial weakness**

Upper motor neuron facial weakness
- Cerebrovascular disease
- Tumour

Lower motor neuron facial weakness
- Bell's palsy
- Ramsay Hunt syndrome
- Trauma
- Parotid tumour
- Sarcoid
- Multiple sclerosis

Examination

Facial asymmetry is common, as is an asymmetry of movement of the lower face during conversation. Carefully observe the movements of the patient's face while you are taking the history. An asymmetry of blinking is a useful indicator of mild weakness of orbicularis oculi. Decide whether the nasolabial folds are equally well defined. Note any difference in the position of the angles of the mouth but remember that in a long-standing facial weakness fibrotic contracture of the muscles can elevate the angle of the mouth, suggesting that the facial weakness is on the other side. Bilateral facial weakness is easily overlooked. The face lacks expression and appears to sag (Fig. 11.82).

Ask the patient to elevate the eyebrows (Fig. 11.83) then close the eyes tightly. Normally, the eyelashes virtually disappear. A useful sign of a mild weakness is a

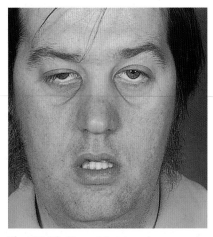

Fig. 11.82 Bilateral facial weakness.

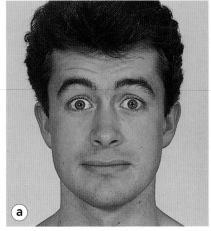

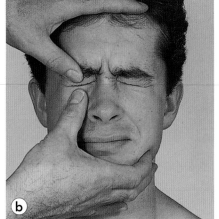

Fig. 11.83 The patient has been asked to elevate the eyebrows, then to close the eyes tightly.

more marked protrusion of the eyelashes on the affected side (Fig. 11.84). Try to open the eyes by pressing the eyelids apart with your thumbs. If there is no weakness, the patient can prevent the eyelids separating. Now ask the patient to blow out the cheeks, then purse the lips tightly together (Fig. 11.85). Finally, ask the patient to tighten the neck muscles in order to assess platysma. Weakness of stapedius is suggested if the patient complains of an undue sensitivity (hyperacusis) to noise in the affected ear.

Many patients who complain of an altered sensation of taste are found to have a disturbance of olfaction. Taste is difficult to test. Simply applying drops of a test solution on the protruded tongue seldom produces a consistent response. For assessing seventh nerve function, the stimulus should be confined to the anterior two-thirds of the tongue, each side of which is tested separately. Sweet (sugar), salt, bitter (quinine) and sour (vinegar) solutions are applied in turn, the mouth being washed out with distilled water between testing. Taste assessment is seldom justified for routine diagnostic purposes. Ask the patient if there has been any loss of lacrimation.

The area of skin around the ear that is supplied by the seventh nerve receives overlapping innervation from the fifth and ninth nerves. Nothing is gained, therefore, by testing sensation in this area.

Clinical application

UPPER MOTOR NEURON FACIAL WEAKNESS

An upper motor neuron facial weakness results from interruption of descending fibres passing from the contralateral motor cortex to the ipsilateral facial nerve nucleus. There is minimal asymmetry of frontalis contraction on the two sides but substantial asymmetry of the lower face (Fig. 11.86). Causes include cerebrovascular disease, tumour and head injury.

LOWER MOTOR NEURON FACIAL WEAKNESS

In a lower motor neuron facial weakness, all the facial muscles are equally affected unless the lesion lies so distally that it involves individual branches of the nerve. The site of the lesion can be deduced from the presence or absence of certain symptoms and signs. If it lies at or beyond the stylomastoid foramen, there will be no disturbance of taste, hearing or lacrimation. Involvement of the nerve immediately proximal to the origin of chorda tympani will result in loss of taste over the anterior two-thirds of the tongue; involvement proximal to the departure of the nerve to stapedius will result in hyperacusis. Loss of lacrimation is added to these other symptoms if the nerve is damaged at or proximal to the gasserian ganglion.

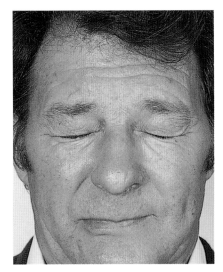

Fig. 11.84 The patient has been asked to close the eyes tightly. The eyelashes on the right are slightly more prominent than those on the left.

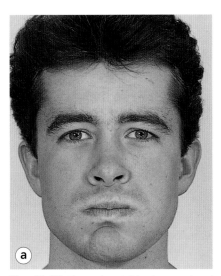
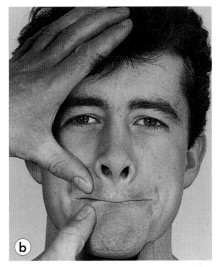
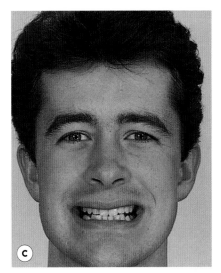

Fig. 11.85 The patient is blowing out the cheeks, pursing his lips and baring his teeth.

BELL'S PALSY

Bell's palsy is an idiopathic paralysis of the facial nerve. When the resulting facial weakness is substantial, there is loss of forehead furrowing, eye closure and mouth elevation (Fig. 11.87). If denervation occurs, regrowth of fibres may extend to muscles not originally part of their innervation (aberrant reinnervation). In such patients blinking can result in synkinetic contraction of muscles in the lower face (Fig. 11.88) and misdirection to the lacrimal gland of fibres originally destined for the salivary glands results in eye watering when a food stimulus appears (crocodile tears).

RAMSAY HUNT SYNDROME

The Ramsay Hunt syndrome is the consequence of herpetic involvement of the geniculate ganglion. A vesicular eruption can occur at a number of sites, including the pinna (Fig. 11.89).

FACIAL MOVEMENT DISORDERS

- *Fasciculation* – virtually confined to patients with motor neuron disease.
- *Myokymia* – produces a fine, more or less continuous, shimmering contraction of some or all of the muscles supplied by the facial nerve. Multiple sclerosis is the most common cause.
- *Hemifacial spasm* – involuntary, haphazard contraction of facial muscle, often initially confined to orbicularis oculi (Fig. 11.90). Eventually a mild facial weakness appears.

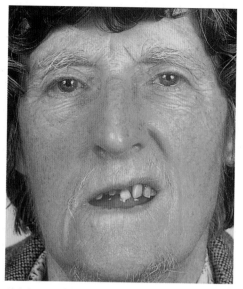

Fig. 11.86 Upper motor neuron facial weakness. The patient has been asked to bare her teeth.

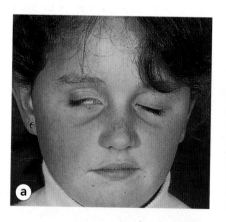

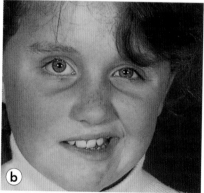

Fig. 11.87 A right Bell's palsy in a girl aged 11 years.

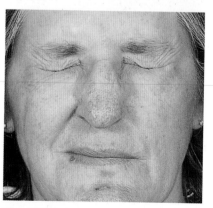

Fig. 11.88 Aberrant reinnervation. The right angle of the mouth elevates during eye closure. Previous right Bell's palsy.

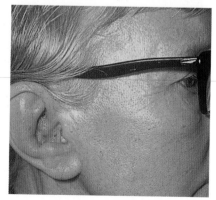

Fig. 11.89 Vesicular eruption in a case of the Ramsay Hunt syndrome.

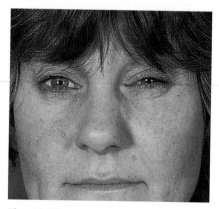

Fig. 11.90 Left hemifacial spasm. The left palpebral fissure has narrowed during the contraction.

- *Blepharospasm* – forced involuntary repetitive blinking.
- *Tics* – stereotyped repetitive movements, at least in part under voluntary control.
- *Orofacial dyskinesia* – involuntary semirepetitive contraction of muscles round the mouth, often with abnormal movements of the tongue. Occurs spontaneously and with certain drugs, particularly phenothiazines.

The acoustic (eighth) nerve

STRUCTURE AND FUNCTION

Vibration of the tympanic membrane, triggered by a sound stimulus, is transmitted through a chain of three ossicles (the malleus, incus and stapes) situated in the middle ear (Fig. 11.91). The movements of the ossicles are also influenced by the tensor tympani and stapedius muscles. The base of the stapes is attached to the oval window. Vibration of the oval window sets up movement in the perilymph which occupies the bony labyrinth, comprising the cochlea, the vestibule and the semicircular canals. Lying within the bony labyrinth and containing endolymph is the membranous labyrinth comprising the cochlear duct, the saccule, the utricle and three semicircular ducts. The semicircular canals, each surrounding a semicircular duct, are arranged in planes roughly at right angles to each other. The canals open into the vestibule which contains the saccule and utricle. Specialised receptor areas (maculae) are found in the saccule and utricle. At one end of each semicircular canal is a receptor organ (crista ampullaris).

The inferior part of the bony labyrinth contains the osseous canal of the cochlea. A bony spur, the osseous spiral lamina, projects into the canal, dividing it into two corridors: the scala vestibuli and the scala tympani (Fig. 11.92). In the wall of the cochlear duct, resting on the basilar membrane, is the spiral organ of Corti, which is innervated by the cochlear component of the auditory nerve. The vestibular component innervates the specialised receptor areas of the utricle and the semicircular canals. The saccule and part of the posterior semicircular canal receive fibres from the cochlear division.

The vestibular and cochlear components unite within the internal auditory canal. The nerve then crosses the subarachnoid space and enters the brainstem at the junction of pons and medulla, lateral to the facial nerve. In the brainstem the acoustic nerve projects predominantly to the contralateral inferior colliculus. From here, fibres pass to the medial geniculate body and then in the auditory radiation to the auditory cortex in the upper aspect of the temporal lobe (Heschl's gyrus). The fibres of the vestibular nerve terminate in four separate nuclei. A projection from the lateral vestibular nucleus forms the vestibulospinal tract, which descends, mainly ipsilaterally, to the cervical and lumbar motor neurons. The medial vestibular nucleus has connections to the contralateral abducens nucleus and the cerebellum. These pathways are important in gaze-holding and for the control of smooth pursuit eye movements.

Sound waves, transmitted through the perilymph, reach the organ of Corti via the ossicular chain, by vibration of the round window or by bony transmission. High-frequency waves produce a maximal response in the basal part of the cochlea; low-frequency waves at its apex. Activity in the components of the auditory brainstem

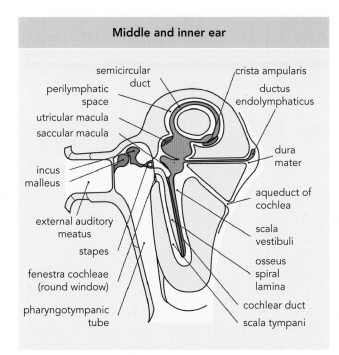

Fig. 11.91 Organisation of the middle and inner ear. The endolymphatic system is coloured purple.

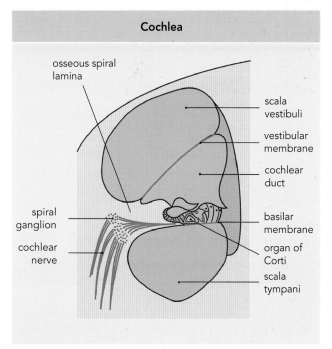

Fig. 11.92 The cochlea.

pathway is reflected in a succession of negative potentials recorded from mastoid and scalp electrodes following a click stimulus. Seven potentials occurring within the first 10 ms of the stimulus are thought to relate to specific anatomical sites.

The nerve endings in the cristae and maculae are triggered by movements of the endolymph, either from stimulation of the hair processes of the cristae or by movements of small calcific particles (the otoliths) embedded in a membrane of the maculae of the utricle and saccule. Head position is coded by the receptors of the utricle and saccule. Head tilt shifts the otoliths, displaces the hair cells and initiates an action potential in the fibres of the vestibular nerve. The semicircular canals are responsible for the detection of rotational head movements, via patterns of flow produced in the endolymphatic system.

Overall, the vestibular system provides information on head posture and movement, integrated with visual data and proprioceptive information arising from neck muscle receptors.

SYMPTOMS

Deafness

If the patient complains of deafness, determine the mode of onset, whether progressive or static, and whether unilateral or bilateral. Other important factors include the family history and noise exposure.

Vertigo

If the patient has vertigo, ascertain whether symptoms can be induced by certain postures or movements.

Questions to ask
Dizziness

- Does the patient describe dizziness or giddiness or is there an experience of rotation, either of the patient or of the environment (vertigo)?
- Is the dizziness accompanied by an unsteadiness when walking?
- Is any vertigo triggered only by a certain movement or head posture?

Examination and clinical application

See Chapter 4.

The glossopharyngeal (ninth) nerve

STRUCTURE AND FUNCTION

The ninth, tenth and eleventh cranial nerves share a motor nucleus (nucleus ambiguus) that innervates the striated muscle of the pharynx, larynx and upper

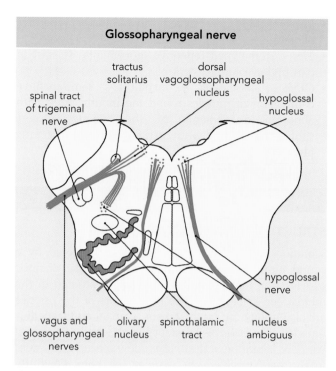

Glossopharyngeal nerve

Fig. 11.93 Relationship of the central components of the glossopharyngeal nerve.

oesophagus (Fig. 11.93). Corticobulbar fibres destined for each nucleus ambiguus originate in both cerebral hemispheres. The glossopharyngeal nerve emerges from the upper part of the medulla, bounded above and below by the facial nerve and the vagus respectively. It leaves the skull through the jugular foramen in company with the vagus and the accessory nerves. The general visceral efferent and special visceral afferent fibres are not readily testable. Somatic afferent components in the glossopharyngeal nerve supply a number of structures, including the tonsillar fossa and parts of the pharynx. Arterial baroreceptors in the carotid sinus are innervated by the glossopharyngeal nerve, while those in the aortic arch are innervated by the vagus.

Differential diagnosis
Ninth cranial nerve disorders

- Jugular foramen syndrome
- Chiari malformation
- Lateral medullary syndrome
- Glossopharyngeal neuralgia

The gag reflex

The gag reflex is triggered by applying a stimulus to the tonsillar fossa. The end-result is midline elevation of the palate. The afferent arc probably travels in the glossopharyngeal nerve only if the stimulus is painful. The efferent arc, supplying levator palati, passes in the vagus.

The gag reflex

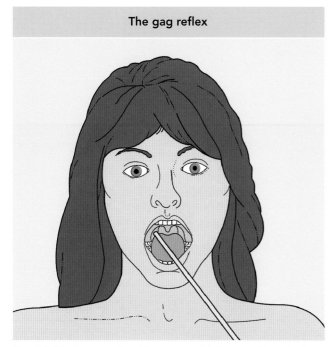

Fig. 11.94 The gag reflex. The orange stick is pressed into the base of the tonsillar fossa.

Examination

The motor innervation of the ninth nerve cannot be tested, nor can the cutaneous distribution in the region of the pinna be separated from the overlapping contributions of the seventh and tenth nerves.

Testing the gag reflex is an uncomfortable experience and should be performed only if there is a suspicion of a disturbance of the lower cranial nerves. Clearly indicate to the patient what is involved. Press the end of an orange stick first into one tonsillar fossa then the other (Fig. 11.94). Besides confirming that the palate rises in the midline, ask the patient if the sensation is comparable on the two sides. In the presence of a glossopharyngeal lesion, the gag reflex is depressed or absent on that side.

Clinical application

Isolated lesions of the ninth nerve are almost unknown. A destructive process in the region of the jugular foramen, most commonly a nasopharyngeal carcinoma, disrupts the ninth, tenth and eleventh cranial nerves. In the Chiari malformation, stretching of the ninth nerve can lead to depression of the gag reflex on one or both sides. Glossopharyngeal neuralgia usually results from distortion of the nerve by a tumour or a vascular anomaly. Paroxysms of pain in the tongue, soft palate or tonsil are triggered by swallowing, chewing or protruding the tongue. Involvement of fibres from the carotid sinus can result in syncopal attacks occurring at the time of the painful paroxysms or triggered independently by swallowing.

The vagus (tenth) nerve

STRUCTURE AND FUNCTION

The roots of the vagus leave the medulla immediately below the glossopharyngeal nerve. Both nerves pass through the jugular foramen alongside the accessory nerve. The components of the vagus mirror those of the glossopharyngeal nerve. The special efferent fibres innervate the striated muscle of the pharynx, larynx and upper oesophagus. The recurrent laryngeal branch of the vagus supplies all the intrinsic muscles of the larynx except for cricothyroid, which is supplied by the external branch of the nerve.

In the heart, fibres from the right vagus end principally around the sinoatrial node, while fibres from the left end principally around the atrioventricular node. Vagal fibres innervating the aortic arch are concerned with the baroreceptor reflex.

Differential diagnosis

Tenth cranial nerve disorders

Bilateral supranuclear palsy (pseudobulbar palsy)
- Stroke
- Motor neuron disease

Unilateral nuclear lesions
- Lateral medullary syndrome

Bilateral nuclear lesions (bulbar palsy)
- Motor neuron disease

Recurrent laryngeal palsy
- Aortic aneurysm
- Malignancy
- Post-thyroid surgery

Examination

Evaluation is confined to assessment of spontaneous and reflex movements of the uvula and posterior pharyngeal wall. A unilateral lesion of the vagus produces paralysis of the ipsilateral soft palate. At rest, the palate lies slightly lower on the affected side then deviates to the intact side during phonation or on testing the gag reflex (Fig. 11.95). An accompanying deviation of the median raphe of the posterior pharyngeal wall is more characteristic of a glossopharyngeal, rather than a vagal, lesion. Minor deviations of the uvula, particularly if not consistent, should be ignored. The accompanying unilateral vocal cord paralysis, leading to hoarseness, is not confirmable by bedside examination.

Bilateral palsies of the vagus produce severe palatal palsy, with nasal regurgitation and aphonia.

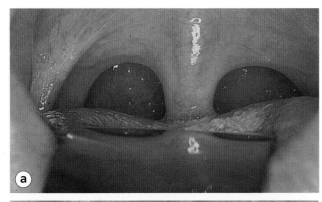

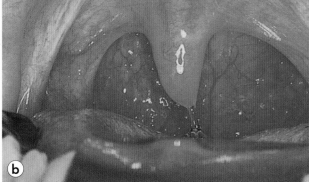

Fig. 11.95 Palsy of the left vagus. The palate deviates to the right on phonation (b).

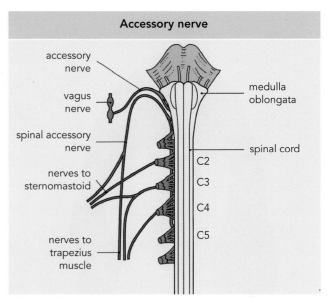

Fig. 11.96 Distribution of the components of the accessory nerve.

Clinical application

A unilateral disturbance of the corticobulbar projection to the nucleus ambiguus is usually without consequence. However, bilateral supranuclear lesions, for example caused by cerebrovascular disease, are symptomatic. Nuclear vagal lesions occur in polio and after lateral medullary infarction. The main branch of the vagus is seldom affected in isolation. Recurrent laryngeal palsies are more common and are usually left-sided because of the longer course of the nerve on that side. Causes include aortic aneurysm, thyroid surgery and malignant invasion of the mediastinum. Isolated laryngeal palsies are often of unknown aetiology.

STRUCTURE AND FUNCTION

The accessory nerve has both cranial and spinal components. The cranial part originates from the nucleus ambiguus and exits from the medulla in line with the ninth and tenth cranial nerves (Fig. 11.96). The spinal part is formed by a series of rootlets that emerge from the lateral aspect of the cervical spinal cord down to the fifth segment. The rootlets form a single trunk that ascends alongside the cord, passes through the foramen magnum and unites with the cranial component. The combined nerve leaves the skull through the jugular foramen.

The cranial root joins the vagus, while the spinal root receives contributions from the second, third and fourth cervical roots (Fig. 11.96) before innervating sternomastoid and the upper fibres of trapezius. The fibres from the second and third cervical roots passing to the sternomastoid are probably proprioceptive, while the fibres from the third and fourth roots to the lower part of trapezius are purely motor.

The spinal accessory nucleus receives innervation from both cerebral hemispheres. The fibres concerned with the innervation of sternomastoid possibly undergo a double decussation within the brainstem.

Differential diagnosis
Accessory nerve disorders

- Involvement in jugular foramen tumours
- Accessory palsy of unknown cause

Examination

There is no way of assessing the innervation of the cranial component of the accessory nerve but that of the spinal component can be assessed by examining trapezius and sternomastoid. The function of trapezius is assessed by asking the patient to elevate the shoulder, first without, then with, resistance (Fig. 11.97). The strength of contraction of sternomastoid can be gauged by asking the patient to rotate the head to the relevant side against resistance (Fig. 11.98).

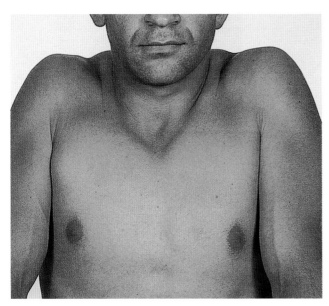

Fig. 11.97 Testing the trapezius muscles. The shoulders are elevated first without, then with, resistance.

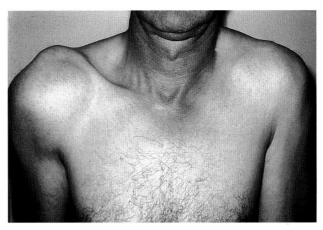

Fig. 11.99 Right accessory nerve lesion.

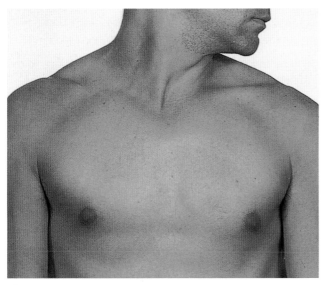

Fig. 11.98 Testing head rotation.

Clinical application

Isolated lesions of the eleventh cranial nerve are rare. Tumours in the region of the jugular foramen are likely to produce a combined palsy of the ninth, tenth and eleventh nerves (Fig. 11.99). In the presence of a hemiplegia, the trapezius muscle on the hemiplegic side is affected. A delay in shoulder shrug may be an early sign. The same hemiplegia, however, will affect the contralateral sternomastoid, that is the muscle rotating the neck towards the hemiplegic limbs. The weakness in such patients is incomplete. Spasmodic torticollis is a focal dystonia particularly affecting the sternomastoid muscle. Typically, there are repetitive rotatory movements

of the head and neck, which lead to hypertrophy of the relevant muscles in longstanding cases (Fig. 11.100).

The hypoglossal (twelfth) nerve

STRUCTURE AND FUNCTION

The hypoglossal nucleus lies close to the midline in the floor of the fourth ventricle and receives supranuclear fibres from both but principally the contralateral hemisphere. The hypoglossal nerve leaves the skull through the anterior condylar canal and supplies all the intrinsic muscles of the tongue, and all its extrinsic muscles except palatoglossus.

Differential diagnosis
Tongue paralysis

- Malignant invasion of the skull base
- Chiari malformation
- Pseudobulbar palsy with cerebrovascular disease or motor neuron disease

Examination

First inspect the tongue as it lies in the base of the oral cavity. In many patients there are tremulous movements that are often hard to distinguish from fasciculation or true involuntary movements. Fasciculation imparts a shimmering motion to the surface of the tongue. Involuntary movements include a coarse tremor, for example in Parkinson's disease, and complex, unpredictable movements found in such conditions as Huntington's disease and orofacial dyskinesia. While assessing the tongue for spontaneous contractions, observe its bulk. As the tongue wastes it becomes thinner and more wrinkled. Now ask the patient to protrude the tongue. Minor deviations from the midline are sometimes

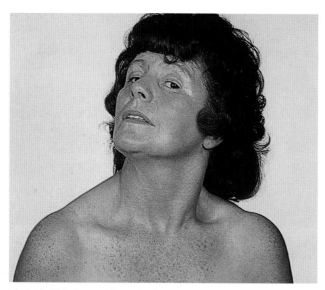

Fig. 11.100 Spasmodic torticollis associated with contraction of the left sternomastoid.

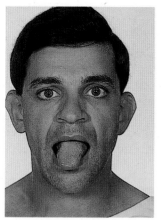 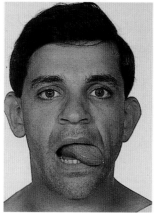

Fig. 11.101 Examination of the tongue. Protrusion (a) and lateral movements (b).

seen in normal individuals. Finally, ask the patient to move the tongue rapidly from side to side and assess its power by instructing the patient to push the tongue against the side of the cheek (Fig. 11.101). A disturbance of the speed of tongue movement occurs in extrapyramidal diseases, including Parkinson's disease.

Clinical application

UNILATERAL AND BILATERAL LOWER MOTOR NEURON LESIONS

In a unilateral hypoglossal nerve lesion, there is focal atrophy, fasciculation and deviation to the paralysed side (Fig. 11.102). Such a lesion can occur in isolation or as the consequence of malignant invasion of the skull base. Bilateral involvement of the lower motor neuron projections to the tongue is usually part of a bulbar palsy. There is additional involvement of the other lower

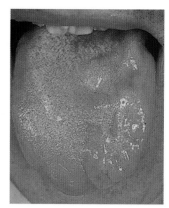

Fig. 11.102 Left hypoglossal nerve lesion.

brainstem motor nuclei, resulting in dysphagia and dysarthria. The tongue is wasted and immobile.

UNILATERAL UPPER MOTOR NEURON LESION

A unilateral upper motor neuron lesion has little effect on tongue function, although it may protrude slightly to the side of the hemiparesis.

BILATERAL UPPER MOTOR NEURON LESION

Bilateral involvement of the pyramidal projections to the brainstem nuclei, usually the consequence of cerebrovascular disease, results in a pseudobulbar palsy. There is dysphagia, dysarthria and emotional lability. The tongue is stiff and immobile and there is weakness of palatal elevation combined with a brisk gag reflex and jaw jerk.

	Review
	Cranial nerve examination
I	Examine smell in each nostril
II	Examine visual acuity, visual field, fundus and pupillary light response
III, IV, VI	Examine eye movements and near reaction. Check for nystagmus
V	Examine motor and sensory innervation plus the jaw jerk and the corneal response
VII	Examine the muscles of facial expression (plus buccinator) and taste over the anterior two-thirds of the tongue
VIII	Examine hearing and perform Rinne's and Weber's tests
IX	Examine pain sensation in the tonsillar fossae
X	Examine palatal movement plus the gag reflex
XI	Examine sternomastoid and the upper fibres of trapezius
XII	Examine tongue movements and appearance

Red flag – urgent referral
Cranial nerve symptoms

- Visual obscuration with posture change. Suggests papilloedema. If confirmed – urgent referral.
- Diplopia. Numerous causes, but all require neurological or ophthalmological appraisal.
- Facial numbness. In isolation, may be the first sign of an isolated trigeminal neuropathy, but skull base metastases need to be considered.
- Lower motor neuron facial paresis. Usually due to a Bell's palsy. If so, may benefit from steroids and aciclovir.
- Dysarthria. In isolation, may be part of a cranial neuropathy, but not uncommonly the presenting feature of motor neuron disease.

The motor system

STRUCTURE AND FUNCTION

The major supraspinal influences on motor activity are the sensorimotor cortex (exerting its role primarily through the pyramidal system), the basal ganglia, a number of tracts descending from the brainstem and the cerebellum. The upper motor neuron defines that part of the motor pathway between the cerebral cortex and the anterior horn cell. The lower motor neuron consists of the anterior horn cell and its motor axon.

The pyramidal tract

The motor cortex is situated in the precentral convolution, anterior to the rolandic fissure (area 4). Movements of the contralateral half of the body are represented inversely, with a large area responsible for the hand, thumb and fingers, and a much smaller area, on the medial aspect of the hemisphere, responsible for the lower limb (Fig. 11.103). Corticospinal neurons originate in the premotor association area (6), the motor area (4), the sensory area and part of the sensory association area. The medial aspect of area 6 is called the supplementary motor area.

The motor cortex sends approximately a million pyramidal tract axons to the medulla. Less than 50% of the neurons providing the fibres traversing the medullary pyramids are located in the precentral primary and supplementary motor areas, with the rest coming from the postcentral cortex. The fibres from the cortex pass through the corona radiata and internal capsule before traversing the midbrain and pons on their way to the medulla (Fig. 11.104). Approximately 75% of the fibres reaching the medulla continue into the spinal cord, forming the lateral and ventral corticospinal tracts. Approximately three-quarters of the fibres decussate. Some pyramidal fibres terminate directly on anterior horn cells but most synapse with internuncial neurons in the spinal grey matter, which, in turn, transmit to the anterior horn cells.

The motor cortex is particularly concerned with skilled activities requiring finely tuned movements of the hand and fingers. Less than 25% of the corticospinal neurons conduct at a velocity exceeding 25 m/s. The majority are small and slowly conducting, influencing fine gradations of force by being recruited early in the performance of a motor task. The larger, more rapidly conducting neurons are recruited late when larger movements are required.

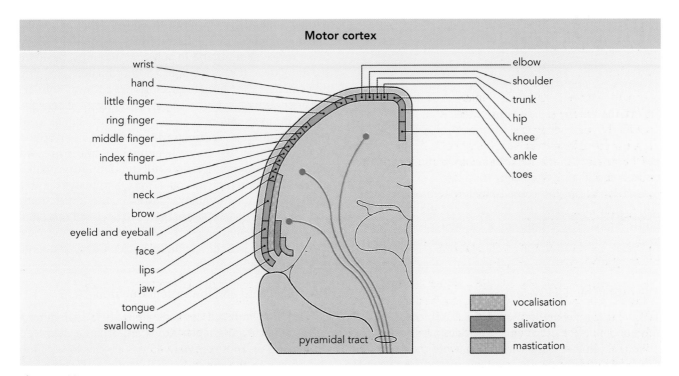

Fig. 11.103 Organisation of the motor cortex.

Pyramidal system

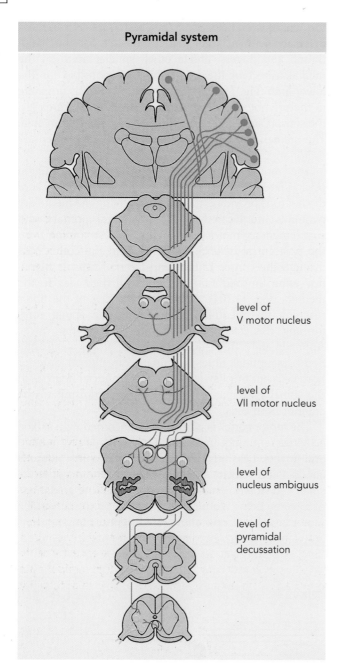

level of
V motor nucleus

level of
VII motor nucleus

level of
nucleus ambiguus

level of
pyramidal
decussation

Fig. 11.104 Pathway of the pyramidal system.

Discharge rates in the neurons relate to the force being exerted and its rate of change.

Activity within the corticospinal system also releases limbs from the postures imposed by gravity. In the upper limbs, this results in inhibition of flexors and facilitation of extensors, with the reverse effects in the lower limbs.

The extrapyramidal system

The basal ganglia are located in the basal forebrain and the midbrain. They include the nucleus accumbens, the putamen, globus pallidus and caudate nucleus, the substantia nigra and the subthalamic nucleus. Major inputs to the basal ganglia come from the cortex, the

thalamus and the reticular formation. Major outputs pass from the globus pallidus to the thalamus and pons and from the substantia nigra to the thalamus, superior colliculus and reticular formation. Finally, there are multiple interconnections between the various components of the system. The pigmented structures of the basal ganglia give rise to dopaminergic driven pathways passing from the pars compacta of the substantia nigra to the striatum (caudate nucleus and putamen) and from the ventral tegmentum to the nucleus accumbens and the frontal cortex.

The basal ganglia integrate the individual components of skilled motor tasks and are important in the control of heavily learned motor activity.

The tracts descending from the brainstem

Vestibulospinal tract The vestibulospinal tract descends uncrossed from the lateral vestibular nucleus. Its principal projection is to the cervical cord.

Reticulospinal tracts Inhibitory and facilitatory reticulospinal tracts descend from the region of the midbrain and pons (Fig. 11.105). There are four inhibitory pathways, two of which are monoaminergic. The pathways of the monoaminergic tracts are uncertain. A dorsal reticulospinal system passes from the pontomedullary reticular formation to the dorsolateral column of the spinal cord. The fourth inhibitory pathway originates in the medulla and descends ventral to the lateral corticospinal tract. The facilitatory reticulospinal tract passes from the pons and runs in the anterior column of the cord close to the ventral sulcus.

The initiating signals for locomotion are largely the responsibility of the reticulospinal and vestibulospinal tracts. The two monoaminergic inhibitory reticulospinal pathways alter the effects of the flexor reflex afferents. The dorsal reticulospinal tract inhibits segmentally active flexor reflex afferents and Ib polysynaptic paths. By doing so, it allows the activation of coordinated stepping movements. The ventral reticulospinal pathway inhibits the monosynaptic reflex arc, particularly of extensors, again in preparation for the release of spinal cord structures from their antigravity function. Interruption of this pathway results in hypertonicity and increased reflexes. The antigravity reflexes for standing are promoted by the facilitatory reticulospinal tract. Stimulation of this pathway tonically augments flexors in the upper limbs and extensors in the lower limbs. The vestibulospinal pathway has similar properties. The cerebellum has major inputs to the lateral vestibular nucleus and hence its descending pathway.

The spinal cord and lower motor neuron

The anterior horn cell contains alpha, beta and gamma motor neurons. The alpha axons are of large diameter, conducting at approximately 45 m/s in the lower limb and 55 m/s in the upper limb. A motor unit comprises the anterior horn cell, its axon and the muscle fibres it innervates, which may range from 10 to several hundred.

The stretch reflex The afferent limb of the stretch reflex arc is contained in Ia fibres innervating the muscle spindle. The fibres synapse with anterior horn cells that supply alpha motor neurons to the skeletal muscle containing that spindle. The muscle spindle is innervated by gamma fibres. Ib afferent fibres, originating from the Golgi tendon

organ have an inhibitory effect on the stretch reflex via interneurons (Fig. 11.106).

Other reflexes Flexor reflex afferents (FRA), contained in small fibres, are excited by painful stimulation of the skin and deeper structures. They reach the motor neurons by polysynaptic pathways through interneurons within the spinal cord. For the lower limb, these polysynaptic pathways innervate the segments needed to evoke a flexor withdrawal reaction to a painful stimulus. Connections to the other side of the cord facilitate extensor tone there.

Muscle The fibres of skeletal muscle consist of myofibrils bounded by a sarcolemmal membrane. There are at least two types of muscle fibre with differing histochemical characteristics. Type 1 fibres are slow contracting, type 2 fast contracting.

The reflexes and abnormal muscle tone The stretch reflex has phasic and tonic components. The tendon reflexes are phasic. Tonic stretch reflexes result in a sustained muscle contraction that has both dynamic (velocity-dependent) and static (length-dependent) components. Patients who relax poorly are activating tonic stretch reflexes that then hinder displacement of the limb.

Spasticity Spasticity is a feature of an upper motor neuron lesion, although its appearance owes more to disruption of the ventral reticulospinal pathway than to altered pyramidal tract function. Indeed, selective damage of the latter results in hypotonia rather than spasticity. In spasticity the increase in muscle tone is velocity-dependent. As the speed of displacement is increased, a critical velocity is reached at which muscle tone suddenly increases and resistance appears. After a pyramidal tract lesion, the development of increased tone in antigravity

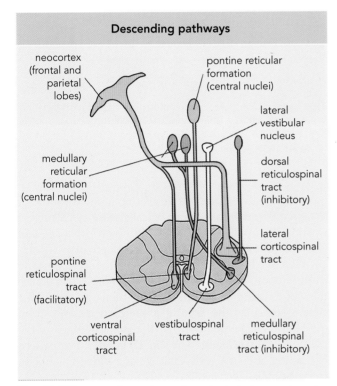

Fig. 11.105 Descending pathways from the brainstem concerned with movement.

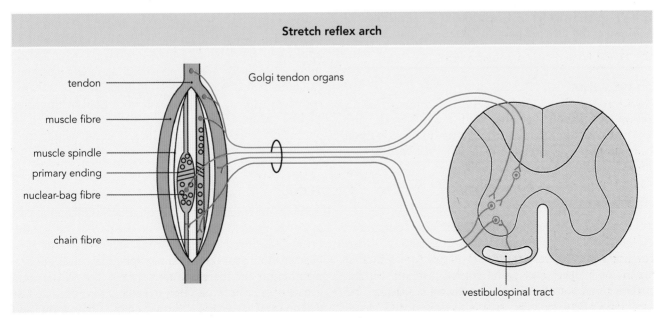

Fig. 11.106 The stretch reflex arc.

muscles results in extension of the lower limbs. At a certain point of flexion of the extended limb, the hypertonicity suddenly resolves because of a length-dependent inhibition of the quadriceps stretch reflex: the clasp-knife effect. The phenomenon is less evident in the upper limbs and is particularly evident in spinal lesions. The inhibition of lower limb extensors at a critical level of stretch results from facilitation of the flexor reflex afferent system due to loss of its inhibition by interruption of the dorsal reticulospinal tract. The degree of loss of flexor inhibition determines the likelihood of flexor spasms emerging.

Rigidity The rigidity of Parkinson's disease and other extrapyramidal disorders is more uniformly distributed between flexors and extensors and is not velocity-dependent. Furthermore, a clasp-knife effect does not occur. In some cases, the rigidity is fluctuant, producing a cogwheel effect. The frequency of the cogwheeling is more closely linked to the frequency of the action than to the resting tremor found in parkinsonian patients.

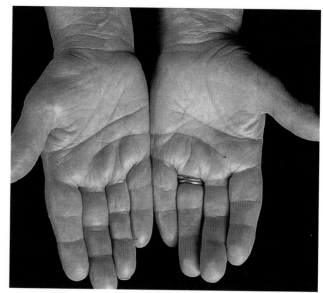

Fig. 11.107 Focal wasting of the right thenar eminence secondary to median nerve compression.

| **?** | Questions to ask |
| | **Muscle weakness** |

- Is the weakness confined to one limb or to one side of the body?
- Is the weakness static, progressive or fluctuant?
- Is the weakness accompanied by a feeling of stiffness or is the affected limb floppy?

SYMPTOMS

When recording a complaint of weakness, determine its mode of onset, it distribution, whether it fluctuates in severity and whether it is associated with feelings of stiffness in the affected part.

Examination

A detailed outline of the limb muscles and their examination is contained in Chapter 10. This section concentrates on an overview of patterns of weakness and how that pattern is helpful in diagnosis.

APPEARANCE

Some thinning of the small hand muscles is common in elderly people but is not associated with weakness. When assessing muscle wasting, do not neglect areas hidden when the patient lies in the supine position. Sit the patient forward to look at the periscapular muscles and turn the patient over to assess the bulk of the glutei, hamstrings and calves. A global loss of muscle bulk is

more likely to be the result of impaired nutrition or malignancy rather than neurological disease. Focal muscle wasting can rapidly follow injury of a joint with consequent immobilisation. If you suspect a discrepancy in size between two limbs, use a tape measure to record the limb cirumference. Choose a suitable landmark, for instance the joint margin of the knee, then measure the circumference of the limb at a specified distance from the landmark. Remember that the circumference of the dominant limb is likely to be slightly greater. The pattern of wasting often suggests a particular peripheral nerve or root disorder (Fig. 11.107).

While inspecting the muscle, look for spontaneous contractions. Fasciculation is caused by spontaneous contraction of the fibres belonging to a single motor unit. Depending on the size of the motor unit, the fasciculation appears either as a fine flicker (e.g. in a hand muscle) or as a coarse twitch (e.g. in the thigh). Fasciculation often appears in short bursts before disappearing for several minutes. Muscles may hypertrophy as well as atrophy. Pseudohypertrophic muscles are infiltrated by fat and connective tissue and are weak on formal testing (Fig. 11.108). Muscle palpation provides little information, although ischaemic, fibrotic muscle feels harder than normal and acutely inflamed muscle is tender.

TONE

Assessment of muscle tone requires both skill on the part of the examiner and relaxation on the part of the patient. Ensure that the patient is comfortable and warm. First observe the limb posture, as this may indicate the distribution of altered tone between the flexors and extensors of the limb. For screening purposes, assess flexion and extension at the elbow, pronation and supination of the forearm and flexion and extension at

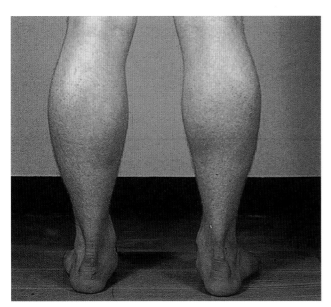

Fig. 11.108 Pseudohypertrophy of the calf muscles.

the knee, using a range of speeds rather than a fixed velocity. Remember to take account of any painful limb or joint.

Spastic limbs

In spastic limbs, at a critical velocity a catch appears that is absent during slower displacements. Subsequently, the hypertonus fades away as stretch continues. Spasticity is selectively distributed. In the upper limbs it predominates in flexors and is more evident when the forearm is supinated than when it is pronated. In the lower limb it is greater in quadriceps than in the hamstrings. This selectivity may vary, particularly in spinal cord disease but the finding is highly suggestive of a disorder affecting the upper motor neuron. In spinal cord disease, release of flexor reflex afferents may be so prominent that mild stimulation of the lower limb produces a flexor reaction at the hip and knee. In longstanding spasticity, you may find that the limb can no longer be fully displaced at the affected joint. For example, in the leg, persistent hypertonia in the plantar flexors can lead to shortening of the tendo Achilles.

Rigidity

Rigidity is more uniformly distributed in the limb. It may begin unilaterally and is sometimes easier to detect in one joint than another. The resistance is felt at low speeds of displacement and does not 'melt away'. Rigidity is activated by contraction of muscle in an unaffected limb. If you have doubts regarding an increase in tone, ask the patient either to clench the teeth or grip the hand not being tested. In patients with rigidity, the increased tone becomes more evident during this procedure. At times rigidity is not uniform but fluctuates in a phasic manner, aptly described as cogwheeling.

Many tense, nervous patients will appear to have a fluctuant increase in tone but the variability should suggest there is no significant pathology.

Gegenhalten

A more diffuse increase in tone, Gegenhalten, can be found in patients with an altered level of consciousness and in individuals with frontal lobe lesions.

Hypotonia

Reduced tone is more difficult to detect. The limb is floppy and is liable to show abnormal excursions when moved passively. Hypotonia occurs in the presence of a lower motor neuron lesion and in cerebellar disease.

MUSCLE POWER

Muscle weakness is often suggested by lack of spontaneous movement in the affected part during conversation or when the patient walks. In Parkinson's disease, however, certain automatic movements can disappear even in the absence of weakness. The UK Medical Research Council system of classification is recommended for grading muscle weakness. To apply this system to a muscle, test its strength as shown for biceps in Figure 11.109. Remember to take account of the patient's age, occupation and your own physical development. In practice grades 4 and 5 are separated by a wide range of strength but as you gain experience you can overcome this problem by using the grades 4+, 4++ and 5–.

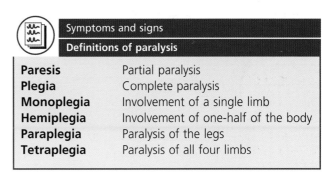

Symptoms and signs	
Definitions of paralysis	
Paresis	Partial paralysis
Plegia	Complete paralysis
Monoplegia	Involvement of a single limb
Hemiplegia	Involvement of one-half of the body
Paraplegia	Paralysis of the legs
Tetraplegia	Paralysis of all four limbs

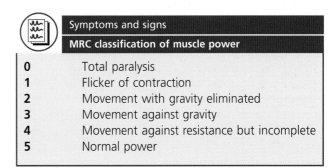

Symptoms and signs	
MRC classification of muscle power	
0	Total paralysis
1	Flicker of contraction
2	Movement with gravity eliminated
3	Movement against gravity
4	Movement against resistance but incomplete
5	Normal power

A description of the methods of assessing individual muscles is given in Chapter 10. Looking at a limited number can screen for many neurological disorders. In the upper limbs, first ask the patient to shrug the shoulders. In an early pyramidal lesion above the level of

Testing biceps

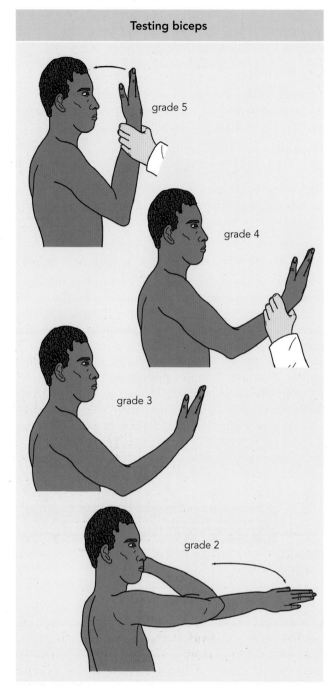

grade 5

grade 4

grade 3

grade 2

Fig. 11.109 The application of the MRC system of grading muscle power to the examination of biceps.

C2 (but also in unilateral Parkinson's disease), the affected shoulder lags behind its fellow (Fig. 11.110). Next, test deltoid, biceps, triceps, then the first dorsal interosseous and abductor pollicis brevis. Score each muscle on the MRC scale. Test one arm at a time rather than trying to test both arms together. In the lower limb, look at hip flexion and extension, knee flexion and extension and dorsiflexion and plantar flexion of the feet.

If the degree of muscle weakness fluctuates during the course of the examination, test for fatiguability. In the upper limb first attempt to depress the arms when

Early pyramidal lesion

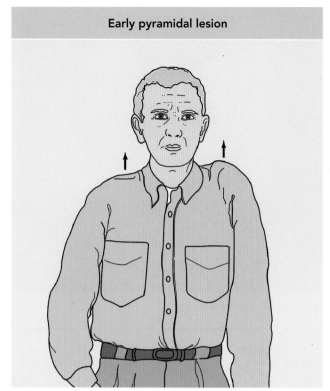

Fig. 11.110 Delayed right shoulder shrug in a patient with an early pyramidal lesion.

abducted to 90°. Then ask the patient to maintain this posture for a minute and retest. In the lower limb, hip flexion can be tested in a similar fashion. Remember that a fluctuating performance is also often prominent in nonorganic weakness.

Myotonia results in impaired relaxation of skeletal muscle after contraction. Ask the patient to clench the fists tightly then release them; if the patient has myotonia, there is a significant delay before the fingers can be fully extended. There is likely to be abnormal dimpling of muscle after percussion. Tap the thenar eminence with the patella hammer. In the presence of myotonia, the muscle dimples and stays dimpled for several seconds. The same sign can be elicited in the tongue (Fig. 11.111).

 Emergency
Rapidly developing limb weakness

Consider: Guillain–Barre syndrome, cord compression

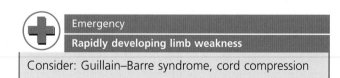 Emergency
Acute hemiplegia

Consider: most likely CVA (cerebrovascular accident), but other possibilities include abscess, cerebral tumour and encephalitis

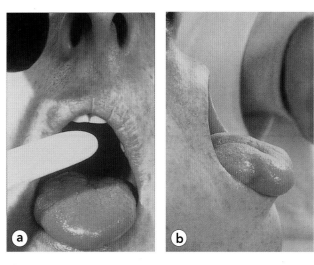

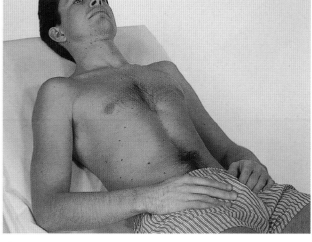

Fig. 11.111 Percussion myotonia of the tongue.

Fig. 11.112 Posture of the upper limbs for testing the biceps and supinator reflexes.

DEEP TENDON REFLEXES

Testing the reflexes assesses the reflex arc and the supraspinal influences that operate on it. Each reflex is graded according to strength of response, as shown in the 'symptoms and signs' box.

Reflexes are remarkably variable in normal individuals. Some patients have very brisk reflexes, although unaccompanied by clonus. Others have very depressed responses that often appear better preserved at the ankle than elsewhere, the opposite of what one would find if a neuropathy was the cause of the hyporeflexia.

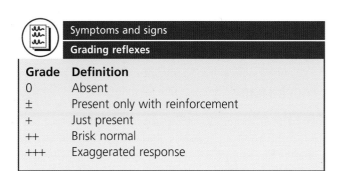

	Symptoms and signs
	Grading reflexes

Grade	Definition
0	Absent
±	Present only with reinforcement
+	Just present
++	Brisk normal
+++	Exaggerated response

THE UPPER LIMB

The reflexes of the upper limb routinely tested are the biceps, triceps and supinator (the roots subserving each reflex are shown in brackets). The biceps and supinator reflexes are tested first, with the patient in the posture shown in Figure 11.112.

Biceps (C5/6)

The whole arm must be exposed when testing this reflex. Place the thumb or index finger of your left hand on the biceps tendon then strike it with the patella hammer using a pendular motion by extending then flexing your wrist. Grasp the hammer at the end rather than halfway down the shaft (Fig. 11.113). The response consists of

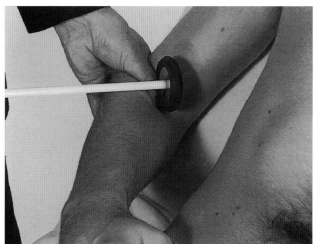

Fig. 11.113 Testing the right biceps reflex.

contraction of the biceps muscle. If there is no response, ask the patient to clench the teeth or grip the fingers of the other hand shortly before testing (Jendrassik manoeuvre). Now examine the reflex in the left arm. Lean over and use your inverted thumb to mark the position of the tendon.

Supinator (C5/6)

With the patient's arm in the semipronated position, strike the radial margin of the forearm approximately 5 cm above the wrist (Fig. 11.114). You can if you wish interpose your finger. The response is a contraction of brachioradialis and biceps. When eliciting the biceps and supinator reflexes, observe also the fingers of the hand. A brisk reflex is accompanied by finger flexion. In certain instances, despite a depression of the direct reflex, flexion of the fingers still occurs (inversion). This physical finding, usually due to cervical spondylosis, suggests the combination of a depression of the reflex arc at the C5/C6 level, together with an exaggeration of

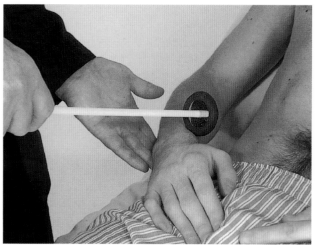

Fig. 11.114 Testing the right supinator reflex.

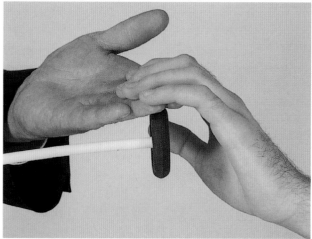

Fig. 11.116 Eliciting a finger jerk.

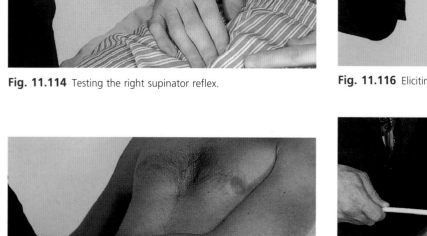

Fig. 11.115 Testing the left triceps reflex.

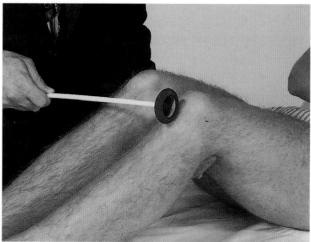

Fig. 11.117 Eliciting the knee reflexes.

reflexes at a lower level due to a coexistent pyramidal tract disorder.

Triceps (C6/7)

To test the right triceps jerk, bring the patient's right arm well across the body, with the elbow flexed at approximately 90° so that the triceps tendon is adequately exposed (Fig. 11.115). Strike the tendon with the patella hammer. A normal response is contraction of the triceps. Having tested the reflex on the right, bring the left arm over and test the reflex on that side.

Finger (C8)

The finger jerk is usually present only when there is a pathological exaggeration of the reflexes. With the patient's arm pronated, exert slight pressure on the flexed fingers with the fingers of your left hand. Now strike the back of your own fingers with the hammer. A positive response leads to a brief flexion of the fingertips (Fig. 11.116).

LOWER LIMB

Knee (L2/3/4)

To test the knee jerks insert your left arm underneath the patient's knees and flex them to approximately 60° (Fig. 11.117). If the patient is properly relaxed, the legs will sag when you remove your arm. Tap first the right patella tendon and then the left. If one or both reflexes is particularly brisk, test for knee clonus by fitting your thumb and index finger along the upper border of the patella with the knee extended (Fig. 11.118). Exert a sudden, downward stretch and maintain it. Any repetitive contraction of the quadriceps (i.e. clonus) even if only two or three beats, is strongly suggestive of a pyramidal tract disorder.

ANKLE (S1)

The patient's leg is abducted and externally rotated at the hip, flexed at the knee and flexed at the ankle. If hip abduction is limited, rest the leg on its fellow to allow adequate access to the Achilles tendon (Fig. 11.119). If

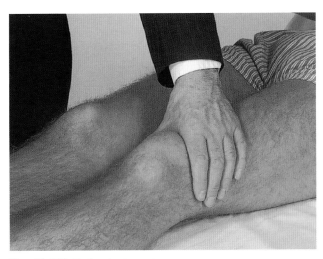

Fig. 11.118 Testing for knee clonus.

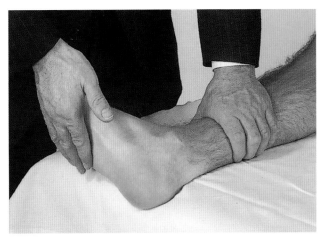

Fig. 11.120 Testing for ankle clonus.

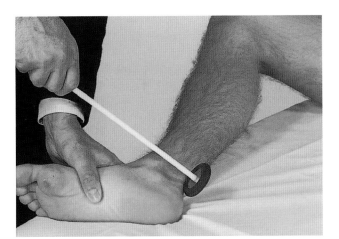

Fig. 11.119 Eliciting the ankle reflex.

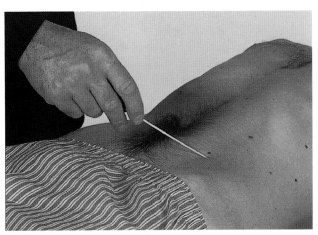

Fig. 11.121 Testing the abdominal responses.

the reflex is brisk, look for clonus. With the limb in the same position, forcibly dorsiflex the ankle and maintain that position (Fig. 11.120). Three to four beats of symmetrical ankle clonus is acceptable in normal individuals but asymmetric or more sustained clonus is pathological.

OTHER REFLEXES

Abdominal responses

The abdominal responses diminish with age and are more difficult to elicit in the obese or in women who have had children. They are cutaneous reflexes whose latency suggests mediation through a spinal reflex arc. Before you can assess the abdominal reflexes, the patient must be relaxed and lying flat. Lightly draw the end of an orange stick across the four segments of the abdomen around the umbilicus (Fig. 11.121). Normally there is a reflex contraction in each segment. To summarise the findings in your notes draw a cross with an o, ± or + in each segment according to response.

Cremasteric reflex

The cremasteric reflex is elicited by stroking the upper inner aspect of the thigh. It is mediated through segments L1 and L2 and leads to retraction of the ipsilateral testicle.

Plantar response

The plantar response is elicited by applying firm pressure (use an orange stick) to the lateral aspect of the sole of the foot, moving from the heel to the base of the fifth toe, then, if necessary, across the base of the toes (Fig. 11.122). While you do this observe the metatarsophalangeal joint of the big toe. In the normal adult, the toe plantar flexes. In the presence of a pyramidal tract lesion, the toe dorsiflexes. The same dorsiflexion appears in normal individuals if a sharp stimulus is applied to the big toe and in infants if the stimulus is applied over a wider area. The reflex is considered to be part of a flexor withdrawal response to a noxious stimulus. With the development of the upright posture, descending pathways, one of which is the pyramidal tract, inhibit the reaction except when stimulation is applied directly to the big toe. Damage to descending pathways, particularly the corticospinal

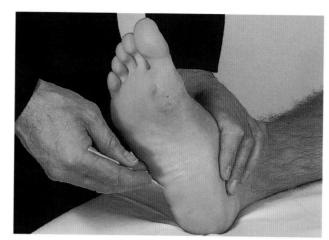

Fig. 11.122 Testing the plantar response.

system, releases the inhibition and allows the appearance of the pathological response. In certain spinal cord disorders, in which the flexor withdrawal response is totally disinhibited, minor stimulation of the foot or other part of the leg results in flexion at hip, knee, ankle and toe. There is no point in testing the plantar response if the big toe is immobile or if there is severe loss of S1 cutaneous innervation. Summarise your findings with arrows: for flexor ↓, for extensor ↑ and for equivocal ↓↑.

Anal reflex

The anal reflex is assessed by pricking the skin at the anal margin. Normally, there is a brisk contraction of the anal sphincter. The tone of the anal sphincter can be assessed by inserting a finger into the anus and asking the patient to bear down.

THE EXTRAPYRAMIDAL SYSTEM

Examination of tone has already been considered and the interpretation of abnormal movements including tremor will be considered later.

Bradykinesia

Bradykinesia is particularly associated with Parkinson's disease. The problem may be confined to one limb, at least initially, or it may be generalised. Initiation of movement is delayed, the actual movement slowed and its adjustment insensitive. Muscle power remains intact. To look for bradykinesia in the upper limbs, ask the patient to tap repetitively the back of one hand with the other. Ask the patient to use such force that the tapping is audible. Typically, if the movement is bradykinetic, its sound diminishes and falters. Now ask the patient to 'polish' the back of one hand with the other. In bradykinesia, a movement of reduced amplitude is seen that eventually may cease completely. To assess bradykinesia in the lower limbs, ask the patient to tap your hand repetitively, first with one foot, then the other. Many individuals find it difficult to sustain a rhythm but

with bradykinesia the movement will again fade away. There are many ways of assessing bradykinesia without recourse to formal examination. Watch the patient dressing or using a knife and fork. Ask them to write and examine the size of the script and its legibility. See how easily they stand from a sitting posture and time how long they take to walk a set distance.

Involuntary movement

Begin by detailing the characteristics of the movement. Is it present at rest, with the limb completely supported or when the limb takes up a particular posture or only when the patient carries out a skilled activity? Ascertain the frequency of the movement and its distribution. Is the problem mainly proximal or distal? Are the movements brief or sufficiently prolonged to cause an abnormal posture?

Tremor

Tremor is a rhythmic movement that, at a particular joint, is usually confined to a single plane. Physiological tremor is a normal finding, usually detectable only with electromyography. Enhanced physiological tremor is triggered by agitation, the use of sympathomimetic agents and thyrotoxicosis. Its frequency is around 9 Hz in younger people. Stimulation of β_2-adrenergic receptors in muscle accounts for enhanced physiological tremor.

| **Questions to ask** |
| **Tremor** |

- Is the tremor mainly present at rest, when the hands are held out, or when they are used?
- Is the tremor relieved by alcohol?
- Is there a family history of tremor?

Myoclonus

Myoclonus is characterised by rapid, recurring muscle jerks. The movement is similar to the startle reaction described as 'jumping out of one's skin'. The movements are either generalised or confined to one part of the body. In some patients they appear only when the limb is activated.

Chorea

Patients with chorea appear to fidget. They show brief, random movements that do not have the shock-like quality of myoclonus. Typical movements include furrowing of the eyebrows, pursing of the lips, elevation of a shoulder and random contraction of the fingers. Both proximal and distal limb muscles can be affected. As the movements are short-lived, sustained postures do not occur. Ask the patient to grip your hand: you will find that the grip waxes and wanes with the fluctuations of the chorea. The tendon reflexes may be prolonged because of the superimposition of a late, sustained contraction on the phasic reflex. The choreiform movements tend to be accentuated by a skilled action.

Athetosis

Athetoid movements are slower still than chorea and become prominent during the performance of voluntary activity. The distal parts of the limbs are predominantly affected. In the hand, the posture oscillates between hyperextension of the fingers and thumb, usually with pronation of the forearm and flexion of the digits associated with supination (Fig. 11.123). In some patients, the movements are superimposed on more sustained postures. In the hand, this combines flexion of the wrist with extension of the fingers and, in the foot, flexion of the toes associated with inversion at the ankle. In progressive disease states, the abnormal sustained postures become dominant. Assessment of the plantar response is difficult if athetosis is affecting the foot. Stimulation of the sole is liable to produce extension of the toes whether or not there is a pyramidal tract disorder. A combination of choreiform and athetoid movements is called choreoathetosis.

Hemiballismus

Hemiballismus results in violent swinging movements of the contralateral arm and leg. The movements, in which rotation is prominent, are of maximal amplitude at the shoulder and hip. The affected limbs are relatively flaccid.

Dystonia

In dystonia, abnormal postures result from contraction of antagonistic muscle groups. It is exacerbated by attempts at voluntary movement. The dystonia may be generalised or localised to one area.

Tics

Tics are repetitive movements that appear, at least briefly, to be under voluntary control. They predominate in younger people. Typical examples are head nodding and jerking. The movement is easily mimicked.

Dyskinesia

Brief, involuntary movements around the mouth and face are relatively common in elderly people (orofacial dyskinesia). Similar movements can be induced by long-term phenothiazine therapy and in patients on L-dopa. The former problem tends to persist whatever adjustment is made to the medication but the latter is dose-dependent.

Differential diagnosis	
Movement disorders	

- Parkinson's disease
- Multisystem atrophy
- Huntington's disease
- Essential tremor
- Palatal myoclonus
- Hemiballismus
- Generalised torsion dystonia
- Focal dystonia
- Facial myokymia

Myokymia

Myokymia confined to the eyelid is a common experience in normal individuals and is felt as a fine twitching. In pathological myokymia, this fine movement extends to other parts of the facial musculature. The movements are easily missed but on examination a continuous, fine flickering motion can be seen. If the movements are extensive, the eye may close slightly and the mouth retract (Fig. 11.124).

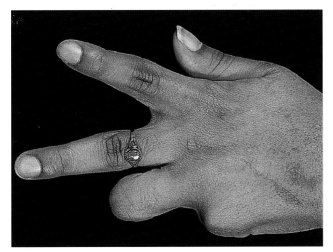

Fig. 11.123 Athetoid hand posture.

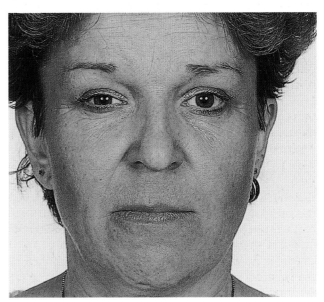

Fig. 11.124 Facial myokymia. The right eye is slightly narrowed.

Asterixis

In certain metabolic disorders, particularly hepatic and renal failure, there is a defect of limb posture control. If the patient is asked to extend the arms and hold the fingers in the horizontal plane, a downward drift of the fingers and hands is interrupted by a sudden, upward, corrective jerk.

Clinical application

UPPER MOTOR NEURON LESION

An upper motor neuron lesion results from disruption of the pyramidal pathway at any point between the motor cortex and the anterior horn cell. Its characteristic features are shown in the 'symptoms and signs' box.

The pattern of weakness is influenced by the site of the lesion but generally it predominates in the upper limb extensors and the lower limb flexors.

Differential diagnosis
The motor system

Upper motor neuron syndrome
- Cerebrovascular disease
- Head or spinal injury
- Tumour

Lower motor neuron syndrome
- Motor neuron disease
- Spinal root or peripheral nerve disorder

Fluctuating weakness
- Myasthenia gravis

Myotonia
- Dystrophia myotonica

Symptoms and signs
Features of upper motor neuron lesion

- Muscle weakness
- Increased deep tendon reflexes
- Depressed abdominal responses
- An extensor plantar response
- Spasticity

LOWER MOTOR NEURON LESION

The characteristic findings in a lower motor neuron lesion secondary to disruption of the pathway between the motor nucleus and the neuromuscular junction are shown in the 'symptoms and signs' box.

The weakness is found in all the muscles supplied by the affected motor neuron. Wasting results from interruption of the nerve axon or its parent cell but can take several weeks to emerge. Fasciculation is particularly prominent when the anterior horn cells or cranial nerve motor nuclei are disrupted. If the lesion is at the anterior horn cell level, for example in motor neuron disease, there will be no sensory signs. If the lesion affects the combined nerve root or the peripheral nerve, sensory signs will almost certainly accompany the motor deficit.

Symptoms and signs
Features of lower motor neuron lesion

- Muscle weakness
- Depressed deep tendon reflexes
- Fasciculation
- Wasting
- Flaccidity

Nerve root disorders are commonly the result of degenerative disease of the spine. Lesions of a single peripheral nerve are usually the consequence of abnormal angulation, stretch or compression. A diffuse disorder of peripheral nerves (although the pattern of distribution can vary) is called a peripheral neuropathy. In most instances, both sensory and motor components of the nerves are affected, resulting in weakness, distal sensory loss and reflex depression.

Myasthenia gravis

In myasthenia gravis, deposition of antibody on the postsynaptic acetylcholine receptor site interrupts the function of the neuromuscular junction. Fatiguable weakness can affect any skeletal muscle. Diplopia and ptosis are particularly common (Fig. 11.125). Muscle wasting is a late and inconsistent feature. The tendon reflexes are preserved.

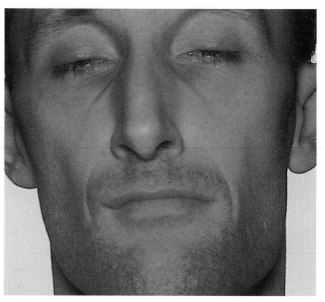

Fig. 11.125 Myasthenia gravis.

EXTRAPYRAMIDAL DISORDERS

A combination of tremor, rigidity and bradykinesia occurs in Parkinson's disease. The distribution can sometimes be disconcertingly focal and often a patient with unilateral Parkinsonism is believed to have a hemiplegia. Postural problems are common; the neck and trunk become flexed. When walking, arm swing is reduced on one or both sides and turning is difficult, the patient taking more steps than usual. Eye movements are slowed and convergence and upward gaze tend to be diminished in range. Some patients have an associated dementia. An identical clinical (and pathological) pattern can coexist with degeneration of the intermediolateral columns of the spinal cord, producing profound autonomic failure. Multisystem atrophy causes extrapyramidal features but also affects pyramidal, cerebellar and autonomic pathways. Many patients with rigidity and bradykinesia have had their symptoms induced by drugs affecting the release of dopamine or its receptor sites, for example, a phenothiazine. Another disorder affecting the extrapyramidal pathways disrupts first the supranuclear, then the nuclear, gaze pathways: progressive supranuclear palsy (Steele–Richardson–Olsczewski syndrome).

MOVEMENT DISORDERS

Tremor

- *Essential (familial tremor)* – absent at rest. Can affect the head, neck and voice as well as the upper and lower limbs. Inherited as an autosomal dominant. Alcohol responsive in 50%.
- *Parkinsonian tremor* – classically a resting tremor at 4–5 Hz, with flexion–extension movements at the wrist and fingers, together with pronation–supination of the forearm. Inhibited briefly by a skilled activity. Sometimes an action or postural tremor is also found.

Myoclonus

- *Palatal myoclonus* – affects the palate, larynx and face. Frequency is 2–3 Hz. Associated with brainstem pathology, usually vascular.
- *Segmental myoclonus* – occurs with spinal cord disease.
- *Generalised myoclonus* – many causes, including familial cases, subacute sclerosing panencephalitis and Creutzfeldt–Jakob disease.

Chorea

- *Sydenham's (rheumatic) chorea* – rare. Sometimes reappears in adult life, either spontaneously or during pregnancy.
- *Huntington's disease* – usually a prominent feature, although not in juvenile-onset cases.
- *Other causes* – thyrotoxicosis, systemic lupus erythematosus, polycythaemia and the oral contraceptive.

Hemiballismus

- Usually due to a vascular lesion in the contralateral subthalamic nucleus.

Dystonia

- *Torsion dystonia* – familial, generalised dystonia predominating in either axial or limb muscles.
- *Drug-induced* – e.g. dopa.
- *Focal dystonia* – e.g. blepharospasm, spasmodic torticollis and writer's cramp.

Myokymia

- *Facial myokymia* is associated with brainstem tumours and multiple sclerosis.

Review

Examination of the motor system

- Inspect muscle bulk and assess any fasciculation
- Examine muscle tone
- Examine power using MRC classification
- Perform the deep tendon reflexes, along with the abdominal and plantar responses
- Assess any involuntary movement

Red flag – urgent referral

Motor or sensory symptoms

- Fatiguable muscle weakness – may indicate myasthenia gravis, but often not linked to neurological disease
- Fasciculation – if isolated, particularly to the calves, is usually benign; if more diffuse, suspect motor neuron disease
- Rest tremor – highly suggestive of Parkinson's disease
- Exercise-induced sensory or motor symptoms – very suggestive of multiple sclerosis
- Lhermitte's phenomenon – shock-like sensations in the spine triggered by neck flexion indicate a cervical cord lesion

The cerebellar system

STRUCTURE AND FUNCTION

The cerebellum comprises two hemispheres and a midline structure, the vermis. Between the vermis and each hemisphere lies the paravermis (intermediate zone). From above downwards, the cerebellar cortex is divided into the anterior and posterior lobes and the flocculonodular lobe. Phylogenetically, there are three components: the archicerebellum, palaeocerebellum and neocerebellum. The archicerebellum (principally the flocculonodular lobe) receives its major input from the vestibular nuclei. The palaeocerebellum (predominantly the vermis) receives projections from the spinal cord, while the neocerebellum, located mainly in the cerebellar hemispheres, lies on a circuit incorporating the cerebral cortex and the pons. The fibres projecting in and out of the cerebellum pass through the superior, middle or inferior cerebellar peduncles.

Embedded in the white matter of each cerebellar hemisphere is the dentate (lateral) nucleus. The fastigial nucleus lies medially, beneath the vermis. Lateral to the fastigial nucleus is the nucleus interpositus.

Risk factors
Cerebral haemorrhage

- Hypertension
- Vascular malformations
- Bleeding disorders
- Sympathomimetic agents
- Cerebral amyloid angiopathy
- Intracranial tumours

Risk factors
Cerebral infarction

- Hypertension
- Diabetes mellitus
- Cardiac disease
- Atrial fibrillation
- Cigarette smoking
- Oral contraceptives
- Lipoprotein abnormalities
- Haematological abnormalities

The cerebellar cortex is supplied by three vessels: the upper surface is supplied by the superior cerebellar arteries and the lower surface is supplied by the anterior inferior cerebellar arteries, with a contribution from the posterior inferior cerebellar arteries. The first two pairs of vessels arise from the basilar artery, the last pair from the vertebral artery.

Dentate neurons discharge before the onset of motor activity and even before the relevant motor cortical discharge. The nucleus interpositus is active during the control of movement and at its termination. Both nuclei are concerned with posture control but activity in the interpositus nucleus appears more closely related to the force of muscle contraction and its velocity. Discharge in fastigial neurons relates partly to velocity and partly to force.

The cerebellum exerts an influence on muscle tone through an effect on motor neuron output to the muscle spindle. Efferents from the flocculus exert an inhibitory effect on the vestibulo-ocular reflex via the fastigial nucleus.

SYMPTOMS

The symptoms of a disruption of the cerebellar system include dysarthria, limb clumsiness and gait ataxia.

Dysarthria

Patients with dysarthria have a defect of pronunciation, although speech content remains normal.

Limb clumsiness

A unilateral cerebellar disorder results in an ipsilateral limb ataxia. If the dominant limb is affected, the patient may well have noticed an alteration in writing. Sometimes the patient may refer to an ataxic limb as being weak rather than clumsy.

Gait ataxia

If the cerebellar problem is confined to one hemisphere, the patient often complains of deviating to that side when walking. With disruption of midline cerebellar structures, however, unsteadiness when walking is the main complaint rather than a tendency to deviate to a particular side. In such cases, the limbs are relatively spared.

Examination

SPEECH

Dysarthria will be apparent while you take the history. Remember to take account of accent. There is no need to give the patient set phrases to pronounce, a brief conversation suffices. In cerebellar dysarthria, speech volume and pitch are typically erratic, so that the rhythm of speech is lost, with pauses then accelerations. If the disorder is severe, speech is shot out in a staccato fashion.

EYE MOVEMENTS

In patients suspected of having cerebellar disease, you need to look for nystagmus and for abnormalities of either saccadic or pursuit movements. The assessment of eye movement has been discussed on pages 337–340.

Symptoms and signs
Eye signs in cerebellar disease

Location	Sites
Flocculus	Abnormal smooth pursuit
	Gaze-evoked nystagmus
Flocculus/nodulus	Down-beat nystagmus
Vermis/fastigial nucleus	Ocular dysmetria
Lateral zones	Ocular dysmetria
	Gaze-evoked nystagmus

LIMB EXAMINATION

The reduced limb tone associated with a cerebellar lesion is difficult to detect. If the problem is unilateral, ask the patient to hold the arms in the position shown in Figure 11.126. If the limb is hypotonic, the hand tends to sag below the horizontal. If there is a severe cerebellar disturbance, the outstretched hands may oscillate. More likely, however, is the presence of an intention tremor. To test this ask the patient to touch first his or her nose, then your finger held approximately 0.5 m away (Fig. 11.127). In a cerebellar ataxia, a tremor emerges that becomes more apparent as the target is approached. If you are undecided, continue but now move your target finger in a random fashion. A mild ataxia may then become more evident.

Occasionally, in disease of the cerebellar pathway, a severe swinging tremor appears as a result of interruption of the corticocerebellar circuit at the level of the red nucleus (rubral tremor). While testing for intention tremor, observe whether the patient's finger reaches the target accurately. It may reach beyond the target (hypermetria), fall short (hypometria) or even bounce against it in an uncontrolled fashion.

Now assess alternating movements in the upper limbs. Ask the patient to hold one hand steady, in the horizontal plane, with the fingers closed. Next ask the patient to tap first the dorsal then the palmar surface of one hand with the fingers of the other, pronating and supinating the forearm in the process. The patient with cerebellar ataxia is clumsy and there are fluctuations in both the speed and amplitude of the movement (dysdiadokokinesis) that are both visible and audible.

Ask the patient to raise the arms rapidly from the sides but stop them abruptly in the horizontal plane. In cerebellar disease, the affected arm oscillates about its intended resting place because of a failure of the damping mechanism. You will already have examined the limb reflexes as part of the motor system examination. They may be unusually sustained in cerebellar disease ('hung up' reflexes).

To assess lower limb coordination, ask the patient to slide the heel of one foot in a straight line down the shin of the other leg: the heel–knee–shin test (Fig. 11.128). In the presence of cerebellar ataxia the heel wavers around the intended pathway. When the heel has reached the bottom of the shin, ask the patient to flex the leg then bring the heel back down on to the shin just below the knee. If there is cerebellar incoordination, the heel may fall short of its target or thump into the shin rather than landing gently. Finally, ask the patient to tap your hand repetitively using first one foot then the other. Be aware, however, that the performance of this test is variable in normal individuals and tends to be less smooth in the nondominant limb.

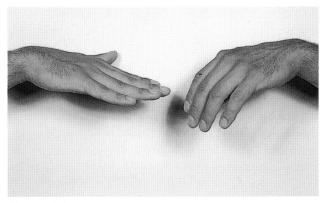

Fig. 11.126 Hypotonia of the left hand in a left cerebellar lesion.

Finger–nose test

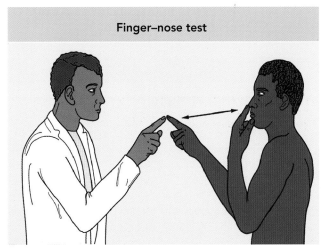

Fig. 11.127 The finger–nose test.

Differential diagnosis
Cerebellar disorders

Hemisphere lesions
- Stroke
- Primary and secondary tumours
- Multiple sclerosis
- Degenerative disorders

Vermis lesions
- Alcohol-related
- Hypothyroidism

Review
Examination of the cerebellar system

- Assess articulation
- Examine pursuit and saccadic eye movements and analyse any nystagmus
- Examine the finger–nose and heel–knee–shin tests
- Assess gait

Heel–knee–shin test

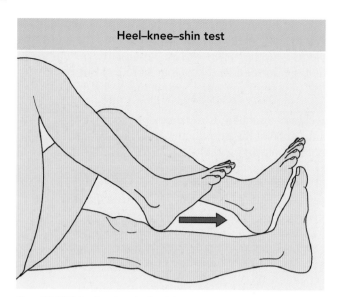

Fig. 11.128 Performing the heel–knee–shin test with the right leg.

Heel–toe walking

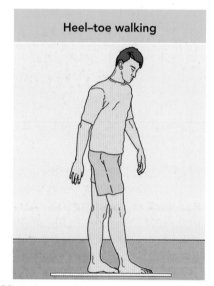

Fig. 11.129 Heel–toe walking.

GAIT

Unless there is a substantial disturbance of midline cerebellar structures, patients do not display any instability of the trunk while sitting but, on standing, oscillations of the body may occur even before gait is initiated. When walking, the patient will use a wide-based gait and is likely to show caution when turning. Attempts to turn quickly will result in problems with posture control. Be prepared to support ataxic patients when you ask them to walk independently. If the patient has a lesion of one cerebellar hemisphere, then deviation to that side occurs on walking. To detect a more subtle disturbance of cerebellar function, ask the patient to walk heel–toe (Fig. 11.129). Again you need to appreciate how variably normal individuals perform this test. People lacking confidence in walking, for any reason, are likely to perform badly.

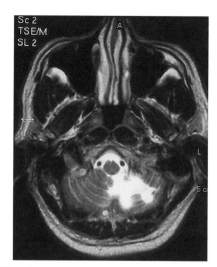

Fig. 11.130 Left cerebellar infarct. T$_2$-weighted MRI.

Clinical application

LESIONS OF THE CEREBELLAR HEMISPHERE

The lesions most commonly affecting the cerebellar hemisphere are infarcts (Fig. 11.130), haemorrhage and tumour. In adults, a tumour involving the cerebellum is usually metastatic. Characteristic symptoms include an ipsilateral limb ataxia, a gait which tends to deviate to the affected side and ocular dysmetria.

MIDLINE CEREBELLAR LESIONS

The predominant complaint in patients with lesions of the vermis or paravermis is a gait ataxia. Tumours are sometimes confined to this area but more often the syndrome is due to selective atrophy secondary, for example, to alcohol. The familial cerebellar atrophies tend to produce a more diffuse atrophy readily detectable by scanning (Fig. 11.131).

Cerebellar signs are very common in patients with established multiple sclerosis but the triad of tremor, dysarthria, and nystagmus, described by Charcot, is rare as an isolated clinical feature. More often it is accompanied by other features of the disease.

The sensory system

STRUCTURE AND FUNCTION

The sensory nerve endings

The majority of the sensory nerve endings in the skin are located in the epidermis. They are more numerous in the face, hands and feet than in the trunk. The individual cutaneous receptors do not respond solely to a specific stimulus but their sensitivity for one usually far exceeds that for the others. Cutaneous receptors include those responding to a deformity of the skin (mechanoreceptors), those responding to temperature (thermoreceptors),

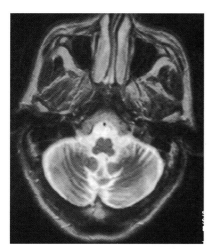

Fig. 11.131 Cerebellar atrophy. T$_2$-weighted MRI.

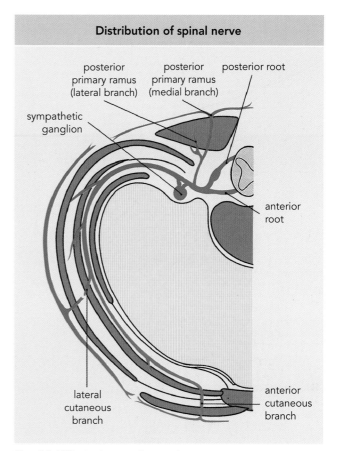

Distribution of spinal nerve

posterior primary ramus (lateral branch)

posterior primary ramus (medial branch)

posterior root

sympathetic ganglion

anterior root

lateral cutaneous branch

anterior cutaneous branch

Fig. 11.132 Distribution of a spinal nerve.

and those responding to pain (nociceptors). Light touch responses are perceived principally by the pacinian corpuscle and the hair follicle receptors. Pacinian corpuscles also identify a vibrating stimulus when applied to the skin. Information about the position and posture of the limbs (proprioception) is derived from end organs in muscle, the muscle spindle and the Golgi tendon organ. The nerve fibres issuing from these various receptors are either myelinated or nonmyelinated.

The spinal roots

At each segmental level, the dorsal root (purely sensory) and the ventral root (predominantly motor) join to form a mixed spinal nerve that produces two branches: the posterior primary ramus and the anterior primary ramus. The brachial and lumbosacral plexuses, responsible for the nerve supply of the upper and lower limbs, are each supplied by the relevant anterior primary rami. In the trunk, the anterior and posterior primary rami are distributed to the hypaxial (ventral) and epaxial (dorsal) musculature, respectively, and to the corresponding overlying skin (Fig. 11.132). The areas of skin supplied by the branches of the dorsal roots are called dermatomes. The arrangement of dermatomes is straightforward in the trunk but more complicated in the limbs (Fig. 11.133). The cutaneous distribution of some of the peripheral nerves is summarised in Figure 11.133. Considerable overlap of distribution exists both for adjacent dermatomes and peripheral nerves.

The posterior columns

All sensory fibres have their first cell station in the dorsal root ganglion. Proprioceptive fibres tend to run the whole length of the cuneate fasciculus but fibres in the gracile fasciculus leave in the upper lumbar segments of the cord, synapsing in Clarke's column before passing into the dorsal spinocerebellar tract. Above this level, the fasciculus gracilis is occupied by fibres solely concerned with cutaneous sensation. Initially, as successive fibres enter the dorsal columns, distal segmental fibres are

displaced medially. Immediately above the gracile nucleus is nucleus Z, believed to receive proprioceptive information from the ipsilateral lower limb. Second-order neurons from the gracile and cuneate nuclei and from nucleus Z decussate to form the medial lemniscus, which in turn projects to the ventroposterior nucleus of the thalamus. Vibration sense is principally conveyed in the posterior columns but also in the spinothalamic system.

The spinothalamic tract

Another group of fibres enters the spinal cord and terminates in the posterior horn. The majority of the axons within the spinothalamic tract originate from layer V (Fig. 11.134). The fibres then pass ventral to the spinal canal before ascending in the anterolateral quadrant. Here the fibres from the sacral segments come to lie laterally and superficially as they are displaced by fibres from higher segmental levels. There is no firm evidence that the ascending spinothalamic tract is divided into discrete ventral and dorsal components. Fibres conveying temperature sense and pain travel in the spinothalamic tract.

The spinocervical tract

The third ascending pathway begins with cells from laminae IV and V of the dorsal horn that send fibres ipsilaterally in the spinocervical tract to the lateral cervical nucleus, which is situated lateral to the dorsal horn of the

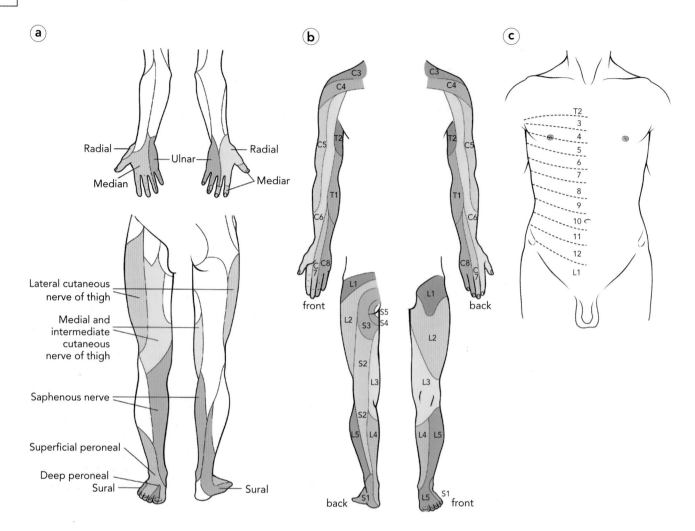

Fig. 11.133 Sensory examination. Distribution of (a) some peripheral nerves, (b) limb dermatomes and (c) thoracic dermatomes.

upper segments of the cervical cord (Fig. 11.134). From here fibres decussate and join the medial lemniscus. The spinocervical tract contains axons that respond principally to light pressure but also contains fibres responding to noxious thermal and mechanical stimuli.

The thalamus

In simplified terms, the medial part of the ventroposterior nucleus of the thalamus receives information from the face and the lateral portion from the medial lemniscus and the spinothalamic tract.

Symptoms and signs		
Sensory disturbances		
	Light touch	**Pain**
Reduced	Hypaesthesia	Hypalgesia
Lost	Anaesthesia	Analgesia
Exaggerated	Hyperaesthesia	Hyperpathia
Exaggerated (at normal threshold)	—	Hyperalgesia

The cortex

Areas of the cortex concerned with the processing of ascending sensory information include the primary somatic area (S1), the secondary somatic area and the adjacent cortex. Most of the afferent fibres to S1 arise from the ventroposterior nucleus of the thalamus. Representation is parallel to that of the motor cortex.

Pain

According to the gate control theory of pain perception, the activity level of certain cells in the substantia gelatinosa (lamina II and III) can inhibit conduction of impulses in the central pain pathways. These inhibitory cells are activated by impulses in large diameter peripheral afferent fibres and switched off by impulses in small diameter myelinated and unmyelinated fibres.

Visceral pain is transmitted by sympathetic or parasympathetic fibres. Impulses emanating from free nerve endings in the gut pass into the posterior root via the splanchnic nerves. Their central connections are similar to those of the spinothalamic fibres. In some instances pain from a viscus is interpreted as arising from

Spinal sensory pathways

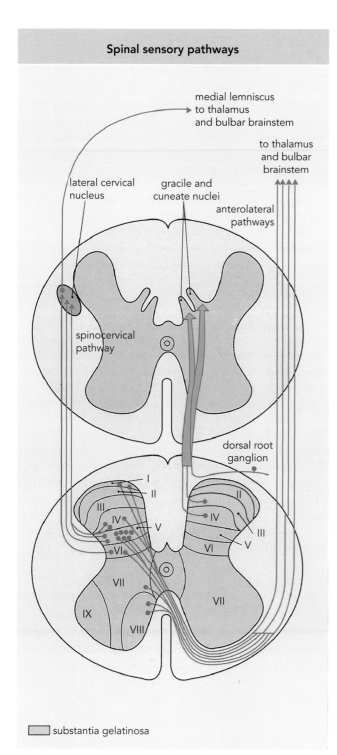

Fig. 11.134 Sensory pathways in the spinal cord.

SYMPTOMS

Sensory symptoms include pain, paraesthesiae (tingling) and numbness. Frequently the patient's understanding and use of these terms differ from that of the physician. Clearly establish what the patient means. Many use

a superficial body part possessing the same segmental innervation (referred pain).

Questions to ask

Sensory disturbances

- When numbness is described, does that mean actual loss of cutaneous sensation?
- Does the distribution of any numbness or tingling follow the distribution of a peripheral nerve or nerve root?
- Does any loss or altered sensation ascend onto the abdomen or thorax?

numbness to describe a lack of use of a limb, rather than a defect of sensation.

Pain

Only rarely does the particular quality of a pain serve to identify its likely source. In peripheral nerve injury, signs of nerve damage may be accompanied by a distressing, persistent burning sensation known as causalgia. Pain related to peripheral nerve disease usually localises to the distribution of the affected nerve. In nerve root disorders, the pain is not referred in a dermatomal distribution but follows a distribution corresponding to the muscles (myotome) or to other deep structures (sclerotome) supplied by that root. A particular type of pain can emerge after damage to the spinothalamic tract or the thalamus itself (thalamic pain). It is persistent, with a very unpleasant burning or scalding quality and is exacerbated by painful or tactile contact.

Paraesthesiae and numbness

Patients often struggle when describing the nature of sensory disturbances. They tend to resort to a previous experience to assist their description (e.g. the recovery of sensation after a dental anaesthetic).

Examination

Sensory examination is difficult. There are few objective criteria, assessment being largely dependent on the patient's subjective responses, which may well falter as the patient fatigues. It is seldom necessary to test all sensory modalities and even then certainly not in all parts

Differential diagnosis

Conditions affecting sensation

- Mononeuropathies, e.g. carpal tunnel syndrome
- Radiculopathies, e.g. cervical spondylosis
- Transverse myelitis
- Brown–Séquard syndrome
- Syringomyelia
- Multiple sclerosis
- Spinal cord compression
- Cerebrovascular disease of the cerebral hemisphere

Review

Sensory examination

- Light touch
- Two-point discrimination
- Proprioception
- Vibration sense
- Pain and temperature
- Cortical sensory function
- Sensory suppression

of the body. The areas tested and the modalities used should be influenced by the type of sensory disturbance suggested by the history. If the patient has an area of reduced cutaneous sensation, start testing within that area, moving out gradually to determine the zone of transition to normal sensation.

Avoid being overpersuasive when attempting to confirm a preconceived area of sensory deficit.

LIGHT TOUCH

Use a wisp of cotton wool to test light touch sensation (Fig. 11.135). The distal parts of the limb are more sensitive than the proximal and hair-containing skin is more sensitive than smooth skin. Do not drag the cotton wool along the surface of the skin but apply it at a single point. Ask the patient to keep the eyes closed and to respond when contact is made.

If the patient complains of unilateral sensory change, compare equivalent parts on the two sides of the body. If the history suggests a cortical lesion but cutaneous sensation appears intact, assess the effect of simultaneous stimulation of equivalent body parts. In parietal lesions, the half-body supplied by the damaged cortex may fail to register a stimulus when there is competition from the intact opposite side, even though a stimulus, applied in isolation, is appreciated (sensory suppression or extinction). In hemisensory loss, the change to normal appreciation will occur strictly at the midline.

TWO-POINT DISCRIMINATION

Two-point discrimination is tested with a pair of compasses specifically designed for this purpose, with gradations in centimetres indicating the separation of the tips, which are blunt rather than pointed. Apply the tips with equal, gentle pressure (Fig. 11.136) while the patient's eyes are closed and establish the minimum separation at which two points are confidently identified. As an approximate guide, a young adult will detect a separation of approximately 3 mm on the finger tips, 1 cm on the palm of the hand and 3 cm on the sole of the foot. The sensation is conducted in large myelinated fibres via the posterior columns to the cortex.

PROPRIOCEPTION

While assessing joint position sense ensure that the patient's eyes remain closed. Begin by testing the patient's ability to appreciate passive movements of the joints. It is rare to find a loss of proximal joint position sense; more often the problem is confined to the digits. During testing avoid pressing on the digit in such a way that the patient appreciates the direction of movement. To test the terminal interphalangeal joint of the index finger grip the sides of the phalanx with the thumb and forefinger of your right hand using your left to stabilise the proximal joints of the finger (Fig. 11.137). The movement appreciated will be barely perceptible to the naked eye. If the responses are inaccurate, move proximally until the movements are accurately perceived. Indicate your findings in the notes as 'JPS – intact to movement of the distal interphalangeal joint of 10°' or whatever range you have chosen.

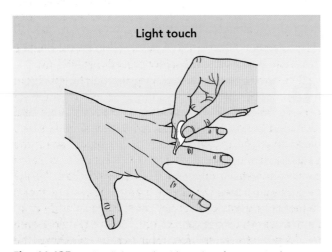

Light touch

Fig. 11.135 Testing light touch with a wisp of cotton wool.

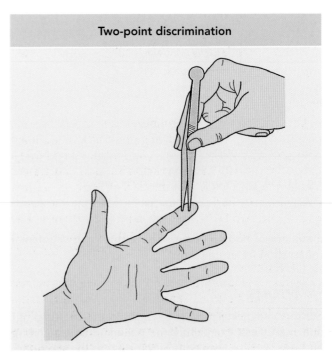

Two-point discrimination

Fig. 11.136 Testing two-point discrimination.

Joint position sense

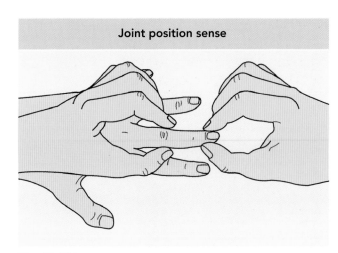

Fig. 11.137 Testing joint position sense.

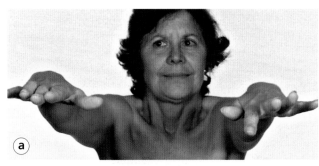

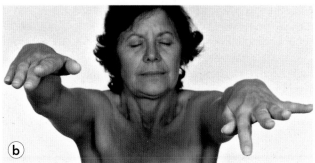

Fig. 11.138 Pseudoathetoid posturing.

You can test active proprioception by asking the patient, with the eyes closed, to locate a digit of one hand with the index finger of the other limb. Alternatively, move the limb with intact sensation into a certain posture and then ask the patient to mimic that position with the affected limb. Finally, ask the patient to hold the hands outstretched while the eyes are closed. With severe loss of distal proprioception, the fingers move in an irregular, purposeless fashion, as if exploring their environment (pseudoathetosis) (Fig. 11.138).

To test the quality of the proprioceptive information coming from the lower limbs, ask the patient to stand with the feet together and the eyes closed. Where there is loss of proprioception, the patient immediately loses stability (positive Romberg's test). Be ready to support the patient.

Vibration sense

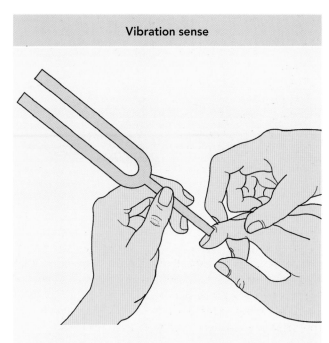

Fig. 11.139 Testing vibration sense in the right index finger.

VIBRATION SENSE

Vibration sense is tested using a 128 Hz tuning fork. To test in the finger, apply the gently vibrating base of the fork to the pulp of the finger or the knuckle of the distal interphalangeal joint (Fig. 11.139). For the foot, start with the pad of the big toe or the dorsum of the interphalangeal joint. If vibration sense is absent there, test more proximally. The chest wall acts as a resonator and a more accurate level of vibration loss on the trunk is obtained by applying the fork to a fold of skin pulled away from the underlying rib. In practice, this is seldom necessary. Semiquantitative testing is achieved by waiting until the perception of vibration has ceased on one limb then transferring the tuning fork to the other limb.

PAIN

Pain is best tested using a sharp pin or needle (Fig. 11.140). Venepuncture needles are unsuitable as they readily puncture the skin, particularly in elderly people. Purpose made 'sharps' are now available and should be discarded using standard safety procedures after use.

Remember that you are testing the painful quality of the stimulus, rather than merely an appreciation of contact. Either ask the patient to close the eyes and identify if the contact is painful or present the sharp and blunt ends of the pin in a random fashion, asking the patient to distinguish one stimulus from another. In some pathological states, diffuse pain radiates out from the site of contact. Remember that certain areas, for instance callouses, are liable to show diminished sensitivity to pain. Deep pain sense can be tested by applying pressure to deeper structures, for example, by pinching the tendoachilles.

Pin-prick

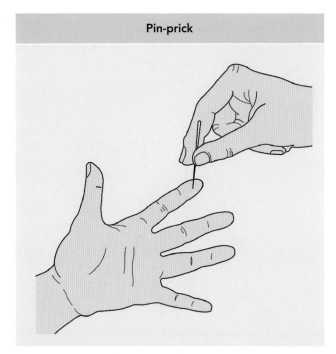

Fig. 11.140 Testing pin-prick sensation.

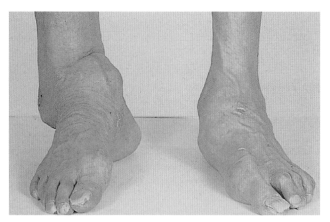

Fig. 11.141 Charcot joint – right ankle.

TEMPERATURE

A reduced or exaggerated response to a thermal stimulus can exist over a fairly narrow band of temperature but to test temperature sense it generally suffices to use two metal tubes, one containing water mixed with ice chips, the other containing hot water. Test the tubes on yourself before testing the patient. Ask the patient to distinguish hot from cold on comparable parts of the two sides of the body. You will need to renew the tubes if the examination is protracted.

WEIGHT, SHAPE, SIZE AND TEXTURE

Certain sensory modalities are worth testing if a disturbance of cortical function is suspected. To test weight appreciation put an object in the patient's palm, allowing the hand to move up and down so that the patient appreciates both the pressure exerted by the weight and the resistance experienced when the hand is moved against gravity. Compare the effect of the same weight in the other hand or alternate differing weights between the two hands and ask the patient to distinguish them.

Shape recognition is also heavily dependent on cortical function. Ask the patient to assess the shape of a coin and also (although this involves other sensory modalities) whether it possesses a milled edge. If the hand is paretic, the patient will experience great difficulty in manipulating the object but in this case you can guide the patient's finger over the surface and edge of the coin. Watching the patient manipulate the coin gives you valuable information about both the motor and sensory status of the digits. Another problem arises if the patient is aphasic or agnosic. Such patients will face difficulties in describing the object, even in the absence of any sensory loss. Coins can also be used for testing size recognition. You can use materials of different form (velvet, wool, linen and so on) to test the patient's appreciation of texture.

Clinical application

NERVE AND ROOT DISORDERS

Considerable anatomical variation exists in the classical cutaneous distributions. For example, the median nerve can supply three or four digits, rather than three and a half. Within an affected nerve or root distribution all sensory modalities will be equally affected, with a boundary zone of partial loss in which appreciation of light touch is more disturbed than that of pain and temperature. In a peripheral neuropathy affecting sensory fibres, there will be a distal disturbance of sensory function which gradually merges into normality. A large-fibre neuropathy will tend to spare pain and temperature sensitivity. A small-fibre neuropathy, predominantly affecting pain and temperature, is rare. If pain fibres to the skin and joints are affected, consequences include painless skin ulceration, sometimes leading to amputation or a severe derangement of joint function which remains painless – Charcot joint (Fig. 11.141).

SPINAL CORD DISORDERS

- *Transverse cord lesion* – sensory level around the site of the lesion, often with a small zone in which cutaneous stimulation can evoke a painful reaction. Causes include transverse myelitis and trauma.
- *Unilateral cord lesion (Brown–Séquard)* – produces contralateral loss of pain and temperature to a level slightly below the lesion, with ipsilateral weakness and depression of vibration and joint position sense (Fig. 11.142). Causes include trauma and multiple sclerosis.
- *Central cord lesion* – disrupts crossing spinothalamic fibres, leading to bilateral, selective loss of pain and temperature over the affected segments (Fig. 11.143).

Brown – Séquard lesion

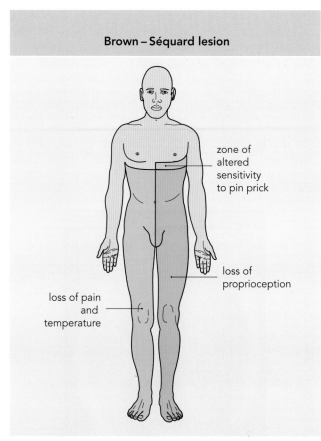

zone of altered sensitivity to pin prick

loss of proprioception

loss of pain and temperature

Fig. 11.142 Distribution of sensory and motor deficit in Brown–Séquard lesion.

Central cord lesion

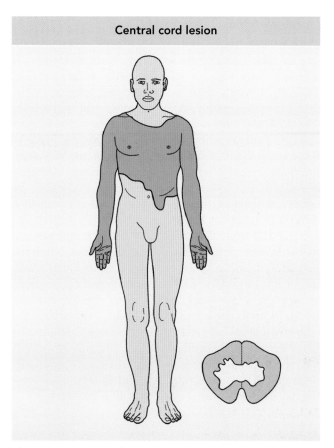

Fig. 11.143 'Cape' of selective pain and temperature loss due to a central cord lesion extending from approximately C3 to D10.

Causes include central cord tumours and syringomyelia.

- *Dorsal column lesion* – interferes with vibration sense, proprioception and two-point discrimination. A cervical cord lesion will predominantly affect upper limb joint position sense. Some patients with cervical dorsal column lesions describe a shock-like sensation radiating down the spine when the neck is flexed (Lhermitte's sign).
- *External compression* – tends to spare the deeper fibres in the spinothalamic tract coming from the segments immediately below the level of compression. Conversely, a tumour spreading from the centre of the cord is likely to spare the superficial fibres emanating from the sacral segments.
- *Brainstem and thalamic disorders* – in the medulla, lateral lesions predominantly affect contralateral pain and temperature sensation, while medial lesions disrupt sensation served by the dorsal columns. Above this level, pathological processes usually disturb all sensory modalities in the contralateral half of the body and cause ipsilateral facial sensory loss if the relevant part of the trigeminal nucleus is involved. Thalamic lesions affect all aspects of sensation on the opposite side of the body. In some cases, spontaneous pains occur, accompanied by intense burning sensations when certain cutaneous stimuli are applied (thalamic syndrome). The cause is almost always vascular.

CORTICAL LESIONS

The cortex is concerned principally with the finer aspects of sensory appreciation. It allows definition of object size, shape, weight and texture. Loss of this facility is called astereognosis. The cortex allows both accurate definition of the site of contact and discrimination of single or multiple stimulation. It is closely concerned with the appreciation of joint position. Sensory suppression is a particular feature of cortical lesions. In nondominant parietal lobe lesions, neglect of the contralateral limbs can be so profound that the patient denies their existence and tries to remove them as if belonging to another person.

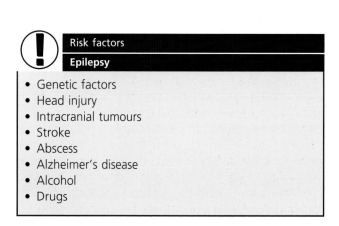

Risk factors

Epilepsy

- Genetic factors
- Head injury
- Intracranial tumours
- Stroke
- Abscess
- Alzheimer's disease
- Alcohol
- Drugs

NONORGANIC SENSORY LOSS

The most common pattern of nonorganic sensory loss is one in which cutaneous sensation to all modalities is affected, with little or no change in proprioception. Typically, a single limb is involved but sometimes the problem occupies one side or the lower half of the body (Fig. 11.144).

Many patients with nonorganic sensory loss perceive it as confined strictly to the limb. Consequently, sensation returns to normal at the shoulder or above an approximately horizontal line at the level of the groin. Typically, the transition is sudden with the patient reacting adversely if a painful stimulus is being used. Rarely, the patient will respond to a stimulus in the intact limb by saying yes and in the defective limb by saying no. Sometimes, when the patient turns into a prone position, the previously numb leg regains sensation on its extensor surface, having been transposed, so to speak, to the other side of the bed. Levels of nonorganic loss can fluctuate, even within the course of a single examination. Hemisensory loss virtually never ceases at the midline, either straying beyond or falling short. Facial sensory loss, when not organically determined, has a tendency to be purely facial, following the hair line superiorly and the jaw line inferiorly.

The unconscious patient

SYMPTOMS

Lesions confined to one cerebral hemisphere seldom interfere with consciousness. Coma is the consequence either of extensive bilateral hemisphere disease, a unilateral hemisphere mass lesion or a more discrete pathology confined to certain parts of the brainstem.

Mass lesions in one cerebral hemisphere affect the conscious level by causing downward herniation of brain tissue through the tentorial notch, with secondary compression of the brainstem (Fig. 11.145). Two types of herniation are described: a central form, usually associated with slowly expanding, medially placed masses, and an uncal form, in which masses in the middle cranial fossa,

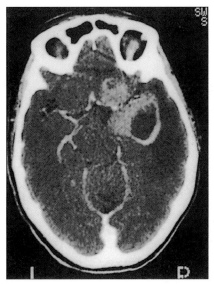

Fig. 11.145 CT scan showing herniation of a right temporal mass with distortion of the upper brainstem.

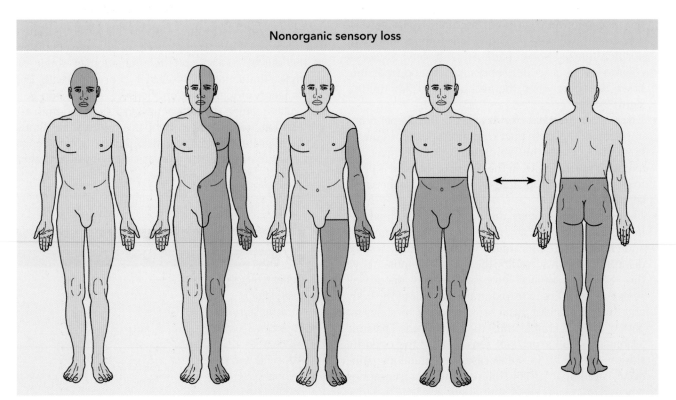

Fig. 11.144 Patterns of nonorganic sensory loss (shaded blue).

particularly of the temporal lobe, cause displacement of the medial aspect of the uncus over the free edge of the tentorium. Pathological consequences of this herniation include ipsilateral third nerve compression, distortion of the contralateral cerebral peduncle, and paramedian brainstem haemorrhages.

Examination

Many aspects of the general examination can be performed in the unconscious patient. The posture may be of value in diagnosis. Carefully examine the skin for signs of injury, petechial haemorrhages or evidence of drug abuse.

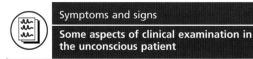

Symptoms and signs

Some aspects of clinical examination in the unconscious patient

- Boggy scalp swelling
- Alcoholic fetor
- Spider naevi
- Venepuncture marks
- Hepatomegaly
- Hypotension

SKELETAL SYSTEM

Palpate the long bones for evidence of fracture. Note the presence of any localised scalp swelling indicating focal

trauma and inspect the external auditory meati for signs of bleeding, suggesting the possibility of a basal skull fracture.

CARDIOVASCULAR SYSTEM

Perform a routine cardiovascular assessment, looking particularly for hypotension or hypertension, pulse abnormality and abnormal heart sounds or murmurs.

RESPIRATORY SYSTEM

Assess respiratory rhythm and rate. Sometimes the patient's fetor, for example of alcohol, gives a clue to the diagnosis but remember that in an individual who has been drinking the coma may have another cause (e.g. a head injury).

GASTROINTESTINAL SYSTEM

Palpate the abdomen. Is there hepatomegaly, suggesting primary liver disease, perhaps resulting in gastrointestinal haemorrhage from oesophageal varices? Look for other markers of liver disease, such as spider naevi.

LEVEL OF CONSCIOUSNESS

Do not use terms such as stupor or coma to describe the patient's conscious state. Record the best level of response of which the patient is capable (Fig. 11.146). Having performed other aspects of the examination, you can then proceed to grade the conscious level using the Glasgow Coma Scale (Fig. 11.147). Note that this scale assesses neither eye movements nor the pupils.

Grading of coma

1. Alert

2. Drowsy but responds to verbal stimulation

3. Unconscious – no response to verbal stimulation, but withdrawal response to pain

4. Unconscious – decorticate responses to pain (flexion of upper limb and extension of lower limb)

5. Unconscious – decerebrate responses to pain (hyperextension of both upper and lower limbs)

6. Unconscious – no response to pain

Fig. 11.146 Grading of coma.

Glasgow coma scale

	Patient's response	Score	08.00	10.00	12.00
Eye opening	spontaneous	4			
	to speech	3			
	to pain	2			
	none	1			
Best verbal responses	orientated	5			
	confused	4			
	inappropriate	3			
	incomprehensible	2			
	none	1			
Best motor responses	obeying	6			
	localising	5			
	withdrawing	4			
	flexing	3			
	extending	2			
	none	1			

Fig. 11.147 Glasgow coma scale.

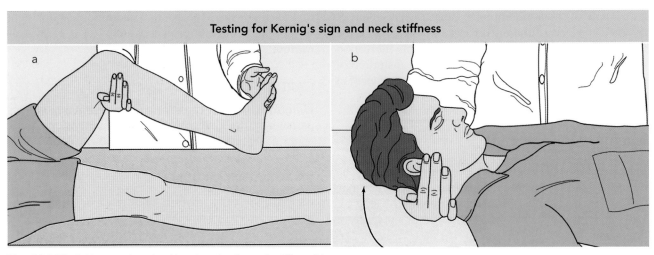

Fig. 11.148 Eliciting Kernig's sign (a) and testing for neck stiffness (b).

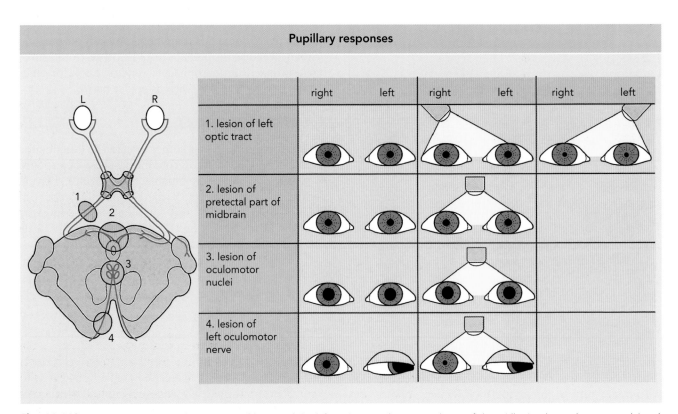

Fig. 11.149 Pupillary responses in the presence of lesions of the left optic tract, the pretectal part of the midbrain, the oculomotor nuclei and the left oculomotor nerve.

SIGNS OF MENINGEAL IRRITATION

Flex the neck to see whether there is any abnormal resistance to the movement or a reaction on the part of the patient (Fig. 11.148). Neck stiffness suggests meningeal irritation. Kernig's test is performed by flexing the leg at the hip with the knee flexed, then extending the leg at the knee. The patient may react as the leg is extended or there may be an obvious reflex spasm in the hamstring muscles. With deepening levels of coma, these signs of meningeal irritation disappear.

THE PUPILS

Examine the pupils for symmetry and size then test the direct light response using a bright pencil torch (Fig. 11.149). The presence of an optic tract lesion can sometimes be confirmed by finding a lack of response when light is shone into the eyes from the affected half field. A pathological process in the region of the pretectum will interrupt the pupillary light response. The pupils are midposition in size and fixed to light. Lesions of the oculomotor complex itself are likely to produce slightly irregular pupils fixed to all forms of stimulation. Disruption of the third nerve beyond the nucleus produces a characteristic eye position associated with a fixed dilated pupil.

In metabolic coma, the pupils remain reactive and symmetric, although often relatively small. Only in profound metabolic coma do the pupils become fixed. Certain drugs can influence pupil size or reactivity. Atropine will cause pupillary dilatation, as will overdosage of amphetamines or tricyclic antidepressants. Morphine derivatives, in excessive dosage, result in pinpoint pupils that retain their reactivity.

OCULAR MOVEMENTS

First note any spontaneous eye movements. In many unconscious patients the eyes roam from side-to-side. The movements are usually conjugate but may occasionally become disconjugate. At other times the eyes should remain in the midposition. Any deviation of one or both eyes implies a defect of oculomotor function unless there is a pre-existing strabismus.

Now assess eye movements. Having gently elevated the upper lids, firmly rotate the head laterally, then vertically (doll's head manoeuvre). If reflex eye movements are intact, the eyes move so as to leave them directed forwards. A more potent stimulus for reflex eye movement is achieved by caloric stimulation. Clear the external auditory meatus of any wax then inspect the tympanic membrane to ensure it is intact. Position the patient so that the head is elevated to approximately 30° above the horizontal and, using a soft rubber catheter, gently instil ice-cold water into the external auditory meatus. A total volume of about 50 ml suffices. If the brainstem reflexes are intact the eyes will tonically deviate to the side of the irrigated ear. It is usually not necessary to test reflex vertical movements. In order to do so, both ears have to be simultaneously irrigated with cold water (for down gaze) or warm water (for up gaze). Nystagmus is an unlikely finding in the comatose patient but a variety of vertical movements can occur. Commonly a rapid downward or upward conjugate movement followed by a gradual return to the midposition (ocular bobbing and reverse bobbing respectively) is observed.

Sustained horizontal ocular deviation indicates a frontal or brainstem lesion. In the former, the eyes deviate away from the side of the accompanying hemiplegia. In a brainstem lesion below the decussation of the supranuclear pathway for horizontal gaze, the eyes deviate to the opposite side and hence to the side of an accompanying hemiparesis. Failure of upgaze occurs in the early stages of central transtentorial herniation.

MOTOR RESPONSES

Motor function in the limbs can be assessed partly by observing the patient's posture and partly by assessing the response to pressure over the sternum or, for assessing the limb response by squeezing the nail bed of a digit or

the tendoachilles. Always test bilaterally; an absent response from one side alone suggests the likelihood of an interruption of the pyramidal tract supplying that side of the body. An appropriate response is one that withdraws the limb from the stimulus. The two principal inappropriate responses are decorticate and decerebrate posturing. In the former, the upper limbs flex and adduct, the lower limbs extend and plantar flex. This response typically follows an acute vascular event affecting the cerebral hemisphere or internal capsule. In decerebrate rigidity, the upper limbs are extended, adducted and hyperpronated, with the lower limbs fully extended. This pattern appears with lesions in the region of the pons that separate lower brainstem structures from descending pathways but it can also occur in some of the metabolic comas.

| **Differential diagnosis** |
| **Coma** |

Metabolic coma
- Hypoglycaemia
- Hyperglycaemia
- Uraemia
- Hepatic encephalopathy
- Hypercapnoea
- Drugs

Structural coma
- Hemisphere mass lesions: tumour, extradural haematoma, subdural haematoma
- Brainstem stroke

RESPIRATORY STATUS

A number of abnormal respiratory patterns in the unconscious patient may allow localisation of the lesion responsible for the coma (Fig. 11.150).

In Cheyne–Stokes respiration the respiratory rate waxes and wanes, with intervening periods of apnoea. The pattern is seen in metabolic coma but also with bilateral deep hemisphere lesions. Central neurogenic hyperventilation consists of a persistently increased rate of relatively deep breathing. It is triggered by lesions lying between the lower midbrain and the lower pons. Apneustic breathing results in short periods of respiratory arrest on inspiration. Pontine infarction is the usual cause. Ataxic respiration is erratic in timing and depth and is triggered by disturbances of the respiratory centres of the medulla.

Clinical application

There are significant differences between the neurological findings in patients whose coma has a metabolic basis and the findings in patients who have a structural lesion affecting the cerebral hemispheres or brainstem.

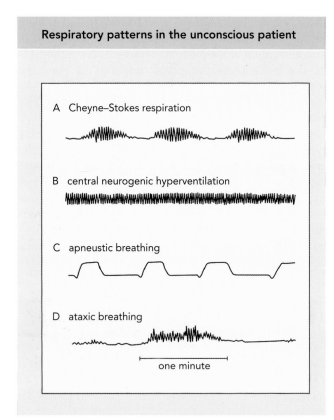

Respiratory patterns in the unconscious patient

A Cheyne–Stokes respiration

B central neurogenic hyperventilation

C apneustic breathing

D ataxic breathing

one minute

Fig. 11.150 Respiratory patterns.

METABOLIC COMA

Patients in metabolic coma usually pass through phases of waning consciousness during which they become less alert, apathetic and disorientated. The pupils remain reactive until the late stages of metabolic coma. The eyes remain central but reflex movement, even that elicited by caloric stimulation, may eventually be lost. The visual axes remain parallel and undeviated. Both generalised and focal motor seizures can occur. Decorticate or decerebrate posturing are seen and some patients (e.g. those with hypoglycaemia or hepatic coma) will display a hemiplegia that recovers when the metabolic abnormality is corrected. Myoclonic jerks occur in uraemia and in patients with hypercapnoea. In Wernicke's encephalopathy, the altered mental state is accompanied by ophthalmoplegia, nystagmus and ataxia. Papilloedema with intense retinal venous congestion is found in a small proportion of patients with respiratory failure. In drug-induced coma, although the doll's head and cold caloric responses are eventually lost, the pupils usually remain reactive until the very late stages.

STRUCTURAL CAUSES OF COMA

When supratentorial lesions cause coma, the pattern of development of physical signs allows differentiation between central and uncal herniation. The pattern may alter according to the speed with which the size of a supratentorial mass increases.

With central herniation, as the conscious state alters, the first eye movement abnormality observed is impairment of reflex upward gaze. The pupils remain reactive. As a hemisphere lesion is present, there is likely to be a contralateral hemiplegia. The ipsilateral limbs may show a diffuse increase in tone and the most likely respiratory arrhythmia is Cheyne–Stokes respiration (Fig. 11.151). Further signs appear as the transtentorial herniation proceeds. Horizontal eye movements become increasingly difficult to elicit, even using caloric stimulation. The pupils become fixed to light but remain midposition in size. Decorticate posturing of the unaffected side becomes decerebrate and the most likely breathing pattern to emerge is central neurogenic hyperventilation.

Uncal herniation produces a different picture, at least initially. The pupil of the eye ipsilateral to the lesion becomes dilated and this is followed by the development of an ophthalmoplegia. Initially, the contralateral pupil remains reactive and the eye moves fully with reflex stimulation but subsequently reflex movements are lost. The limbs ipsilateral to the lesion can develop a hemiplegic posture relatively early, due to compression of the contralateral cerebral peduncle against the tentorial edge (Fig. 11.152). Later bilateral decerebrate posturing appears. Central neurogenic hyperventilation is the most likely respiratory dysrhythmia.

The final stages of the two types of herniation are similar. Respiration becomes erratic and signs of cardiovascular instability emerge. Pupillary dilatation is a terminal event.

Supratentorial masses producing coma are usually vascular rather than neoplastic. Causes include extradural, subdural and primary intracerebral haemorrhage. The

Symptoms and signs

Assessment of coma

- Take history if possible
- Assess level of consciousness – use Glasgow coma scale but remember its limitations
- Look for signs of meningeal irritation
- Assess pupils
- Assess ocular movements, if necessary using doll's head manoeuvre
- Assess motor responses
- Assess respiration
- Perform a general physical examination, including the heart, the abdomen and the skull

Emergency

Coma

Consider myriad causes but specialist appraisal is mandatory

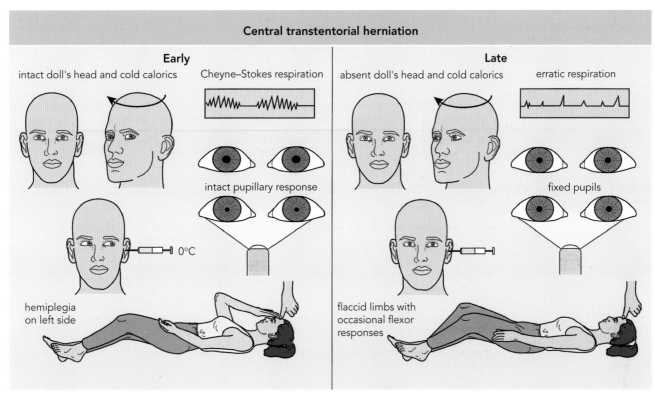

Fig. 11.151 Central transtentorial herniation.

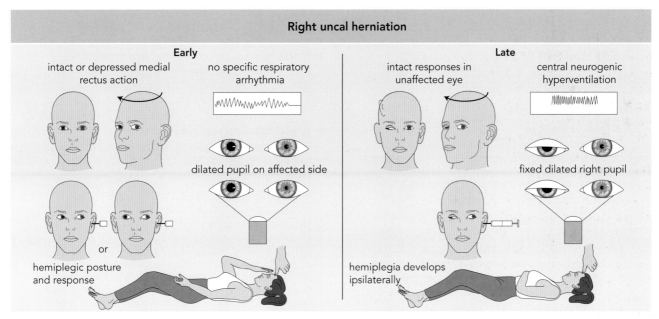

Fig. 11.152 Right uncal herniation.

spectrum of pathological processes in the brainstem producing coma is considerably wider and includes infarction, tumour and haemorrhage.

BRAIN DEATH

The end point of many structural and metabolic insults to the brain is a state in which a deeply comatose patient maintains circulatory function providing that respiration is supported by artificial means. There is good evidence to suggest that if brainstem function can be shown to have ceased in such patients, there is no prospect for recovery (Fig. 11.153). Criteria of brainstem death have been devised to appraise this state, in order to identify patients in whom further attempts at life-support are of no value (Fig. 11.154).

Brainstem reflexes

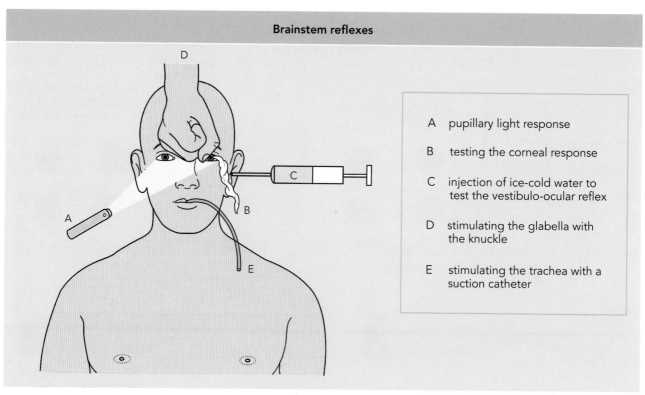

A   pupillary light response

B   testing the corneal response

C   injection of ice-cold water to test the vestibulo-ocular reflex

D   stimulating the glabella with the knuckle

E   stimulating the trachea with a suction catheter

Fig. 11.153 Testing brainstem reflexes.

Criteria for brain death

1. Pupillary response
Use a bright torch (not an ophthalmoscope) to confirm that the pupils fail to respond.

2. Corneal response
Gently apply a wisp of cotton wool to the cornea. There should be no response. Note that repeated testing can readily traumatise the cornea.

3. Vestibulo-ocular reflex
Inspect the tympanic membrane to ensure that it is intact and not obscured by compacted wax. Insert a soft rubber catheter into the external auditory meatus and slowly inject approximately 50 ml of ice-cold water. Repeat the test in the other ear. There should be no ocular deviation.

4. Motor response in cranial nerve distribution
This is most readily assessed by applying a painful stimulus to the glabella. The patient fails to respond.

5. Gag or tracheal response
Either stimulate the palate or pass a suction catheter into the trachea. The patient fails to show any response.

6. Respiratory reaction to hypercapnia
First administer a combination of 95% O_2 and 5% CO_2 via the respirator until the P_{CO_2} has risen above 6.0 kPa (40 mmHg). Disconnect the respirator but administer 100% oxygen through a tracheal catheter at around 6 l/min. Observe if any respiratory reponse occurs when the P_{CO_2} exceeds 6.7 kPa (50 mmHg).

Fig. 11.154 Criteria for diagnosing brain death.

The first essential, when applying these criteria, is to ensure that the coma is not the consequence of a metabolic or drug-induced state that is potentially reversible. Usually retesting is performed after a period of at least 24 h. This allows confirmation of the clinical diagnosis by another doctor and the positive exclusion of reversible factors. The responses to testing of brainstem function are likely to be depressed in the presence of hypothermia. The patient's body temperature must be above 35°C before testing is carried out. It must be clearly established that the patient's respiratory failure is not the consequence of neuromuscular blocking agents.

Stimulation of a peripheral nerve can be carried out to confirm that neuromuscular conduction is intact. Finally, a specific cause for the patient's coma must be identified. For most neurological disorders this will be evident from the patient's history or imaging. Identification of drug-induced or metabolic coma is likely to take longer.

There are certain spinal reflexes that can persist in the presence of brainstem death. These include the stretch reflexes, plantar responses or withdrawal and flexion of the upper or lower limb triggered by neck flexion. The United Kingdom criteria for brain death no longer include the presence of an isoelectric electroencephalogram recording, although this criterion still receives support in other countries, for instance the United States of America.

Examination of elderly people
The nervous system

Primitive reflexes
- Glabellar tap
  - found with increasing frequency with age
- Palmomental reflex
  - bilateral responses found with increasing frequency with age
- Snout and suckling reflexes
  - seldom, particularly the latter, found in normal, elderly, individuals
- Grasp reflex
  - the presence of grasp reflexes correlates with evidence of cognitive impairment

Cranial nerve function
- Smell
  - sensitivity declines after the age of 65 years
- Eyes
  - mild ptosis common in elderly people
  - upgaze declines with age
  - the light and accommodation responses decline with age and the pupils become more miosed

- Taste
  - sensitivity declines with age, with a higher threshold
- Hearing
  - declines with age

Motor system
- Reflexes
  - contrary to established teaching, the ankle jerks are preserved in old age
  - the abdominal responses diminish and their latency increases with age
- Movements
  - lingual–facial–buccal dyskinesias are found in elderly people without a history of neuroleptic drug exposure

Sensation
- Vibration
  - threshold for appreciation increases with age
- Two-point discrimination
  - threshold increases with age

Gait
- Becomes increasingly cautious with increasing age

Review
Framework for the routine examination of the nervous system

- Assess higher cortical function including orientation, memory, intelligence, speech and praxis, together with appraisal of the primitive reflexes
- Assess the patient's psychiatric status if that appears relevant
- Assess cranial nerve function (see p. 358)
- Assess motor function – appearance, tone, power, reflexes and involuntary movements

- Assess cerebellar function – speech, eye movements, limb coordination and gait
- Assess sensory function – as appropriate, testing light touch, two-point discrimination, proprioception, vibration sense, pain and temperature, and cortical sensory function
- Where relevant, carry out a standard protocol for assessing the unconscious patient

Infants and children

One of the challenges of paediatric medicine and child health is dealing with a range of patients, from the preterm newborn weighing less than 1 kg to the postpubertal 15-year-old weighing 55 kg. The younger the child, the more often he or she is brought to see the doctor, and the more different the consultation is from that described in previous chapters.

> 'Children are not just small adults – their needs are different and have to be recognised.'
>
> Professor James Spence, 1943

When examining children, the general principles of history-taking and examination also apply, although the manner and order in which they are approached differ: the convention of taking a history, inspecting, palpating, percussing and auscultating remain the cornerstones of all consultations but the emphasis is different in children.

Trainee doctors need basic skills to begin to feel confident in dealing with the child patient and their families.

For convenience, this chapter divides the child patient into five age categories, although these groups tend to merge into one another:

- Newborn and very young baby (0–8 weeks)
- Older baby and toddler (2–24 months)
- Preschool child (2–5 years)
- School child (5–10+ years)
- Adolescent (10+ to approximately 16 years).

In each section of this chapter, the discussion of growth, development, history-taking and examination of systems will take into account important age-related differences.

Taking a history

History-taking is the key part of an assessment of a child's condition. The diagnosis is often revealed by a well-taken history, with the examination findings confirming or refuting the working diagnosis revealed during the history. In previous chapters, advice was given on how to approach patients who provide their own histories of complaints and symptoms; children come to the doctor with their parents and it is the parents who usually supply these details, although older children will often make important contributions.

Listen to the parents: they know their child best and, generally, if they describe a problem then there is a diagnosis to be made. The younger the child the more reliant you will be on the parents' account of the problem. Sometimes acute anxiety about a child's well-being, coupled with parental exhaustion, leads to difficulties in effective communication between parent and doctor but if you can empathise with the parents' perspective it will help you to be a more understanding and compassionate doctor.

The older the children, the more you can communicate with them. The challenges lie in communicating effectively with children of different ages and abilities. This skill takes time to acquire; some will acquire it faster than others.

It is important to establish a rapport with the child and his or her parents and siblings. Introduce yourself to the child and other family members as you welcome them into the consulting area. Try and allow the children (including the siblings) to feel relaxed and comfortable during the consultation; this is more likely if there are a variety of toys and games lying about the room. Children up to and including school age may well prefer to be on a parent's lap, eventually feeling confident enough to explore the room during the history-taking.

After the presenting complaint has been defined, information about the child's previous well-being and that of the family and their circumstances need to be recorded.

In the very young child, history-taking should include information about the pregnancy, labour and delivery as well as the condition at birth and early feeding progress, details of immunisations and a developmental history. These details may become less relevant in the older child.

Previous illnesses, hospital or doctor attendances as well as recent and previous medications are required in any child's history.

The family history is important and can be clearly presented by using a two- or three-generation family tree. Include details about parents' and siblings' medical histories and make direct queries in line with the presenting problems. Include history of previous pregnancies and relevant pregnancy and prenatal problems (Fig. 12.1). If an autosomally recessive condition is being considered, it may be necessary to ask if the parents are consanguineously related. Although a large proportion of the world's families involve cousin marriages, this is a delicate subject that should be dealt with in a tactful way. One approach is to enquire if the parents have any relatives in common (e.g. grandparents or cousins) (Fig. 12.2).

At first it can seem intrusive to ask about the child's family and any surrounding issues. One approach is to tell the child and family that you are going to ask a number of routine questions about the child's background after hearing about the presenting complaints. The initial history-taking is the most 'natural' opportunity to collect this information, as having to go back and ask more questions out of the context of history-taking is more awkward.

The social history is separate from but allied to the family history. It is important to understand the composition of the household in which the child lives. The two-generation family tree can be further annotated with names, occupations and other details, helping to fill in details of the child's social history. It should include details about the parents' occupations and whoever else is helping with child care. Children old enough to be

Pedigrees and family trees

The pedigree chart is preferred by geneticists and uses specific symbols to demonstrate information about that family. This pedigree demonstrates an X-linked condition (e.g. G6PD deficiency) and an autosomal recessive inheritance

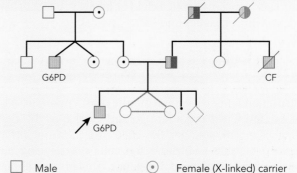

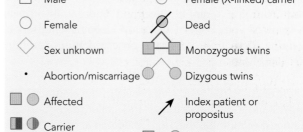

More social details about the family can be added. Some colleagues find this addition of information 'graffiti', others find it helpful as a 'map' of the child's family, helping the doctor to understand how the family and the diseases have interacted

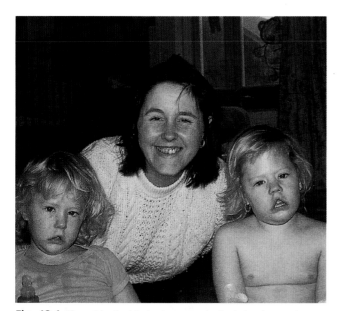

Fig. 12.1 These identical twins have myotonic dystrophy, as does their mother. This picture shows the phenomenon of 'anticipation', in which the condition is worse in each successive affected generation.

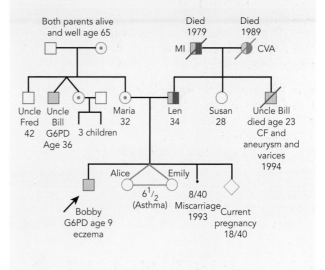

Fig. 12.2 The three-generation family tree.

attending nursery or school should be asked the name of the establishment as well as how they are getting on.

Child abuse is a common problem. Children can be harmed by adults in a number of different ways: emotionally, physically, neglected, sexually or, rarely, by induced illnesses and poisoning. The nature of any injury or illness in any child, from any background, must be explained satisfactorily in the history and be a plausible cause of the findings seen on examination. If you have any such concerns about a child or family you must share them with colleagues and social services.

The examination

Inspection and observation are the most important skills to be developed if you are going to arrive at the right diagnosis. The younger the child, the more important it is to be able to observe the child's well-being and any physical signs from a distance. This process should start from the moment the child and family appear in front of you. Do not wake up sleeping children to examine them until you have observed them carefully first (Fig. 12.3).

How one approaches a child to be examined is determined by the child's age, level of development and understanding. The younger the child (except in the youngest of infants), the more imaginative one may have to be to ensure a satisfactory consultation but remember it is easy to make older children and adolescents feel patronised.

Whenever possible try not to allow your eye level to be higher than that of your patient. If necessary, get down on the floor; this may be very basic psychology but it works. If you are approaching a child seated on its parent's lap or on a bed or couch, when you are within 1 metre of the patient the child should see you are coming down to eye level. This is especially important when several doctors congregate around a bed, for example, on ward rounds. Always remember what it is like from the child's perspective, especially when being surrounded by a group of unfamiliar adults.

It may take some time to win the confidence of young children. Sometimes the pyrexial, irritable child may not allow you any physical contact without crying and, despite a friendly approach, it may also be impossible to observe the child at rest. Once a child starts crying it may be difficult to continue with the examination.

Palpation and auscultation may be important parts of the physical assessment. The order in which you perform them depends on where the problem is, what the problem is likely to be and how ill and how cooperative your young patient is. Whenever possible start peripherally with the hands or feet, making it clear to the child that you are a friendly doctor. Percussion is rarely a rewarding process in the very young.

Young patients should think the examination is fun. If you present yourself as playing a game, they will be relaxed and you will gain more information; if a child is frightened or in pain, then this can be impossible to achieve. Make the child comfortable first. Ensure your hands are clean and warm and that your stethoscope will not be too cold on the child's skin.

Avoid unpleasant procedures if at all possible (e.g. rectal examinations). Think of what implications your actions may have in the future: if your examination and care of a child does not cause upset, and you relieve pain and discomfort effectively, that child is more likely to tolerate future examinations. It is better to have a limited but tolerable examination than to try and complete a full

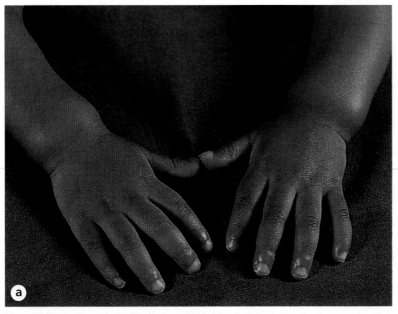
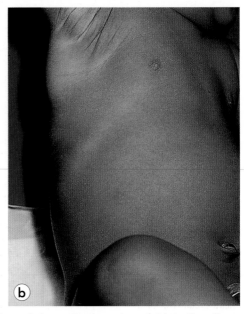

Figs 12.3 Swollen wrists (a) and rib ends (b) seen in rickets. Observation may be all that is needed to notice these signs of rickets. Sometimes these findings are coincidental to the presenting problem.

examination that results in an inconsolable child because the child is more likely to be uncooperative next time.

Growth and development

Growth involves an increase in size and concludes when an individual has acquired full size and reproductive capabilities. Development parallels growth and leads to individuals acquiring all the skills and attributes that enable them to achieve full independence from their parents and to raise their own children.

GROWTH

Compared with other mammals and primates, human offspring are very immature and dependent. A human newborn is completely dependent for most of its first year until weaned and walking. Our newborns have a head that is only just small enough to be delivered through the average woman's pelvis. The cerebral neuronal network is almost complete at birth, but is more or less devoid of myelin, whereas most other species have completed this essential 'wiring' before the end of gestation, hence the more advanced abilities of their newborns. If the growth in head (or occipital frontal) circumference (Fig. 12.4) of

a child in the first year of life is extrapolated into the volume of brain growth, it is clear why humans cannot have more developed newborns – this is the price *Homo sapiens* pays for being bipedal with a narrow pelvis and large brain.

The continuum of growth from baby to adult has been described by three main phases (Fig. 12.5):

- Infant phase: a continuation of the exponential fetal growth rate that slows down in the second year of life. Critical factors are nutrition and hormones controlling metabolism (e.g. insulin-like growth factors such as IGF_1).
- Childhood phase: this extends from the second to beyond the 10th year. Critical factors are the pituitary hormones (especially growth hormone).
- Adolescent (pubertal) phase: this extends from the onset of puberty until the achievement of final adult stature and fully mature reproductive capabilities. Critical factors are the sex steroids (androgens and oestrogens).

Each of the phases is interdependent on a large number of factors such as genetics, nutrition, hormones and the environment (including love and affection) (Fig. 12.6).

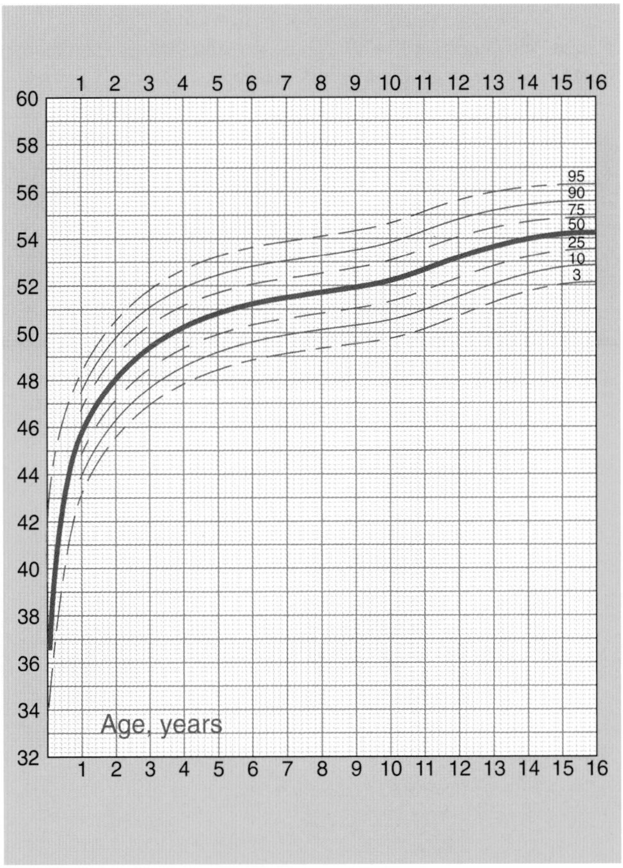

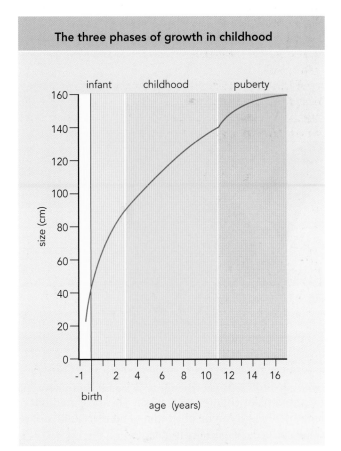

The three phases of growth in childhood

Fig. 12.4 Head circumference chart. The phenomenal growth in head circumference seen during the first years of life is as a result of brain myelination, without which the infant's development cannot advance. (© Child Growth Foundation, adapted with permission.)

Fig. 12.5 Three phases of growth in childhood (after Professor J. Karlberg). The growth velocity varies at different ages – this is as result of many variable influences. Karlberg summarised the continuum into three phases, each with their own principal factors.

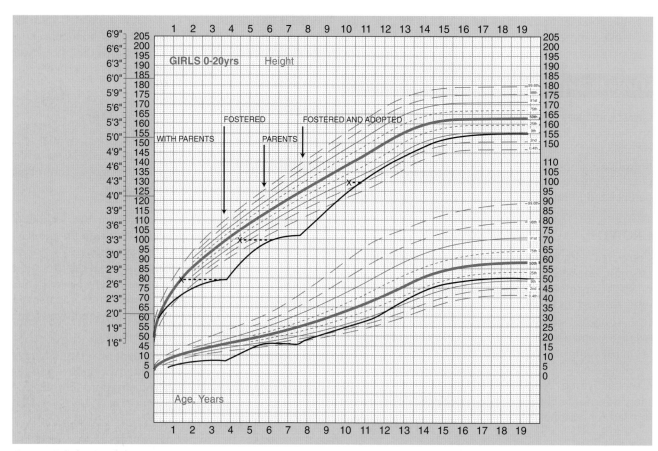

Fig. 12.6 Nonorganic failure to thrive. For some children who are not growing as well as expected, no organic cause can be identified. If they are removed from their home environment, their growth velocities may accelerate. The importance of an affectionate and loving environment for normal growth and development cannot be over estimated. (© Child Growth Foundation, adapted with permission.)

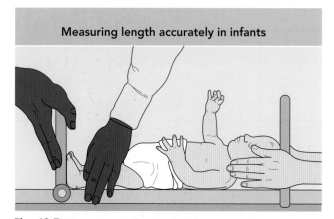

Fig. 12.7 Measurement of supine length.

Any examination of a child is incomplete without an assessment of growth and development. It is usual to assess weight in all ages, supine length (Fig. 12.7) and head circumference in infants (<2 years), and standing height in older children (Fig. 12.8). The measurement of length or height can be misleading and inaccurate unless done correctly, especially in infants.

Growth charts are used to help determine the expected range at any given age; there are standards derived for most developed nations and by the World Health Organization. Either the standard deviation scores either

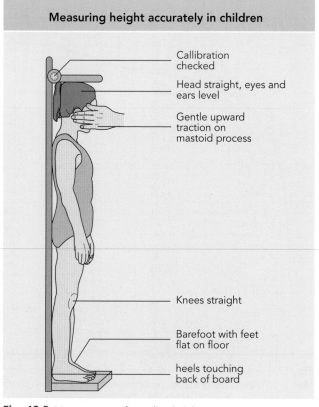

Fig. 12.8 Measurement of standing height.

side of the mean, or centiles are used to recognise the different normal variations in growth and growth velocity. The more serial measurements there are available to plot, the more certain one can be about whether the pattern of growth falls within an expected range (Figs 12.9, 12.10).

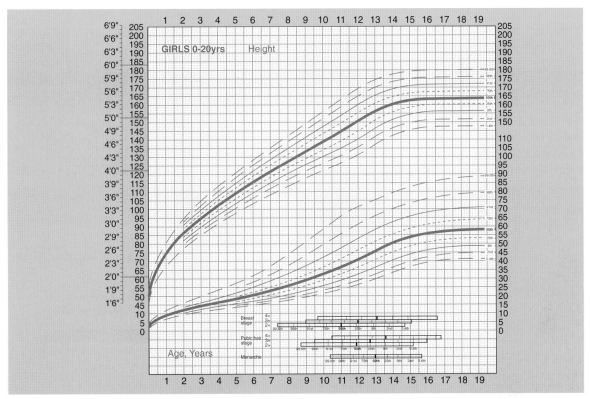

Fig. 12.9 Childhood Growth Foundation (UK) growth charts for girls. (© Child Growth Foundation, adapted with permission.) For pubertal stages see Figs 8.1, 8.3 and 12.44.

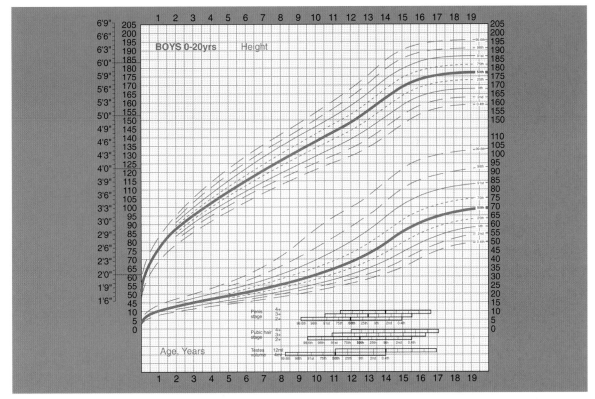

Fig. 12.10 Childhood Growth Foundation (UK) growth charts for boys. The charts for boys and girls are British standards derived from longitudinal data observed in cohorts of British children with cross-sectional observations used in updating them. (© Child Growth Foundation, adapted with permission.) For pubertal stages see Figs 9.4 and 12.44.

DEVELOPMENT

Evaluation of a child's development is more complicated than assessment of growth because of the large variation in the normal patterns of development. Furthermore, an individual child's rate of development can vary, and there are also confounding transcultural and transracial differences.

Although newborn babies are dependent, they can hear, smell, taste, feel and see. By the end of their development they will be able to think and solve problems, be mobile and agile, develop innumerable skills and be capable of rearing their own children.

For convenience, development is usually considered under eight main headings, which can be easily remembered as four sets of pairs:

* Gross motor   Motor skills
* Fine motor   Motor skills
* Vision   Special senses
* Hearing   Special senses
* Expressive language   Communication

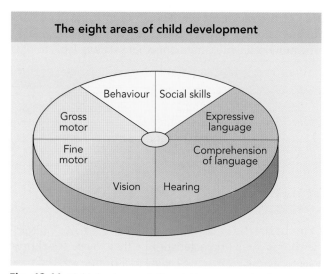

The eight areas of child development

Fig. 12.11 Child development. The eight areas are closely interdependent. To reflect this, some group hearing with speech and vision with fine motor.

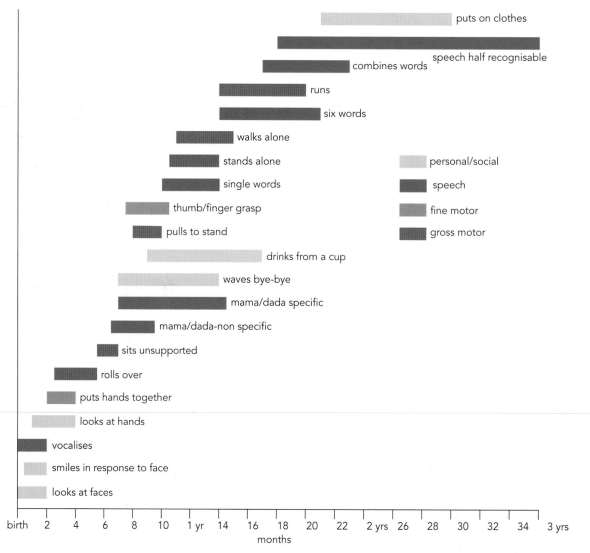

Fig. 12.12 Outline of some important common developmental milestones. The bar represents the typical age of acquisition, the right-hand end representing when >90% of healthy normal children should have acquired these skills.

- Comprehension   Communication
- Social skills   Psychosocial
- Behaviour   Psychosocial

Various schemes have been elaborated to help health professionals determine whether a child is developing along an expected pattern of 'normality'. Some of these schemes are merely screening devices; others are more elaborate and describe an infant or an infant's abilities more thoroughly (Figs 12.11, 12.12).

The newborn and very young baby

Only babies born at term are discussed here; preterm newborns have characteristics of their own. Newborns (called neonates when <4 weeks old) are extraordinary patients to be involved with. At birth they are 'untried' in terms of most homeostatic processes. They have recently completed the transition from the relatively hypoxic environment of the uterus, where they were dependent on the placental circulation (Fig. 12.13), and have had to cope with the stress of delivery, including huge adaptations in their cardiorespiratory physiology to enable them to breathe air.

Newborns and young babies are examined routinely at birth, at approximately 6–8 weeks of age and when receiving immunisations. They are usually seen by doctors (e.g. general practitioners, paediatric resident staff or specially trained midwives) trained in their care. They are also seen if they are acutely ill by doctors unaccustomed to young babies (e.g. accident department staff).

Specific aspects about the 'routine neonatal examination' are discussed at the end of this section.

GROWTH

Newborns appear on the steepest part of the infant growth curve. They tend to lose 5–10% of their birth weight in the first week but then steadily gain an average of 25–30 g/day over the next 6 months. The length measurement of newborns and infants is likely to be unacceptably inaccurate unless a supine stadiometer is used (see Fig. 12.7). The head circumference is a valuable measurement during this period. Care needs to be taken when measuring the true head circumference: use a nonstretchable tape, applied closely around the scalp and take the largest circumference obtained around the occiput and forehead. With correct technique a reliable interobserver measurement to within ±0.1 cm can be obtained (Fig. 12.14).

DEVELOPMENT

At birth, the newborn can hear, smell, taste, feel and see (but only up to approximately 30 cm). The social smile (smiling in response to smiling and cooing parents) is a very important milestone of higher cortical function. Most behaviour observed in newborns before this event is the result of responses initiated by the brainstem and spinal cord, for example, startling to sound and the primitive reflexes.

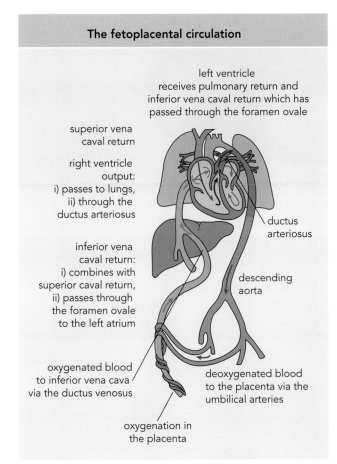

The fetoplacental circulation

left ventricle receives pulmonary return and inferior vena caval return which has passed through the foramen ovale

superior vena caval return

right ventricle output:
i) passes to lungs,
ii) through the ductus arteriosus

ductus arteriosus

inferior vena caval return:
i) combines with superior caval return,
ii) passes through the foramen ovale to the left atrium

descending aorta

oxygenated blood to inferior vena cava via the ductus venosus

deoxygenated blood to the placenta via the umbilical arteries

oxygenation in the placenta

Fig. 12.13 The fetoplacental circulation. The fetal cardiorespiratory blood flow is in parallel rather than in series after birth with the closure of the foramen ovale and the ductus arteriosus.

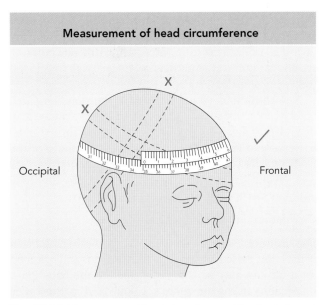

Measurement of head circumference

X

X

Occipital   Frontal

✓

Fig. 12.14 Measurement of head circumference. The simplest 'investigation' in paediatric neurology.

HISTORY

The feeding history is important because feeding is the most strenuous action the newborn has to do. Any compromise in cardiorespiratory function is revealed in difficulty in taking or completing feeds. In breastfed babies, it is difficult to be certain how well the feeding is progressing because the quantities of feed are unknown. Mothers breastfeeding for the first time may not be sure how well they (both) are doing. Ask the mother how often and for how long her baby breastfeeds, how she feels the feeds are progressing, and whether she has any subjective feelings of let down of milk. Documented weight gain in the baby and the mother feeling that her breasts empty are helpful indicators. With bottle-fed babies it should be easy to ask about quantities of infant formula taken.

Details about maternal health, the pregnancy and delivery, as well as the baby's condition and birth weight, are important to record. Apart from any parental concerns, ask about vitamin K administration, jaundice, stools and how the baby responds to handling. Pay close attention to what an experienced mother's observations have to say about her baby: she will have spent a great deal of time observing the baby closely; if she perceives something different about this baby then it may be an important diagnostic clue.

EXAMINATION

Newborns and young babies are examined when they are acutely ill or, more commonly, during routine checks. The observation and skills used are common to both the acute and routine situations. You should plot the progress of weight and head circumference on a centile chart. The baby must be undressed to be fully examined.

The very young (like the very old) often have nonspecific symptoms and signs even when they are seriously ill. Doctors in training need to know the most important signs and symptoms of serious ill health in the very young. To help less experienced carers of newborns, a scoring system for symptoms and signs was developed (see 'symptoms and signs' box).

Newborns and young babies can become very sick quickly. Infections should be included in the differential diagnosis of any sick baby. These infections can often be bacterial and serious. It is good practice to think of the likely infection and how it was acquired and to complete a full septic screen and give broad-spectrum parenteral antibiotics until the culture results are known.

Circulation and cardiovascular

The order of examination will depend on the condition of the baby. Auscultation of the heart sounds and listening for murmurs may be the priority before the baby cries. Inspection of the newborn's colour and perfusion is crucial. Peripheral cyanosis is common in the first days of the newborn period (acrocyanosis) because of vasoconstriction and relative polycythaemia (haemoglobin range 14.9–23.7 g/dl at birth): capillary refill time may therefore be more sluggish. Central cyanosis is best observed in the tongue and mucous membranes; these may be the only sites that are noticeably blue in cyanosed nonwhite babies. On inspection, the only signs of congenital heart disease may be respiratory distress at rest. A pale baby may be anaemic or even hypoxic.

The rate, rhythm and character of the brachial and femoral pulses (Fig. 12.15) need to be assessed. Weak or absent femoral pulses may suggest coarctation of the aorta, as would four-limb blood pressure measurements demonstrating an upper limb to lower limb gradient in blood pressure. Large volume pulses are found with a patent ductus arteriosus. The precordium should be palpated and the presence of an apex beat (usually on the left) and heaves or thrills noted (Fig. 12.16).

The separation of the two components of the second heart sound on auscultation may be difficult because of the baby's fast heart rate (Fig. 12.17). A single second heart sound may indicate pulmonary outflow obstruction. Innocent (non-pathological) systolic murmurs are

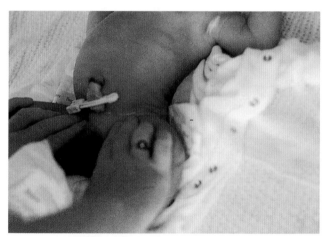

Fig. 12.15 Palpating femoral pulses. The femoral pulse can be difficult to feel; use a point halfway from pubic tubercle to anterior superior iliac spine as a guide and do not press so firmly as to occlude the pulsation.

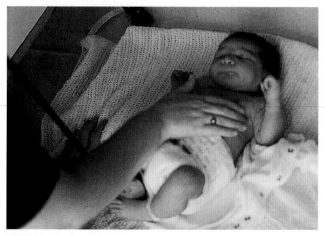

Fig. 12.16 Palpating the apex beat. Palpate the whole precordium, left and right. The apex beat is usually palpated in the left fifth intercostal space in the midclavicular line.

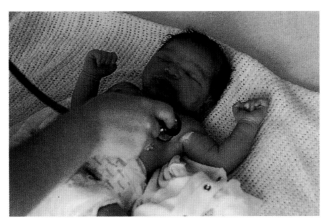

Fig. 12.17 Auscultating the heart sounds and listening for murmurs. Even when the baby is asleep, it can be hard at first to differentiate the first and second heart sound; palpating a brachial or femoral pulse simultaneously may help you.

Symptoms and signs

The baby check

Baby check* is a system to help parents, health professionals and carers assess the seriousness of a baby's illness. It uses 19 signs and symptoms with scores which, when added together, give a total score which correlates with the seriousness of the baby's illness. The scoring system has been validated for use by parents, doctors and nurses in babies under 1 year old.

Signs	Symptoms	Score
1. Unusual cry	e.g. high-pitched, weak, moaning or painful	2
2. Fluids taken in previous 24 h	Less than normal	2
	Half normal	4
	Very little	9
3. Vomiting	Vomiting at least half of a feed in the three previous feeds	4
4. Vomiting bile	Any green bile in vomit	13
5. Wet nappies (urine output)	Less urine than normal	3
6. Blood in nappy	Large amount of blood in nappy	11
7. Drowsiness	Occasionally drowsy	3
	Drowsy most of the time	5
8. Floppiness	Baby seems more floppy than normal	4
9. Watching	Baby less watchful than normal	2
10. Awareness	Baby responding less than normally to the surroundings	2
11. Breathing difficulties	Minimal recession visible	4
	Obvious recession visible	15
12. Looking pale	Baby more pale than normal, or been pale in last 24 h	3
13. Wheezing	Baby has wheezing breath sounds	2
14. Blue nails	Apparent blue nails	3
15. Circulation	Baby's toes are white, or stay white for 3 s after squeezing	3
16. Rash	Rash over body, or raw weeping area >5 cm × 5 cm	4
17. Hernia	Obvious bulge in scrotum or groin	13
18. Temperature (rectal)	Temperature >38.3°C by rectal thermometer	4
19. Crying during checks	If baby has cried during checks (more than a grizzle)	4

Total scores

0–7 Baby is only a little unwell, medical attention is not necessary

8–12 Baby is unwell but not seriously; seek advice from doctor, health visitor or midwife

13–19 Baby is ill; contact your doctor and arrange to be seen

>20 Baby is seriously ill and needs to be seen by a doctor immediately

If the baby appears to be worse after a low score, re-examine the baby and re-score.

*Adapted from the 'BabyCheck' booklet with permission.

Review

Normal range for newborns

- Heart rate: 110–160 beats/min (>180 tachycardia)
- Systolic blood pressure: 50–85 mmHg (very variable, depending on age, gestation and weight)
- Respiratory rate: 30–50 breaths/min (>60 tachypnoea)

Questions to ask

Jaundice in young babies

- Was the baby jaundiced in the first 24 hours of life?
- Was the baby still jaundiced during the third week of life?
- Is the baby well, thriving and gaining weight?
- What is the colour of the stools and the urine?

Symptoms and signs

Respiratory distress

- Tachypnoea (normal upper limit varies with age)
- Recession (includes subcostal, intercostals or tracheal tug)
- Grunting (an end-expiratory groaning noise, breathing out against partially adducted vocal cords and providing self-positive end expiratory pressure)
- Flaring of nostrils (the alae nasi are accessory muscles of respiration)
- Cyanosis (may be subclinical, so check oxygen saturation with pulse oximeter)
- Apnoea (may be how a very young baby presents with a respiratory disorder, associated with a colour change – pallor or cyanosis)
- A periodic breathing pattern may be noted in preterm or very young babies and is physiological, often with pauses of 3–5 seconds being observed (especially during sleep) without a change in colour being seen

The presence of jaundice is very common. When seen in the first 24 hours of life it is usually due to a pathological haemolytic process. A physiological jaundice is extremely common after the second day, continuing into the second week. It is usually related to breastfeeding. If jaundice is in association with pale stools, dark urine or failure to thrive, then pathological hepatic or obstructive cause is much more likely. Bilirubin in the urine requires investigation.

The gastrointestinal tract starts at the mouth and ends at the anus. Both ends need to be looked at. The palate must be inspected for clefts and palpated for clefts (Fig. 12.18). The position and patency of the anus needs to be checked (Fig. 12.19). While viewing the perineum, the external genitalia should be inspected. In boys, both

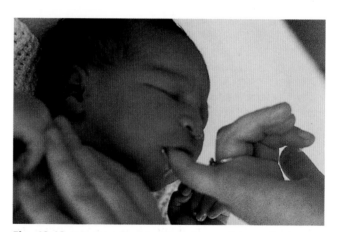

Fig. 12.18 Palpation of palate. The palate needs inspection by direct vision and palpation.

common in the newborn and may be heard on day 1 in over 20% babies who have structurally normal hearts. Pansystolic and continuous murmurs are suspicious, as are ejection systolic murmurs that radiate to the back or neck. Many babies with structural congenital heart disease may not have a murmur, although they may have symptoms and other signs of cardiovascular disease.

Breathing and respiration

The presence of respiratory distress is the most important observation to be made. Auscultatory signs are usually far less significant than the observation one makes as a baby is undressed.

Remember that all babies are obligate nose-breathers during feeding and nasal obstruction may manifest as a feeding problem. The presence of audible inspiratory stridor or a hoarse cry warrants further evaluation.

Abdomen

Observing a feed and inspection of stools can be important parts of the evaluation. The vomiting or 'posseting' of small quantities of milk is common but bile-stained vomiting warrants urgent assessment.

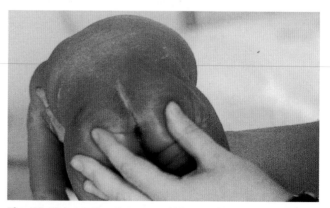

Fig. 12.19 Inspecting the anus. Ask if meconium has been passed during the first 24 hours.

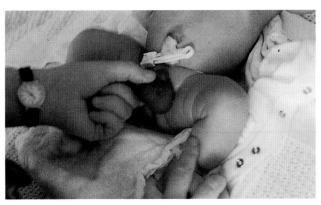

Fig. 12.20 Palpation of male genitalia. At term both testes should be well in the scrotum. Hydroceles are common. If the testes are not in the scrotum, can you feel them in the inguinal canal?

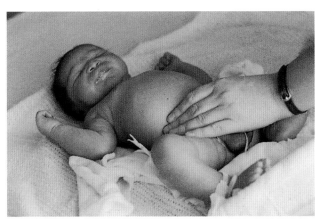

Fig. 12.22 Palpation of liver edge. Most babies and infants have a 1 cm palpable liver edge.

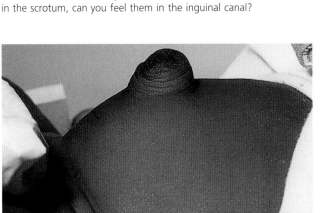

Fig. 12.21 Umbilical hernia. Umbilical hernias are very common (especially in some racial groups). They do not obstruct, they resolve spontaneously and need no treatment. Paraumbilical hernias, however, will require surgery.

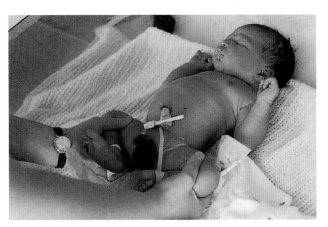

Fig. 12.23 Examining the hips (abduction). Ortolani manoeuvre may detect relocation of dislocated hips.

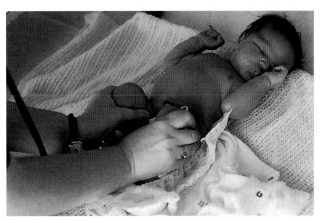

Fig. 12.24 Examining the hips (adduction). Barlow's manoeuvre may detect dislocatable hips.

testes should be in the scrotum (Fig. 12.20). Small hydroceles are common and need no action. If hernias are suspected then make a prompt referral to a paediatric surgeon. The penis should have a normally sited urethral orifice with a foreskin adherent to the glans (this adherence is physiological and should not be interfered with). In girls there should be an introitus and a normally sized clitoris. Any ambiguity in the genitalia requires urgent assessment by a paediatric endocrinologist before sex is assigned.

The abdomen should not be distended. Divarication of the rectus abdominis muscles is common, as are umbilical hernias (Fig. 12.21); neither require any treatment. The umbilical stump has usually separated by the 10th day.

A liver edge is usually palpable (approximately 1 cm below the costal margin) (Fig. 12.22) and the lower pole of the right kidney and a spleen tip are sometimes palpable.

Examine the hips while the nappy is off. The Ortolani and Barlow manoeuvres are used to detect abnormalities in the hip joint. These manoeuvres must be done very gently and should not cause the baby distress. A unilateral dislocated (subluxed) hip may be found on inspection,

with apparent shortening of the thigh. This might be confirmed when abduction is restricted and when anterior pressure on the greater trochanter (Fig. 12.23) results in feeling a 'clunk' as the femoral head relocates in the acetabulum (Ortolani's test). With the hip flexed and the thigh adducted and with pushing posteriorly in the line of the femur, a posterior dislocation of the femoral head will 'clunk' back out of the acetabulum as the thigh is abducted (Barlow's manoeuvre) (Fig. 12.24). Do not

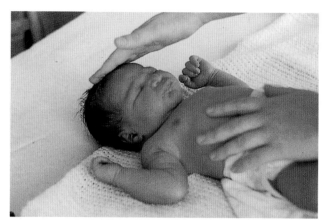

Fig. 12.25 Palpation on the fontanelle. Note the tone and size of anterior and posterior fontanelles.

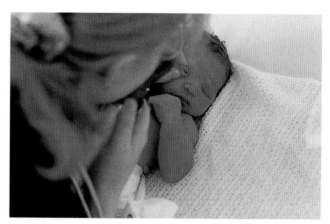

Fig. 12.27 Ophthalmoscopy of the red reflex. Never omit this check; if eyes are closed, come back later.

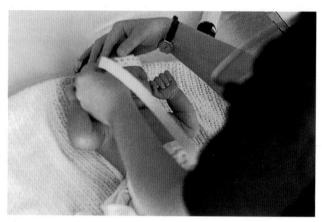

Fig. 12.26 Measuring the head circumference. Be accurate because this measurement may need to be referred to at a future date.

tone or movement must only be considered if the baby's head is in the neutral position in the midline. The asymmetric tonic neck reflex is a strong influence on posture and movement. The rest of the primitive reflexes may then be helpful if there are concerns about movement. The Moro (startle) reflex is an unpleasant stimulus to the baby and should not be done without a good reason (e.g. in evaluating a potential Erb's palsy).

The baby should be able to fix on and follow an object through 90°. Using an ophthalmoscope, look for the presence of a red reflex in each eye (Fig. 12.27). Any absent red reflex may be due to a cataract and warrants an urgent expert ophthalmological assessment. Squints can be normal when under 8 weeks old but should diminish with age.

Young babies should startle to loud noises (e.g. telephone ringing or door slamming) and should quieten to sounds that are loud and constant (e.g. vacuum cleaners).

attempt this examination unless you have been trained in it.

Neurology and development

A feel of the anterior fontanelle (Fig. 12.25) is part of the ritual of a paediatrician's assessment of a newborn baby. Fontanelle size is very variable and its tone is altered by crying. Bulging fontanelles indicate raised intracranial pressure, as in hydrocephalus, meningitis or other causes of space-occupying lesions. A cranial ultrasound scan will quickly and easily demonstrate enlarged ventricles and may show other causes of bulging fontanelles.

Inspection and palpation of the baby's head is always warranted. Moulding or caput is common in the first 24 hours, as is a 'chignon' after a ventouse delivery. Swelling over either parietal bones is usually caused by cephalohaematomas (subperiosteal bleeds), which are bounded by suture lines and which may persist for weeks. The head circumference should be measured (Fig. 12.26).

The best way to assess a newborn's nervous system is to observe the baby. Eliciting all the primitive reflexes is less helpful than observation. Any asymmetry of

Review

Low birth weight (LBW) babies

- Important because of the increased morbidity and mortality seen in the affected infants
- You must differentiate between babies who are preterm, normal for gestation or small for gestational age
- LBW defined as <2.5 kg birth weight; about 7% of UK births
- Babies >2.5 kg birth weight may be at risk of similar complications because of antenatal growth retardation such babies appear emaciated.
- Very low birth weight (VLBW) defined as <1.5 kg; about 1% of UK births (mostly all preterm)
- Extreme low birth weight (ELBW) defined as <1.0 kg; about 0.5% of UK births (almost exclusively very preterm)

Review

Gestation and weight at gestation

- Term – born 37–42 completed weeks gestation from last menstrual period (LMP)
- Preterm – born before 37 completed weeks (259 days) gestation from LMP – note that a preterm baby's age can be expressed as either a chronological (uncorrected) age or an age postconception (corrected); the latter is important when considering growth and development in the first 2 years
- Post-term – born after 42 completed weeks (294 days) gestation from LMP
- Small for gestational age or 'small for dates' – birth weight below 10th centile for gestational age
- Large for gestational age or 'large for dates' – birth weight greater than 90th centile for gestational age

THE ROUTINE NEONATAL EXAMINATION

Most developed countries have a policy of examining all neonates in the first few days of life. This examination has a number of objectives. It is a form of screening, attempting to identify congenital abnormalities that may benefit from intervention. It also provides an opportunity to answer whatever questions the parents may have about their new baby.

This examination is best performed at or beyond 24 hours of age. This is often not possible with earlier discharge from delivery units. The older the baby, the more confident one can be in diagnosing 'normality'.

Examine neonates in front of the parents. The examiner can review the mother's notes and take a history of maternal and family health, the progress during pregnancy, the results of antenatal tests (such as ultrasound anomaly scans) and an account of the delivery and condition of the newborn at birth. Subsequent feeding history and whether the baby has passed meconium and urine normally are important.

Dysmorphology terms

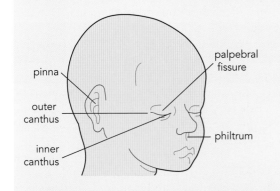
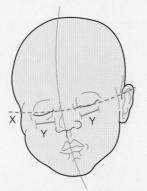
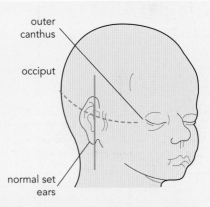

The proportions of a baby's face when viewed from the front, with a line through the eyes is about half way from vertex to chin (x), the **palpebral fissures** (the slits through which your eyes look) should be of equal length (y) measured from inner to outer **canthus**. There is usually a very mild slant to the palpebral fissures, if this slant is exaggerated then it is described as **upward slanting** (as may be seen in Trisomy 21, Down syndrome). Alternatively, the slant may be in the opposite direction and is described as **downward slanting** (as may be seen in many syndromes).
The distance between the eyes is approximately that of the palpebral fissures (y).
Hypotelorism is when this distance is too short and **hypertelorism** is when this distance is too long and the eyes appear too far apart.
The **philtrum** leads from the nostrils to the edge of the upper lip.
A line from the outer canthus towards the occiput should cross the attachment of the upper helix of the **pinna** (ear lobe) to the side of the head. Where this does not occur then the ear is described as **low set** and may appear **simple** (poorly formed helix) and **rotated** as well.

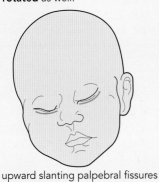
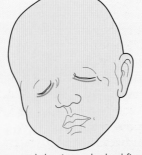

upward slanting palpebral fissures   downward slanting palpebral fissures   low set and rotated ear

Fig. 12.28 Facial dysmorphology vocabulary explained. A few of the commonly referred to anatomical terms used in describing facial features are demonstrated.

Neonatal examination

Here is an approach to help you remain systematic in your approach to examining newborns. The more important congenital anomalies tend to occur on or near the midline, so using a constant point of origin (e.g. the mouth) start examining the neonate along the midline, circumnavigating the entire baby and arriving back at your point of origin. At some points you may stray from the midline (e.g. to look at the eyes, or auscultate the heart). At the end do not forget the hands, feet and hips need checking.

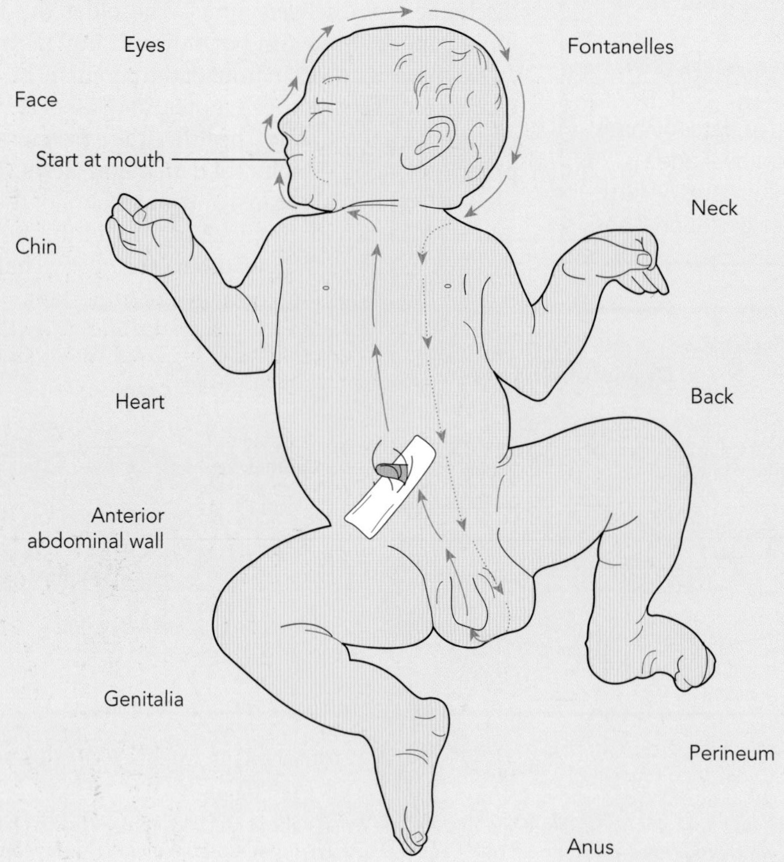

Eyes

Face

Start at mouth

Chin

Heart

Anterior abdominal wall

Genitalia

Fontanelles

Neck

Back

Perineum

Anus

Fig. 12.29 Scheme for examining newborns. By 'circumnavigating' the baby in a systematic way, most visible congenital abnormalities will be detected.

As neonates are 'new and untested', this examination, more than any other at a later date, is more likely to reveal congenital abnormalities. Single minor congenital abnormalities occur with a frequency of up to 14% of live births. The greater the number of congenital abnormalities, the greater the possibility that there may be more serious congenital abnormalities present. Severe and lethal congenital abnormalities are seen in about 1.5% of live births. It is worth understanding the descriptive terms used to describe dysmorphic signs (Fig. 12.28). The examiner needs to develop a systematic method of looking for and excluding dysmorphic features and congenital abnormalities. You must examine the undressed baby in a warm environment (Fig. 12.29).

There are a great number of minor findings that may be found on examination that are remarkable because they either are present at birth and resolve on their own or because they appear after birth but need further attention (Fig. 12.30).

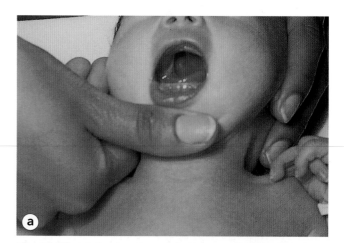

Fig. 12.30a Cleft palate. Inspect the palate and palpate for any clefts.

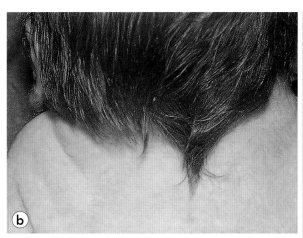

Fig. 12.30b Low hairline. Examine the scalp and hair and hairline. This may be indicative of a syndrome, a low hairline is seen in Turner's syndrome.

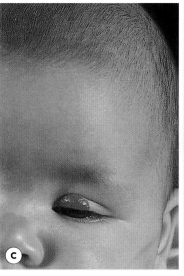

Fig. 12.30c Cavernous haemangioma. Cavernous haemangiomas ('strawberry naevus') can occur anywhere and are more common in preterm babies; they get bigger during the first year and eventually regress. Treatment is only indicated if the naevus interferes with breathing, feeding or vision or if otherwise problematic.

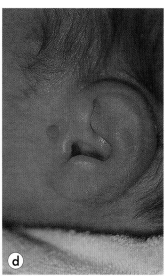

Fig. 12.30d Preauricular tags. Preauricular tags are common and often there is a family history. They may represent a cosmetic problem requiring plastic surgery or they may be associated with other otological abnormalities.

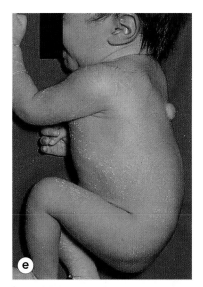

Fig. 12.30e Thoracic myelocele. Neural tube defects are now less prevalent in developed countries. Examine the back carefully by inspection and palpation from occiput to coccyx. If a neural tube defect is detected, remember to examine for signs of hydrocephalus and bladder and bowel function as well as dislocated hips.

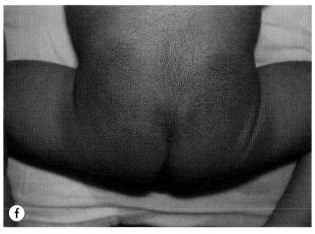

Fig. 12.30f Blue spots. These 'Mongolian' blue spots are common in all racial groups (except those of Northern White European origin). They are present from birth and may persist beyond the third year.

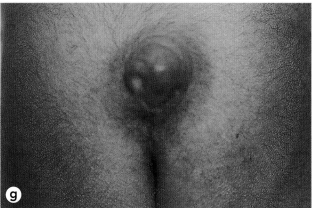

Fig. 12.30g Lumbar meningomyelocele. Lumbosacral neural tube defects are the most common. Folic acid supplements before conception and in early pregnancy have helped to reduce the incidence of these serious malformations.

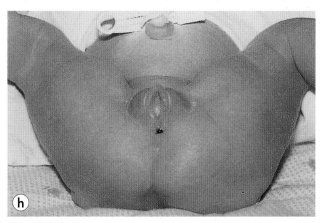

Fig. 12.30h Imperforate anus. Anogenital abnormalities need to be excluded by careful history and inspection. Meconium can be passed via a fistula into any other cloacal structure (e.g. the vagina). These abnormalities are seen associated with other congenital abnormalities.

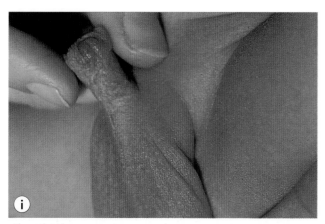

Fig. 12.30i Hypospadias. Check that the foreskin has fused normally on the ventral surface of the glans. If it has not, then note where the external urethral meatus is sited. Hypospadias occurs when the urethral meatus is not at the tip of the glans; commonly it is mild and on the glans, or rarely, more severe and on the shaft of the penis or perineum. Check for fixed flexion of the penis (chordee).

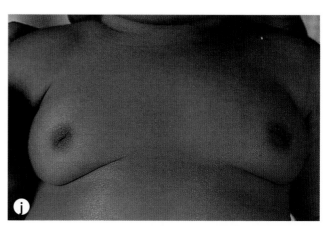

Fig. 12.30j Neonatal breast development. The influence of maternal hormones may result in palpable breast tissue of babies of either sex. No action is required and this resolves spontaneously.

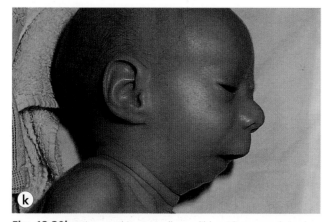

Fig. 12.30k Micrognathia. A small mandible with a normal-sized tongue represents a potential hazard to this baby's airway. A cleft palate can be associated. Breathing and feeding may need some assistance.

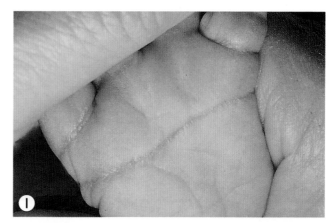

Fig. 12.30l Single palmar crease. A single palmar crease can be a normal finding. However, it can be part of a series of minor observations which can add up to a more important diagnosis, such as Down's syndrome.

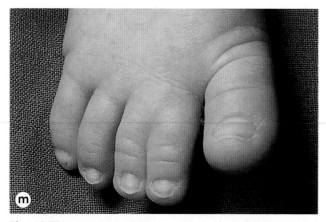

Fig. 12.30m Syndactyly of the second and third toes. Minor congenital abnormalities like this, when isolated, are common and often familial. Noticing one minor finding should prompt you to ensure there is not another to be observed.

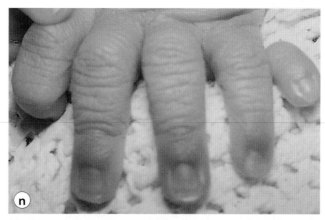

Fig. 12.30n Postaxial extra digit. Also very common and often familial. Refer for a plastic surgery consultation, rather than having them 'tied off'.

- Newborns have to adapt from an aqueous, thermally-regulated environment to the outside world. They have to keep their skin moist and stay warm. There are a variety of cutaneous phenomena that are benign and self-limiting.
- Confusion can occur when trying to differentiate between staphylococcal septic spots (not common but serious) (Fig. 12.31) and erythema toxicum, a transient eosinophilic infiltration of the skin (very common and completely benign) (Fig. 12.32). The former spots are often in skin creases and get bigger and 'more angry', the latter look red but are transient and appear anywhere on the baby.

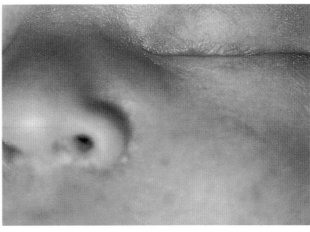

Fig. 12.31 Staphylococcal skin infection. The appearance of pustules in moist skin creases that do not spontaneously go away may herald the collapse of the baby with staphylococcal sepsis.

Review
Examination of newborns and young babies

- Babies are routinely seen by doctors for checks at birth and at 6–8 weeks old
- All newly qualified doctors should be able to perform a routine neonatal examination and define a baby as normal or otherwise
- Babies can become ill at an alarming rate and all healthcare professionals seeing them can benefit from scoring systems to help them to evaluate symptoms and signs
- Observation is the most important skill that paediatricians and children's nurses use to assess babies

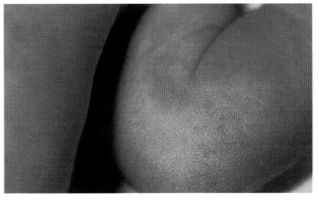

Fig. 12.32 Erythema toxicum. These spots can look a lot like staphylococcal pustules except that they spontaneously disappear and reappear in another area of skin. The rash is caused by eosinophilic infiltrates that are of no serious significance.

By the time of qualification, students should be confident in examining babies and diagnosing 'normality'.

Older babies and toddlers

The term 'infant' has been used previously to describe children under 2 years of age. We prefer to think of 'older babies' as being infants that are not yet walking and 'toddlers' as babies who have only recently acquired this skill. These children are frequently brought to their doctor. They attend for routine immunisations and developmental checks and are most likely to be seen by doctors in various settings (e.g. primary care, accident and emergency departments, community clinics, paediatric departments).

This period involves very rapid changes in growth and especially in development. During this period, the child progresses from being primarily supine and unable to move around, to becoming a toddler who is able to run and talk.

At the beginning of this period the effects of passively acquired maternal immunity (transplacental immunoglobulin G) mean that babies are not as prone to intercurrent viral illnesses as they will be later (Fig. 12.33). From the age of 3 or 4 months this passive immunity is diminishing and immunologically the baby is now on his or her own. On average, the healthy older baby and toddler will have to deal with eight self-limiting viral illnesses per year. Sometimes two or three of these illnesses will occur 'back to back', causing a great deal of anxiety in the parents, and the infant may temporarily fail to thrive. This acquisition of active immunity to the common viruses prevalent in the child's community is a part of normal growth and development.

In many developed countries, a comprehensive immunisation programme from birth to 2 years aims to prevent up to nine or more important infectious diseases

Serum immunoglobulin levels

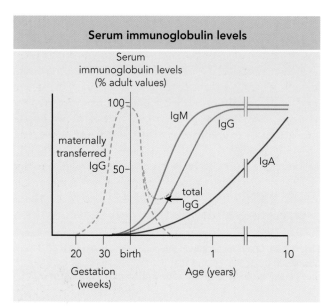

Fig. 12.33 Immunoglobulin levels vary with age. At birth babies have had a transplacental transfusion of maternal IgG that wears off by the end of the first 6 months. This provides passive immunity to the newborn baby; afterwards the child must develop his or her own active immunity after infection or immunisation.

Palmar and pincer grip

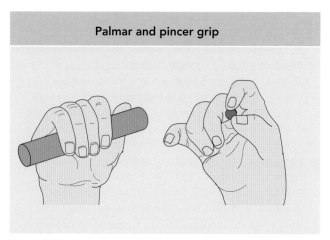

Fig. 12.34 Palmar and pincer grasp. The development of palmar and then pincer grasp represents a great step forward in fine motor skills and relies heavily on visual feedback.

(e.g. diphtheria, tetanus, pertussis, polio, *Haemophilus* type B infections, pneumoccal infections, meningococcal group C infections, measles, mumps and rubella). Visits for primary immunisation provide an opportunity for the infant's primary care physician to observe an infant's growth, development and general health.

GROWTH

Babies in this phase are still growing rapidly. There is a distinct deceleration in their growth velocity in the latter part of the first year and into the second year. The 'average infant' will have doubled birth weight by approximately 5 months and trebled it by just after a year.

The most dramatic changes are seen in head growth. This is as a result of myelination of cortical tracts and pathways leading to rapid brain growth, which are crucial in enabling developmental advances in this period.

DEVELOPMENT

At the beginning of this phase, a baby's cortical function has only recently demonstrated the important milestone of social smiling (6–8 weeks age). By the end of this phase (aged 2 years) the child will be walking, communicating wants and needs verbally and nonverbally, and will have developed sophisticated hand function and coordination.

The key question in this age group is: *Are the parents concerned about their child's developmental progress?* Only

occasionally do parents seem truly unaware of their child's significant developmental problem.

The first areas to develop rapidly are vision and the control of hand movements and the next are the gross locomotor skills needed to roll over and sit without support. During this time visual acuity and hand dexterity are continuing to improve. Fine and gross motor development rely heavily on the progression of visual development. The child listens to adults and siblings intently. He or she starts to babble and to understand more and more of what is said. Once confidence is gained when prone with hips flexed, the baby finds him- or herself teetering on hands and knees and then begins to crawl. Soon after that, the toddler is pulling up to stand and cruising around the furniture: the prelude to solo walking. Fine motor skills include the continued refinement of grasp until the pincer grip (Fig. 12.34) is achieved. At around the same time, vocalisations have become more and more specific and 'dada' and 'mama' are said with meaning. Comprehension of language now includes following some instructions and commands. This is all usually achieved in the first year.

In the following year, continued improvements in walking (with the feet less far apart) are followed by running at speed, kicking a ball and rapid changes in direction. Fine motor skills are seen in manual dexterity (tower of six cubes) and improved self-help abilities (feeding with a spoon, drinking from a cup and beginning to undress themselves). Communication continues to advance with the increase in vocabulary and the combination of words to make short phrases. Comprehension of language is still greater than expressive language abilities.

HISTORY-TAKING

During a consultation the parents are the usual historians. The baby or toddler will often arrive with siblings in tow. By involving the whole family in the consultation, the child may be put at ease and a more satisfactory result obtained.

The history should cover the same areas as with the newborn and very young baby and include points particularly relevant to this period, for example, current feeding, weaning, developmental abilities, immunisations received.

EXAMINATION

During the history it is often best to keep the child on the parent's lap and play with them. Depending on how well you are getting on, you may be able to start examining the child. If the child is wary, it may be necessary to demonstrate your intentions by examining an elder sibling, teddy or parent. Try and show the child that whatever you are going to do is more of a game, rather than anything threatening to them.

It is important, as with newborns, to examine the most relevant system indicated by the history first because this may be your only chance. Make sure that you have examined the whole child undressed by the end of your examination. This should be done in stages. Save the more unpleasant parts of the examination (e.g. looking at the ears and throat) until last.

Circulation and cardiovascular system

Look at the child's colour and ask if there have been any dramatic changes in this. Infants are now no longer polycythaemic; indeed they are likely to be 'physiologically' anaemic (lower end of expected range for haemoglobin is 9.4 g/dl at 2 months and 11.1 g/dl at 6 months). Central cyanosis can be missed if a 'dummy' (or pacifier) is not removed from the mouth.

Capillary refill time is a very sensitive sign and should be the same as for adults (less than 2–3 s). Environmental cold stress can prolong the capillary refill time in otherwise well babies. As in newborns, the cardiac output is mostly regulated by rate rather than stroke volume. Tachycardia is an important physical sign that needs evaluation, e.g. febrile, unwell, upset and crying?

Blood pressure should be measured in any sick infant or when cardiovascular, renal, endocrine or neurological diagnoses are being considered. The interpretation of a single blood pressure measurement requires knowledge of three factors: what size of cuff was used relative to the child's upper arm; the size of the child; and what emotional state the child was in at the time of measurement. The cuff size is critical, as blood pressure measurements may be spuriously high if too small a cuff is used or the infant is crying. Normal ranges are published according to size and age.

Palpation of the apex beat is helpful because some murmurs may be palpable as heaves or thrills. During auscultation of the heart sounds, normal splitting of the second heart sound may be difficult to hear in a tachycardic child.

Nearly one-third of children will have a murmur heard at some point of their lives. Less than 1% of children will have a structural heart lesion. Innocent murmurs have particular characteristics: ejection systolic flow murmurs are either 'short and buzzing' (caused by turbulent aortic flow) or 'soft and blowing' (caused by turbulent pulmonary flow); venous hums are low pitched and more noticeable after exertion or inspiration and they are abolished by lying supine.

True pathological murmurs are usually louder, harsher and longer and may radiate or have a diastolic component to them. Look for other symptoms and signs of cardiovascular disease.

> **Review**
>
> **Measuring children's blood pressure**
>
> Children's blood pressure measurements can be obtained using:
> - Oscillometry (dynamap)
> - Sphygmomanometry (using a stethoscope or Doppler probe or by palpation)
> - Direct (invasive) measurement (in intensive care)
>   *Remember the two-thirds rule:*
> - Cuff width must be at least two-thirds of the distance from shoulder to elbow
> - Cuff (bladder) length must be at least two-thirds of the limb circumference

> **Review**
>
> **Normal cardiovascular and respiratory ranges for older babies and toddlers**
>
> - Heart rate: 110–150 beats/min (>160 tachycardia)
> - Systolic blood pressure: 80–95 mmHg (depends on age and height)
> - Respiratory rate: 25–35 breaths/min (>40 tachypnoea)

Breathing and respiration

Watching and listening to the child's respiratory pattern is the most useful part of the examination of the respiratory system. Auscultation may add some more information, but is frequently 'drowned' by loud transmitted upper respiratory tract breath sounds.

Look at the upper respiratory tract (in the ears, nose and throat) at the end of the examination. Coryza (profuse discharge) and pink inflamed mucous membranes in the throat and ears are most likely to be caused by a viral upper respiratory infection. Antibiotics are not required unless a true secondary bacterial infection is suspected.

Differential diagnosis

Childhood rashes

- Rashes in childhood are very common and all you need is a simple and logical approach to make a diagnosis most of the time.
- The most clinically important rashes to recognise promptly are ones that are purpuric (nonblanching)
- If the rash is erythematous (blanching) and is associated with an intercurrent illness, then it is most probably related to an infection: often viral and self-limiting
- Any chronically itchy rash is likely to be eczema and should be treated with emollients

Red flag – urgent referral

Nonblanching (purpuric) rashes

- Meningococcal septicaemia (Fig. 12.35)
- Idiopathic thrombocytopenic purpura (Fig. 12.36)
- Fingertip bruises in non-accidental injury (Fig. 12.37)
- Henoch–Schönlein purpura (Fig. 12.38)

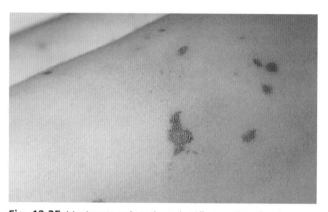

Fig. 12.35 Meningococcal septicaemia. All purpuric rashes in childhood need careful evaluation. The lives of patients with meningococcal disease depend on their doctor recognising this purpuric rash as early as possible. Note that the rash may start off as erythematous and then progress to nonblanching purpura. It is the speed of the rash's progression and the patient's degree of illness that are the hallmark of this infection. Treat immediately with an appropriate parenteral antibiotic.

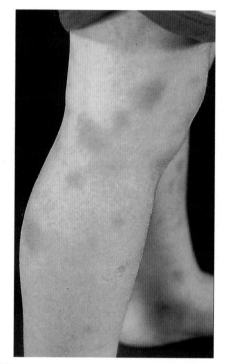

Fig. 12.36 Idiopathic thrombocytopenic purpura (ITP). ITP in childhood differs from the adult condition by being more benign and is self-limiting. Acute leukaemia is a very important differential diagnosis to be rapidly excluded by a full blood count and blood film.

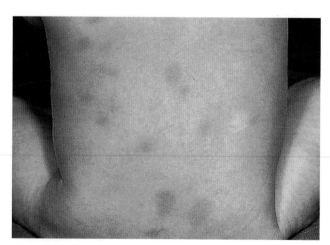

Fig. 12.37 Fingertip bruising; nonaccidental injury. All children have falls and minor injuries that result in bruises. Most bruises occur in areas of likely accidental impact (e.g. shins and elbows). Any bruise in a usually protected site is a worry. Ask how it happened. Is the injury consistent with the history? If you are worried, discuss immediately with senior staff.

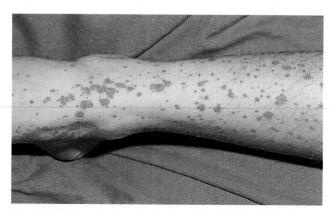

Fig. 12.38 Henoch–Schönlein purpura (HSP). HSP is an 'allergic' vasculitis that has a characteristic distribution along the back of the legs, extending up to the buttocks. It is associated with many systemic symptoms, such as joint swelling and (uncommonly) may result in permanent renal impairment.

Lymphadenopathy (localised or generalised) is common in association with frequent upper respiratory tract infections and viral illnesses. It may appear to persist if there is little or no interval between these infections. Acutely tender lymphadenopathy can be associated with bacterial infections. Persisting, asymmetrical large and nontender lymphadenopathy in association with constitutional symptoms needs accurate diagnosis and prompt treatment.

Abdomen

Bile-stained vomiting, pallor, excessive inconsolable crying, a distended abdomen, lumps in the groin and blood in the stool are all indicators of an acute abdominal problem. Children with peritonitis will lie very still, with their knees flexed, and breathe without moving the diaphragm. A diagnosis needs to be established and the child treated promptly.

After careful inspection, palpation can be attempted with warm hands. This will be a fruitless exercise if the infant is crying. Patience is needed and more than one attempt at palpation may be required, perhaps when the child is sleeping on a parent's lap.

Examine the anogenital area. In boys, always check that the testes are in the scrotum (a visual check will do, if they are obviously present). Do not attempt to retract the foreskin (it is physiologically adherent to the glans). In girls the external genitalia are less visible than when they are newborn. The labia majora are fleshy and obscure the introitus, clitoris and urethral opening. The vulval area in young girls is consequently infrequently observed by doctors. It is often preferable to ask someone more used to examining girls' perineums when this area is the focus of the presenting problem in young girls.

The hip joint is a frequent cause for concern (in many age groups) because of an acquired limp. As in abdominal palpation, if the child is not relaxed then the chances of a meaningful examination are limited. With the child on the parent's lap, gently explore the passive range of movements the child will tolerate. Look at the child's expression, to know when to stop. Internal and external rotation of the hip (with the hip and knee both in 90° of flexion) is one of the most reproducible and sensitive ways to pick up hip joint pathology.

Neurology and development

The neurological assessment of infants relies heavily on history (for developmental skills) and inspection and observation for confirmation of the reported abilities and the presence of any focal signs. The history is the key in many neurological diagnoses. When dealing with possible fits or 'funny turns', a first-hand account is best of all; a parent's video of the episode may be most valuable. Observation is more important than testing reflexes. Flexibility and improvisation are needed to extract whatever physical sign you are trying to elicit. Save the cranial nerve examination until last and check behaviour,

movement, gait and coordination by observation while the child plays.

Observation of gross motor skills will enable posture, power and, when the child is picked up, tone to be assessed. In younger babies antigravity power should be demonstrable by lifting the limbs or, when prone, the head off the bed. Assessment of truncal tone is important in the youngest of babies upwards. The limbs can be inspected and palpated in play to ascertain tone, muscle bulk, power and sensation (by gently tickling). Deep tendon reflexes can be elicited with patience. In an easily distracted child, reinforcement can be employed in play (squeeze the toy) if necessary. Coordination is hard to test formally in this age group and the observation of fine motor skills and gait are the most one can rely on.

The cranial nerves can be assessed by observation of behaviour and facial expression.

The olfactory (first) nerve This is rarely tested but smell can be assessed by asking the toddler to find a mint hidden in a handkerchief.

The optic (second) nerve In babies and toddlers visual acuity can be checked formally by a variety of techniques in a visual laboratory. Examining the visual fields and employing fundoscopy is often difficult in this age group. However, in the older (preschool age) child this is more straightforward and acuity can be checked beyond the age of 2 years with shape or letter matching.

The oculomotor, trochlear and abducens (third, fourth and sixth) nerves For assessing these nerves, eye movements can be observed when the child follows a toy or light in the vertical and horizontal plane. Nystagmus is normally seen in extremes of lateral gaze or may be pendular in a severely visually impaired child.

The trigeminal (fifth) and facial (seventh) nerves The trigeminal nerve can be tested when the jaws are clenched on a bottle or biscuit, and the facial nerve by encouraging the child to smile or shut their eyes.

The acoustic (eighth) nerve In some places hearing is still routinely screened in children from 7 to 8 months of age. Many places have now introduced universal Oto-Acoustic Emission (OAE) Hearing Screening in the neonatal period.

The glossopharyngeal (ninth), vagus (tenth) accessory (eleventh) and hypoglossal (twelfth) nerves Testing the function of these nerves is slightly more difficult in this age group, a history of regurgitation or choking on feeds may be relevant.

When inspecting the throat, at the end of your examination, you may be lucky and notice the following: movement of the uvula as you inspect the throat (ninth nerve intact); no hoarseness in the cry (tenth nerve intact); shrugging of the shoulders and turning of the head using the sternomastoid (eleventh nerve intact); waggling of the tongue as the spatula is used (twelfth nerve intact).

Differential diagnosis

Cranial nerve lesions in children

Cranial nerve lesions are not very common. Here are three important ones:

- Probably the most common cranial nerve to malfunction is the eighth nerve. Sensorineural hearing impairment occurs in approximately 0.1% live births and has a variety of congenital and acquired causes
- A lower motor seventh nerve lesion, as seen in a Bell's palsy, or after birth injury (forceps), is reasonably common. Remember that there are a number of causes, some more benign than others. With Bell's palsy check blood pressure and perform an audiogram
- A sixth nerve palsy may be a sign of raised intracranial pressure (the affected eye looks medially or convergently.) Most childhood squints are convergent (or alternating) and are due to refraction differences or ocular muscle imbalances

Review

Child development

This is a difficult subject to summarise because of the large degree of normal variation in acquisition of skills (milestones). Always correct age for prematurity. Some warning signs in the first year of life include:

- Any child whose parent expresses specific concerns about his or her development
- The loss of any acquired skills (developmental regression)
- Persistence of adducted thumbs from the neonatal period
- No social smile by age 8 weeks
- No startling to sound or responding to nearby voices by 8 weeks
- Not visually fixing and following from before 8 weeks
- Definite asymmetry of tone and movement (with head in midline) during the first year
- Not sitting unsupported by 8 months
- No polysyllabic babbling by 8 months

The preschool child

The preschool age group, 2–5 years of age, are the next most frequent attenders of their doctors. In common with younger children they will have a similar frequency of viral illnesses and potential for accidental self-poisoning. These viral illnesses will be more frequent as the child

Review

Examination of older babies and toddlers

- Young children are frequently brought to see their doctor
- Young children are undergoing the most rapid changes in development
- From the age of 4 months, a child is immunologically 'solo' and is prone to have frequent viral illnesses (average 8–10 per year)
- When examining this age group, it is important to engage the child in play if you are to be successful

mingles with peers at playgroup and nursery. Their cooperation with your examination can be extremely variable and if you can make their visits to you fun, then all the better.

GROWTH

Growth during this phase appears almost linear on the growth chart. In fact, the growth rate is decelerating by approximately 30% over this period. It should be possible now to estimate the midparental height centile and compare it with that of the child's height centile.

Review

Midparental height

- This calculation enables a prediction of the child's adult target height range
- The mean difference in final adult height is 14 cm between men and women
- For boys add 14 cm to mother's height
- For girls subtract 14 cm from father's height
- The midpoint between the parents' corrected heights is the midparental height

DEVELOPMENT

This period is characterised by advances in communication and the use and understanding of language and involves the transition from a mobile toddler, who communicates only a little verbally, to the chattering 4-year-old, using sentences and telling long, involved stories. Social and behavioural landmarks include the general behaviour of the child in relation to other adults and children, as well as specific abilities, for example, potty training. The advances in language, speech and communication mean that certain tests and facets of the clinical examination are approaching those used in adults.

HISTORY

Most of this age group start off on their parent's lap. Ask the siblings questions as well during your history-taking. The confident and relaxed child will begin to explore the room before too long and will be happy to supply small pieces of the history (e.g. siblings' names). The history may need to contain all of the details noted for a younger child but details about the pregnancy and so on are becoming less relevant.

The history should include details about developmental skills acquired and whether the parents or health visitor have any concerns. Other specific points include diet (peak age for incidence of dietary iron-deficiency anaemia), exercise tolerance and coughing (asthma is commonly underdiagnosed).

EXAMINATION

Generally this is best done on the parent's lap. Even the most apparently confident child may become upset when placed alone on an examination couch. Focus on the area of interest first and save the less pleasant parts until last. Make a game of it all and satisfy any curiosity expressed by the child (e.g. by letting them listen to mummy's heart or look in daddy's ear).

Circulation and cardiovascular system

An opportunity to auscultate the heart is now less of a priority and checking the perfusion (capillary refill time) pulse and blood pressure (if indicated) can be done before then.

The fall in heart rate means that the first and second heart sounds can be more carefully assessed. Innocent, benign flow-related murmurs are also common in this age group.

Breathing and respiration

Observation of the chest shape and respiratory pattern are again invaluable. Auscultation is seldom rewarding in the absence of observed respiratory distress. Peak flow measurements are not reproducible until age 4–5 years.

Review
Normal cardiovascular and respiratory ranges for preschool children

- Heart rate: 110–160 beats/min (>160 tachycardia)
- Systolic blood pressure: 80–100 mmHg (depends on age and height)
- Respiratory rate: 25–30 breaths/min (>30 tachypnoea)

Abdomen

All of the points made previously about acute abdominal problems can occur but now much less commonly. If the child is on a bed or couch it is important to make sure that a parent is near the head end. It is worthwhile kneeling down, making sure the child's eye level is above yours and looking at the child's face, not the belly.

It is likely that an abdominal examination will be successful as long as one does not mention whether the child is ticklish, otherwise it can all become hopelessly 'giggly'. Sometimes this can be avoided by allowing the child to palpate his or her own tummy, with your hand on top.

Leg posture and gait are a frequent source of parental anxiety as the toddler gains confidence on his or her feet. Genu varus (bow legs) is normal early on and there is then a tendency to genu valgus (knock knees) before a more straight leg grows in school-age children (Fig. 12.39).

Again the hip joint may be a focus of concern because of a limp or leg, thigh or knee pain. The limits of external and internal rotation can help decide what needs further evaluation.

Neurology and development

Gait and gross motor abilities are assessed as the child is playing in the room. Fine motor abilities can now be readily assessed with a pencil and paper, by asking the child to copy various shapes: a circle by age 3 years, a cross by 4 years, a square by 4 years 6 months and triangles by 5 years. Language and speech can be harder to assess. Hearing can be checked using free field audiometry. Vision can be tested with shape- or letter-matching by the age of approximately 3 years. Social and behavioural skills are either observed or enquired about with the history.

The neurological examination is now somewhere between what was described for toddlers and a more adult format. Reflexes, fundoscopy, visual fields and

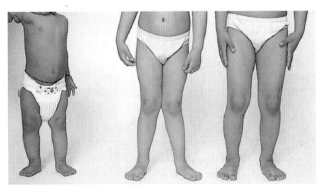

Fig. 12.39 Three boys' legs – which legs are normal? These three brothers all have normal legs. The youngest has mild genu varus (bow legs), which is physiological in the toddler. The middle brother has genu valgus (knock knees), which is physiological in the preschool-aged child. The eldest brother has 'straight' legs.

specific motor and coordination tasks are all possible, as long as the child perceives your examination as fun.

Review
Examination of preschool children

- The preschool child is usually very healthy
- Thoughtful examination is needed, assessing the most relevant system first
- The examination should be fun for both patient and doctor

The school-aged child

The school-age group, 5–10+ years of age (until the onset of puberty), are seen less often by their doctors. It is also the age at which psychological factors are beginning to play a bigger role in how and what the child may complain of to their parents and doctors.

GROWTH

The growth in this age group is steady but slowly decelerating. The height will usually be following near the midparental centile. Accelerations in height velocity may be attributed to an excessive weight gain (not uncommon) or more importantly (and rarely) to endocrine causes (e.g. precocious puberty). Decelerations may be due to inadequately managed or unrecognised chronic illness (e.g. asthma or coeliac disease) or endocrine problems (Figs 12.40, 12.41).

DEVELOPMENT

These children are spending the majority of the day away from home, at school. They will become more independent from their parents and carers but more dependent on their peer group. Social and behavioural aspects of development are now more important. Language and cognitive skills, literacy and numeracy are further developed in class and at home. Vision, hearing and motor skills are approaching adult abilities.

HISTORY

It is a good idea to invite the child to be the historian and rely on the parent for back-up. Some will want their parents to give all the history, whereas others may be very capable historians. This will depend on the child's character, previous (good or bad) experience of a doctor

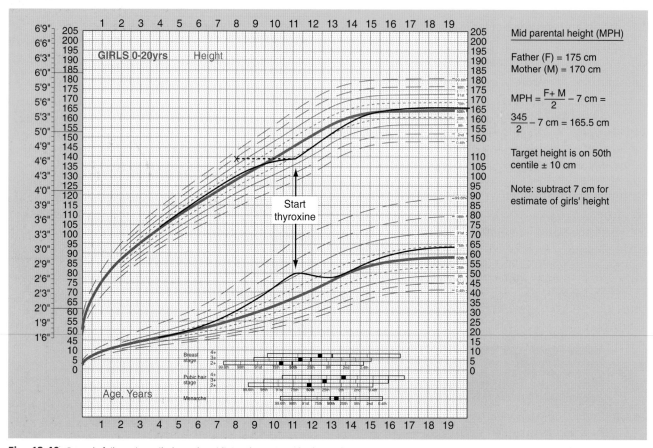

Fig. 12.40 Growth failure: juvenile hypothyroidism. These growth charts demonstrate an 11-year-old girl diagnosed with hypothyroidism. Note how her height velocity has decelerated with a retarded bone age. After starting thyroxine she loses weight, her height catches up and her puberty progresses rapidly (see Figs 12.43 and 12.44). (© Child Growth Foundation, adapted with permission.)

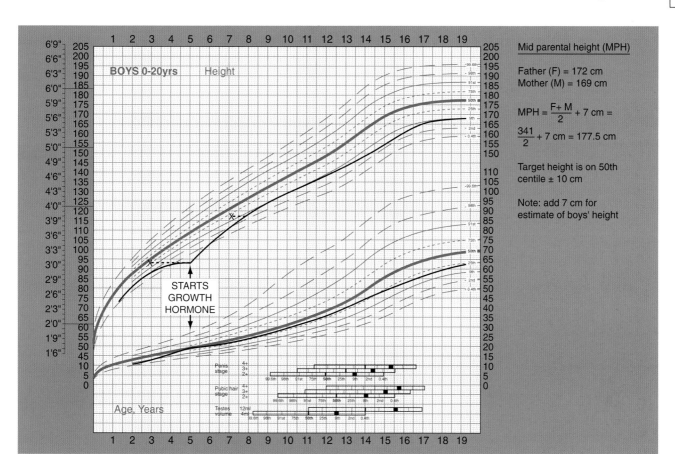

Mid parental height (MPH)

Father (F) = 172 cm
Mother (M) = 169 cm

$$MPH = \frac{F+M}{2} + 7 \text{ cm} =$$

$$\frac{341}{2} + 7 \text{ cm} = 177.5 \text{ cm}$$

Target height is on 50th
centile ± 10 cm

Note: add 7 cm for
estimate of boys' height

Fig. 12.41 Growth failure: early idiopathic growth hormone deficiency. This boy's infant growth appears reasonably normal, although perhaps less than his midparental height may suggest. His height velocity decelerates drastically by the age of 5 years and the diagnosis is made. Growth hormone supplementation through the rest of childhood and adolescence provides catch-up growth and a reasonable final adult height. His puberty is a little later than average (see Fig. 12.44 for pubertal stages). (© Child Growth Foundation, adapted with permission.)

and how ill they are. Children with chronic diseases are often poor at the long-term history but more reliable with the acute story. It is important to pitch the questions in terms the child understands and which are not patronising (e.g. using the family's terms for faeces, penis, bottom and so on).

Background information about the home and especially school is important. Establish how much the presenting complaint affects the child's life at school and at home. If only school time is affected then the problem may not be an organic one. Hobbies, sports and pastimes give other clues to the seriousness of the illness and its impact on the child's life.

EXAMINATION

The sequence of the examination is now more or less dictated by you. There are very few differences in technique from examining adults, except that the examination should continue to be fun. Peak flow can be used as a reproducible way of monitoring asthma (Fig. 12.42).

Review

Normal cardiovascular and respiratory ranges for school-age children

- Heart rate: 80–120 beats/min (>120 tachycardia)
- Systolic blood pressure: 90–110 mmHg (depends on age and height)
- Respiratory rate: 20–25 breaths/min (>25 tachypnoea)

Review

Examination of school-age children

- School-age children are usually very healthy and do not see their doctors much
- Examination is in a manner similar to adults, as long as everything is explained adequately
- Psychological factors are becoming increasingly relevant

Peak expiratory flow rate: normal paediatric values

height (m)	height (ft)	predicted **EU** PEFR (l/min)
0.85	2'9"	87
0.90	2'11"	95
0.95	3'1"	104
1.00	3'3"	115
1.05	3'5"	127
1.10	3'7"	141
1.15	3'9"	157
1.20	3'11"	174
1.25	4'1"	192
1.30	4'3"	212
1.35	4'5"	233
1.40	4'7"	254
1.45	4'9"	276
1.50	4'11"	299
1.55	5'1"	323
1.60	5'3"	346
1.65	5'5"	370
1.70	5'7"	393

Fig. 12.42 Normal peak expiratory flow (PEF) values in children correlate best with height; with increasing age, larger differences occur between the sexes. These predicted values are based on the formulae given in: Cotes J. E. 1979 Lung function, 4th edn. Blackwell Scientific, London. Adapted for EU scale Mini-Wright peak flow meters by C. Clarke.

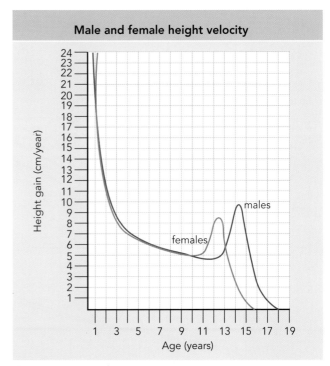

Fig. 12.43 Height velocity in girls and boys. Note how before the pubertal growth spurt there is little difference in girls' and boys' height velocities. Also note that girls' pubertal height velocity peaks are earlier and less tall than those for boys. These are thought to be the main factors determining the difference in adult male and female height.

Adolescents

The adolescent group of patients is not usually very well served by the medical profession, particularly in the latter half of adolescence.

Paediatricians and general practitioners usually feel confident with the initial part of adolescence but this wanes towards the middle and end of adolescence. There are many reasons for this:

- Adolescents seldom consult their doctor, so neither is very familiar with each other.
- Adolescents are in the transition from childhood to adulthood and are uncertain as to how to behave as adults, but do not want to behave as children.
- Doctors need to allow them to be adolescent and accept that the adolescent is easily embarrassed and often anxious.
- The presenting problems can have a psychological basis.
- Adolescents with a chronic illness (e.g. diabetes, cystic fibrosis, sickle cell disease) will demonstrate normal adolescent rebellion, which can have serious long-term health consequences.
- Risk-taking behaviour (cigarettes, alcohol, drugs, sex, etc.) is normal and when it does go wrong, in health terms, it is hard not to appear judgemental and authoritative as the doctor.

- Deliberate self-harm (overdoses especially) in adolescents is becoming more prevalent. Understanding the reasons for this behaviour can be challenging.
- Confidentiality and consent are sometimes a source of conflict between patient, parent and doctor.

The adolescent's doctor needs to be aware of, and open-minded about, the nature and cause of the complaint and sensitive to the patient's need to be seen with (or without) a parent. Adolescents are usually able to give informed consent for examination and treatment if the reasons are explained to them in a way they can understand. They are still their parent's (or carer's) legal responsibility and problems can arise when there is a disagreement. It is good practice to communicate effectively with both the adolescent and parents.

GROWTH

During the first 10 years there is remarkably little difference between the height and weight velocity in the growth of girls and boys. Both have a slowly decelerating growth until puberty, then there is a growth spurt that lasts for 2–3 years. This will complete the child's physical transformation into a young adult (Figs 12.43, 12.44 and see Figs 8.1, 8.3 and 9.4).

The adolescent phase of growth is initiated by sex steroids that are produced by the gonads, stimulated by gonadotrophins from the anterior pituitary. Along with

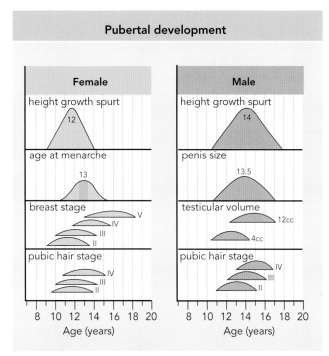

Fig. 12.44 Pubertal staging in males and females. These standard puberty stagings are important to note whenever you plot children's growth in the second decade (see Figs 8.1, 8.3 and 9.4).

the dramatic increase in size and growth, these sex steroids will promote the development of secondary sexual characteristics and fertility.

PUBERTY

The onset of puberty is less than 1 year apart in girls (mean age 11.4 years) and boys (mean age 12.0 years) but the pubertal growth spurt occurs in girls approximately 2 years before boys. The first physical sign of puberty in a girl is the development of breast tissue under the nipples (mean age 11 years); the first physical sign in boys is the enlargement of the testes from their prepubertal volume of less than 2 ml to an endocrinologically active volume of greater than 4 ml (mean age 12 years). However, a boy's growth spurt does not occur until the testicular volume is approximately 10 ml.

A delay in growth and puberty can be a source of great unhappiness for the adolescent who is endocrinologically normal but, because of an inherited tendency, develops and matures more slowly than peers (Fig. 12.45).

A constitutional delay in growth and puberty is more of a problem for boys than girls because boys have their pubertal growth spurt 2 years later than girls and because boys' growth spurts are larger than girls', so its absence is more apparent.

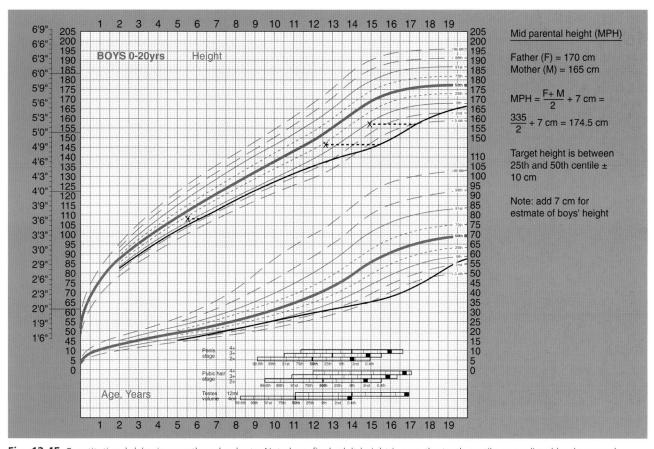

Fig. 12.45 Constitutional delay in growth and puberty. Note how final adult height is near the tenth centile as predicted by the growth velocity observed between age 4 and 10 years. He was most psychologically stressed in his 16th year (see Figs 12.43 and 12.44). (© Child Growth Foundation, adapted with permission.)

Differential diagnosis

Constitutional delay in growth and puberty

- This condition is most common in boys
- Patients usually have a history of growing in the lower quartile of the normal range but by the middle teenage years are very much shorter than their peers (at this time they present to a specialist clinic)
- Severe psychological stress may result from this genetic and physiological delay in puberty
- Pharmacologically inducing puberty is an effective way of relieving the stress suffered by these patients

Over the next 2 years in girls, and 3 years in boys, there are changes in body shape and composition (lean mass and distribution of body fat) along with growth of pubic hair (and facial and body hair in boys).

In girls, when the growth spurt (height velocity) decelerates to less than 4 cm per year, the menarche can occur; height continues to increase for 1.5–2 years after the menarche. Final adult height is achieved when the bony epiphyses fuse in the vertebrae and along the long bones of the leg. It is impossible to evaluate an adolescent's growth without knowledge of what stage of pubertal development they have reached.

DEVELOPMENT

Development continues long after growth has finished. It is mostly in the spheres of social and behavioural development that adolescents are still progressing. This age group is requesting and gaining more independence from their parents and carers. They have completed their primary education and will be completing their secondary education by the end of this phase. Interests will change and relationships with peers are crucial to the adolescent's self-image.

The gap between the end of growth and the end of development into a fully independent adult is apparently widening. The mean age for pubertal milestones appears to have come down from that of a century ago. In the developed world, there is a decreased need for unskilled workers and an increased need for skills and higher education to be a successful provider. Thus the end of 'development' is often only complete after the age of 20 years.

HISTORY

Depending on the presenting problem, it may be necessary to agree who remains in the consulting room. This is one area in which confidentiality and consent may become a point of conflict. When taking the history, it is important to direct your questions primarily to the patient, and only when necessary to the parent or carer.

Details about the family and relationships between members of the household are important. Details about school, progress with school work, hobbies, sports, pastimes and friendships can all help give an indication of how the adolescent is coping with the increasing stresses of the real world. Again, it is easier to take a quick trip through this part of the history at the beginning because, if problems of psychosocial issues arise later, it can seem awkward to 'go back' and ask the straightforward questions.

EXAMINATION

Most adolescents are very self-conscious of their appearance, so make sure they have suitable facilities to prevent undue embarrassment (e.g. blankets and screens around the examination couch). The examining doctor will need to decide during the history-taking whether the parent is to be invited alongside the patient. Which side of the screens should the parent stay? This can be difficult to get right every time. When an adolescent is seen alone during the physical examination, it is advisable to include a chaperone in the examination room.

Apart from the assessment of growth and puberty and attention to the adolescent and parent relationship, the rest of the examination will be similar to that for an adult patient.

Review

Normal cardiovascular and respiratory ranges for adolescents

- Heart rate: 60–100 beats/min (>160 tachycardia)
- Systolic blood pressure: 100–120 mmHg (depends on age and height)
- Respiratory rate: 15–20 breaths/min (>25 tachypnoea)

Review

Examination of adolescents

- Adolescents are usually very healthy and do not see their doctors much
- They are generally not well served by their doctors
- Psychological factors are important
- Risk-taking is normal but hazardous (sex, drugs and so on)
- Deliberate self-harm is increasingly common and must be properly assessed by a trained counsellor on a case by case basis

Red flag – urgent referral

Presentations, symptoms and signs in paediatric medicine

There are so many presentations, symptoms and signs to take a special note of in paediatric medicine. The contents of this chapter and this list are no substitute for a standard text in clinical paediatrics and the clinical experience gained in the clinic, emergency department or on the wards. The following are some that are considered to be important.

History

- When the parents express grave concern about the rapidity of their child's illness. This is a finding in children with evolving bacterial septicaemia
- Any child with any injury where the history is not consistent with the examination findings. This could be a child protection problem; refer to senior colleagues.
- Jaundice in babies under 48 hours old. This is a haemolytic neonatal jaundice until proven otherwise.
- Persisting jaundice in neonates who have pale stools and dark urine. This is caused by biliary/liver disease until proven otherwise.
- Vomiting that is bile stained. This is a surgical cause (obstruction/intussusception/ appendicitis) until proven otherwise.
- Passage of blood per rectum. Cause may be surgical or infective, but can also be due to local causes.
- Persisting and ongoing fever for more than 5 days. Diagnosis of Kawasaki's disease needs to be considered.

Growth

- Children whose plotted height, weight or head circumference are crossing centiles in a dramatic way (deviation may be upwards but more often downwards). Deviation in previous growth patterns require evaluation of accurate longitudinal data.
- Development of secondary sexual characteristics before age 8 years in girls and age 10 years in boys. Suggests precocious puberty.

Development

- Any history suggestive of regression (i.e. loss of previously acquired skills). Indicates possible neurodegenerative condition.
- At 8 weeks (corrected) old, act if any of the following is present/absent:
  - failure to fix and follow a visual stimulus
  - failure to startle to sound
  - failure to smile responsively.
- Any obvious asymmetry of neonatal reflexes or persistence of head lag. Requires expert developmental examination.

- At 6–8 months (corrected) old, act if any of the following is present/absent:
  - obvious hand preference
  - fisting of hands
  - squint (strabismus).
- Persistence of primitive reflexes. Requires expert developmental examination.
- At 12 months (corrected) old, expert developmental examination is required if any of the following is present/absent:
  - unable to sit or bear weight
  - persistence of hand regard
  - absence of babbling and cooing
  - absence of saving reactions.
- At 18 months (corrected) age, expert developmental examination is required if any of the following is present/absent:
  - inability to stand without support
  - inability to understand simple commands
  - no spontaneous vocalisation
  - no pincer grip
  - casting (throwing) still present.

Examination

- Young children who appear 'too good/quiet' (e.g. not crying/complaining) may be more ill than at first appears, as may children who are 'inconsolable' (i.e. too irritable) to their parent's attempts at soothing them. The seriously ill child can easily be overlooked because of their lack of interaction.
- Nonblanching (purpuric) spots in a child with fever. Meningococcal bacteraemia can be easily overlooked in the early stages of the illness.
- Bulging fontanelle. May suggest raised intracranial pressure (ICP) or even meningitis.
- Abnormal posture (e.g. opisthotonus, or tripod stance). Children will always adopt positions of comfort; if they appear not to, ask yourself why, what is the discomfort due to?
- Children whose heart rate and/or respiratory rate is sustained and above the normal range for age (out of proportion to their fever). Refer to age-specific normal ranges. Persistent tachycardia suggests bacteraemia and tachypnoea suggests lower respiratory tract infection (LRTI).
- Any child with central cyanosis (look at the tongue) and any child with oxygen saturation <92% in air. Always look at central mucous membrane colour (remove the pacifier), use pulse oximeter if available.

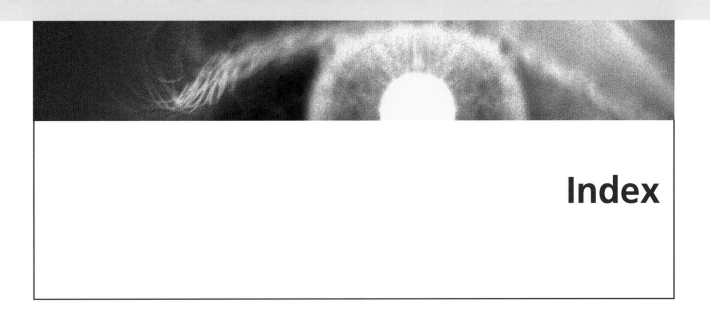

Index

Note: Page numbers in **bold** refer to figures.

Index

Index

Index

Index

Index

Index

Index

Index